INTRODUCTION TO
NUTRITION

INTRODUCTION TO
NUTRITION

THIRD EDITION

HOME ECONOMICS AND NUTRITION DEPARTMENT
NEW YORK UNIVERSITY

Macmillan Publishing Co., Inc.
NEW YORK

Collier Macmillan Publishers
LONDON

Macmillan Publishing Co., Inc.
866 Third Avenue, New York, New York 10022

Collier Macmillan Canada, Ltd.

Library of Congress Cataloging in Publication Data

Fleck, Henrietta Christina, (date)
    Introduction to nutrition.

    Includes bibliographies and index.
    1. Nutrition.   I. Title.   [DNLM: 1. Nutrition.
QU145 F593i]
TX353.F54 1976   641.1   75–4726
ISBN 0–02–338430–1

Printing: 2 3 4 5 6 7 8   Year: 6 7 8 9 0 1 2

Preface to the Third Edition

College students in an introductory course in nutrition seek answers to many questions that reflect their heightened interest in the subject. Examples are related to the safety of food; vegetarianism; nutritional labeling, nutritive contributions of specific foods; vitamin supplements; the value of a single nutrient, such as vitamin C in the treatment of colds; appropriate diet for athletes; the effect of cholesterol on health; and problems of feeding the hungry world. An attempt has been made in this book to scientifically answer these and other questions.

To give a total picture of nutrition, the subject is discussed from personal and social concerns. Students are encouraged to broaden their knowledge and to clarify their attitudes about nutrition by becoming familiar with the nutrients essential to health. Dietary needs, underload and overload, sources in foods, the effect of food preparation and other influences on deterioration, the nutritional status of the American population, and a review of the pertinent research are some of the topics emphasized. The nutritional needs for various age levels and for both sexes are covered, and a discussion of the particular problems and situations that may influence nutritional intake of individuals at various age levels is presented. This provides a background for the student to analyze his or her own food habits in light of possible changes.

Many forces determine food habits. Lifestyles, for instance, and their effect on nutritional adequacy are explored in a chapter that includes a section on vegetarianism. Economic stress affects food expenditures and information about purchasing food for home consumption and for eating out is supplied. Psychological and sociological aspects of nutrition, such as personal meanings attributed to food, the impact of geography and culture, and value systems, have an impact on nutritional adequacy. The effect of drugs, alcohol, and a lack of exercise on nutritional status is treated. Students will gain insights into the complexities of factors that shape why or how they eat.

World conditions, such as inflation, recession, and high food prices; the energy crises; the problems of ecology; the effect of drouth, flood, and weather conditions on crops; war and conflict; and the slow movement toward attacking world hunger or planning a national nutrition policy are important considerations for the social aspect of nutrition. Our country, with the largest resources of food in the world, has been beset by criticism. Americans are accused of overeating and excessive food waste when millions are hungry, including many in the United States. The answer is not simple, but the serious student of nutrition will find information in this text that will be helpful in reaching conclusions.

This book assists a student to place information from both social and personal angles in proper perspective and in relation to pertinent facts. Judging the accuracy or competency of sources of information is an important skill. How, for example, can nutritional claims highlighted in newspaper or magazine columns or on radio and television programs be evaluated? Finally, a student should emerge from his or her study of nutrition with confidence in planning a personal program for optimal nutrition.

Many people have aided in the production of this book. Special recognition is given to many friends in business, to staff members of professional publications, to the Department of Agriculture, to the Nutrition Statistics Branch of the Health and Nutrition Examination Survey, to the Food and Nutrition Board of the National Research Council, and to personnel of scientific and international organizations for supplying illustrations, charts, maps, reports, and other materials. Staff and graduate students in nutrition at New York University have assisted in many ways. Lastly, my husband deserves particular appreciation for his encouragement, assistance, and advice.

H. F.

Contents

The Meanings of Food

Food has many meanings. A food may arouse feelings of gladness, sadness, femininity, masculinity, poverty, prosperity, pleasure, power, sophistication, revolt, or comfort. These and a host of other associations arise from the culture in which a person lives, the family in which he grew up, and his experiences of everyday living. How people respond to different foods can reveal a great deal about their origin.

Family Foods

Eating has an intimate association with the family unit, according to Cussler and De Give,[1] and implies kinship. Lewin[2] talks of the feeling of security engendered by the particular foods served by one's family. These are the foods that fit within the range of the

family's likes, that are readily available in the home, and that meet the family's purse demands. These foods have an intimate appeal. The family eats them when it is alone and does not usually serve them to guests. Lewin calls them "foods for us."

When the family is planning its own meals, the "foods for us" or the way they are served may reflect the individual preferences of the family members. For example, one person might like his soup or coffee very hot; others might prefer it only slightly hot or lukewarm. Some might like their toast crisp, others soft. In many families the husband or father may be given the choice servings of all foods, but this custom is not so prevalent among younger married couples, with whom the masculine and feminine roles are tending to merge.

Different family members may have strong preferences in seasonings. Some automatically reach for extra salt, cover their meat or vegetables with catsup, or are particularly fond of the flavor of garlic in salads or meat dishes.

Sometimes the preparation of a food in the kitchen has definite rituals. A mother may insist on using a special utensil for preparing a certain dish; if it is not available, she does not make that dish. Some people insist on cer-

---

[1] Margaret Cussler and Mary L. De Give, *'Twixt the Cup and the Lip*, Twayne Publishers, Boston, 1952.

[2] Kurt Lewin, "Forces Behind Food Habits and Methods of Change," in Carl E. Guthe and Margaret Mead (eds.), *The Problem of Changing Food Habits*, Bulletin No. 108, National Academy of Sciences—National Research Council, Washington, D.C., 1943.

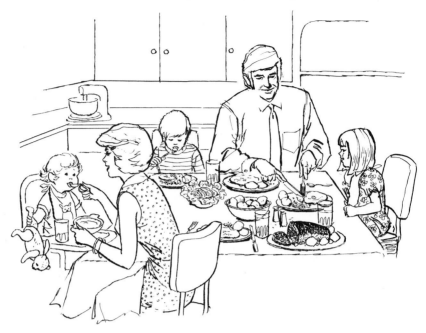

FIGURE 1–1. *"Foods for us" have an intimate appeal.*

tain ingredients in preparing family meals—the fat used may have to be butter, margarine, lard, bacon fat, or chicken fat. In some parts of the South, only white cornmeal is used; in others, only yellow.

When guests come, there is a change in the family eating pattern—how much of a change will depend on the importance of the guest. Some kind of fowl, roast meat, or game may become the main dish for a company meal, to be followed, perhaps, by an elaborate dessert. Special china may be used, and the meal will probably be served in the dining room, patio, or some place other than the kitchen, which is used for many family meals. This concern for guests may reflect a need to demonstrate status, to show that the head of the family is a good provider. Even for the casual guest dropping in for a brief visit, food is given a social connotation, for he is usually offered at least a beverage. Food is a symbol of hospitality and friendship.

Meals

Food may be eaten at certain times of the day for the sole purpose of satisfying hunger.

Some meals, however, have a strong significance, according to Fathauer.[3] Much more sentiment is associated with dinner than with lunch in most societies, for example. Lee,[4] an anthropologist, offers an explanation for the difference between the meaning of dinner and other meals by the concentration on a main dish—platter or casserole with a special arrangement of food to which all other dishes are subsidiary—a procedure that reflects values. With the marked trend toward casual meals, new meanings are emerging in relation to the choices of foods and types of service. One meaning is that eating facilitates interpersonal relations.

Certain foods are also associated with each meal of the day. Fruit juices, cereals, eggs, bacon, and sausage belong to breakfast. Although cereals may be used in preparing a

[3] George H. Fathauer, "Food Habits—An Anthropologist's View," *Journal of the American Dietetic Association*, Vol. 37, No. 4 (October 1960), pp. 335–338.

[4] Dorothy Lee, "Why Do People Eat What They Eat?" *Proceedings of the Fourth Annual Food Forum*, Sponsored by the United Fruit Company, New York, November 5, 1954.

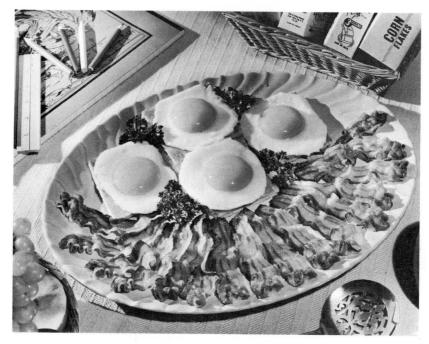

FIGURE 1–2. *Bacon and eggs spell breakfast to many people.*

dish for another meal—in breading meats, in casseroles, or in desserts—they are never served as cereal dishes at lunch or dinner. And if a luncheon dish—sandwiches or certain salads—is served as the main course at dinner, a person may feel cheated because the dinner menu should be more substantial and consist of meat, vegetables, and a dessert. If a food steps out of its assigned role, people can find it disturbing. Or sometimes an unusual combination of foods can cause bewilderment, as shrimp with bananas. However, sharp distinctions are no longer as prevalent (for example, among certain groups soups have become identified with breakfast), and there is a growing tendency to accept different combinations and to be creative about foods.

Great importance is attached to the order in which food is eaten, and this, too, cannot be disturbed without causing a certain amount of insecurity. Soup is served at the beginning of the meal, not at the end (although in some countries it is served after the main course). In China, a delicious soup terminates a banquet. And even though children beg for desserts at the beginning, they are served at the close of the meal. The time at which a beverage is served may be a matter of family ritual. Mothers teach their children to eat foods in a certain order, according to Lee. They must learn the foods to be eaten first and those eaten last. Eating dessert first is out of order. Each family develops its own customs in serving foods, and any deviation can be disturbing. The dinner hour is usually set at a fixed time each day—say, six or eight o'clock. Linen napkins may customarily be used, or paper napkins—tablecloths or place mats. Flowers or other table decorations may be important. And some foods may demand particular types of dishes; for example, many families always serve fruit in a glass dish. If the food is served at the table, the father might do the serving, or the mother; sometimes the children help. Saying grace may be an integral part of family living. In some families, there might be rituals with particular dishes, like carving fowl or lighting a flaming dessert.

The attitude of the family toward certain meals can be significant: Does everyone make an effort to be present? Do they dress in a

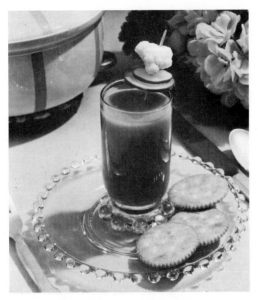

FIGURE 1–3. *The order for appetizers is at the beginning of the meal. (Courtesy Campbell Soup Company)*

certain manner? Is mealtime important? Or, specific mealtimes are completely ignored in favor of casual eating. These situations will vary from family to family, but they are an important aspect of daily living.

Age Preferences

We think of some foods as being childish, adult, or for older people. Milk, soft foods, or foods in small pieces are often considered childish. Frequently, a person in an emotional turmoil who unconsciously wishes to go back to the days of his childhood may resort to such foods. A psychologist can sometimes determine, to a certain extent, the maturity of a person, as well as signs of emotional difficulty, by the type of food he eats.

Grown-up foods or beverages signify maturity, which may be why children clamor for tea or coffee at an early age. Adolescents, on the other hand, may scorn cereals because they feel that these are for younger brothers and sisters.

Soft foods are sometimes assigned to elderly people because they are easily chewed. In fact, foods for the elderly resemble those for children in the minds of many. That is why companies have had difficulty selling foods with a geriatric label. Older people do not want to be identified with these soft, childish foods.

Sex Roles

Family custom even assigns masculine and feminine roles to food and its service. For example, while the wife still carries the major responsibility in preparing food, the husband may have the job of carving the meat; he may even cook the meat outdoors in the barbecue pit. In addition, certain foods themselves are considered masculine—meat, potatoes, pie, and the like. Others, such as light fluffy desserts, salads, and tea, seem more feminine.

In most countries of the world, according to Mead,[5] women's concept of themselves and men's sense of women depend on the way wives select, prepare, and serve food. Women attempt not only to reproduce the foods served by their mothers but also to perpetuate memories of foods served by their mothers-in-law. In the trend toward the blending of sex roles, the masculine and feminine attributes of food are less sharply defined.

Religious Customs and Moral Values

For centuries the religion of an individual has had a bearing on the way he feels about food. In most homes there are still vestiges of feasts and fast days and the kinds of food that are encouraged or forbidden by religious rule. If an individual does adhere to these religious regulations about food, he may feel very virtuous; if he ignores them, he may have a serious feeling of guilt. Overeating may be a sin. Opera and theatrical stars often pack kosher and other foods of religious connotations to take with them on tours.

Foods may also take on moral values. People may feel very strongly that something is or is not good for them. It may be morally good to eat green vegetables and liver. Moth-

[5] Margaret Mead, *Food and the Family*, A UNESCO Project, Manhattan Publishing, New York, 1950.

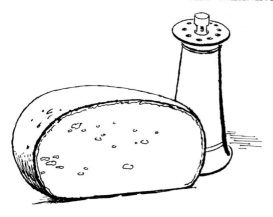

FIGURE 1–4. *An old Israeli custom is to bring salt and bread to a new home, signifying peace and welcome.*

ers praise children for eating these foods but seldom commend a child who eats ice cream.

Symbolism

Each family will consciously or unconsciously assign certain symbolic values to foods. The color of food has a symbolic meaning. White meat of chicken and white bread are symbols of status or even prosperity. Dark bread is associated with peasants. Bread and salt brought into a new home are symbols of welcome and peace in Israel.

Terms like heavy, light, or rich are assigned to foods. The heavy foods are those believed to be difficult to digest—elaborate desserts, dishes with sauces, and meats with gravy. The light foods, on the other hand, are those that do not give a feeling of stuffiness, like salads, toast, or tea. The rich ones are creamed soup, whipped cream, fried foods—foods associated with considerable fat.

A culture defines the foods that are edible or inedible. People may have strong guilt feelings about eating a food considered inedible by their group. Long ago a Frenchman, M. Serrel, pointed out that there are over 2 million known species of animals and only 50 are domesticated and eaten. Of the 250,000 known species of vegetables, only about 600 are cultivated.

Foods are categorized as "hot" or "cold" in many Latin-American countries, parts of China, in East Pakistan, among peasants in the Peruvian Andes, and among other cultures.[6] These designations do not refer to the temperature of the food but to beliefs about a health, nutritional, medicinal, or other quality attributed to the food. Cold foods are fruits, vegetables, milk, and pork. Examples of hot foods are cereals, sugar, some meats, and alcohol. These preferences have nutritional implications. The Peruvian Indians, for example, reject available turnip greens because it is a cold food. Their vitamin A deficiency could be alleviated seasonally if these greens were included in their diet.[7,8]

Since time began, food has probably been used as a device for punishment as well as a token of affection. A mother may refuse a child certain food unless he eats other foods first, or she may threaten to withhold it for some reason that has nothing to do with the food, such as asking him to be a good boy while she is away, or no dessert. People frequently reward themselves with certain foods. A salesman who has made an excellent sale may order a steak dinner. And the student who has made a good grade in a quiz may indulge himself in a hot chocolate sundae.

Another way in which food is used is to relieve tension. When persons are worried, afraid, or concerned in some manner, they may eat more food than usual. Sometimes quantities of food are eaten at one time after a very upsetting experience—a serious quarrel, worry about loss of a job, or concern about family matters. The food itself usually gives little pleasure but individuals claim the emotional disturbance is eased. Another example of how food relieves tension or frustration is

[6] E. Neige Todhunter, "Food Habits, Food Faddism, and Nutrition," in Miloslav Rechcigl, Jr. (ed.), *Food, Nutrition, and Health,* Vol. 16, S. Karger, Basel, 1973, pp. 297–298.

[7] R. B. Mazees and P. T. Baker, "Diets of Quechua Indians Living at High Altitudes. Nunoa, Peru," *American Journal of Clinical Nutrition,* Vol. 15, No. 3 (March 1964), pp. 341–351.

[8] R. B. Mazees, "Hot–Cold Beliefs Among Andean Peasants," *Journal of the American Dietetic Association,* Vol. 53, No. 1 (January 1968), pp. 109–113.

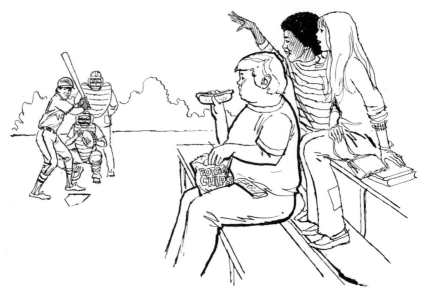

FIGURE 1–5. *A fat boy watching a school baseball game is eating food to compensate for his lack of participation.*

that of the rejected child who compensates with hot dogs and ice cream sodas while watching others play.

From the day of birth, foods convey meanings and feelings related to security, protection, love, and strength. Hamburgers and ice cream give feelings of "home" to Americans abroad. Conversely, there are connotations of fear, pain, rejection, and deprivation.[9] Motherhood is interpreted for a child through his associations with food, according to Fathauer.[10] A baby's sense of security reflects the manner in which he is fed.

In short, many customs and traditions—and the emotional associations attached to food—are developed in the family. These all become part of the children's heritage. The young bride going into her kitchen for the first time brings with her a complex fund of information that she has gathered in her parents' home. Much of this she will pass on to her children.

---

[9] Charlotte G. Babcock, "Attitudes and the Use of Food," *Journal of the American Dietetic Association*, Vol. 38, No. 6 (June 1961), pp. 546–551.

[10] Fathauer, op. cit.

Communication Through Food Ways

There are various ways in which family members may communicate through the use of food. One member may transmit to the others such feelings as indifference, anger, resentment, or sadness by the way he dawdles or picks at his food. A wife may wheedle her husband into certain purchases she feels are very important either for herself or for her home by resorting to the device of serving his favorite foods.

A person's enjoyment of his food can be transformed into happiness, interest, affection, and other positive feelings. Everyone has had the experience of seeing someone who was very unpleasant before a meal change his attitude when presented with a food he liked very much.

And feelings can be reflected in the way food is prepared. A mother can show her pleasure with her children or her husband by the extent to which she makes an effort to serve them some of their favorite foods. A young woman can transmit feelings of indifference or annoyance to her male companion by the dissatisfaction she expresses about the food they are eating. The kind of food that is served or given to others may indicate the degree of affection and respect held for them, and their response to it is equally significant. Old friends may reminisce about the foods of their childhood. Gifts of these favorite foods, such as a particular cheese, bread, or wild fruit may be exchanged. Chairman Mao, for example, presented a Chinese boyhood friend on a visit from America with a scarce green vegetable called *Tung hsien tsai*, eaten only by people from Hunan and Szechwan.[11]

Food symbols may engender feelings of inadequacy as shown by the comment, "Tea sandwiches are only for ladies," made to a male athlete. Many Americans expressed disapproval when "hot dogs" were served to visiting royalty because they felt these communicated disrespect for the visitors.

Special Occasions

By group custom, foods become symbols for certain occasions or situations. Although turkey is widely distributed and used under many other circumstances, it will probably always be associated with Thanksgiving in the minds of Americans. Other countries have similar symbols for their harvest holidays. Many Czechs serve mushrooms on their day of thanksgiving, according to Du Bois,[12] as a commemoration of their ancestors' being saved from starvation over 700 years ago. One morning they found the fields covered with edible mushrooms, which they called "Jesus Bread" because they felt the mushrooms came from the Lord. *Hutsput* is the name of a stew served by the Dutch along with other holiday fare for their day of giving thanks. The origin of this food dates back to the 1500's when the Dutch were starving and besieged by the Spaniards. When hope seemed lowest, the enemy left in the middle of the night, leaving pots of stew on the battlefield. The grateful Dutch have made stew a traditional dish for their feast of thanksgiving. Large moon cakes are typical for the Chinese Moon Festival, which is similar to our Thanksgiving Day. The feasting of the Mardi Gras comes before the fasting of Lent. During the fall of 1973, the scarcity of *vanispati* or cooking oil in India dimmed the celebration of Duvali, the advent of winter.

Cookies are generally symbolic of Christmas or other occasions. Fruitcake is also associated with Christmas in many homes. A birthday calls for a certain type of cake, which will vary from family to family. In some families chicken is the Sunday meat. Champagne is synonymous with gay celebrations or with the rich. The Pennsylvania Dutch had a cake called "funeral cake" because it was frequently taken to the homes of bereaved families. Many families treasure certain recipes or modes of preparing foods that may be symbolic of a certain occasion, such as a wedding or the birth of a child. Steak may be served with mushrooms if father has had a raise or a child has brought home a good report card.

Status Values

Many foods have status value and are identified with homes on different rungs of the social ladder. These status foods vary from one country to another. In England, for example, someone of the lower class, or at least marked as lower class, may order kippers or tripe, spread sweet marmalade on his toast, and complete his meal with some kind of "gooey" dessert. If he is upper class, he will use bitter marmalade, have his coffee without milk, and end his meal with savories (pastries filled with cheese, bacon, mushrooms, or oysters).

A segment of our population known as upwardly mobile is constantly looking for foods that are not attributed to their own group but are typical of social groups above them. In this way they can identify themselves with a social status superior to their own. Moore[13] points out that in America

---

[11] Frank Ching, "A Boyhood Friend Pays Call on Mao," *The New York Times*, September 9, 1973, p. 8.

[12] Rachel Davis Du Bois, "An All-American Thanksgiving," *Forecast for Home Economics*, Vol. 75, No. 1 (September 1959), pp. 23–25,

[13] Harriet Bruce Moore, "Psychological Facts and Dieting Fancies," *Journal of the American Dietetic Association*, Vol. 28, No. 3 (September 1952), pp. 789–794.

foods have snob appeal if they are rare, expensive, exceptionally difficult to prepare, or extreme in flavor or taste. Forcing oneself to acquire a taste for status foods may be a part of the strategy of status-seekers.

Some persons who have improved their socioeconomic status may feel insecure and offended if offered food they consider low in status, such as boiled cabbage or hamburger. These or other foods may remind them of poverty or certain aspects of low-income living. A character in *Plutus*, a play by Aristophanes, remarked about a newly rich acquaintance, "Now, he doesn't eat lentils anymore." By the same token a man of new wealth may order asparagus instead of commonplace peas.

Advertising has done a great deal either to change or to inculcate certain ideas about foods. Although margarine, for example, makes a significant nutritional contribution, many people rejected it because they said they did not like the taste, it did not spread properly, or it was particularly objectionable when melted on hot vegetables. Actually, these individuals were rejecting it because they felt that people of upper status used butter. Later, advertising projected a new image of margarine by stressing that "nice" people used it, and overcame some of this difficulty. Recently some margarines have achieved a different appeal because of the unsaturated fatty acid content.

The social status ascribed to certain foods may be much more important to some people than any nutritive value they contain. Foods like Persian caviar or pheasant under glass have high social status. In some areas of our country, if a food is packaged, wrapped, or preserved in some manner, it has greater status. Certain persons feel that foods purchased directly from the source of supply, such as fruits and eggs from the farm, have special value. On the other hand, people who live on farms often place a high value on foods from the city. Most imported foods have high status value for Americans.

Other foods may be symbols of prosperity or success in another culture. In a section of the West Indies, if the Sunday meal does not have rice and beans, the husband has not been a good provider that week. In some families,

a heavily laden table is a symbol of affluence. There are other socioeconomic labels on food. Hamburger or stew, for example, lacks status. Cereals have strong meanings for most nationalities. Cornmeal for some Italians means *polenta*. Scots have a passion for oatmeal. North Africans relish *couscous*.

National and Regional Preferences

One of the strongest influences on food habits is the nationality of the family group. Sometimes the use of certain national foods is very firmly entrenched and a person will go to great lengths to secure them. If they are impossible to get, he may become very unhappy. For example, students from the Far East who come to America to study and have to eat in American restaurants complain that it is difficult to get an adequate amount of rice or that it is not cooked to their liking. In other countries—for instance, Greece and Italy—food means bread, and all other foods are a complement to bread.[14] To American Indians, food meant corn. It would be interesting to speculate which food of a given nationality group would be the last one to disappear when its families were being acculturated.

Although regional lines are fast disappearing in America because of rapid transportation and wider distribution of food, nevertheless, each region of the country may still harbor a fondness for certain foods typical of that area. This fact is exemplified by the New Englander who still has a strong taste for seafood, the Southerner who likes hot breads and grits, and the West Coast resident who likes salads. The extensive mobility of families in this country is helping to spread these regional preferences. The homemaker who has picked up some ideas about food in Texas may introduce them to neighbors in Illinois or in Oregon or wherever she may reside. The result is that many families today have eating patterns that reflect the foods of many different parts of the country and, especially in urban areas, of other countries. Rice means prosperity and stability

---

[14] Lee, op. cit.

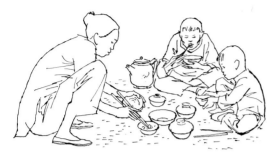

FIGURE 1–6. *Oriental families traditionally use chopsticks in eating their food.*

in China. In a Chinese revolutionary opera, *Sha Chia Pang*, about a future Chinese Utopia, there is a song, "I wish you one day . . . nine bowls of rice."[15]

Food in America reflects stratification along political, philosophical, and other lines. The blacks are proudly eating soul foods, the white-collar liberals are eating fish and chicken to keep down their cholesterol, and the "hard hats" are eating red meat to connote their degree of affluence. Youth are becoming vegetarians with almost a religious zeal and insist upon foods grown without chemical fertilizers or pesticides. Counterculture food such as mixtures of oats, sunflower seeds, peanuts, and dates and similar combinations may be preferred to hot dogs and carbonated beverages.[16]

Cultural Taboos and Dislikes

Certain foods are considered delicacies by some people but scorned by Americans. In Siam, Indochina, and some parts of India, spiders are considered fine food. The peasants of central Europe have used June bugs for making soup. The Arabs and other Orientals have been eating locusts for centuries. Where monkeys are plentiful, they have been eaten. Bats and mice are eaten in several parts of the world.

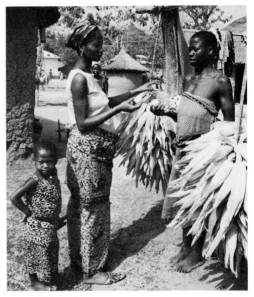

FIGURE 1–7. *A social worker in the Ivory Coast urges a village woman to use eggs in the family diet, a food against which there is a taboo.* (UNICEF)

Simoons[17] argues that eating habits do not reflect rationalization or instinct but the food ways of a group. The strongest aversions are to flesh foods. Hindus refuse to eat beef. Indians in Guiana abhor chicken, and Americans are averse to dog meat. In the Tiv tribe of Nigeria, men eat pork but it is taboo to their women. Many of these food meanings are associated wth religious observance. Starving Africans have thrown away gifts of American powdered milk because it harbors evil spirits.

Some Europeans consider corn and oats fit only for cattle. Many Puerto Ricans consider fruit to be unhealthy. Some vegetarians in India refuse to eat milk and eggs. The Jains of India believe that grains and seeds contain the germ of life and avoid their use in the diet. Ugandans regard milk as a carrier of leprosy.

The food eaten every day by people reflects complex psychological and sociological meanings. Persons concerned with nutrition must bear this fact in mind.

[15] Peggy Printz, "The Chen Family Still Has Class," *The New York Times Magazine*, October 14, 1973, pp. 43–70.

[16] Modern Living, "The Kosher of the Counterculture," *Time*, November 16, 1970, pp. 59–61.

[17] Frederick J. Simoons, *Eat Not This Flesh*, University of Wisconsin Press, Madison, Wis., 1967.

SELECTED REFERENCES

Cussler, Margaret, and Mary L. De Give, *'Twixt the Cup and the Lip*. Twayne Publishers, Inc., Boston, 1952.

Eppright, Ercel S., "Factors Affecting Food Acceptance," *Journal of the American Dietetic Association*, Vol. 23, No. 7 (July 1947), pp. 579–587.

Galdston, Iago, "Nutrition from the Psychiatric Viewpoint," *Journal of the American Dietetic Association*, Vol. 28, No. 5 (May 1952), pp. 405–409.

Ginsburg, Sol Wiener, "The Psychological Aspects of Eating," *Journal of Home Economics*, Vol. 44, No. 5 (May 1952), pp. 325–328.

Guthe, Carl E., and Margaret Mead (eds.), *Manual for the Study of Food Habits*, Bulletin No. 111, National Academy of Sciences—National Research Council, Washington, D.C., 1945.

Lewin, Kurt, "Forces Behind Food Habits and Methods of Change," in Carl E. Guthe and Margaret Mead (eds.), *The Problem of Changing Food Habits*, Bulletin No. 108, National Academy of Sciences—National Research Council, Washington, D.C., 1943, pp. 44–49.

Pumpian-Mindlin, E., "The Meaning of Food," *Journal of the American Dietetic Association*, Vol. 30, No. 6 (June 1954), pp. 576–580.

Star, Jack, "Why You Choose the Foods You Do: The Psychology and Physiology of Eating," *Today's Health*, Vol. 51, No. 2 (February 1973), pp. 33–37.

Stiebeling, Hazel, and Thelma A. Dreis, "Habit—And More," *Food, the Yearbook of Agriculture, 1959*, U.S. Department of Agriculture, Washington, D.C., 1959, pp. 631–635.

Todhunter, E. Neige, "Food Habits, Food Faddism and Nutrition," in Miloslav Rechcigl, Jr. (ed.), *Food, Nutrition and Health*, Vol. 16, S. Karger, Basel, 1973, pp. 287–314.

———, "Food Is More Than Nutrients," *Food and Nutrition News*, Vol. 43, Nos. 6–7 (March–April 1972), pp. 1–4.

Trager, James, *Foodbook*, Grossman Publishers, New York, 1970.

2

Nutrition— Yesterday and Today

Food is a basic need of the human race because it contains the nutrients essential to life. The importance of an adequate diet can be dramatized when one realizes that his eyes, blood, muscles, bones, and teeth—every part of his body—were once food.

Food *does* make a difference if adequate amounts of nutritious foods are eaten. A good diet has a tremendous bearing on a person's vitality, health, emotional stability, and enthusiasm for life. One who is well-nourished will reflect this fact in his personal appearance. Generally his posture is good, his muscles are firm, his complexion is clear, and his eyes sparkle. He is prepared to meet life with equilibrium.

By contrast, those who are undernourished are inclined to tire easily, to be irritable, and to worry. They generally lack stamina and purpose; they are much more susceptible to illness than the well-nourished; and their life often appears to be a drudgery. These people frequently are not aware that poor eating habits may be one root of their difficulty.

Not only is day-to-day living affected by the type of food one eats, but there are long-term effects as well. Young men and women of America are about 2 inches taller and are stronger on the whole than their grandparents in their youth. Scientists say that one of the major reasons is that the eating habits of Americans have improved. Consider, for example, the children of Orientals in California, who are larger than their parents. This tendency of youth to grow faster and taller has also been found true in several other countries. Children who have been undernourished make striking improvments in health and the quality of living when nutritious food is made available, as demonstrated by Austrian children after World War I and the success of the UNICEF program. Unfortunately, some effects of malnutrition are irreversible.

Other observations and research have strengthened the proof that good nutrition makes a difference in the health and appearance of people. In the late 1800's and the early 1900's, Wilbur Olin Atwater, the first director of research in the United States Department of Agriculture noted in the Appalachian highlands the contrast between the attractive children and the prematurely aged

11

women who were only thirty. He attributed the condition of the women to the poor quality of the diets.

Robert McCarrison,[1] a British physician, studied the health of people in different sections of India. Great differences in stature and well-being were attributed to diet. Lord John Boyd Orr,[2] a Scottish physician and scientist noted for his work with the Food and Agriculture Organization of the United Nations, had similar impressions when studying various tribes in Africa. Greater vigor and stature were associated with a diet that included meat and milk in contrast to a diet composed entirely of cereals and other plant foods.

Margaret Ohlson[3] and co-workers did research on the dietary practices of 100 Midwestern women ranging in age from 30 to 70 years. The women who were in good health, with no history of chronic or other weakening diseases, drank more milk and ate more eggs, vegetables, and whole grain cereals and bread than the women who had chronic diseases and who were in general ill health.

These observations and research point to the important conclusion that the *kind* and *amount* of food eaten by a person have an influence on his well-being.

Consequently, it is essential to distinguish between *food* and *nutrition*. People often have the false impression that if they eat just any food they are nourished. It is not as simple as that. Foods are merely the conveyors of the nutrients necessary to well-being, and the particular food eaten may not contain the required nutrients. The terms *well-fed* and *well-nourished* may not be synonymous. *Well-fed* connotes quantity or economic quality of

food, whereas *well-nourished* implies receiving adequate food containing the required nutrients for good health. In addition, it is important that the proper proportion of these various essential nutrients be supplied.

With this background, how might *nutrition* be defined? *Nutrition* has been defined by experts as the combination of processes by which all parts of the body receive and utilize the materials necessary for performance of their functions and for the growth and renewal of all components. The study of nutrition is closely related to other sciences, such as chemistry, especially biochemistry, physiology, physics, endocrinology, and anatomy. Social sciences are related to nutrition, particularly in its practice. It is an integral part of the study for such professions as medicine, public health, dietetics, and dentistry.

History of Nutrition

The knowledge that nutrition is essential to well-being presents a dramatic story that took centuries to evolve. Although often referred to as a twentieth-century science, nutrition has been an integral part of science and the practice of medicine for more than 2000 years. During the early period, physicians were the nutritionists. Hippocrates, known as the "father of medicine," was the first great physician to indicate an interest in nutrition. In his earlier years he was a physiologist and consequently was concerned about the functioning of the body. Some of his famous quotations are interesting: "I think of the stomach as a kind of stewpot in which food gets cooked or stewed by body heat," and "Children produce more heat and need more food than adults."

Another famous Greek physician was Galen, who lived in Rome in the second century A.D. He was noted for his work in experimental physiology. Since human dissection was frowned upon in Rome, Galen did his experiments in anatomy and physiology on cattle, pigs, and apes and demonstrated that blood vessels carried blood and not air, as previously believed. He recorded the results of his experiments in some 16 books, which served as medical texts for many years.

[1] Robert McCarrison, "Faulty Food in Relation to Gastro-intestinal Disorders," *Journal of the American Medical Association*, Vol. 78, No. 1 (January 1922), pp. 1–8.

[2] J. B. Orr and J. L. Gilks, "Studies of Nutrition: The Physiques and Health of Two African Tribes," *Medical Research Council Special Report Series No. 155*, His Majesty's Stationery Office, London, 1931.

[3] Margaret Ohlson et al., "Food Selection and Well-being of Aging Women," *Journal of the American Dietetic Association*, Vol. 33, No. 5 (May 1957), pp. 566–570.

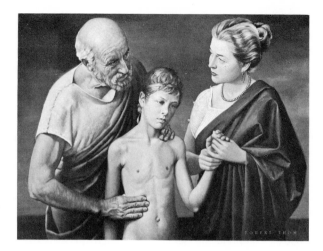

(*Figures 2–1, 2–2, and 14–1 are from a continuing series, "A History of Medicine in Pictures." They are reproduced by special permission of Parke, Davis and Company, who commissioned the original oil paintings, and by whom they are copyrighted. The project was written and directed by George A. Bender, painted by Robert A. Thom.*)

FIGURE 2–1. *A mother brings her ailing son to Hippocrates, the Father of Medicine, who was the first physician to indicate an interest in nutrition.*

One of the most colorful and original experimenters in nutrition was Sanctorius, a young Italian doctor of the late sixteenth century. He was noted for devising a huge scale, one arm of which held a chair. At times he would sit on the chair, eat his meals, and even sleep there. He took his weight in the morning, before and after eating; he weighed all the food that he ate and the waste material that was excreted. Since the results did not match, he was curious about what had happened to the food. These experiments continued for 30 years, and he kept very careful records of his work, but never did find the answers to the difference in weight.

In the seventeenth century, the scientist with his experimental methods complemented the physician as nutritionist. An Englishman, William Harvey, made revolutionary discoveries concerning circulation. And the development of the microscope by Anton van Leeuwenhoek, a Dutchman, enabled scientists to study blood cells as well as other physiological phenomena.

Modern physiology and chemistry had their beginnings in the eighteenth century. René de Réaumur, a distinguished French scientist who lived in the middle of the century, learned the scientific steps in digestion. From his experiments he concluded that the stomach did not

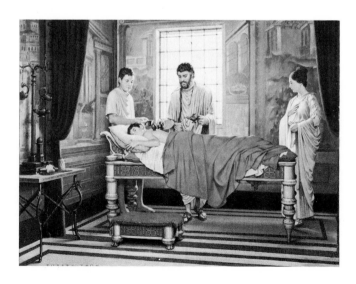

FIGURE 2–2. *Galen, a Greek physician, in Rome (2nd century A.D.) contributed to advances in nutrition through experimental physiology.* (*Parke Davis*)

grind food but, rather, that it produced chemicals that affected food. Spallanzani, a famous Italian investigator, concentrated on studying the digestion of the food in the stomach and the function of gastric juice.

Boyle, an English scientist known as the "father of chemistry," demonstrated, in experiments on mice placed in jars, that there was something in air that is necessary for life.

These experiments to determine what air contained that was essential to life were continued by Mayow, an English physiologist and chemist. As a result of certain experiments, he claimed that this essential part of the air after being breathed into the lungs was taken up by the blood and carried to all parts of the body. This statement was quite an advance over the older theory of the air and lungs being simply a cooling system for the heart and body. These findings, however, were not accepted for more than 100 years.

Joseph Priestley, an English scientist of the eighteenth century, performed some of Mayow's experiments as well as other research, and is credited with discovering the gas later called oxygen.

Antoine Lavoisier, a French scientist living at the time of the French Revolution, repeated the experiments of Boyle, Mayow, and Priestley and gave the name *oxygen* to this part of the air. Later he showed that another component of air was carbon dioxide. His experiments disclosed the fact that the food that is eaten is like a fuel in the body and that the more a man worked, the more food he needed. Lavoisier is often called the "father of nutrition."

The nineteenth century was noted for chemical investigations, plus respiration and energy studies.

In 1834, William Prout, a London physician, was the first scientist to classify food into three groups. He believed that all foods were made up of the following classifications: foods of an animal or albuminous nature, foods of a vegetable or saccharine nature, and a group of fatty or oily foods. Involved and lengthy names were given to each group. Prout did not demonstrate the amount of each of these classes that should be eaten, but emphasized that it was important to eat some of each kind.

François Magendie, a French physician and physiologist, demonstrated that there was a nutritional difference between foods that contained nitrogen and those that did not. Using dogs as experimental animals, he fed them various types of foods lacking in nitrogen, such as sugars or oils, and found that the dogs grew weaker and soon died. As a result, he believed that foods containing nitrogen were essential to life. Gerrit Jan Mulder, a Dutch chemist, gave foods with nitrogen the name of *protein*, which means "to take first place." Carl Voit, a famous German physiologist, was responsible for the first work on nitrogen-balance studies. Using dogs as experimental animals, he demonstrated that the use of protein is to build and maintain tissues.

Wilbur Olin Atwater, a student of Voit, while working at the Office of Experiment Stations of the U.S. Department of Agriculture, published the first analysis of an American food—corn—and prepared the first food composition tables in this country. His work on animal respiration led to the development of the calorimeter. F. G. Benedict, following Atwater's experiments, was able to devise a portable apparatus for measuring metabolism.

At the beginning of the twentieth century, research on protein was emphasized. Atwater, in addition to his other interests in nutrition, studied the protein requirements of man. He recommended 125 grams of protein daily for a laboring man. Russell H. Chittenden, on the faculty at Yale University and the first university teacher of physiological chemistry in America, was also interested in protein and published reports of his unusual studies in 1904. He was noted not only for his research but also for his role as teacher of many professional men.

Yale made another outstanding contribution through the famous team of Thomas Osborne and Lafayette Mendel, scientists who cast considerable light on differences of proteins in various types of food. They demonstrated that casein could be used as a sole source of proteins to promote growth in animals and that grain proteins were not always adequate.

Frederick G. Hopkins, an English scientist, believed that there were certain "accessory

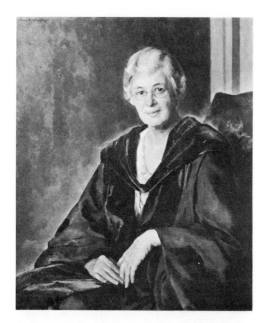

FIGURE 2–3. *Mary Swartz Rose, the first professor of nutrition in the United States.*

food substances" whose deficiency would cause certain diseases, and mentioned rickets and scurvy specifically. His work was a forerunner of the research done on vitamins in the twentieth century, as discussed in Chapters 11–14.

Henry Clapp Sherman, a chemistry professor at Columbia University, did a great deal to supply quantitative knowledge of nutritional requirements of man, work that had been started by Atwater. Mary Swartz Rose was the first professor of nutrition in the United States. She was appointed professor in 1921 at Teachers College, Columbia University, and wrote a number of outstanding books in the field and performed important experiments on energy metabolism. She is also noted for many contributions to nutrition education.

Elmer V. McCollum, a student of Mendel, published *The Newer Knowledge of Nutrition* in 1918. In this book he introduced the term *protective foods*, meaning milk, eggs, and leafy vegetables, and claimed that these foods could contribute to the preservation of youthful qualities.

Within the last 60 years, vitamins have been discovered and active research has un-

covered human needs for a number of macrominerals and microminerals.[4] During the same period Rose[5] made an outstanding contribution to the establishment of the amino acid and protein needs of man. The advent of clinical nutrition advanced nutrition knowledge and many types of nutrition research, according to Sebrell.[6]

Other facets of nutrition have been gaining emphasis. Iago Galdston[7] believed that during the period of great emphasis on particular knowledge about nutrients interest in the human being was lost or at least decreased. He said, "We became so preoccupied with subject matter that we forgot the man to whom the subject relates." This observation led to the addition of another dimension to the study of nutrition, namely, its psychological and sociological aspects. These, no doubt, mark a new era in the history of nutrition.

Origin of Nutrition Standards

Although much information had been contributed by research in the past, the question of amounts and kinds of food to be consumed daily had not been answered. Dietary standards, therefore, are an innovation of comparatively recent times. The first standards were established in 1936 through the League of Nations and were based on the limited information available at that time. Variations in the requirements of different nutrients were very pronounced. Sherman had established standards for protein, calcium, phosphorus, and iron for adults, and Lucy Gillette had

[4] Charles Glen King, "Foods and Nutrition Through Fifty Years," *American Journal of Public Health*, Vol. 58, No. 11 (November 1968), pp. 2015–2020.

[5] William C. Rose, "The Sequence of Events Leading to the Establishment of the Amino Acid Needs of Man," *American Journal of Public Health*, Vol. 58, No. 11 (November 1968), pp. 2020–2027.

[6] William H. Sebrell, Jr., "Clinical Nutrition in the United States," *American Journal of Public Health*, Vol. 58, No. 11 (November 1968), pp. 2035–2042.

[7] Iago Galdston, "Nutrition from the Psychiatric Viewpoint," *Journal of the American Dietetic Association*, Vol. 28, No. 5 (May 1952), pp. 405–409.

worked out caloric standards for children that were utilized in developing the League of Nations standards. No standards covering all the nutrients for all ages were available.

Pett,[8] the prominent Canadian scientist, is of the opinion that the use of a dietary standard was influenced by the concepts held by its innovator. The first standards were developed to indicate amounts of food necessary to keep people from starving. Next, they were related to agricultural production, that is, the kinds and yields of crops required for adequate energy needs of the population. It was Hazel Stiebeling of the Institute of Home Economics of the Department of Agriculture who suggested in 1933 the first standards for minerals and vitamins in addition to energy and protein. She used the word *optimal*. This gave emphasis to health rather than minimal standards for existence or for preventing dietary deficiency diseases.

American dietary standards were developed prior to our entry into World War II. Health experts recommended that the latest nutritional knowledge be applied for the purpose of maintaining health and productivity during a time of great national stress. Therefore, in 1940 the National Research Council organized a Food and Nutrition Board, which was composed of outstanding scientists and physicians concerned with nutrition. This board accepted the responsibility for developing and proposing a dietary standard for the United States.

A very important step was taken by the Food and Nutrition Board in planning these *Recommended Dietary Allowances,* which were first published in 1943. The result was a marked and wise departure from former thinking in regard to standards. At specified periods the Food and Nutrition Board revises the dietary allowances in light of new discoveries and research. Revisions were made in 1945, 1948, 1953, 1958, 1964, 1968, and 1974. These allowances serve as a guide in planning and evaluating the daily diet.

Table 2–1 cites the recommended dietary allowances (1974 revision) for the indicated nutrients.

The major objective of the Food and Nutrition Board of the National Research Council in the development of the recommended dietary allowances is to encourage the development of food habits by the population of the United States that will allow for maximum returns in the maintenance of health. The recommended dietary allowances[9] are recommendations for the amounts of nutrients to be consumed daily and are not to be confused with requirements. Individuals differ in nutrient requirements, so the recommended dietary allowances are planned to exceed requirements, except for kcalories; thus the needs of nearly all are met for both sexes and all ages, and including pregnant and lactating women.

The 1974 recommended dietary allowances include kcalories, protein, vitamin A, vitamin D, vitamin E, ascorbic acid, folacin, niacin, riboflavin, thiamin, vitamin B_6, vitamin B_{12}, calcium, phosphorus, iodine, iron, magnesium, and zinc as the nutrients essential for the maintenance of good nutrition of practically all healthy people in the United States. The amounts of these nutrients are expressed in terms of scientific measures, such as grams (g), milligrams (mg), micrograms (μg), or international units (IU).

The nutrients included have had human requirements established as a basis for determining allowances. The present knowledge about many other nutrients is incomplete as to requirement. To assure that possible unrecognized nutritional needs are met, emphasis should be given to as varied a selection of foods as is practical. Another suggestion is to consider the importance of an awareness of the psychological and social values of food. Diets are more than combinations of nutrients. Selection should be made from the foods that are considered acceptable and palatable by individuals and family members.

Because the allowances provide for a safety

---

[8] L. B. Pett, "Limitation in the Use of Dietary Standards," *Journal of the American Dietetic Association,* Vol. 27, No. 1 (January 1951), pp. 28–31.

[9] Food and Nutrition Board, *Recommended Dietary Allowances,* 8th ed., National Academy of Sciences—National Research Council, Washington, D.C., 1974.

TABLE 2–1

Food and Nutrition Board, National Academy of Sciences—National Research Council Recommended Daily Dietary Allowances,[a] Revised 1974.

Designed for the maintenance of good nutrition of practically all healthy people in the United States

	AGE (years)	WEIGHT (kg)	WEIGHT (lb)	HEIGHT (cm)	HEIGHT (in.)	ENERGY (kcal)[b]	PROTEIN (g)	Vit A Activity (RE)[c]	Vit A (IU)	Vit D (IU)	Vit E Activity (IU)[e]	Ascorbic acid (mg)	Folacin[f] (µg)	Niacin[g] (mg)	Riboflavin (mg)	Thiamin (mg)	Vit B12 (mg)	Vit B12 (µg)	Calcium (mg)	Phosphorus (mg)	Iodine (µg)	Iron (mg)	Magnesium (mg)	Zinc (mg)
Infants	0.0–0.5	6	14	60	24	kg × 117	kg × 2.2	420[d]	1400	400	4	35	50	5	0.4	0.3	0.3	0.3	360	240	35	10	60	3
	0.5–1.0	9	20	71	28	kg × 108	kg × 2.0	400	2000	400	5	35	50	8	0.6	0.5	0.4	0.3	540	400	45	15	70	5
Children	1–3	13	28	86	34	1300	23	400	2000	400	7	40	100	9	0.8	0.7	0.6	1.0	800	800	60	15	150	10
	4–6	20	44	110	44	1800	30	500	2500	400	9	40	200	12	1.1	0.9	0.9	1.5	800	800	80	10	200	10
	7–10	30	66	135	54	2400	36	700	3300	400	10	40	300	16	1.2	1.2	1.2	2.0	800	800	110	10	250	10
Males	11–14	44	97	158	63	2800	44	1000	5000	400	12	45	400	18	1.5	1.4	1.6	3.0	1200	1200	130	18	350	15
	15–18	61	134	172	69	3000	54	1000	5000	400	15	45	400	20	1.8	1.5	2.0	3.0	1200	1200	150	18	400	15
	19–22	67	147	172	69	3000	54	1000	5000	400	15	45	400	20	1.8	1.5	2.0	3.0	800	800	140	10	350	15
	23–50	70	154	172	69	2700	56	1000	5000		15	45	400	18	1.6	1.4	2.0	3.0	800	800	130	10	350	15
	51+	70	154	172	69	2400	56	1000	5000		15	45	400	16	1.5	1.2	2.0	3.0	800	800	110	10	350	15
Females	11–14	44	97	155	62	2400	44	800	4000	400	12	45	400	16	1.3	1.2	1.6	3.0	1200	1200	115	18	300	15
	15–18	54	119	162	65	2100	48	800	4000	400	12	45	400	14	1.4	1.1	2.0	3.0	1200	1200	115	18	300	15
	19–22	58	128	162	65	2100	46	800	4000	400	12	45	400	14	1.4	1.1	2.0	3.0	800	800	100	18	300	15
	23–50	58	128	162	65	2000	46	800	4000		12	45	400	13	1.2	1.0	2.0	3.0	800	800	100	18	300	15
	51+	58	128	162	65	1800	46	800	4000		12	45	400	12	1.1	1.0	2.0	3.0	800	800	80	10	300	15
Pregnant						+300	+30	1000	5000	400	15	60	800	+2	+0.3	+0.3	2.5	4.0	1200	1200	125	18+[h]	450	20
Lactating						+500	+20	1200	6000	400	15	80	600	+4	+0.5	+0.3	2.5	4.0	1200	1200	150	18	450	25

SOURCE: Food and Nutrition Board, *Recommended Dietary Allowances*, 8th ed., National Academy of Sciences—Washington, D.C., 1974.

a The allowances are intended to provide for individual variations among most normal persons as they live in the United States under usual environmental stresses. Diets should be based on a variety of common foods in order to provide other nutrients for which human requirements have been less well defined.

b Kilojoules (kJ) = 4.2 × kcal.

c Retinol equivalents.

d Assumed to be all as retinol in milk during the first 6 months of life. All subsequent intakes are assumed to be half as retinol and half as beta-carotene when calculated from international units. As retinol equivalents, three fourths are as retinol and one fourth as beta-carotene.

e Total vitamin E activity, estimated to be 80 per cent as alpha-tocopherol and 20 per cent other tocopherols.

f The folacin allowances refer to dietary sources as determined by *Lactobacillus casei* assay. Pure forms of folacin may be effective in doses less than one fourth of the recommended dietary allowance.

g Although allowances are expressed as niacin, it is recognized that on the average 1 mg of niacin is derived from each 60 mg of dietary tryptophan.

h This increased requirement cannot be met by ordinary diets; therefore, the use of supplemental iron is recommended.

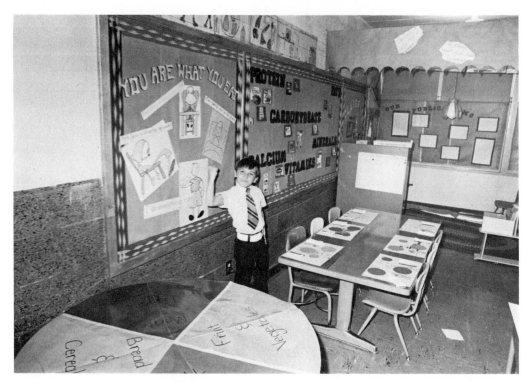

FIGURE 2–4. *Understanding nutrition is an important requisite to adequate nourishment of an individual.*

factor, an individual cannot assume that it is feasible to reduce the nutrients by one fourth or one third and still maintain adequate nutritional status. The techniques for making such precise determinations of dietary needs are not available. No individual can know if he happens to be among the ones that may need less. It is possible that he or she may benefit from the full quota. Information is not available for each individual about the exact amount of specific nutrients that are required. Security can come only from using the recommended dietary allowances as an effective guide.

The knowledge available in the recommended dietary allowances, food guides, and food composition tables must be supplemented by an understanding of nutrition that includes the factors which influence the way individuals select and consume their food. More is known about food acceptability, flavor, taste, mouth feel, and the like than about

potent influences such as food beliefs and attitudes, religion, social, cultural, and economic background, and environment. Understanding nutrition is paramount to adequate nourishment of an individual and reflects the need for an appropriate nutrition education program.

Use of Recommended Allowances

The Recommended Dietary Allowances have value in planning and obtaining food supplies for population groups, for evaluating food consumption records in relation to nutritional status, in establishing policy guidelines for health and welfare programs, as assessment techniques for government nutrition surveys, for nutrition education programs, and for product development, nutrition labeling, and regulation of nutritional labeling.[10]

---

[10] Ibid., pp. 13–20.

A number of questions arise about the use of the Recommended Dietary Allowances. Consideration must be given, according to Darby,[11] to the biological availability of nutrients in certain foods and in combinations, the influence of food processing, the effect of food preparation, patterns of diet, and the effects of additives. Individuals must recognize that Recommended Dietary Allowances are based on existing knowledge and change consequently with new knowledge.

Development of Food Guides

The next important step was the translation of the standards with their scientific measures—grams, milligrams, micrograms, and other units—into terms of foods that are eaten daily. From time to time, different types of food guides have been developed. All of them have limitations.

The genesis of the first attempt to develop food guides is unknown.[12] World War I stimulated the dissemination of considerable food and nutrition information. The efforts of Caroline L. Hunt, a specialist in food and nutrition in the Bureau of Nutrition and Home Economics, are reflected in the historic bulletin, "A Week's Food for the Average Family," published by the Department of Agriculture in 1921. This was followed by another bulletin, "Good Proportions in the Diet," released in 1923.[13]

The rationale of Hunt's plan was that the number of different foods available in the United States was great. New plants and other food sources were constantly being introduced, and improved agricultural and manufacturing processes were invented. All these foods, however, could be divided into a small number of categories, and foods within

a group could be interchanged, such as the various green vegetables.

Hunt classified the common foods into five groups according to their composition and consequent nutritive contribution, as follows: (1) fruits and vegetables, (2) meat, milk, and other foods that contributed complete and efficient protein, (3) cereals, (4) sugar and sugar foods, and (5) fats and fatty foods. Representatives of these five groups should be found in a daily meal, a day's ration, or a weekly food supply to provide the nutrients for a wholesome diet. These early guides were general in nature and did not indicate specific amounts or attempt to evaluate nutritive contributions within a group. The purpose of the guide was educational, especially in the selection of foods and in the planning of meals.

The rationing of such food items as meat, sugar, butter, and canned goods during World War II demanded the development of a new guide, according to Hill. The "Basic 7" food guide was developed as a part of the National Nutrition Program under the agency that became the War Food Administration, that is, the U.S. Department of Agriculture. Nutritionists in the Bureau of Nutrition and Home Economics worked with nutritionists of other agencies and with the Advertising Council in the development of a useful food guide. The "Basic 7" was first published in 1943 as "The National Wartime Food Guide." Suggestions were made for ways to correct common dietary shortages and for alternative choices for foods in limited supply.

After the war, the "Basic 7" was reviewed by nutritionists. A decision was made to change this general guide to one that included the number of servings needed for each group. This revision, known as the "National Food Guide" was issued in 1946. The seven food groups with daily requirements are as follows:

Group 1. Leafy green and yellow vegetables—one or more servings
Group 2. Citrus fruit, tomatoes, raw cabbage—one or more servings
Group 3. Potatoes, other vegetables, and fruits—two or more servings
Group 4. Milk, cheese—for children: three to four cups of milk; for

[11] William J. Darby, "Nutrition in the 1970's," *Nutrition Reviews*, Vol. 30, No. 2 (February 1972), pp. 27–29.

[12] Mary M. Hill, "Food Guides—Their Development and Use," *Nutrition Program News*, U.S. Department of Agriculture, July–October 1970, pp. 1–5.

[13] Caroline L. Hunt, *Good Proportions in the Diet*, Farmer's Bulletin No. 1313, U.S. Department of Agriculture, Washington, D.C., 1923.

adults: two or more cups or the equivalent

Group 5. Meat, poultry, fish, eggs, dried peas or beans—one to two servings

Group 6. Bread, flour, cereal (whole grain, enriched)—at least three servings

Group 7. Butter or fortified margarine— at least one tablespoon

The basic assumption underlying this food guide is that, if these seven groups are included, then adequate amounts of essential nutrients are represented and other foods may be eaten in sufficient quantity to maintain weight. This list also gives a person an op-

portunity to include those foods he likes very much but that do not contribute some of the important nutrients. If a person is overweight, attention must be given to foods that are not so high in kcaloric value. But if he is underweight, more emphasis must be given to foods that are high in kcalories.

One limitation in using the basic seven guide concerns the size of a serving. Individuals vary greatly in their concept of a serving. Many homes do not have a standard measuring cup, so that an idea of even a cup measure may be somewhat nebulous. Generally speaking, however, a serving of fruit or vegetable refers to at least a half-cup portion (standard measuring cup).

In teaching, the basic seven are generally

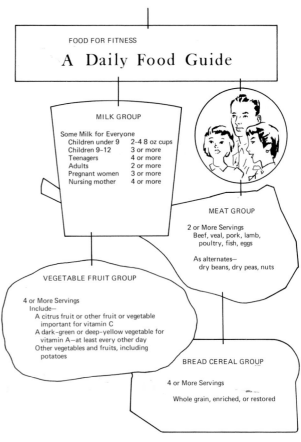

FIGURE 2–5. *A mobile depicting the Food for Fitness Guide.* (*Adapted from* Daily Food Guide, *U.S. Department of Agriculture*)

portrayed in the shape of a wheel or pie-shaped graph, which helps an individual realize that each group is equally important. Another advantage is that this guide does help an individual feel secure about the adequacy of his diet. He can readily check to see if he has had the indicated amount of food from each of these groups, and then he is free to eat other foods. The only additional factor he needs to watch is his weight.

The most recent food guide developed by the Institute of Home Economics of the Agricultural Research Service is called *Food for Fitness, a Daily Food Guide.*[14] The four food groups in this guide, with the recommended daily consumption, are as follows:

MILK GROUP Foods included are milk—fluid whole, evaporated, skim, dry, buttermilk; cheese—cottage, cream, cheddar-type, natural or processed; ice cream. Cheese and ice cream may replace part of the milk in equivalent amounts. See Chapter 16 for a table of equivalents. Amounts recommended—some milk everyday for everyone. Recommended amounts are given in terms of whole fluid milk:

Children under 9	2 to 3 8-oz cups
Children 9 to 12	3 or more
Teenagers	4 or more
Adults	2 or more
Pregnant women	3 or more
Nursing mothers	4 or more

VEGETABLE–FRUIT GROUP Foods included are all vegetables and fruit. Amounts recommended are four or more servings each day, including a good source of vitamin C or two servings of a fair source; one serving, at least every other day, of a good source of vitamin A. If the food chosen for vitamin C is also a good source of vitamin A, the additional serving of a vitamin A food may be omitted. The remaining one to three or more servings may be any vegetable or fruit, including those that are valuable for vitamin C and vitamin A. Count as one serving: ½ cup of vegetable or fruit; or a portion as ordinarily served, such as

one medium apple, banana, orange, or potato, half a medium grapefruit or cantaloupe, or the juice of one lemon.

MEAT GROUP Foods included are beef; veal; lamb; pork; variety meats, such as liver, heart, kidney; poultry and eggs; fish and shellfish; and, as alternatives, dry beans, dry peas, lentils, nuts, peanuts, peanut butter. Amounts recommended are two or more servings every day. A serving is counted as 2 to 3 oz of lean cooked meat, poultry, or fish—all without bone; two eggs; 1 cup cooked dry beans, dry peas, or lentils; or 4 tbs peanut butter.

BREAD–CEREAL GROUP Foods included are all breads and cereals that are whole grain, enriched, or restored; check labels to be sure. Specifically, this group includes breads, cooked cereals, ready-to-eat cereals, cornmeal, crackers, flour, grits, macaroni and spaghetti, noodles, rice, rolled oats, and quick breads and other baked goods if made with whole-grain or enriched flour. Parboiled rice and wheat may be included in this group. Amounts recommended are four or more servings daily. Count as one serving: one slice of bread; 1 oz ready-to-eat cereal; ½ to ¾ cup cooked cereal, cornmeal, grits, macaroni, noodles, rice, or spaghetti. If no cereals are chosen, add an extra serving of breads or baked goods to make at least five servings from this group daily.

The advantage of this particular guide is its simplicity. It is believed that people can remember a few food groups more easily. This is especially true with foreign-speaking groups, elementary school children, or persons with limited education. However, this guide has its limitations, too. Each food group must have definite interpretations so that wise selections may be made. There is also the same problem about size of servings. In using any of these food guides, it is important to know the nutritive values of foods within a group. For example, are all citrus fruits equally high in vitamin C value? If not, what compensations are necessary? What substitutes, if any, can be made for milk? Some have doubted the

---

[14] *Leaflet No. 424,* U.S. Department of Agriculture, Washington, D.C., revised 1967.

22   INTRODUCTION TO NUTRITION

value of using the Basic Four because so many foods are processed, according to Leverton.[15] Actually only 6 per cent of the money spent for food could not be placed in the four food groups. The value of these food guides is that they form a kind of blueprint in planning a day's meals, with the possibility of making adaptations for individual needs and preferences.

Status of American Nutrition

The nutritional status of the nation is difficult to assess, according to Henderson,[16] because it is related to certain social, educational, and economic conditions. Prominent on the list are (1) elimination of extreme poverty, (2) the difficulty in educating the consumer so that he will be sufficiently nutrition conscious and informed to eat nutritious meals, and (3) the development of realistic nutrition standards and guidelines to keep the consumer up to date about convenience, prepared foods, new foods, and snacks.

Nutrition Surveys

Two important surveys of nutritional status have been undertaken by the government; the first was the *Ten-State Nutrition Survey*[17] in 1968–1970 and the second was the *First Health and Nutrition Examination Survey*[18] in 1971–1972.

[15] Ruth Leverton, "Tools for Teaching Food Needs," *Journal of Home Economics*, Vol. 65, No. 1 (January 1973), pp. 37–39.

[16] L. M. Henderson, "Nutritional Problems Growing out of New Patterns of Food Consumption," *American Journal of Public Health*, Vol. 62, No. 9 (September 1972), pp. 1194–1198.

[17] *Highlights, Ten-State Nutrition Survey, 1968–1970*, DHEW Publication No. (HSM) 72–8134, Center for Disease Control, Health Services and Mental Health Administration, U.S. Department of Health, Education, and Welfare, Atlanta, Ga., 1972.

[18] National Center for Health Statistics, *Preliminary Findings, First Health and Nutrition Examination Survey, United States, 1971–1972*, DHEW Publication No. (HRA) 74–1291–1, Health Resources Administration, Public Health Service, U.S. Department of Health, Education, and Welfare, Rockville, Md., 1974.

Ten-State Nutrition Survey

The *Ten-State Nutrition Survey* was limited to ten states because of constraints of time and money. Washington, California, Texas, Louisiana, South Carolina, Kentucky, West Virginia, Michigan, Massachusetts, and New York were chosen. About 40,000 individuals were involved. The largest percentage of persons in the sample was white, and, second, black; the smallest percentage was Spanish-Americans (Puerto Ricans, predominantly from New York City, and Mexican-Americans from Texas and California).

Income status was another population characteristic. Careful evaluation was made of this factor because adequate nutrition is related to adequate income. Income level was expressed in terms of a poverty income ratio (PIR) as developed by Orshansky.[19] This ratio related certain income characteristics of a given family to a defined poverty level. A large number of the families included in the survey were living below or slightly above the poverty level. Mean values for PIR varied widely from state to state. It was possible to divide the ten states and New York City into two large groups based on PIR. One group, Kentucky, Louisiana, South Carolina, Texas, and West Virginia, were identified as low-income-ratio states because more than half the families in the sample were living below poverty levels. In the five remaining states, California, Washington, Michigan, New York and New York City, and Massachusetts had more than 50 per cent of the families living above the poverty level and were designated as high-income-ratio states.

The distribution of ethnic groups varied widely from state to state. Generally, the proportion of black families was greatest in the low-income-ratio states, followed by Spanish-Americans, and then whites. The median years of school completed by individuals in the study were lower in the low-income-ratio states.

When malnutrition of people of similar ethnic background was compared, the nutri-

[19] Mollie Orshansky, "The Shape of Poverty in 1966," *Social Security Bulletin*, March 1968.

tional inadequacies were higher in the low-income-ratio group, indicating that factors other than income, such as social, cultural, and geographic differences, also affect the nutritional status of a group. For example, there was a high prevalence of low vitamin A values among Mexican-Americans in the low-income-ratio states as contrasted to the absence of vitamin A problems among Puerto Ricans in the high-income-ratio states, primarily in New York City.

Although the primary interest in each state was malnutrition among the poor, the sample population did not include all this lower-income group within a state, nor was it restricted to only the poor. The income characteristics of some of the districts had changed since 1960 (date of the last census). Some middle- and upper-income familes resided in districts having a low average income. The sampling procedure appears to yield a representative sample of low-income families, but those with higher incomes living within these areas who were included may have special characteristics and not be representative of the middle- and high-income population. Therefore, the two income groups cannot be considered representative of the entire population within a county or state, and the findings cannot be extrapolated and applied to the overall population of the states from which samples were drawn.

There was a heavy representation of children in the sample. More than 50 per cent of the persons examined were 16 years of age or less; 30 per cent were 17 to 44 years of age, and the remaining 17 per cent were 45 years of age or older. Certain subgroups received more detailed biochemical and dietary evaluation. Among these groups were high-risk populations such as infants and young children, adolescents, pregnant and lactating women, and persons over 60 years of age. All individuals had a clinical evaluation, which included medical history, physical examination, anthropometric measurements, X-ray examination of the wrist, dental examination, and collection of blood for hemoglobin and hematocrit determinations. Dietary data included information about nutrient intakes, food habits, and methods of food preparation.

Findings of interest (see Table 2–2) in regard to specific nutrients included the high prevalence of low hemoglobin and hematocrit values in all segments of the population. Low levels of serum iron and serum transferrin saturation and, to a lesser extent, low levels of serum and red-blood-cell folic acid were also revealed. There was a tendency for lower hemoglobin levels to be associated with lower dietary iron intakes. This evidence indicates a widespread problem of iron deficiency.

A comparatively large proportion of pregnant and lactating females gave evidence of low serum albumin levels, which suggested marginal protein levels in their diets. In all other groups, the dietary protein intakes were generally above levels believed to be adequate.

In regard to vitamin A, young people in all groups indicated high prevalence of low vitamin A levels. Spanish-Americans of all ages in low-income groups had a major problem, especially in low-income-ratio states.

Vitamin C nutriture was not a major problem among any of the groups studied. More males had lower vitamin C levels than females. With an increase in age there was a greater prevalence of poor vitamin C status. Riboflavin status was poor among blacks and among young people of all groups. Thiamin nutriture did not appear to be a problem. The survey showed no evidence of an iodine deficiency. Although not anticipated, goiter was prevalent, but no relationship could be found between goiter and the deficiency of iodine. Iodized salt was not readily available or used in all of the communities surveyed.

This survey was limited to a study of some 12 of the nutrients known to be essential for good health. No information, for example, was secured on such poorly studied nutrients as zinc, magnesium, and vitamin E. Other studies must be designed to secure information on these and other problems of nutriture.

Health and Nutrition Examination Survey

The National Health Survey Act of 1956 provides for the establishment and continuation of a National Health Survey to obtain information about the health status of the popu-

TABLE 2–2

Relative Importance of Nutritional Problems in the Ten-State Nutrition Survey, 1968–1970

Low-Income-Ratio States: Kentucky, Louisiana, South Carolina, Texas, West Virginia

ETHNIC GROUP	AGE	SEX	Iron	Protein	Vitamin A	Vitamin C	Riboflavin	Thiamin	Iodine	Growth and development	Obesity
BLACK	0–5 years	Both	●	○	●	○	●	○	○	●	○
	6–9 years	Both	●	•	•	○	●	○	○	●	—
	10–16 years	Females	●	•	•	○	●	○	○	•	•
		Males	●	○	•	○	●	○	○	•	•
	17–59 years	Females	●	•	○	•	●	○	○	—	●
		Males	●	○	○	●	●	○	○	—	○
	Over 60 years	Females	●	•	○	○	●	○	○	—	●
		Males	●	•	○	●	●	○	○	—	○
WHITE	0–5 years	Both	●	○	•	○	•	○	○	●	—
	6–9 years	Both	●	○	•	○	•	○	○	●	—
	10–16 years	Females	●	○	•	○	•	•	○	•	•
		Males	●	○	•	○	•	•	○	•	●
	17–59 years	Females	●	○	○	○	○	○	○	○	●
		Males	●	○	○	●	○	○	○	—	•
	Over 60 years	Females	●	○	○	○	○	○	○	—	●
		Males	●	○	○	●	○	○	○	—	○
SPANISH-AMERICAN	0–5 years	Both	●	○	●	○	●	○	○	●	—
	6–9 years	Both	●	○	●	○	●	○	○	●	—
	10–16 years	Females	●	•	●	○	●	○	○	•	—
		Males	●	○	●	○	●	○	○	•	—
	17–59 years	Females	●	•	●	○	•	○	○	—	—
		Males	●	•	●	○	•	○	○	—	—
	Over 60 years	Females	●	•	●	○	•	○	○	—	—
		Males	●	•	●	●	•	○	○	—	—
	Pregnant and lactating women		●	●	—	—	—	—	—	—	—

24

High-Income-Ratio States: California, Massachusetts, Michigan, New York (and New York City), Washington

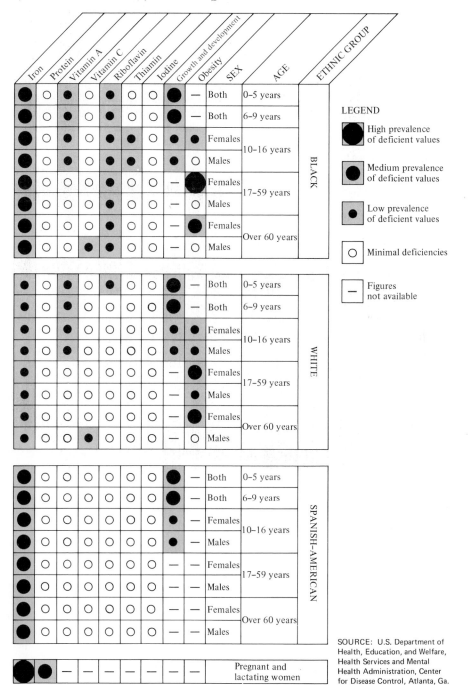

LEGEND

⬤ High prevalence of deficient values

◉ Medium prevalence of deficient values

• Low prevalence of deficient values

○ Minimal deficiencies

— Figures not available

SOURCE: U.S. Department of Health, Education, and Welfare, Health Services and Mental Health Administration, Center for Disease Control, Atlanta, Ga.

25

lation of the United States. The preliminary results of the *Ten-State Nutrition Survey* plus an evaluation of the various programs carried on by a number of federal agencies to combat hunger and malnutrition highlighted the need for data on the magnitude and distribution of these problems in the total population of the nation. In 1969 the Department of Health, Education, and Welfare established a continuing national nutrition surveillance system under the authority of the 1956 Act for the purposes of measuring the nutritional changes in the population and monitoring the changes over time. The responsibility for this task was assigned to the National Center for Health Statistics (NCHS).[20]

The task force of NCHS recommended that the National Nutrition Surveillance Survey (NNSS) be a continuing national probability sample to provide baseline distributional and trend data on the nutritional status of individuals 1 year and over—later established at 1 to 74 years of age—and with special emphasis on those segments of the population classified as at or below the poverty level, women of childbearing age, preschool and young school children, and the aged. It was further recommended that the NNSS become an integral part of the National Health Survey because of similar and compatible objectives.

The amalgamation of the Health Examination Survey and the NNSS led to a renaming of this new enterprise as the Health and Nutrition Examination Survey (HANES). Specifications include that each cycle of HANES cover approximately a 2-year period and be based on a sample of about 30,000 persons 1 through 74 years of age. All persons would receive a specifically designed nutrition examination to consist of a general physical examination; dermatological, ophthalmological, and dental examinations; body measure-

ments; biochemical assessments; and dietary intake measures. A one fifth subsample, aged 25 to 74 years, would receive a more detailed examination. Additional information for the entire sample, such as demographic, health history, health-care needs, and data on participation in food programs such as food stamps, would be obtained.

A discussion of the preliminary findings of dietary intakes in the first survey indicated that race and income levels do not appear to be associated in mean iron intakes in the age groups less than 18 years of age. With few exceptions, the subgroups studied had mean iron intakes below the standards. In the age groups above 45 years, income was an important demographic variable without regard to race. Both white and black adults in the lower income level had iron intakes below the standards. White and black adults in the income group above poverty level approached the standards. Sex was an important variable without regard to race or income. All females of ages 18 to 44 years of both races and income levels had mean iron intakes below the standards. All males of similar age for both race and income groups had mean iron intakes that exceeded the standards.

Mean calcium and vitamin A and C intakes in relation to standards did not vary by race or income levels. These mean nutrient levels either approached or met the standards. Generally, males and females of ages 18 to 44 years of both races and income groups had mean nutrient intakes above the standards. The exceptions were black females of ages 18 to 44 years in both income groups who showed mean calcium levels below the standard, and white females of similar ages in the low income group who had vitamin A levels below the standard. On the whole, all population groups had adequate mean calcium and vitamins A and C intakes in relation to the standard. Yet a substantial proportion of individuals had intakes less than standard; the percentages for calcium ranged from 12 to 75 per cent, for vitamin A from 37 to 74 per cent, and for vitamin C from 39 to 72 per cent.

Biochemical tests reinforced the dietary intake analysis that an iron deficiency existed at all age levels, although more prevalent in

---

[20] Henry W. Miller, *Plan and Operation of the Health and Nutrition Examination Survey, Vital and Health Statistics, Programs and Collection Procedures,* Series 1—Number 10a, DHEW Publication No. (HSM) 73–1310, National Center for Health Statistics, Health Services and Mental Health Administration, Public Health Service, U.S. Department of Health, Education, and Welfare, Rockville, Md., 1973.

the younger age groups. Whites had a higher prevalence of low serum protein values for all age groups regardless of income level. Black children in the 1- to 5-year age group showed the highest prevalence of low serum vitamin A values.

Even these preliminary findings reveal evidence of relative deficiency of specific nutrients in particular age, sex, race, and income subgroupings. Basic data were provided on the distribution of the U.S. population with respect to various biochemical test values and nutrient intakes.

World Nutrition

Nutrition must be regarded as an integral aspect of the total context of the social and cultural reality of the world, according to Knutsson.[21] Although there has been some progress, the twentieth century has failed to eliminate the tragedy of hunger in the world.[22]

Many factors have contributed to this condition, according to Goldsmith.[23] The developing countries account for more than 85 per cent of the population increase over the last 5 years. This situation has a strong impact on the amount of food available, as well as family income. If families cannot buy food and furthermore have less money to do so, the stage is set for hunger and malnutrition. Other influences are the lack of education, ignorance about nutrition, and dietary habits that do not encourage optimal nutrition, such as taboos, religious beliefs, or cultural patterns. The lack of technology is reflected in inadequate food production, distribution, experimentation, and storage. Rodents and insects are responsible for huge losses of food that could alleviate some of the hunger.

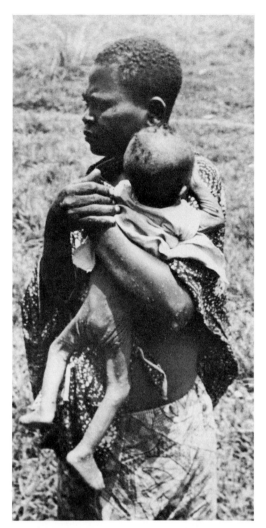

FIGURE 2–6. *Hunger is one of the most serious problems facing the world.* (UNICEF)

Marketing systems and transportation facilities may interfere with the distribution of food. Sometimes food is unequally distributed within a family, such as men being given preferences and pregnant women and children subsequently being deprived of nourishment for their needs. Food has political and social overtones, as evidenced in Biafra and East Pakistan. Sorely needed food may be exported, heightening a scarcity. The government may believe that other national needs and problems have higher priorities than nutrition.

Foods that are necessary for an adequate

[21] Karl Eric Knutsson, "Malnutrition: Macrolevels and Microlevels," in Alan Berg, Neven S. Scrimshaw, and David L. Call, *Nutrition, National Development, and Planning*, MIT Press, Cambridge, Mass., 1973, p. 29.

[22] Lyle P. Schertz, "Nutrition Realities in the Lower Income Countries," *Nutrition Reviews*, Vol. 31, No. 7 (July 1973), p. 201.

[23] Grace A. Goldsmith, "Hunger and Malnutrition—Whose Responsibility?" *Nutrition Today*, Vol. 7, No. 1 (January–February 1972), pp. 16–19.

TABLE 2-3

Recommended Intakes of Nutrients (FAO/WHO)

AGE	BODY WEIGHT	ENERGY (1)		PROTEIN (1,2)	VITAMIN A (3,4)	VITAMIN D (5,6)	THIAMIN (3)	RIBO-FLAVIN (3)	NIACIN (3)	FOLIC ACID$_2$ (5)	VITAMIN B$_{12}$ (5)	ASCOR-BIC ACID (5)	CAL-CIUM (7)	IRON (5,8)
	(kg)	(mJ)	(kcal)	(g)	(µg)	(µg)	(mg)	(mg)	(mg)	(µg)	(µg)	(mg)	(g)	(mg)
Children														
<1	7.3	3.4	820	14	300	10.0	0.3	0.5	5.4	60	0.3	20	0.5–0.6	5–10
1–3	13.4	5.7	1360	16	250	10.0	0.5	0.8	9.0	100	0.9	20	0.4–0.5	5–10
4–6	20.2	7.6	1830	20	300	10.0	0.7	1.1	12.1	100	1.5	20	0.4–0.5	5–10
7–9	28.1	9.2	2190	25	400	2.5	0.9	1.3	14.5	100	1.5	20	0.4–0.5	5–10
Male adolescents														
10–12	36.9	10.9	2600	30	575	2.5	1.0	1.6	17.2	100	2.0	20	0.6–0.7	5–10
13–15	51.3	12.1	2900	37	725	2.5	1.2	1.7	19.1	200	2.0	30	0.6–0.7	9–18
16–19	62.9	12.8	3070	38	750	2.5	1.2	1.8	20.3	200	2.0	30	0.5–0.6	5–9
Female adolescents														
10–12	38.0	9.8	2350	29	575	2.5	0.9	1.4	15.5	100	2.0	20	0.6–0.7	5–10
13–15	49.9	10.4	2490	31	725	2.5	1.0	1.5	16.4	200	2.0	30	0.6–0.7	12–24
16–19	54.4	9.7	2310	30	750	2.5	0.9	1.4	15.2	200	2.0	30	0.5–0.6	14–28
Adult man (moderately active)	65.0	12.6	3000	37	750	2.5	1.2	1.8	19.8	200	2.0	30	0.4–0.5	5–9
Adult woman (moderately active)	55.0	9.2	2200	29	750	2.5	0.9	1.3	14.5	200	2.0	30	0.4–0.5	14–28
Pregnancy (later half)		+1.5	+350	38	750	10.0	+0.1	+0.2	+2.3	400	3.0	30	1.0–1.2	(9)
Lactation (first 6 months)		+2.3	+550	46	1200	10.0	+0.2	+0.4	+3.7	300	2.5	30	1.0–1.2	(9)

SOURCE: *Handbook on Human Nutritional Requirements*, FAO Nutritional Studies No. 28, WHO Monograph Series No. 61, published by FAO and WHO, Rome, 1974.
1 Energy and protein requirements. Report of a Joint FAO/WHO Expert Group, FAO, Rome, 1972.
2 As egg or milk protein.
3 Requirements of vitamin A, thiamin, riboflavin and niacin. Report of a Joint FAO/WHO Expert Group, FAO, Rome, 1965.
4 As retinol.
5 Requirements of ascorbic acid, vitamin D, vitamin B, folate and iron. Report of a Joint FAO/WHO Expert Group, FAO, Rome, 1970.
6 As cholecalciferol.
7 Calcium requirements. Report of a FAO/WHO Expert Group, FAO, Rome, 1961.
8 On each line the lower value applies when over 25 per cent of calories in the diet come from animal foods, and the higher value when animal foods represent less than 10 per cent of calories.
9 For women whose iron intake throughout life has been at the level recommended in this table, the daily intake of iron during pregnancy and lactation should be the same as that recommended for nonpregnant, nonlactating women of childbearing age. For women whose iron status is not satisfactory at the beginning of pregnancy, the requirement is increased, and in the extreme situation of women with no iron stores, the requirement can probably not be met without supplementation.

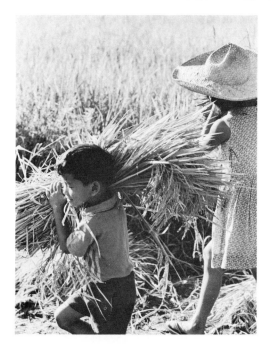

FIGURE 2–7. *Harvesting a new strain of high-yielding rice. (The Rockefeller Foundation, photo by Ted Spiegel)*

diet are often not available in these developing countries. Inadequate protein is one of the most serious problems in many parts of the world. The effect of a diet lacking in

protein is especially critical for young children, who become malnourished. At least 50 per cent of the children in developing countries are suffering from protein-kcalorie malnutrition as well as other deficiency diseases. The future social and economic development of a nation depends on healthy children.

Expert groups of FAO/WHO have contributed suggestions for requirements for important nutrients. The *FAO/WHO Handbook on Nutritional Requirements* (1974)[22] (see Table 2–3) represents a composite summary and commentary of all the recent publications by FAO/WHO on these nutrients. This handbook is recommended by these agencies to be used as a practical guide for agricultural planning and should be helpful in nutritional surveys and nutrition education in the world.

The answers for solving the condition of malnutrition in the world are not simple. Research, emergency measures, and long-term projects in relation to critical problems seem imperative. The question is to what extent can nutrition be given attention when the world is grappling with political, economic, ecological, and other crises of prime importance.

[22] *Handbook on Human Nutritional Requirements*, FAO Nutritional Studies No. 28. WHO Monograph Series No. 61, published by FAO and WHO, Rome, 1974.

SELECTED REFERENCES

Berg, Alan, *The Nutrition Factor*, The Brookings Institution, Washington, D.C., 1973.

———, Nevin S. Scrimshaw, and David Call, *Nutrition, National Development, and Planning*, The MIT Press, Cambridge, Mass., 1973.

Center for Disease Control, Health Services and Mental Health Administration, *Ten-State Nutrition Survey, 1968–1970*, Dietary, Vol. 5, DHEW Publication No. (HSM) 72–8133, U.S. Department of Health, Education, and Welfare, Atlanta, Ga., 1972.

Darby, William J., "Nutrition in the 1970's," *Nutrition Reviews*, Vol. 30, No. 2 (February 1972), pp. 27–31.

Goldsmith, Grace A., "Hunger and Malnutrition—Whose Responsibility?" *Nutrition Today*, Vol. 7, No. 1 (January–February 1972), pp. 16–19.

Hegsted, Mark, "Dietary Standards," *Journal of the American Dietetic Association*, Vol. 66, No. 1 (January 1975), pp. 13–21.

Hollingsworth, Dorothy, and Margaret Russell, *Nutritional Problems in a Changing World*, John Wiley & Sons, Inc., New York, 1973.

Kallen, David J., "Nutrition and Society," *Journal of the American Medical Association*, Vol. 215, No. 1 (January 4, 1971), pp. 94–100.

Kelsay, June L., *A Compendium of Nutritional Status Studies and Dietary Evaluation Studies Conducted in the United States, 1957–1967*, The American Institute of Nutrition, Bethesda, Md., 1969.

King, Maurice, et al., *Nutrition for Developing Countries*, Oxford University Press, New York, 1972.

Leverton, Ruth, "The RDAs Are Not for Amateurs," *Journal of the American Dietetic Association*, Vol. 66, No. 1 (January 1975), pp. 9–11.

Mayer, Jean, *U.S. Nutrition Policies in the Seventies*, W. H. Freeman and Company, San Francisco, 1973.

Miller, Donald F., and Leroy Voris, "Chronologic Changes in the Recommended Dietary Allowances," *Journal of the American Dietetic Association*, Vol. 54, No. 2 (February 1969), pp. 109–117.

Pearson, Paul, "Nutrition Perspectives in the Seventies," *Nutrition Reviews*, Vol. 30, No. 2 (February 1972), pp. 31–34.

Robbins, Gordon, "Ten-State Nutrition Survey: Educational Implications," *Journal of Nutrition Education*, Vol. 4, No. 4 (Fall 1972), pp. 157–158.

Schertz, Lyle P., "Nutrition Realities in Lower Income Countries," *Nutrition Reviews*, Vol. 31, No. 7 (July 1973), pp. 201–216.

White, Philip L., "The World Stops for the Hungry," *Journal of the American Medical Association*, Vol. 215, No. 1 (January 1971), pp. 110–111.

3

Food Habits

A study of the food habits of individuals and of groups of people can be most enlightening. Basic food choices may last for centuries in certain cultures. Many forces shape the habits that determine people's daily food. The influence of the home—especially the mother—the culture in which a person lives, mass media, the knowledge of nutrition, the impact of friends, income, religion, and inflation, work, money, and other factors are far-reaching. Food habits are very complex, often unreasoned, and symbolic. Consequently, they are difficult to change. However, people can improve their ways of eating and thereby benefit in better living.

Definition of Food Habits

The *Manual for the Study of Food Habits*[1] defines food habits as "the way in which individuals or groups of individuals, in response to social and cultural pressures, select, consume, and utilize portions of the available food supply."

Mead[2] suggests the need for a multidimensional code or model that will facilitate a formal description of a people's dietary pattern. Suggestions are to include a description of food in its physiological sensory terms, such as taste, texture, smell and the like, and its chemistry. The nutritional description would include the methods of calculation of nutritional values and the ratio of nutrients to each other.

Cultural terms of the code would embrace an analysis of the agricultural situation, such as soil conditions, planting, harvesting, use of fertilizers, and also methods of processing, storing, and food preparation. Economic descriptions would cover the economic situation regarding distribution, transportation, facilities, and communication, and would include an analysis of the presence or absence of essential food supplies. Sociocultural descriptions would highlight important aspects of social organization having an impact on nutritional status, such as differential access to food by sex or age, any special state like pregnancy or

---

[1] Carl E. Guthe and Margaret Mead, *Manual for the Study of Food Habits*, Bulletin No. 111, National Academy of Sciences—National Research Council, Washington, D.C., 1945.

[2] Margaret Mead, *Food Habits Research: Problems of the 1960's*, Publication No. 1225, National Academy of Sciences—National Research Council, Washington, D.C., 1964.

31

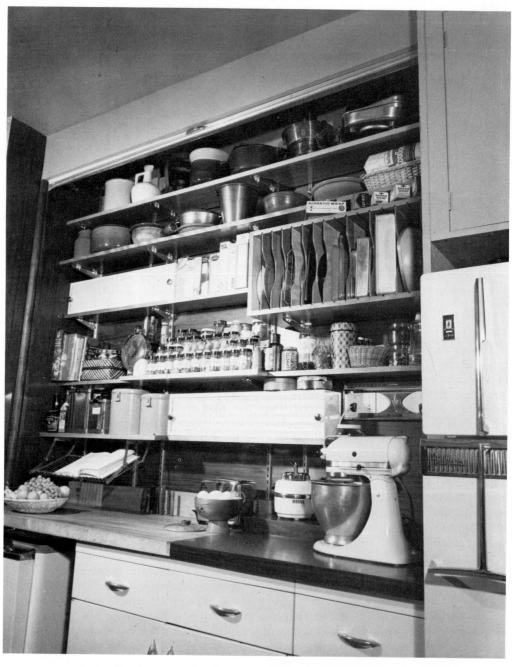

FIGURE 3–1. *Food preparation facilities and equipment have an influence on food habits.*

illness, caste, religion, occupation, or other pertinent influences.

A description of the educational processes would comprise methods of teaching and learning the dietary pattern, whether food is used as a form of discipline, the relation of prestige patterns to weight, height, or age of individuals, effect of social approval and disapproval, and the like. A picture of food handling, such as eating utensils, food combinations, methods of serving, use of color, disposal of leftovers, garbage disposal, and other cultural factors affecting the meal style is important. Finally, a description of dietary pattern that includes geographic and other origins of specific patterns, as well as seasonal characteristics, is important to this code. Mead urges that the model be designed as an open system so that cognizance may be made of new knowledge in every relevant field.

Factors Influencing Food Habits

Culture is one of the most powerful forces that govern the use or nonuse of foodstuffs. Through a complex system of beliefs, prohibitions, rewards, and customs not only is an individual's use of foods determined but his attitude toward certain foods and eating in general. Culture defines not only what is considered food to eat, according to Gifft and others,[3] but for whom, such as for pregnant women, children, or other groups, and the roles that foods play in the lives of the people in a particular culture, such as being only a holiday or festival food or consumed daily.

The scale of values related to food consumption varies from culture to culture. In America, for example, where leanness among many women is highly cherished, food habits are regulated accordingly, sometimes with considerable duress because favorite foods must be foregone. In other cultures women may stuff themselves with rich foods, many of which they may distain, in order to be fashionably plump.

A culture influences the amount of time

and effort devoted to the selection, preparation, and service of food. How people eat reflects their self-cultural concepts. Speed is favored by Americans, as attested by the many hamburger stands or fast-food operations, instant breakfasts, frozen meals, and small kitchens in homes.[4] Work, pleasures, and other demands often place a distance between man and his food.

Guthe and Mead[5] indicate a number of conditions that influence food habits. In each generation, children learn the traditional food habits of their families; these habits, in turn, are passed on to their children. Granted, other influences may change these modes of eating; but each home has vestiges of the past in its eating patterns. The advance of technology is important, particularly in relation to the production, processing, and distribution of food. Advances in nutrition, science, and medicine will have an impact. Changes in the environment, as in housing and household equipment, control of temperature, as by air conditioning, and changes in transportation leave their mark. Educational level and child-rearing practices must be mentioned, too.

Mass media also have an influence. Many individuals cannot resist the glowing descriptions of food on television and radio commercials, in magazines and newspapers, and on bus or subway advertisements. New foods and new ways of preparing old foods are thus brought to the attention of the public.

Changes in the world around people have an effect on the way they eat. When cafeterias were introduced into Paris, for example, the traditional French 2-hour lunch period was disturbed. As lunch is the main repast of the day for the French, many adjustments had to be made when it was eaten at the cafeteria. Here in America, the advent of television meant that many children and even whole families were fed in front of the television screen. The heightened interest in travel and the mobility of families in our country have created an interest in international foods as

[3] Helen H. Gifft, Marjorie B. Washbon, and Gail G. Harrison, *Nutrition, Behavior, and Change,* Prentice-Hall, Englewood Cliffs, N.J., 1972, p. 34.

[4] Tony Jones, "Food: The Spirit Made Flesh," *Harpers* (Wraparound), Vol. 247, No. 1478 (July 1973), p. 3.

[5] Guthe and Mead, op. cit., pp. 13–19.

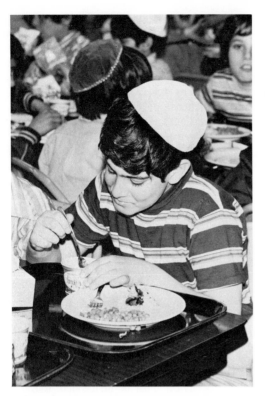

FIGURE 3–2. *Jewish children in a parochial school eating traditional foods that are indicated by their religion.*

well as foods of different sections of the country. The raising or lowering of living standards through increased or decreased incomes has influenced food habits.

Worldwide inflation and recession have brought noticeable changes in food habits. Less meat is consumed and meat substitutes are sought by family food planners. A sharp increase in cereal consumption has replaced many egg and bacon or ham breakfasts. Individuals with fixed incomes, like the elderly, have resorted to desperate solutions, even the use of pet foods. Much more time and effort in buying and preparing food is essential as an aid in spending the food dollar wisely.

The energy crisis has had a number of impacts. Shopping is often less frequent and concentrated in one area because there is insufficient gas to shop around. A reduction in

the use of fuel for food preparation is another consideration. In some instances families are consuming more home-prepared foods, such as baked bread, than formerly.

Other influences are work and leisure patterns of people and the degree to which authorities are recognized. Reference and peer groups are influential. If a famous athlete or entertainer, for example, subscribes to or endorses a food, many young persons may follow the same pattern.

Livingston[6] suggests that food habits are formed by both objective and subjective factors. Objective factors include physical, biological, and technological influences. Subjective factors include cultural, social, and psychological influences.

The Senses and Food Acceptance

Food flavors are important to food acceptance.[7] Flavor is considered to be a blend of all sensory responses to food, including taste, sight, smell, touch, and sound. Children have about 9000 taste buds and generally prefer bland foods. After the age of 10, the taste buds become less numerous and by the age of 20 are at the peak of efficiency. By the age of 45 there is another decrease, and an elderly person may have as few as 3000 taste buds. However, this aged person through appreciation and experience with foods may continue to have a fairly sharp sense of taste.

Temperature may affect the perception of odors. Hot roast beef, for example, has a more pungent aroma than slices of cold beef on a sandwich. The cold of ice cream enhances its flavor. The sight of food can produce pronounced reactions, including suspicions. Off-colored foods tend to produce unusual taste sensations, and orange juice served in a blue glass has less appeal than in a clear glass.

The sense of touch affects the sense of taste. The texture of the food and its pressure

[6] Sally K. Livingston, "What Influences Malnutrition?" *Journal of Nutrition Education*, Vol. 3, No. 1 (Summer 1971), pp. 18–27.

[7] "An Understanding of Flavor Leads to Better Acceptance of School Lunches," *School Nutrition Topics*, Vol. 27, No. 3 (November 1966), pp. 1–2.

in the mouth are contributing factors. Such characteristics as coarseness of cracked wheat bread, smoothness of gelatin or cream cheese, softness of custard, and greasiness of butter are examples. Spices give a feeling of warmth, and peppermint gives a feeling of coolness. Crunching and crackling sounds, such as found in some cereals, have an effect on acceptance, especially by children. Celery has a strong hearing appeal.

Channels and Gatekeepers

The "channel theory" as advanced by Lewin[8] has many interesting implications. Channels are identified as the ways in which food reaches the table, like buying in a store or having groceries delivered, home gardening, cooking, boiling, baking, or other types of food preparation, or preservation, such as freezing or canning. Lewin believed it was essential to know how many food channels existed for a particular family or group in order to understand their food habits. In other words, who moved the food from one channel or another. For example, after food was purchased, was it consumed immediately, stored for various periods of time, used in preparing other forms of food, or was it preserved? If one of these channels was blocked, what did the family do? For example, if certain foods could not be purchased or did not reach the table in some way, what substitutes were used or in what ways did the family meet this situation? Possible solutions might be the omission of the foods, making substitutions, or eating meals away from home in a restaurant or other eating establishment that might have the food desired.

Another important consideration was who controlled these various channels. Lewin referred to this individual or those individuals as the "gatekeeper," usually the mother or homemaker. This person plays a powerful role

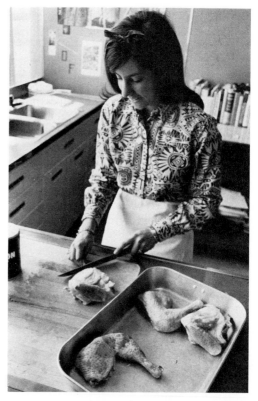

FIGURE 3-3. *The decisions of the family member or members who are the gatekeepers determine which foods will be eaten by the family or group.*

in determining which foods will be utilized by the family. Not only is physical availability considered, but even more important is "cultural availability." Although many foods were accessible, they might be ignored by the gatekeeper because they did not fit into the family's cultural patterns of eating.

A special set of parameters operate in the decisions of a homemaker as a consumer in regard to food choices for her family, according to Bayton.[9] They are the degree of health and nutrition sensitivity to meeting family needs; the sensory aesthetic, or the

[8] Kurt Lewin, "Forces Behind Food Habits and Methods of Change," in Carl E. Guthe and Margaret Mead (eds.), *The Problem of Changing Food Habits*, Bulletin No. 108, National Academy of Sciences—National Research Council, Washington, D.C., 1943, pp. 44-49.

[9] James A. Bayton, "Problems in the Communication of Nutrition Information," in *Proceedings of Nutrition Education Conference*, February 20-22, 1967, U.S. Department of Agriculture, Washington, D.C., 1967.

provision of foods to satisfy the taste–aroma–appearance complex; economics, which involves keeping within the food budget; market knowledge, telling the quality or grade of foods desired; family wishes; time pressures, including the saving of time in preparation and in shopping; preparation pressures, such as using shortcuts whenever possible; and prestige, including her status as a cook, as a shopper, uniqueness of meals, and other achievement satisfactions.

A change in lifestyles has occurred since the days of Lewin's research, and the influence of the wife and mother as the chief gatekeeper has been diluted.[10] Working family members—wife, mother, and teen-agers in addition to the husband and father—have changed this responsibility to one of greater sharing. The masculine members of the family frequently assume a more active role in the purchase and preparation of food. In some homes where mothers are working, school-aged teen-agers may have the task of selecting and preparing the food for the meal or meals that the family eat together.

Patterns in eating styles have altered. Breakfast is omitted or each person prepares his own. Lunch may be taken from home or secured at nursery school or day-care center, school, or at work. The entire family may not be present at dinner because of work, social, or community commitments. Individuals seem to become more and more responsible for the adequacy of their own diet. The family food supply is only one source of an individual's intake. The food eaten away from home has a critical influence on an individual's nutritional adequacy and food habits.

This lessened home control on the dietary intake of family members is a matter of grave concern as related to children. If a mother or parents ignore the overeating or the undereating of children and the rejection of nutritious foods, poor food habits can be quickly established. In severe instances, a child's growth and development may suffer and the quality of his adult health may be diminished.

[10] Mary M. Hill, "Modification of Food Habits," *Food and Nutrition News*, Vol. 44, Nos. 1–2 (October–November 1972), pp. 1, 4.

Impact of Crises on Food Habits

Among other forces affecting the way people eat are the crises they face, such as famines, fire, flood, and widespread disease. With transportation facilities improved and the world better prepared to handle these situations, disasters are not so serious as they were at one time. Not only is it important to consider the kind of food which can best be transported, prepared, and served to disaster victims, but the whole matter of facilities for preparing the food and for keeping it sanitary is another concern.

The tremendous emotional stress on victims of such disasters is sometimes associated with the foods served to them at that time. This factor may affect their future attitudes toward those foods.

Personal crises such as the loss of a loved one, failure in business, or great strain in personal relations can have a strong influence on an individual's food habits. Large quantities of food may be consumed, there may be an urge to return to the food of infancy or childhood for a feeling of security, or food patterns may be altered in other ways to ease the tension.

An economic depression may have serious consequences on people's eating habits. When incomes are reduced, they will be forced to eat less expensive foods. But unless they are well grounded in the best buys nutritionally, it is possible that they will eat food with little nutritive value. In addition, the psychological impact of a scanty table is quite detrimental to the pride of the homemaker as well as to the provider of the family. Complicating this situation are the problems and tensions that accompany an economic dilemma and make it difficult to eat in a relaxed manner because the family is so concerned about its plight.

Modifying Food Habits

Food habits offer great resistance to change, partly because of their complex origin and partly because habits are such an integral part of everyday living. But habits can be modified. The damaging effects of poor food habits should not be taken lightly.

Improvement of food habits can generally

be motivated much more readily through feelings than through logic, according to Galdston.[11] Lewin[12] felt that motivation could be categorized under three major headings: values, food needs, and obstacles to overcome.

Values might vary in degree with different individuals and could occur singly or in combination. The first value that Lewin found in his interviews was money. For example, if a food became too expensive in the estimation of the family, such as oranges at a certain season of the year, they ceased to buy it. Another value was health. Mothers particularly may feel very strongly that their children need to have a quart of milk a day so that they will have good bones and teeth. A third value was taste. Some individuals did not like the taste of certain foods and so they were omitted from the day's diet. The fourth value, which had a very strong impact, is the matter of status. Status might imply the use of particular brands, food that was sent from other regions of the country, or even imported foods. In Lewin's interviews, money and health were more significant than other values. Money, however, was mentioned less frequently by the upper-income participants than by the middle or lower groups. Health seemed to be a much more significant value in the upper-income group than in the lower-income group.

The second item to which Lewin referred in regard to motivation was related to foods that the family considered necessary and satisfying. He felt that these needs might change because of satiety—that is, having an abundance of a particular food because of change in the situation, or because of cultural forces. If a food was consumed over a long period of time, it might lead to a decrease in the desire for that specific food. An eating problem or habit might be difficult to change because a youngster had had a particular food repeatedly at school. Young men who have been in the armed forces might have difficulty in overcoming an aversion for certain kinds of foods that they had to consume in large quantities while in service. When a homemaker uses a wide choice of foods in planning her meals, it is much easier to motivate her family to eat certain important foods.

The third item to be considered in motivation was how to overcome certain obstacles. This might involve distribution of food, lack of adequate help in the home, time necessary for preparing foods, or excessive cost. Plans must be made to overcome these obstacles in the best possible manner.

A typology of change processes is discussed by Bennis[13] that has many implications for adapting food habits. *Planned change* is deliberate and involves goal setting. *Indoctrination* is deliberate, but there is an imbalanced power ratio because something or somebody exerts greater influence than the individual himself. The school lunch program, in a way, indoctrinates children into certain food habits through the food choices offered to them. In *coercive change* there is no mutual goal setting. Limitations on foods that are available during time of war is an example of changing food habits in this manner.

Technocratic change emerges as a result of collecting and interpreting data. In a simplified version, individuals may discover after observations that they feel better if they eat regularly or if they include orange juice in their diet. *Interactional change* is characterized by a lack of deliberate goal setting. Friends or family members unconsciously assist each other in changing a habit. A friend might remind an overweight teen-ager about the kcaloric content of a food about to be consumed. *Socialization change* implies an interactional hierarchical control, such as parent–child, teacher–student, or counselor–camper relationship. The adult is more deliberate than the child in attempting to bring about a change in food habits.

Emulative change is facilitated by the influence of identification. This change is well

---

[11] Iago Galdston, "Nutrition from the Psychiatric Viewpoint," *Journal of the American Dietetic Association*, Vol. 28, No. 5 (May 1952), pp. 405–409.

[12] Lewin, op. cit.

[13] Warren G. Bennis, "A Typology of Change Processes," in Warren G. Bennis, Kenneth D. Benne, and Robert Chin (eds.), *The Planning of Change*, Holt, Rinehart and Winston, New York, 1961, pp. 154–156.

illustrated by the influence of peers on food habits of adolescents. If the leaders of the group, or power figures, scorn milk or other nutritious foods, parents encounter difficulty in altering this situation. *Natural change* is brought about without apparent deliberation or goal setting. The impact of crises, unanticipated consequences, quirks of fate, and the like may alter food habits. The advent of a convenience food, greater availability, or other means of securing nutritious foods with little effort are examples.

Psychologists and nutritionists make certain recommendations for changing food habits. If an individual shows certain undesirable habits, the first step is to examine the total dietary behavior and to highlight the commendable aspects. Nearly everyone has some good habits, and it helps morale to emphasize them. With this positive approach, it is possible to examine less desirable habits with the idea, "Why do I do this?" If, for example, it is discovered that too few fruits and vegetables are eaten, the person desiring to modify his diet might make an earnest analysis of the fruits and vegetables that are enjoyed and include them in his diet. If there is a weakness for very rich desserts, they might be replaced by fruit served in interesting ways or low-calorie desserts that look rich. A low-calorie cookbook might give suggestions. If an individual is careless about milk consumption, an effort might be made to include it at some particular meal or time during the day, for example, on cereal for breakfast, at lunch, during coffee break, or as a nightcap. The point is that the time when milk is to be consumed must be planned so that habit can be established.

If a person does not like milk or eggs, plans can be made to include these foods in other forms in the diet. Sometimes a hard-cooked egg can be enjoyed when combined with a green salad or served chopped on vegetables. Some of the milk may be incorporated in soups, puddings, creamed dishes, cheese, or ice cream. But it is difficult to get the total milk quota into the diet in this way.

Attention may need to be given to other poor food habits, such as an inadequate amount and kind of food, hurried eating, omitting meals, incomplete mastication of food, overindulgence in snacks, irregular meal hours, eating too much candy, and drinking large quantities of tea and coffee. Poor health habits like lack of sleep and too little exercise, decayed teeth, and chronic fatigue have an influence, too. Mental health is also important.

Not only is some kind of planning essential in modifying food habits, but one must also have a strong desire and willingness to do so. One way in which people can be motivated to change their habits is to watch for results. Research has proved that people who eat a good breakfast, for example, work better, think better, react better, and are better adjusted to life itself.

An individual who hesitates to eat breakfast might be encouraged to try it and then to see how he feels in the middle of the morning or at 11:30. The results can be most encouraging. Teen-agers who are not eating adequate food may be helped in improving their diet by the results—a clear complexion, added vitality, or dynamic attractiveness.

Behavior modification cannot rest on one technique or on simple implementation of rewards and punishments as highlighted in the popular literature, according to Kanfer.[14] Todhunter[15] makes some excellent suggestions that might be useful when a person is attempting to change his food habits. The impact of his culture, traditions, and beliefs on the habit should be examined. This influence should be respected and, if necessary, eating should be adapted in a satisfactory manner, such as smaller servings, perhaps, if obesity is the problem. Proposed changes must be examined in relation to lifestyles, such as being compatible to work and home conditions. It is helpful to share behavior modification with others who have the same problem, as is demonstrated in the Weight Watcher's

[14] Frederick H. Kanfer, "Behavior Modification —An Overview," in Carl E. Thoresen (ed.), *Behavior Modification in Education*, The Seventy-second Yearbook of the National Society for the Study of Education, University of Chicago Press, Chicago, 1973, pp. 3–4.

[15] E. Neige Todhunter, "Food Habits, Food Faddism and Nutrition," in Miloslav Rechcigl, Jr. (ed.), *Food, Nutrition and Health*, Vol. 16, S. Karger Basel, 1973, pp. 301–304.

program. Keep the goal simple rather than attempting to make sweeping changes all at one time. Some benefits must accrue to the individual attempting to change so that there is a positive feeling.

Research on Food Habits

Margaret Mead,[16] while a member of the Committee on Food Habits of the National Research Council, made a review of food habits that has many implications for the present day. She observed that systematic additions to knowledge in all fields, such as the physical and social sciences, psychology, and anthropology, must be combined to provide a good background for recommendations toward changing food patterns. She further cautions that any change in food patterns must be considered in the light of the total cultural pattern, because it is possible that desirable nutrition changes would make for undesirable cultural changes. An example would be a gift to people in other countries of certain American foods that might be very good for them nutritionally but about which they have serious taboos or superstitions, such as milk, in some cases.

From a study of various data, she identified certain important social–psychological characteristics of American food patterns. The status given to meat every day, much sugar, and the importance of white bread arise from the European peasant conceptions of status. A mother will tell a child that something is good for him and yet no one in the family seems eager to eat it. Similarly, foods that are considered poor in nutritive quality seem to delight certain family members.

An effect of the Puritan tradition is using food for purposes of reward and punishment. A common example is asking a child to eat his food and promising to reward him with dessert. Other tendencies in American dietary ways, as identified by Mead, are an emphasis on appearance of food rather than the taste, and an increasing preference and emphasis on refined, purified, and highly processed foods. Americans also appear to object to food dishes that are so complex in nature that individual

foods cannot be identified—casseroles, for instance.

Mead also states that the food habits of other cultures are significant sources for understanding the background of certain subcultural groups in America. She believes that it is impossible to think of changes for the total country but that, rather, we must think of ways to change food habits of a community of second-generation Americans of Polish, Italian, Chinese, or other extraction. Another group might be families with limited education or sharecroppers whose food habits are tied to a single crop. Mead suggests that psychiatrists might be helpful in giving nutrition experts insights about the reasons for acceptance or rejection of food.

Eppright,[17] in a study of food preferences of Iowans, discovered that people generally were unable to analyze in a discriminating manner why they liked or disliked certain foods. The knowledge that a food promoted health did not enhance its popularity.

Moore[18] refers to food as the "unspoken language." She states that food is used as an indication of one's social experience, status, and gentility. A homemaker is acclaimed by her neighbors according to her knowledge and skill with food. She states further that food, eating, and diet are highly emotionalized areas and that it is important to acknowledge this fact in trying to understand people's food habits.

Galdston[19] also claims that few individuals are interested in nutrition for the sake of health. He says that greater cognizance must be taken of the fact that eating is identified with cultural taboos, prestige tokens, social regulations, emotions, and ceremonies. Ginsburg[20] believes that eating has psychological

---

[16] Guthe and Mead, op. cit.

[17] Ercel S. Eppright, "Factors Affecting Food Acceptance," *Journal of the American Dietetic Association*, Vol. 23, No. 7 (July 1947), pp. 579–587.

[18] Harriet Bruce Moore, "Psychological Facts and Dieting Fancies," *Journal of the American Dietetic Association*, Vol. 28, No. 9 (September 1952), pp. 789–794.

[19] Loc cit.

[20] Sol Wiener Ginsburg, "The Psychological Aspects of Eating," *Journal of Home Economics*, Vol. 44, No. 5 (May 1952), pp. 325–328.

overtones. The psychological aspects begin in early infancy and last throughout life. He claims that the attitudes, concerns, prejudices, likes, dislikes, and needs of people cannot be fully understood unless this idea is accepted.

Cussler and De Give[21] demonstrated that friends generally were not the best sources for diffusing nutrition information. The possible reason for this fact is that changes in food habits may have been related in moral terms; "it is good for you" or "you must do it." People objected to the exploitation of pleasant friendship relationships to pass on this type of information. When emphasis was placed on helping in some type of adjustment rather than on moral grounds, there was less resistance.

People resist change, according to Patrick.[22] They must first feel a need for change. Change cannot materialize if they are afraid, threatened, forced, or do not understand. To foster change in people's food habits, there must be information about beliefs, relative values, the nature of the community, what they eat and what they think they should eat, foods associated with age, sex, and special occasions, and what they like to eat.

Food habits are closely related to self-image. A person feels he has formed these habits and they are a part of him. This attitude gives him license to eat as he wishes. Mead[23] believes that this connection between self-concept and the food eaten has a reference to the willingness to change. If each day a person eats the food of his class, group, religion, and so on, and then he makes a decision not to eat a familiar food, the change can be disturbing. An example is cited of a group of Indonesians who came to Holland to live. They accepted Dutch food and clothes with enthusiasm.

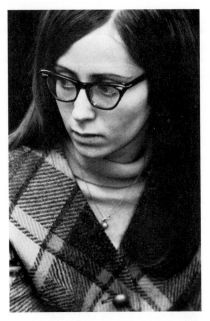

FIGURE 3–4. *Self-concept influences food habits, including modification.*

Whenever difficulties arose with the government, however, they resorted to their former food habits.

Dickens[24] discovered that age is a factor in food preferences. For example, the percentage of women in Mississippi who used instant milk, cake mixes, and instant coffee decreased from middle to old age. Aldrich[25] makes a plea that research be conducted to learn much more about why individuals, ethnic groups, and nations eat as they do.

An examination of the food habits of low-income families in various parts of America can be a fruitful study. Kolasa and Bass[26]

[21] Margaret Cussler and Mary L. De Give, *'Twixt the Cup and the Lip*, Twayne Publishers, Boston, 1952.

[22] Ralph Patrick, "Social and Cultural Determinants of Food Habits," in *Proceedings of Nutrition Education Conference*, February 20–22, 1967, U.S. Department of Agriculture, Washington, D.C., 1967.

[23] Margaret Mead, "The Social Psychology of Food Habits," in Anne Burgess and R. F. A. Dean (eds.), *Malnutrition and Food Habits*, Macmillan, New York, 1962, pp. 79–80.

[24] Dorothy Dickens, "Factors Related to Food Preferences," *Journal of Home Economics*, Vol. 57, No. 6 (June 1965), pp. 427–430.

[25] Robert A. Aldrich, "Nutrition and Human Development," *Journal of the American Dietetic Association*, Vol. 46, No. 6 (June 1965), pp. 453–456.

[26] Kathryn M. Kolasa and Mary A. Bass, "Food Behavior of Families Enrolled in the Expanded Food and Nutrition Education Program and Other Selected Homemakers in Hancock County, Tennessee," reported by Kolasa at the American Home Economics Association Annual Convention at Atlantic City, N.J., June 27, 1973.

studied the food behavior of selected families in Hancock County, Tennessee. Food behavior, including food selection, procurement, and meal planning, differed generally from that of the nationwide, average EFNEP (Expanded Food and Nutrition Education Program) family. The main sources of food supply were home gardens and stores with limited stocks of staple and perishable groceries. Produce from the garden was canned, frozen, or dried. Much wild game, such as ground hog, squirrel, rabbit, and the like, is now scarce and meat purchased did not replace these sources of protein. Wild greens and available berries were gathered. Flour and cornmeal products were widely used in the daily menu, but many of these products were not enriched. The researchers point out that low-income families in the nation vary widely in their food habits.

De Garine[27] suggests that other facets of food habits be researched. For example, it has been demonstrated that there is a correlation between economic factors and food consumption. Although more difficult to quantify, further research into an individual's psychological experiences and his attitudes toward food might be encouraged. Extrapolation of definitions valid in Western industrial and urban societies to traditional and rural societies should be discouraged because characteristics, values, and determinants differ. Observations on food habits in developing countries should not be reduced to measurement against an idealized, scientific concept of nutrition. Geographic limitations should not be placed on which foods are edible and which food habits should be prized.

[27] Igor De Garine, "Food Is Not Just Something to Eat," *Ceres*, FAO Review, Vol. 4, No. 1 (January–February 1971), pp. 46–51.

SELECTED REFERENCES

Burgess, Anne, and R. F. A. Dean, *Malnutrition and Food Habits*, Macmillan Publishing Co., Inc., New York, 1962.

Gifft, Helen H., Marjorie B. Washbon, and Gail G. Harrison, *Nutrition, Behavior, and Change*, Prentice-Hall, Inc., Englewood Cliffs, N.J., 1972.

Grivetti, Louis E., and Rose Marie Pangborn, "Food Habit Research: A Review of Approaches and Methods," *Journal of Nutrition Education*, Vol. 5, No. 3 (July–September 1973), pp. 204–208.

Gussow, Joan, "Counternutritional Messages of TV Ads Aimed at Children," *Journal of Nutrition Education*, Vol. 4, No. 2 (Spring 1972), pp. 48–52.

Guthe, Carl E., and Margaret Mead (eds.), *The Problem of Changing Food Habits*, Bulletin No. 108, National Academy of Sciences—National Research Council, Washington, D.C., 1943.

———, and Margaret Mead, *Manual for the Study of Food Habits*, Bulletin No. 111, National Academy of Sciences—National Research Council, Washington, D.C., 1945.

Lionberger, Herbert F., *Adoption of New Ideas and Practices*, Iowa State University Press, Ames, Iowa, 1960.

Lowenberg, Miriam E., "The Development of Food Patterns," *Journal of the American Dietetic Association*, Vol. 65, No. 3 (September 1974), pp. 263–268.

———, E. Neige Todhunter, Eva D. Wilson, Jane R. Savage, and James L. Lubawski, *Food and Man*, 2nd ed., John Wiley & Sons, Inc., New York, 1974.

Mead, Margaret, *Food Habits Research: Problems of the 1960's*, Publication 1225, National Academy of Sciences—National Research Council, Washington, D.C., 1964.

Parrish, John B., "Implications of Changing Food Habits for Nutrition Educators," *Journal of Nutrition Education*, Vol. 2, No. 4 (Spring 1971), pp. 140–146.

Schultz, Howard G., Margaret H. Rucker, and Gerald F. Russell, "Food and Food-Use Classification System," *Food Technology*, Vol. 29, No. 3 (March 1975), pp. 50–64.

Todhunter, E. Neige, "Food Habits, Food Faddism and Nutrition," in Miloslav Rechcigl, Jr. (ed.), *Food, Nutrition and Health*, Vol. 16, S. Karger, Basel, 1973.

Wenkam, Nao S., "Cultural Determinants of Nutritional Behavior," *Nutrition Program News*, U.S. Department of Agriculture, Washington, D.C., July–August, 1969, pp. 1–4.

4

The Nutrients

The source of nutrients is food. Man cannot be well nourished unless he selects his foods wisely. Foods vary widely in their nutritive contribution and no one food is perfect. Many combinations of foods will lend themselves to a nutritious diet.

Techniques of Nutrition Research

Man's first study was upon himself—man. The earliest records contain references to observations and speculations about the relationship of food to health. Often the ideas expressed are erroneous in terms of current information, but they were confined to the only technique available at the time, noting the results of eating certain foods upon man's behavior and well-being.

A biblical reference illustrates an early experiment that tested two types of diets. When Daniel[1] was brought to the court of Nebuchadnezzar and told to partake of the king's wine and meat, he requested that he and his three companions be given "pulse [legumes] to eat and water to drink [for ten days]. Then let our countenances be looked upon before thee,

and the countenance of the children that eat of the portion of the king's meat: . . . . And at the end of ten days their countenances appeared fairer and fatter in flesh than all the children which did eat the portion of the king's meat [and wine]."

Man has served as a subject for many other types of experiments. From Vesalius'[2] (1514–1564) dissection and consequent publication, *On the Structure of the Human Body*, down to current studies of amino acid needs there are many examples of man used as an essential "tool" for laboratory investigation. Studies on man (and woman) are considered one of the best ways of learning the nutritive needs of the human species.

However, using human subjects often proves too time-consuming, too costly, and perhaps undesirable from a medical point of view, so the scientist has utilized a variety of other methods to help him in his search for information about nutrition. The study of animals and microorganisms and the use of chemical

---

[1] *The Bible* (King James Version), Daniel 1:3–17.

[2] E. Neige Todhunter, "Human Nutrition—Past and Present," *Centennial Symposium: Nutrition of Plants, Animals, Man*, College of Agriculture, Michigan State University, East Lansing, Mich., February 14–16, 1955.

43

analysis and isotopes are techniques employed in nutritional investigations.

Almost every animal has, in some way, contributed to our knowledge and appreciation of nutrition. Bees, fowl, dogs, guinea pigs, monkeys, birds, and farm animals are among those used in the laboratory. However, rats and mice are probably the most widely accepted experimental animal because rats are similar to man in food habits and needs. They are small and easily handled in large numbers; they grow rapidly and are short-lived. In fact, the life cycle is one thirtieth of the human cycle, so that the effect of nutritional variations can be studied for many generations.

The desire to get information even more rapidly than was possible with the rat led to the use of microorganisms. This action proved effective since many of the nutrients required by human beings are also needed by bacteria. Their rapid growth, quickly detectable metabolic changes, and large numbers provide excellent insight into problems of nutrition research.

Another method of investigation that opened doors was the development of chemical techniques of research. Through these means, the scientist was able to measure the effect of varying amounts of different substances on the nutritive status of the individual. Using blood, urine, and tissue slices, a chemical analysis could help to determine the amounts of nutrients necessary for the best health. Also, through chemistry, synthetic nutrients were developed so that purified diets containing specific nutrients could be fed to experimental animals. Another contribution is the creation of structural analogs (see Chapter 11), which facilitated the development of deficiency diseases for laboratory study.

Isotopes have been used in nutritional research and have been particularly instrumental in adding an appreciation of nutritional interrelationships. Stable and radioactive isotopes have been used to label mineral elements, organic compounds, and portions of organic compounds. By tracing these tagged materials, the scientist has increased his understanding of metabolic pathways of nutrition (the successive steps nutrients follow when they participate in body reactions). This research tool is especially valuable in determining information that is difficult, if not impossible, to obtain by traditional research procedures.

Another approach that has provided significant information is a study of the diet of people who, by all accepted standards, appear to be in good health. Methods used in this type of investigation will be discussed later. Atwater, in 1893, published his data on the dietaries of numerous American families of various occupational groups, as described by Sherman.[3] At that time he determined the number of kcalories they consumed, and the amounts of protein, fat, and carbohydrate.

In a different kind of study, a deficiency of a specified nutrient is induced in a subject, laboratory animal, or organism; then, under controlled conditions, the symptoms are observed. This technique has been especially informative about the activity of the "lesser known" vitamins.

A considerable amount of current knowledge relating to many important nutrients has evolved from the use of balance studies. The intake of the nutrient in question and its output are both measured. From these data, plus other corroborative evidence, various observations have been made of the need for and functions of the nutrient according to its behavior. Some nutrients that have been studied this way are calcium, iron, and the amino acids. Reference will be made to these balance studies as each nutrient is discussed.

The study of the nutrition of the cell, the smallest unit of life, has been facilitated by a variety of new methods and techniques,[4] including a knowledge of the fundamental relationship of the nucleic acids deoxyribonucleic acid (DNA) and ribonucleic acid (RNA) to cell division and size of cells. For example, total protein in an organ divided by DNA is an index to cell size. Through biopsy samples, cells can be studied in combination with various other methods for an estimation of body composition.

[3] Henry C. Sherman, *Nutritional Improvement of Life*, Columbia University Press, New York, 1950.

[4] "Nutrition and Cell Growth," *Dairy Council Digest*, Vol. 41, No. 6 (November–December 1970), p. 31.

In nutrition studies, the metric system of weights and measures, instead of the familiar pounds and inches, is commonly used. In addition, metric units are used in most of the world. The Food and Drug Administration prescribed the metric system for nutrition labels because the unit we are most accustomed to, the ounce, is too large to describe conveniently the amounts of nutrients in foods. For instance, 1 gram (g) is about equal to the weight of a paper clip. If a food contains 9 g of protein, this would be expressed in our customary terms as $\frac{9}{28}$ oz. This is an example of how customary measurements used for food composition would not only be very small but appear as confusing fractions.[5]

The basic metric units that consumers will see on nutrition labels are grams (units of mass or weight) and liters (units of volume). The system is based on the decimal system of numbers, and thus involves multiples of 10. It is very easy to go from small units to large, or vice versa, by simply moving decimal points.

We can convert the metric system into the system to which Americans are more accustomed as follows:

$$1 \text{ oz} = 28 \text{ g}$$
$$3\frac{1}{2} \text{ oz} = 100 \text{ g}$$
$$8 \text{ oz} = 227 \text{ g}$$
$$1 \text{ lb} = 454 \text{ g}$$
$$2.2 \text{ lb} = 1 \text{ kilogram (kg)}$$

Once the basic unit is determined, whether grams or liters in the metric system, other multiples are built on it with suitable prefixes. The prefix "kilo" (k) preceding a unit indicates 1000 times that unit. One kilogram equals 1000 grams, for example.

Similarly, the prefix "milli" (m) indicates one thousandth and "micro" (μ) one-millionth of the basic unit. Thus,

$$1 \text{ kg} = 1000 \text{ g}$$
$$1 \text{ g} = 1000 \text{ mg}$$
$$1 \text{ mg} = 1000 \text{ } \mu\text{g}$$

The other basic unit of metric measurement besides the gram that will be found on nutrition labels is the liter, used to measure volume. A liter (l) is a little larger than 1 quart.

$$1 \text{ kl} = 1000 \text{ liters}$$
$$1 \text{ liter} = 1000 \text{ ml}$$

We can translate this system into the one currently used in the United States as follows:

1 gallon	=	3.79 liters
1 quart	=	0.95 liter or 950 ml
1 pint	=	0.48 liter or 480 ml
1 cup (8 fluid oz)	=	0.24 liter or 240 ml
1 tablespoon	=	15 ml
1 teaspoon	=	5 ml

Number of Nutrients

There is an expression "57 from 5," according to Selig,[6] which means that all the 57 nutrients known to be important for life and health can be obtained from the four basic types of food (the *Basic Four*) plus water. Actually, the true number of nutrients is unknown and debatable. Some authorities estimate 40 to 50 nutrients. No doubt there are nutrients that have not been discovered.

Functions of Nutrients

What are some of the important aspects of nutrition discovered throughout the preceding centuries by the combined use of these research techniques? First, the scientist learned that man needs certain substances, named *nutrients*, each day in the diet. What are nutrients? A nutrient may be defined as a substance that is necessary for the functioning of the living organism. Sometimes it is referred to as a material that nourishes the body. The scientist subsequently found that a nutrient can function in the body in three ways:

1. It may provide the body with fuel, which, when oxidized, releases energy for its activities.

[5] "Metric Measures on Nutrition Labels," *Facts from FDA*, Food and Drug Administration, Rockville, Md., 1973.

[6] R. A. Selig, "Fifty-Seven from Five," *February 1971 Supply Letter*, United Fruit and Vegetable Association, p. 7.

2. It may provide materials for the building and upkeep of body tissues, both the skeletal structure and the soft tissues of the body.
3. It may provide the materials that are necessary to regulate body processes or that the body can use to synthesize its own regulatory substances.

A single nutrient may take part in any one of these functions, or two, or even all three. Or a single food may provide nutrients that will participate in one or more of these functions, depending on its composition.

There are five major groups or classifications of nutrients: carbohydrate, protein, fat, vitamin, and mineral. (Strictly speaking, air and water also may be called nutrients, since they participate in the three functions.)

The first nutritive function—providing fuel for energy—is performed by carbohydrates and fats, and also by proteins. This energy function is usually expressed in *kcalories*, a term signifying the potential chemical energy that may be released as heat when food is oxidized. This is what is meant by the kcalorie value of a specific food. The term is also used to express the amount of energy man needs to "do work" or to perform certain tasks. Carbohydrate and protein each supply approximately 4 kcalories per gram, whereas fat provides 9 kcalories per gram.

Performing the second function of nutrients are protein and minerals. They supply the materials for the building and upkeep of body tissue, including the skeletal structure and the soft tissues. However, small amounts of fat are also needed for each body cell. It is possible, too, through the metabolic processes that will be discussed in Chapter 8, that segments of molecules of fat and carbohydrate may become incorporated into the cell structure.

Finally, the nutrient that is most active in regulating body processes is the vitamin group. However, minerals as well as protein deriva-

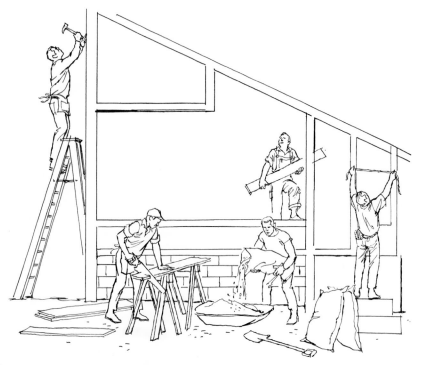

FIGURE 4–1. *The body is much like a house; the finished structure has little resemblance to the materials that go into it.*

tives, such as enzymes and hormones, are also necessary. Carbohydrate and fat, too, may become involved in the same way that they may participate in structural formation.

Obviously, it is impossible rigidly to ascribe certain functions to each type of nutrient. But major classifications can suggest the primary activity of each group. In addition, as will be discussed in the following chapters, there are many interrelationships among individual nutrients.

Food and Nutrients

The food we eat is the sole source of nutrients. Most foods are usually classified as belonging to one of the groups of nutrients. Thus butter is considered as a "fat food" and meat a "protein food." Seldom, however, does a food contain only one nutrient. For example, the primary sources of carbohydrate are sugar, bread, cereals, bread products, and root vegetables. But cereals contain some protein and important vitamins, and the vegetables contain certain minerals as well as carbohydrates. Again, butter may be a prime source of fat, but it also contains vitamin A.

An example of a food with many nutrients is milk. Milk has protein, fat, and carbohydrate. It is an excellent source of calcium and also a good source of vitamin A and riboflavin, plus some thiamin and niacin.

A food, then, is frequently classified according to the nutrient, such as carbohydrate, fat, protein, vitamin, or mineral, that makes its greatest contribution to the diet.

Fiber is sometimes called "the forgotten nutrient." In the past, fiber from vegetables, fruit, and cereals was considered important solely for facilitating elimination. Modern science has suggested other roles for dietary fiber, such as being helpful in dealing with atherosclerosis, diverticular diseases, and cancer of the small intestine, according to Scala.[7] There has been a marked decline in the consumption of whole grains and fresh fruits and vegetables. Scala estimates that consumption

of fiber from fresh fruit and vegetables has declined 20 per cent and that from cereals about 50 per cent. These foods have been substituted for largely by processed foods.

Studies with human volunteers in a low-fiber–high-cholesterol population reduced blood cholesterol significantly with an increase of dietary fiber, especially over a long period of study. Heart disease is relatively rare among people who eat a vegetarian diet.

Diverticular disease is characterized by small "blow-out type" protrusion lesions on the large intestine that become inflamed and often burst, causing infection. In 1973 approximately 500,000 Americans had major surgery for this condition and probably four to six times that many persons had treatment for the condition. In these proportions, the condition is not trivial. Clinical studies indicate that dietary fiber, especially from cereal, is very effective in relieving the conditions of diverticulitis.

Although clearly established correlations do not exist for the relationship of fiber to the alleviation of intestinal cancer, a reasonable hypothesis can be advanced. Since fiber consumption has decreased by a considerable proportion, the frequency and the volume of fecal elimination has undoubtedly decreased in proportion. If cancer is caused by a substance that has access through diet, there is more time for it to produce harm than previously because a longer time may be spent in the intestine. In addition, dietary fiber increases the amounts of water, sterols, bile acids, and fat passing through the large intestine, which has a combined solvent-like effect that could remove some of these undesirable factors.

It appears that a substantial increase of dietary fiber would be beneficial to most Americans. Scala recommends an increase so that the diet would contain 20 to 36 g of dietary fiber daily.

Availability of Nutrients

The consumption of nutrients varies according to availability, cost, preferences, and other factors in the selection of foods, the carriers of nutrients. The expected per capita

[7] James Scala, "Fiber, the Forgotten Nutrient," *Food Technology*, Vol. 28, No. 1 (January 1974), pp. 34–36.

TABLE 4–1

Nutrients Available for Civilian Consumption, per Capita Day, Selected Periods[a]

NUTRIENT	UNIT	AVERAGE, 1957–1959	1967	1972	1973	1974 (PRELIMINARY)	1974 AS A PERCENTAGE OF 1957–1959	1967	1973
Food energy	cal	3140	3210	3320	3300	3350	107	104	102
Protein	g	95	98	101	99	101	106	103	102
Fat	g	143	150	158	155	158	110	105	102
Carbohydrate	g	374	373	381	385	388	104	104	101
Calcium	g	0.98	0.94	0.94	0.95	0.95	97	101	100
Phosphorus	g	1.51	1.52	1.54	1.52	1.54	102	101	101
Iron	mg	16.1	17.2	18.0	17.9	18.3	114	106	102
Magnesium	mg	348	343	346	346	348	100	101	101
Vitamin A value	IU	8000	7900	8100	8100	8200	103	104	101
Thiamin	mg	1.84	1.91	1.94	1.90	1.94	105	102	102
Riboflavin	mg	2.28	2.33	2.35	2.32	2.33	102	100	100
Niacin	mg	20.6	22.4	23.4	22.9	23.4	114	104	102
Vitamin B_6	mg	2.01	2.18	2.29	2.24	2.28	113	105	102
Vitamin B_{12}	μg	8.9	9.5	9.8	9.5	9.7	109	102	102
Ascorbic acid	mg	105	108	115	118	119	113	110	101

[a] Quantities of nutrients computed by Agricultural Research Service, Consumer and Food Economics Institute, on the basis of estimates of per capita food consumption (retail weight), including estimates of produce of home gardens, prepared by the Economic Research Service. No deduction made in nutrient estimates for loss or waste of food in the home, use for pet food, or for destruction or loss of nutrients during the preparation of food. Civilian consumption. Data include iron, thiamin, riboflavin, and niacin added to flour and cereal products; vitamin A value added primarily to margarine, milk of all types, and milk extenders; ascorbic acid added primarily to fruit juices and drinks, flavored beverages and dessert powders, milk extenders, and cereals. Quantities for 1960–1966 were estimated in part by Consumer and Food Economics Institute.

SOURCE: *National Food Situation*, Economic Research Service, U.S. Department of Agriculture, Washington, D.C., November 1974, p. 27.

nutrient levels for 1974 indicate slight gains in all nutrient levels, except calcium and riboflavin, according to Friend and Marston.[8] Greater use of lean pork and beef accounted for higher protein, iron, B vitamins, and phosphorus. Nutrient levels in 1974 were higher by 2 per cent or more than in 1967 for most nutrients. Table 4–1 indicates the nutrients available for civilian consumption per capita per day for selected periods.

In examining Table 4–1, it must be borne in mind that nutrients in these amounts were

available but, obviously, all individuals did not consume these amounts. The table is reassuring to the degree that adequate nutrients are available. Some way must be found for all people to receive an adequate diet.

Seasons appear to have an influence on the adequacy of nutrients in the diet, according to the 1965 Household Food Consumption Survey of the U.S. Department of Agriculture.[9] Amounts of vitamin A and ascorbic acid were lower in spring diets, and calcium shortages were more frequent in summer. Vegetables contribute more vitamin A than any food

[8] Berta Friend and Ruth Marston, "Nutritional Review," *National Food Situation*, Economic Research Service, U.S. Department of Agriculture, Washington, D.C., November 1974, pp. 24–27.

[9] Shirley E. Wegener, "A Diet for All Seasons," *Food and Home Notes*, U.S. Department of Agriculture, March 29, 1971, p. 1.

group in each of the seasons, but green and deep-yellow vegetables made the greatest contribution in the fall.

Nutrient density is another way to examine the nutrients in any given food. The term is related to the concentration of important nutrients, such as vitamins, minerals, proteins, and others, in relationship to kcaloric value. Vegetables and fruits, for example, are noted for their richness of valuable vitamins and minerals and yet do not contribute excessive kcalories. Milk and meat are other foods that have important nutrients in comparison to kcalories. Low nutrient density refers to foods that are high in kcaloric value but carry insignificant amounts of other nutrients. To maintain health, the careful selection and consumption of foods that give evidence of considerable nutrient density is desirable. Carelessness about this responsibility may result in malnutrition.[10]

Deficiency of Nutrients

Jolliffe[11] defined a nutritional deficiency disease as one that is caused by a nutritional inadequacy. At least two kinds of nutritional inadequacies exist. One, caused by an insufficient amount of one or more essential nutrients in the diet, is called a *primary* inadequacy. However, even a person who is consuming an adequate diet can incur malnutrition, nutritional deficiency diseases, or nutritional failure. This happens when factors other than a poor diet, such as a certain type of illness, interfere with the *absorption* of essential nutrients; then a *conditioned* or *secondary* inadequacy results. Thus, in the strictest sense, a nutritional inadequacy develops whenever the tissues are not supplied with adequate amounts of essential nutrients.

In the development of a deficiency disease, the first "line of defense" or adjustment involves the nutrient reserves. These exist so that the tissues may draw upon them during temporary dietary omissions. These reserves are truly temporary in most cases, for the amount of the nutrient that can be stored is exceedingly small. For example, there is only enough available thiamin for a few days, while vitamin A stores are adequate for a few months.

Once these nutrient reserves are exhausted, the next step is a depletion of tissues; again this may be rapid or slow, depending on the former nutritional status and the health of the individual. This stage is the actual beginning of a deficiency condition.

When tissue depletion has reached a critical level, biochemical lesions will occur. These will be reflected in changes in the constituents in the urine and blood.

The fourth step is functional changes, which are manifested by generalized symptoms that might be caused by many things other than a deficiency of nutrients. These complaints include such things as excessive fatigue, inability to sleep, gas, distress, and difficulty with concentration. Other functional changes may be detected by special techniques. Examples of these are measurable changes in work performance and inability to see in dim light.

If the inadequacy persists, the final stage with anatomic lesions develops. At first these lesions are usually subgross and might go undetected, but they can be diagnosed through laboratory techniques. The gross lesions that appear when the condition is greatly advanced are universally recognized. Anatomic lesions include changes in the skin, tongue, cornea, skeleton, and other parts of the body. Nutritional deficiency diseases represent a major problem in public health around the world. These diseases will be discussed and described in subsequent chapters.

As indicated earlier, there are positive indications of good health and nutritional status, but there is a dearth of standards beyond "educated speculation." On the other hand, through surveys and laboratory research, procedures have been developed to evaluate nutritional status from the midpoint of "good" to the outer range of "deficiency state."

---

[10] Philip L. White, "Let's Talk About Food," *Today's Health*, Vol. 48, No. 1 (January 1970), p. 4.

[11] Norman Jolliffe, F. F. Tisdall, and Paul R. Cannon in Norman Jolliffe (ed.), *Clinical Nutrition*, Hoeber, New York, 1950, Chaps. 1–6.

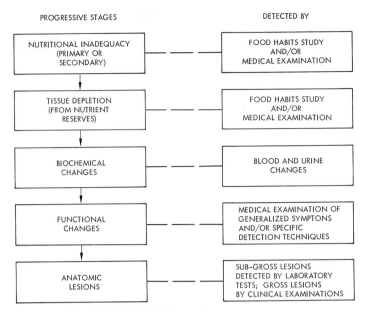

FIGURE 4–2. *The development of nutritional deficiency diseases and methods of detecting them at various stages.*

Methods of Nutritional Assessment

Davidson, Passmore, and Brock[12] believe that nutritional assessment is difficult because there are so many ill defined grades between the obviously well nourished and the ill nourished.

Experts involved in the development of an appropriate design for the Health and Nutrition Examination Survey (HANES)[13] concluded that nutritional status cannot be measured and interpreted by a few simple indexes. A person's nutritional status is reflected in a complex of interrelationships of clinical observations, biochemical assessments, anthropometric measurements, sociological and psychological evaluations, and dietary intake or patterns.

Sandstead and Pearson[14] suggest four major aspects of a clinical appraisal of nutritional status: historical evaluation of the dietary and medical experience: anthropometric measurements of growth, development, and fatness; physical examination for signs consistent with deficiencies; and biochemical assessments. Each of these methods of determining an index of nutritional status will be discussed.

Clinical Observations

Physicians and other health personnel must be especially trained with actual patients to recognize symptoms and conditions associated with nutritional deficiencies, according to the operation of HANES.[15]

Physicians review .the medical history questionnaire before the scheduled examination for possible clues. Physical examinations with an emphasis on nutritional aspects usually include the following: examination of the ears,

[12] Stanley Davidson, R. Passmore, and J. F. Brock, *Human Nutrition and Dietetics,* Williams & Wilkins, Baltimore, 1972, p. 467.

[13] Henry W. Miller, *Plan and Operation of the Health and Nutrition Examination Survey,* DHEW Publication No. (HSM) 73–1310, National Center for Health Statistics, Health Services and Mental Health Administration, Public Health Service, U.S. Department of Education, and Welfare, Rockville, Md., 1973, p. 2.

[14] Harold H. Sandstead and W. N. Pearson, "Clinical Evaluation of Nutritional Status," in Robert S. Goodhart and Maurice E. Shils (eds.), *Modern Nutrition in Health and Disease,* Lea & Febiger, Philadelphia, 1973, Chap. 19.

[15] Miller, op. cit., p. 29.

head, eyes, mouth, and neck (including the thyroid) for possible lesions and abnormalities associated with deficiencies of vitamins A, B complex, and C or minerals, such as iodine and iron. Inspection of the chest and back are made to determine possible deficiencies of vitamins A and D. The scrutiny of deep tendon reflexes and neuromuscular excitability may reveal a lack of thiamin and minerals. Inspection of the skeleton for lesions is undertaken for evidence of deficiences associated with vitamins D or C. The skin of the extremities, especially that of the thighs and the upper outer arms, is checked for indications of deficiences of vitamins A, C, and B_6 or essential fatty acids.

In the dental examination a determination is made of the fluoride content of one tooth and then compared with the number of cavities and fillings. Possible chewing and eating difficulties are noted. All this information can be checked against the dietary history to see if a relationship exists between the kinds of food consumed and the condition of the teeth. Clinical observations are not conclusive on their own but strengthen data gained by other methods of evaluation.

Biochemical Assessments

Laboratory determinations are made from blood and urine samples. From the blood sample, examinations are made of hemoglobin, hematocrit, red cell count, white cell count, vitamin A, iron, folate, vitamin C, total protein, albumin, cholesterol, calcium, phosphorus, and magnesium. The following determinations are made from urine samples: thiamin, riboflavin, iodine, and creatinine. Norms have been established for objectivity of analyses. Techniques are being refined and improved. Some biochemical assessments are more adequate than others, according to Sandstead and Pearson.[16]

Balance studies, a biochemical assessment according to Beal,[17] have the shortcomings of few subjects, expense, and limited duration.

In addition, to interpret the biochemical behavior of the subject, it is necessary to know about his long-time intake, his nutritional state, how he adapts to changes in level of intake, and similar details. This type of study does contribute to an understanding of nutrition but does not measure the incidence of malnutrition.

Anthropometric Methods

Examinations for this method generally include measurement of height and weight, skinfold measurements, and X-rays of the hand and wrist for individuals between 1 and 17 years of age. Sandstead and Pearson recommend that height–weight observations of children be compared with tables of measurements of well-nourished children from the same ethnic and geographic background when available. Caliper measurement of the skinfold is an indirect indicator of fatness, if carefully done. Arm circumference is sometimes meas-

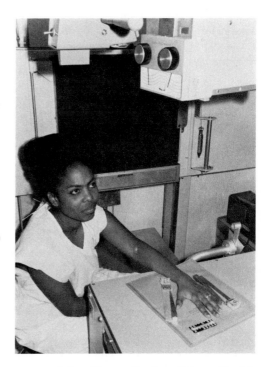

FIGURE 4–3. *One anthropometric method is an X ray of the hand and wrist to determine developmental status and any bone changes in nutrition-deficiency conditions.* (Hanes)

[16] Sandstead and Pearson, op. cit., p. 585.

[17] Virginia A. Beal, "A Critical View of Dietary Study Methods," Part 1, *Food and Nutrition News*, Vol. 40, No. 3 (December 1968), pp. 1, 4.

ured in children as an evaluation of kcalorie and protein reserves. This measurement also indicates muscle mass, which correlates well with linear growth.

Anthropometric measurements are helpful in judging the physical growth pattern of a child—one useful criterion for judging his nutrition.

Evaluation of Nutrient Intake

Another area that can contribute to the evaluation of the nutritional status of the individual is an *appraisal of the food intake.* There are several different ways to obtain a person's food pattern. Each technique has advantages and limitations.

One of the most comprehensive ways of determining the dietary intake of an individual is a diet history, which is obtained by eliciting a detailed report of his usual food patterns. The diet history will reveal his likes and dislikes, factors that influence his diet, and major deviations from the accepted concept of good food habits. It is usually obtained through an interview by a trained nutritionist. The major disadvantage is that it might not reflect the day-to-day deviations found in the normal diet.

The adequacy of the diet history is influenced by the length of time covered by it. Beal indicates that a 3-month period is satisfactory.

The ability of the interviewer can be a definite limitation. He must be able to secure sufficient and accurate information not only on the intake but also on such items as family food purchases, food preparation facilities, and food preferences.

A second technique is to have the person record his food intake on a special form. The diet record may last for 3 days, 1 week, 2 weeks, or any desired period. Morgan,[18] in her discussion summarizing nutrition status studies in the United States, remarked that a 14-day record was needed for a fair estimate of the intake of an individual. There can be con-

siderable variation in the degree of accuracy of the records. The person may forget to include some food, misjudge the portion size, or keep a dishonest record. On the other hand, a conscientious individual can keep a careful and detailed account; then, of course, a good picture of the food habits is obtained.

The "24-hour recall" will reveal many basic food patterns. For example, when the person remembers what he ate in the last 24 hours, his record will indicate important facts: meals that were omitted, favorite foods selected, such as cake or candy, and the frequency of meals and the inclusion of protective foods. The basic error in this type of dietary evaluation is that the day chosen might not be a "typical" day. However, dietary patterns are revealed, for a person will follow many of his usual eating habits in spite of outside pressures.

Morgan points out that the 1-day recall was an effective tool when used to determine the characteristics of the food use of groups of people rather than those of an individual. The number of records obtained would tend to minimize the lack of precision. Sometimes, if only an appraisal is desired, the 24-hour recall is a quick, efficient technique to obtain a working foundation to help with nutrition problems. As the number of 24-hour intakes reported by an individual increases, the possibility of securing a picture of the usual intake improves, according to Beal. The 24-hour recall, plus an inventory of foods eaten during the last 3 months, makes the information more useful. Some indication of frequency of intake is valuable.

Two other methods are used primarily in research studies. One is the "weighing" method. That is, the food to be eaten is weighed, as well as any returned plate waste, and then the actual amount consumed is determined. This is the most accurate method of getting a measure of a diet intake and is frequently used when working with individual subjects in research projects. The other method, the inventory technique, is conducted by a trained nutritionist who makes an inventory of a family's food supply, keeps a record of all food that is brought into the house, either by purchase or by gift, and at the end of a specified period does a closing inventory. From

[18] Agnes Fay Morgan (ed.), *Nutritional Status, U.S.A.,* An Interregional Research Publication, Bulletin No. 769, California Agricultural Experiment Station, Davis, Calif., 1959.

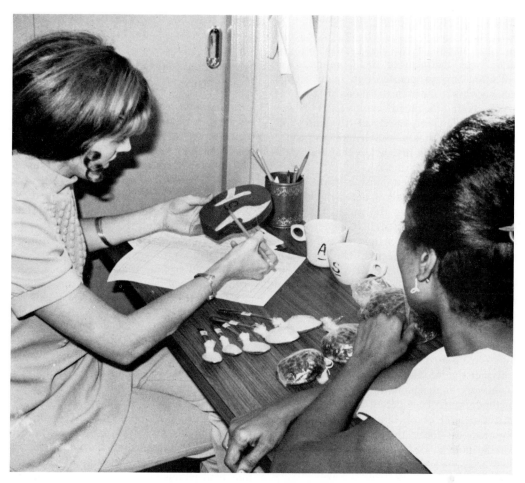

FIGURE 4–4. *A dietary interview by a nutritionist of a participant in a national nutrition survey. Note food models and measuring equipment.*

these data, the food consumed by the family during the time of the study is determined. There are many opportunities for error in this technique, for there is no breakdown among family members of the amount eaten by each. In addition, no allowance is made for plate waste. This method is used when large numbers are surveyed because it gives a clear picture of the foods consumed by a great number of people, and an appraisal can be made about the trends related to people and diet.

Once the diet information is obtained, it must be evaluated by an accepted yardstick to determine if the menus have been adequate. This evaluation may be done in two ways. The first is to compare diet data with the recom-

mendations found in food groups, such as the basic seven or the four groups of the guide to good eating (Chapter 2). This method is not always satisfactory, for little precise information can be derived. A diet might meet all the suggestions enumerated, yet because of its lack of variety within each group, it might not contain the necessary nutrients.

The second way to evaluate nutritional intake is to use an accepted table of food consumption (see Appendix B) to calculate the nutritive value in terms of grams and milligrams of specific nutrients. The total is then compared with the recommended daily allowances for a final evaluation of nutritional adequacy. This method has limitations also, for the food record is only an estimation on the part of the individual as to the amount and preparation of his food. Moreover, as King,[19] the chairman of the Committee on Nutrition Surveys, pointed out, many factors influence the nutritional value of food as expressed in the food composition tables. Seasonal differences, variety of fruit and vegetables, cooking losses, and length and kinds of storage are but a few factors that will result in variability in food values.

Considerable caution must be used if the recommended daily allowance serves as a standard for evaluating the nutrient level of food intake. As discussed in Chapter 2, the allowances include a "margin of sufficiency" above minimal requirements. The suggestion was made that they be used as a point of reference when applied to individuals, and consequently they should be interpreted only in terms of the total observation of the individual's nutritional status.

These techniques for evaluating dietary intake can be used, but care must be taken to interpret the information obtained within the framework of the limitations imposed by the method itself. The dietary intake can show that the level of calcium or the vitamin A reported was lower than that recommended for the individual. However, one cannot say,

[19] Charles Glenn King (chm.), Committee on Nutrition Surveys, *Nutrition Surveys: Their Techniques and Value,* National Academy of Sciences— National Research Council, Washington, D.C., 1949.

on the basis of dietary calculation alone, that a person is deficient in a nutrient.

Sociological and Psychological Evaluations

Information secured from demographic data can be illuminating in judging nutritional status. Income, for example, may indicate if an individual can buy adequate food. Level of education may be an indicator of his knowledge of nutrition and application to his daily food intake. Age may require special attention. Women have nutritional needs that differ from men, particularly during pregnancy and lactation. If ethnic background foods are prized, this must be considered. Other aspects of the environment such as availability of food, work of the individual, family lifestyles, and number of meals eaten away from home may have an impact on nutritional status. An individual's attitude toward food, concern about health, and other psychological characteristics have a bearing.

An individual or a family may wonder how the elaborate methods described here can apply to them. These methods are employed largely for research and health survey purposes as a basis for the development of needed programs. An awareness of the importance of incorporating adequate servings of the basic four food groups into daily food consumption is a major step toward desirable nutritional status. Periodic health checkups are recommended for feedback about nutritional status.

SELECTED REFERENCES

Beaton, George H., and Nelson A. Fernandez, "Surveillance and Evaluation of Nutritional Status," *Proceedings Western Hemisphere Nutrition Congress 111–1971,* Futura Publishing Company, Mount Kisco, N.Y., 1972, pp. 356–363.

Davidson, Stanley, R. Passmore, and J. F. Brock, *Human Nutrition and Dietetics,* The Williams & Wilkins Company, Baltimore, 1972, Chapters 13 and 49.

Friend, Berta, "Nutritional Review," *National Food Situation,* U.S. Department of Agriculture, Washington, D.C., November 1973, pp. 23–24.

Harper, Alfred E., "Recommended Dietary Allowances: Are They What We Think They Are?" *Journal of the American Dietetic Association,* Vol. 64, No. 2 (February 1974), pp. 151–156.

Huenemann, Ruth L., "Interpretation of Nutritional Status," *Journal of the American Dietetic Association,* Vol. 63, No. 2 (August 1973), pp. 123–124.

Miller, Henry W., *Plan and Operation of the Health and Nutrition Examination Survey,* DHEW Publication No. (HSM) 73–1310, National Center for Health Statistics, Health Services and Mental Health Administration, Public Health Service, U.S. Department of Education and Welfare, Rockville, Md., 1973.

Robinson, Corinne H., *Fundamentals of Normal Nutrition,* Macmillan Publishing Co., Inc., New York, 1973, pp. 365–368.

Sandstead, Harold H., and W. N. Pearson, "Clinical Evaluation of Nutritional Status," in Robert S. Goodhart and Maurice E. Shils (eds.), *Modern Nutrition in Health and Disease,* Lea & Febiger, Philadelphia, 1973, Chapter 19.

5

Carbohydrates

Carbohydrate foods comprise the mainstay of the diet of most of the peoples of the world. More than half of their nutrients are derived from carbohydrate foods that vary from one part of the world to another, but are similar in nutritive content. Classic examples are rice, wheat, corn, potatoes, cassava root, bananas, or grain sorghum.

These foods give the highest yield of energy per acre, grow easily, are inexpensive, highly palatable, and can be stored for reasonable periods.

Chemistry and Classification of Carbohydrates

Carbohydrates consist of carbon, hydrogen, and oxygen, with the hydrogen and oxygen in the same proportion as in water, that is, two hydrogen to one oxygen. Carbohydrates are synthesized by plants with the help of sunlight from the carbon dioxide of the air and water.

Carbohydrates can be classified into three major groups on the basis of their chemical structure:

MONOSACCHARIDES The monosaccharides are simple sugars. Glucose, fructose, and galactose are three monosaccharides that are important in human physiology. Glucose (also known as grape sugar, dextrose, and corn sugar) is found in fruits and plant juices, and also in milk and milk products. The second monosaccharide, fructose (sometimes referred to as levulose), is also found in fruits and vegetables, and in honey and cane sugar as well. Galactose, the third type, is found in milk and milk products. In addition to being found in foods, the three monosaccharides are the end products of *all* digestible forms of carbohydrates. Fructose and galactose are then converted to glucose, probably in the liver; from this stage, glucose follows the metabolic pathways and is utilized where needed in the body.

DISACCHARIDES The disaccharides are so called because they yield two simple sugars upon breakdown. The disaccharides are sucrose, lactose, and maltose. Of the three, sucrose, which is composed of one molecule of glucose and one molecule of fructose, is most widely distributed in foods. In its "pure" form, it is found in ordinary table sugar, whether derived from sugarcane or sugar beets. It usually appears mixed with glucose and fructose in fruit and plant juices. Lactose consists of equal parts of galactose and glucose, and is found in varying amounts in the milk of all species of animals. Maltose, which is composed of two molecules of glucose, is the result of the breakdown of starch. During the germination or sprouting of cereal, a specific enzyme acts upon starch and reduces it to maltose. It is also formed as an intermediary product in the breakdown of starch during animal digestion. All three disaccharides are easily digested; they are crystalline, sweet, and easily soluble.

POLYSACCHARIDES The polysaccharides yield more than two simple sugars upon breakdown or digestion. The principal ones we will be concerned with are starch, dextrin, glycogen, and cellulose. Of these, starch is of primary importance to human nutrition. It is found in cereal grains, roots, bulbs, and tubers. (In addition, most plants store their food supply in the form of starch. Then, as ripening takes place, the starch changes into glucose; that is why fruits have a sweet taste when ripe.) When digested, starch is changed first to dextrin, then to maltose, and then into glucose. Cooking makes the starch more available to digestive enzymes: although cold water does not affect it, the starch grains absorb warm water, which causes them to swell and rupture. The second polysaccharide, dextrin, is the intermediate product between starch and sugar. When bread is toasted, some of the starch

becomes dextrin, resulting in a slightly sweet taste. Glycogen, frequently called animal starch, is the form in which animals and man store carbohydrates. It is stored in the human liver, and small amounts are present in every body cell. Cellulose, which is insoluble, is the structural portion of plants; it is also the framework in which the starch granules are deposited. While herbivorous animals are able to get caloric value from cellulose, man cannot utilize its carbohydrate content as there are no enzymes in the body that can digest it. Its chief value for man is that it provides roughage necessary for gastrointestinal health. Other polysaccharides, such as inulin, agar, and pectin, are of little or no nutritional value. As a group, the polysaccharides vary in solubility and digestibility. Figure 5–1 summarizes the classification of carbohydrates.

After being absorbed, carbohydrates exist in the body as glucose and as glycogen. Glucose is a constant constituent of the blood that provides the tissue cells with energy. The amount of glucose circulating in the blood supplies only enough calories for 10 to 15 minutes of normal energy expenditure, and thus has to be constantly replenished from glycogen, the form in which carbohydrate is stored. This store of reserve energy, glycogen, is found in both the liver and the muscles. Most of it is present in the form of a protein

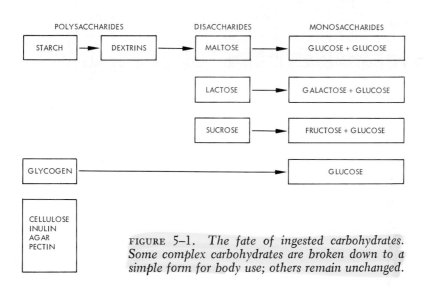

FIGURE 5–1. *The fate of ingested carbohydrates. Some complex carbohydrates are broken down to a simple form for body use; others remain unchanged.*

complex. The amount stored is relatively small. Jolliffe[1] and his associates have estimated that in a 70-kilogram man, the muscle glycogen may be approximately 245 grams and the liver glycogen 108 grams. They further estimated that the blood sugar would be 17 grams of carbohydrate, thus totaling 370 grams of carbohydrate within the body at any one time. This is the equivalent of 1517 calories, or only enough energy to supply the body needs for approximately 13 hours. Consequently, it is very important that the carbohydrate content of the body be constantly replaced by the daily diet.

Function of Carbohydrates

Carbohydrate is an indispensable source of energy, according to Levine,[2] because certain tissues require and use carbohydrate under all physiologic conditions, such as fuel for muscular activity, especially heart muscle. The central nervous system depends upon a continuous supply of glucose for fuel.

In the liver, in addition to being a source of energy, carbohydrate functions in a protective and detoxifying action. For example, the liver is more resistant to various types of noxious agents if adequate glycogen is present. This function of the liver is important to the whole body in removing or destroying toxins and similar substances before they reach vital tissues of the body that are not prepared to cope with them.

In addition, carbohydrate in the liver has a regulating influence on protein and fat metabolism. The liver is partially responsible for carbohydrate's protein-sparing action. Deamination of amino acids in the liver decreases as the availability of carbohydrate increases. Thus, carbohydrate is used for energy and protein is spared. Carbohydrate

intake is important for fat metabolism through facilitating the oxidation of fatty acids. If carbohydrate is severely restricted, as in some faddish diets, fats are metabolized more rapidly and the body has difficulty in handling some of the intermediate products of metabolism known as ketone bodies. The accumulation of ketone bodies leads to ketosis. Thus, carbohydrate is said to have an antiketogenic function.

Carbohydrates tend to conserve water and electrolytes even when the amount in the diet is only 100 g per day.[3] Certain carbohydrates have specific functions. Lactose appears to increase calcium retention in children.[4] The type of dietary carbohydrate has an effect on the level of serum cholesterol, being lower when complex carbohydrates such as dietary fiber and pectin are consumed in preference to sucrose.[5]

The need for specific carbohydrates for certain physiological functioning requires food composition tables that will reveal such sources. Presently, carbohydrate content is usually indicated by "total carbohydrate by difference." This difference is the sum of the percentage of protein, fat, ash, and water subtracted from 100. Both available and unavailable carbohydrates are included. Hardinge, Swarner, and Crooks[6] have prepared such a table of the composition of specific carbohydrates. An additional table of less common carbohydrates has been developed such as the particular carbohydrates in such foods as chick peas, defatted wheat germ, soy sauce, and the sorbitol content of a list of fruits. Food com-

[1] Samuel Soskin and Rachmiel Levine, "Carbohydrate Malnutrition," in Norman Jolliffe (Ed.), *Clinical Nutrition*, Paul B. Hoeber, New York, 1950, Chap. 8.

[2] Rachmiel Levine, "Carbohydrates," in Robert S. Goodhart and Maurice E. Shils (eds.), *Modern Nutrition in Health and Disease*, Lea & Febiger, Philadelphia, 1973, Chap. 3.

[3] W. L. Bloom and G. J. Azar, "Similarities of Carbohydrate Deficiency and Fasting," *Archives of Internal Medicine*, Vol. 112, No. 3 (September 1963), pp. 333–336.

[4] R. Mills et al., "Influence of Lactose on Calcium in Children," *Journal of Nutrition*, Vol. 20, No. 5 (November 1940), pp. 467–476.

[5] Ancel Keys, J. T. Anderson, and F. Grande, "Fiber and Pectin in the Diet and Serum Cholesterol Concentration in Man," *Proceedings from the Society for Experimental Biological Medicine*, Vol. 106 (January–April 1961), pp. 555–558.

[6] Melvyn G. Hardinge, Julia B. Swarner, and Hulda Crooks, "Carbohydrates in Foods," *Journal of the American Dietetic Association*, Vol. 46, No. 3 (March 1965), pp. 197–204.

CARBOHYDRATES

position tables of the future may further develop this important dietary information.

The role of carbohydrate in dental caries is discussed in Chapter 19.

Sources of Carbohydrates

The major carbohydrates may be found in the following four food groups:

1. Cereals and cereal products
2. Vegetables
3. Fruits
4. Concentrated sweets

Of these, the cereals and cereal products form the largest fraction of the human diet. The cereal group includes many forms, such as flour, pastries, bread, cakes, dry cereal, and specialized products. It is interesting to note that the predominant cereal may be influenced by ethnic patterns and agricultural development. For example, wheat is the most popular cereal in the United States, furnishing approximately 25 per cent of the total kcalories consumed, while in the Far East rice might provide as much as 70 per cent of the total. Considerable amounts of oats and corn are consumed by the American people, as well as macaroni, spaghetti, and vermicelli, which are wheat products. Moreover, many processed cereals are available today; these may be in the form of puffed, flaked, or finely ground dry cereals. Many have additional carbohydrate in the form of sugar coating. Cereals also provide small amounts of some of the vitamins and minerals, and varying amounts and kinds of amino acids.

We eat many parts of the vegetable: the root, tuber, leaves, fruit, and seeds. Each part of the plant varies in carbohydrate value. The leaves and stalk of the plant consist largely of cellulose; consequently, the available carbohydrate value is low. The root is the part of the plant that stores food to supply energy and vitamins and minerals for growth. The fruit itself, which usually surrounds the seed, is the reservoir of energy-giving food for the new plant. As a result, these are relatively high in carbohydrate content. For example, leaves such as lettuce, and stalks like asparagus, contain little carbohydrate. But root vege-

tables like beets have a higher content. The variety of the vegetable, and also the season, can affect the carbohydrate content of the food.

Roots and tubers are a popular category of vegetables. Potatoes are the chief food in this group. According to the U.S. Department of Agriculture, the per capita consumption of white potatoes is approximately 118 pounds per year. They are high in starch and relatively low in fiber content. Other commonly used members of this group are sweet potatoes, carrots, turnips, and beets. Closely allied to this group are the squashes—hubbard, acorn, and butternut. These contribute considerable carbohydrate value to the diet, and also vitamin A and small amounts of minerals.

A second group of vegetables is the green leafy variety, which includes cabbage, kale, chard, and so on, all relatively low in carbohydrate content, contributing approximately 3.2 g of carbohydrate for ½-cup cooked vegetable. They contribute sizable amounts of minerals and vitamins to the diet.

Legumes like dried navy and kidney beans, lentils, green or dried peas, and green or dried lima beans are quite high in carbohydrate content, having about 21.2 g per ½-cup cooked legumes. In addition, they are important sources of protein. Thiamin, small amounts of riboflavin, and iron may also be found in legumes.

Fruits also vary in carbohydrate value. Some, like bananas, dates, and figs, have a high content, while others, such as rhubarb, strawberries, and watermelon, are low in carbohydrate. The carbohydrate content may vary as much as from 5 per cent in fresh fruit to 60 to 80 per cent in dried fruit.

Rich sources of vitamins and minerals, fruits are available in many forms—fresh, canned in sugar syrup or water, dried, stewed, frozen, and preserved. In addition they may be purchased as fruit juice. The carbohydrate content may vary according to the processing the fruit has received. Carbohydrate in the form of sugar is often added in processing. For example, sugar syrup is frequently added to canned and frozen fruits, and this will significantly increase the carbohydrate value.

The fourth group of carbohydrate foods is

often referred to as "concentrated sweets," and includes such foods as sugars, syrups, molasses, jams and jellies, beverages, candies, and honey. Sugar consumption in the United States is quite high. Recent surveys indicate 103 pounds per capita yearly consumption of cane and beet sugar. This can be stated another way by saying that we consume almost ¼ pound per day per person. Sugar and its products are used in many ways; for example, as frosting on a cake, to sweeten foods, and in ice cream and beverages.

In the allocation of the consumer dollar, the carbohydrate foods ranked as follows: fruits and vegetables were second to meat, cereals and bread ranked fourth, sugar and sweets were seventh, and potatoes eighth.

An examination of one day's menu will indicate the important role of carbohydrates in the diet. Carbohydrate foods appear in many forms and in varying sized portions.

Frequently nutritionists express concern about the large amounts of carbohydrates of low nutrient density that are consumed. Sugars, many of the concentrated sweets, gum, and syrups are chief offenders. Other carbohydrate foods can supply nutritional benefit in addition to fuel. Cereals, fruits, and vegetables provide protein, vitamins, and minerals in differing amounts, as well as carbohydrates. In an era when the energy needs of the individual are comparatively low, it seems unwise to choose an excessive number of foods from those low in nutrient density.

Although the enrichment program will be discussed in Chapters 11 and 15, it is also pertinent to consider it in relation to carbohydrate foods. Since 1941 the enrichment of flours, breads, and, to some extent, cereals and other grain products has taken place. These foods have been enriched with the B vitamins (thiamin, riboflavin, and niacin) and iron. In some cases, calcium has been added to bread. Because of the prominent place of cereals, flour, and bread in American diet, it is believed that the enrichment program has considerably improved the nutritive content of the nation's food.

Unlike the other carbohydrate foods, cellulose provides no calories, but, as mentioned earlier in this chapter, it serves the necessary function of providing bulk, thus aiding in the elimination of body waste. Green leafy vegetables, like spinach and chicory, stalks of vegetables, such as asparagus, bran, the seeds of fruits and vegetables, and skins of some foods are our major sources of cellulose. In fact, very few foods are residue free. An adequate amount of indigestible fiber is desirable for good health.

Requirements of Carbohydrates

There is a specific need for carbohydrate as a source of energy for the brain and for certain other specialized physiologic purposes. No specific allowances have been established for carbohydrate. It is suggested, however, that some carbohydrate available to the body be included in the diet to prevent ketosis, excessive breakdown of body protein, loss of cations, especially sodium, and involuntary dehydration. The inclusion of 50 to 100 g of digestible carbohydrate daily will offset the undesirable metabolic responses associated with high fat diets or fasting.[7]

Consumption of Carbohydrates

The contribution of major food groups to the carbohydrate supplies available for civilian consumption, according to 1974 data, is as follows: meat (including pork fat cuts), poultry, and fish, 0.1 per cent; eggs, 0.1 per cent; dairy products, excluding butter, 6.6 per cent; fats and oils, including butter, less than 0.05 per cent; citrus fruits, 1.9 per cent; other fruits, 4.7 per cent; potatoes and sweet potatoes, 5.3 per cent; dark-green and deep-yellow vegetables, 0.5 per cent; other vegetables, including tomatoes, 4.5 per cent; dry beans and peas, nuts, soya flour, 2.2 per cent; flour and cereal products, 34.8 per cent; sugars and other sweeteners, 38.4 per cent; and miscellaneous, 0.6 per cent.[8]

Sources of carbohydrate that have decreased

---

[7] Food and Nutrition Board, *Recommended Dietary Allowances*, 8th ed., National Academy of Sciences—National Research Council, Washington, D.C., 1974.

[8] *National Food Situation*, Economic Research Service, U.S. Department of Agriculture, Washington, D.C., November 1974, p. 28.

from 1960 to 1974 in per capita consumption are fresh fruits from 93.4 to 79 pounds and cereals and flours from 133.5 to 128.8 pounds. Increases were in vegetables, fresh, canned, and frozen, from 126.3 to 166.6 pounds and corn syrup and corn sugar from 13.8 to 23.0 pounds.[9]

The important role of carbohydrate in the diet cannot be minimized. It is one of our prime sources of kcalories. In addition, it is closely related to protein and fat metabolism. Among its chief assets is its relatively low cost as a food. And, finally, it must not be forgotten that most carbohydrate foods, such as cereals and cereal products and fruits, are relatively rich in other nutrients. Thus such carbohydrate can bring "dividends" to the diet. The importance of carbohydrate from a health and economic standpoint should not be minimized.

---

[9] Ibid., p. 15.

SELECTED REFERENCES

Davidson, Stanley, R. Passmore, and J. F. Borck, *Human Nutrition and Dietetics,* The Williams & Wilkins Company, Baltimore, Chapter 4.

Food and Nutrition Board, National Research Council, *Recommended Dietary Allowances,* 8th ed., National Academy of Sciences, Washington, D.C., 1974, p. 34.

Hardinge, Mervyn, Julia B. Swarner, and Hulda Crooks, "Carbohydrates in Foods," *Journal of the American Dietetic Association,* Vol. 46, No. 3 (March 1965), pp. 197–204.

Levine, Rachmiel, "Carbohydrates," in Robert S. Goodhart and Maurice E. Shils (eds.), *Modern Nutrition in Health and Disease,* Lea & Febiger, Philadelphia, 1973, Chapter 3.

Pekkarinen, M., "World Food Consumption Patterns," in Miloslav Rechcigl (ed.), *Man, Food and Nutrition,* CRC Press, Cleveland, 1973, pp. 15–33.

Robinson, Corinne H., *Fundamentals of Normal Nutrition,* Macmillan Publishing Co., Inc., New York, 1973, Chapter 5.

6

Fats
and Other Lipids

Fat is an important nutrient for health for all ages. This fact is often deemphasized because the focus of attention is on the role of fat as a risk factor in cardiovascular disease, the number one cause of death in the United States today. An objective review of the information about the role of fat in nutrition is pertinent for the student of nutrition.

Chemistry and Classification of Fats

Fats are composed of the same three elements that are found in carbohydrates: carbon, hydrogen, and oxygen. However, fat is a more concentrated form of fuel, for it contains more carbon and less oxygen than carbohydrates. Thus it supplies two and one fourth times as many calories per given weight.

When a molecule of fat is broken down, it will yield three molecules of fatty acids and one molecule of glycerol. Expressed chemically, fats are simple esters of glycerol and fatty acids. Fatty acids consist of a chain series of carbons attached to a carboxyl group, COOH. It is the presence of this COOH group that confers the acidic property upon the compound. The combinations at each end and the number of carbons in each chain determine the characteristics of each fatty acid. Fats themselves are named according to the fatty acid molecule.

The term *lipid*, which appears frequently in the literature, refers to fats and other compounds that resemble them in physical properties. Lipids are usually classified as simple lipids and compound lipids.

The simple lipids are chemically defined as esters of fatty acids and alcohol. These include two groups: the first, fats, which are esters of fatty acids with glycerol; and the second, waxes, which are esters of fatty acids with an alcohol other than glycerol. The former group, fats, includes the familiar animal and vegetable fats. The waxes include esters of higher fatty acids such as stearic acid and vitamins A and D.

The second group, compound lipids, may be defined as esters of fatty acids containing groups in addition to an alcohol and a fatty acid. This category includes such compounds as the phospholipids. Lecithin, which is a constituent of each cell, is a well-known phospholipid. It is found in egg yolk and milk, to name some sources. A second compound lipid is sterol. One of the most widely distributed and most familiar of this group is cholesterol.

62

Ergosterol, which plays a role in vitamin D metabolism, is another.

The fats found in the American diet are chiefly true fats, or the simple lipids.

Characteristically, fats are not soluble in water. However, they may be dissolved in other substances, often referred to as fat solvents, such as ether, carbon tetrachloride, or chloroform. In the body all the blood lipids —cholesterol, phospholipid, and triglyceride— are bound to specific proteins, the lipoproteins. These proteins solubilize the lipids that are ordinarily not soluble in the plasma and transport them in and out of the plasma. Fats differ in melting points, which are determined by the fatty acid combination with glycerol. Most fats are mixtures of several triglycerides, so the consistency of a fat is not a sharp determinant of its makeup.

The term *oil* refers to the physical state of a fat. Chemically speaking, oil may refer to many different types of organic compounds, such as mineral oil, or lubricating oil from petroleum, or oil of cloves. Oil, when referred to in the context of nutrition, refers to the type of fat that is a liquid at room temperature.

A number of fatty acids are present in foods. Some of these are in a form known as *unsaturated*. This term refers to the fact that the fatty acid molecule contains a double bond between one or more of the carbons in its chain. This double bond permits the compound to receive other elements or radicals, and it is then described as saturated. A saturated fatty acid compound is not as easily oxidized as the unsaturated fatty acid. Commercially, this saturation process takes place when certain oils are hydrogenated (hydrogen is added) to create the popular shortenings used in baking and other forms of food preparation. When the double bonds open and accept hydrogen ions, the fatty acid is more or less solidified, depending on the degree of hydrogenation. Because hydrogenation has markedly reduced the potential for oxidation, these fats may be stored at room temperature.

Certain naturally occurring fats are saturated. These are fats that have all the bonds satisfied. Generally speaking, the fats found in animal sources—beef and lamb fat, for example, or lard—consist of a significantly larger number of saturated than unsaturated fatty acids. On the other hand, vegetable oils, safflower oil, cottonseed oil, and corn oil, to name a few, contain more unsaturated fatty acids. However, one cannot depend on the absolute classification of "animal fat" for designating saturated fats and "vegetable fat" as indicating polyunsaturated fatty acids. Examples are fat from poultry and fish oils, which have a high degree of unsaturated fatty acids, and coconut oil, which has considerable saturated fatty acids.[1]

The P/S is the ratio between polyunsaturated fats (linoleic, linolenic, and arachidonic) to saturated fatty acids (lauric, butyric, myristic, capric, palmitic, caproic, and stearic) in a given food or diet. This ratio is determined by dividing the total polyunsaturated fatty acids by the total saturated fatty acids. For example, the P/S for wheat germ oil is 3.3, which indicates a similar ration of polyunsaturated fatty acids to saturated fatty acids.[2] Monounsaturated fatty acids are palmitoleic, oleic, and erucic acids. Oleic acid is probably the most widely distributed fatty acid in nature. In most fats, oleic acid comprises about 30 per cent or more of the total fatty acids.

Functions of Fats

One of the primary functions of fat is that it serves as a concentrated source of energy. The individual derives 9 kcalories from 1 g of fat, whereas protein and carbohydrate provide 4 kcalories per gram. Fatty acids have been shown to be oxidized for energy directly by the resting muscle, and there is even evidence suggesting that the heart itself depends on them for its energy. Exceptions are erythrocytes and the cells of the nervous system.

Fat, as adipose tissue, is the major source of energy stored in quantity by the body. The end products of the digestion of both carbo-

---

[1] Report of the Food and Nutrition Board, *Dietary Fat and Human Health*, National Academy of Sciences—National Research Council, Washington, D.C., 1966, p. 5.

[2] *P/S Ration*, Bureau of Nutrition, Department of Health, New York City, 1969, p. 1.

hydrate and protein, as well as fat, can be converted to adipose tissue. These reserves are not an inert mass of cells. On the contrary, adipose tissue is active tissue in a dynamic state of change at all times.

The quantity of fat stored, its high kcaloric value, and the convenience of storage with minimum weight and with little amounts of water and minerals make this nutrient an important form of energy storage, according to Mead.[3]

Besides providing a reserve of energy, normal deposits of adipose tissue also protect the individual from outside forces. For example, approximately half the fat deposited in the body is located as a subcutaneous layer that insulates the body from rapid changes in environmental temperature, and it also helps to maintain body temperature at a constant level. In addition, adipose tissue is deposited around organs like the kidneys and reproductive organs and thus cushions them against any sudden injuries. It also serves as a padding in the cheeks, palms of the hands, and balls of the feet.

In addition to the storage depots of adipose tissue, fat is found elsewhere in the body, as in plasma and in each body cell.

Flavors and aromas, which are fat-soluble substances characteristic of certain foods, are one of the many factors determining a person's enjoyment of his diet. The satiety value, or as it is often called "stick-to-the-ribs" value, of the diet is believed to be related to the fat content. The reason might be because fats retard the emptying of the stomach and thus the individual feels satisfied for a longer period of time. The extent to which fats enhance the palatability of the nutritious meals is difficult to determine. However, it is a recognized fact that the attractiveness of the diet is often improved by the addition of such foods as butter, salad dressings, and sauces.

Another important role of fat from a dietary standpoint is that it is frequently the carrier of certain other nutrients. These are primarily the vitamins A, D, E, and K.

In 1929 Burr and Burr[4] demonstrated fatty-acid deficiency symptoms in the rat. The essential fatty acids were later found to be linoleic, linolenic, and arachidonic. These essential fatty acids contain two or more double bonds.

When young rats are kept on a fat-free diet, research shows that they do not grow normally or maintain their weight. In addition, they develop skin disorders and kidney degeneration. Additional investigations on other experimental animals have indicated similar reactions. Consequently, it is believed that these fatty acids are needed for normal growth and reproduction, for healthy skin, and for proper utilization and deposition of fat in laboratory animals.

Arachidonic acid has been shown to be an essential constituent for normal functioning of body cells. This acid can be synthesized from linoleic acid provided that there is an adequate intake of pyrodoxine or vitamin B_6. Thus linoleic acid acts as a precursor of arachidonic acid, so the latter has lost its designation as a true diet essential. Investigators have therefore indicated linoleic as the one essential fatty acid that must be included in the diet.

Essential fatty acids appear to regulate cholesterol metabolism, especially transport, transformation into metabolites, and ultimate excretion. When diets high in polyunsaturated fatty acids, including essential fatty acids, were fed to animals and man, a reduction was shown in serum cholesterol although the ultimate fate of the cholesterol removed from the circulation was not determined.

Essential fatty acids are important in the maintenance of the function and integrity of cellular and subcellar membranes in tissue metabolism. Acting as precursors for a group of hormone-like compounds called prostaglanins, which are important in the regulation of widely diverse physiological processes, is another function of these essential fatty acids.[5]

[3] James F. Mead, "Present Knowledge of Fat," in *Present Knowledge in Nutrition*, 3rd ed., Nutrition Foundation, New York, 1967, Chap. 4.

[4] G. O. Burr and M. M. Burr, "A New Deficiency Disease Produced by the Rigid Exclusion of Fat from the Diet," *Journal of Biological Chemistry*, Vol. 82, No. 2 (May 1929), pp. 345–367.

[5] Roslyn B. Alfin-Slater and Lilla Aftergood, "Fats and Other Lipids," in Robert S. Goodhart and Maurice E. Shils (eds.), *Modern Nutrition in*

The normal American diet seems to provide the minimum, at least, of the essential fatty acid requirement. Coons[6] points out that the average linoleic acid content of all dietary fats is about 10 per cent.

The essential fatty acids are found in common foods. Linoleic acid is quite widely distributed in the vegetable kingdom. It is a major component in various seed oils, such as linseed oil, corn oil, and cottonseed oil, and is also found in vegetable oils. Arachidonic acid is present in very small amounts in liver and fatty tissue of other organs.

The table in Appendix B contains information about the fatty acid content of foods and is subdivided into saturated and unsaturated fatty acids, with the latter further designating the amounts of oleic and linoleic acid.

Foods in the diet must provide sufficient fat to carry adequate fat-soluble vitamins and the essential fatty acids, linoleic and arachidonic acids, the latter of which can be formed from the former. A diet that provides 15 to 25 g of appropriate food fats should meet this need.[7] Appropriate food here indicates the presence of linoleic acid, which is found in edible vegetables oils such as corn, cottonseed, peanut, safflower, and soybean oils, but not in olive or coconut oils.

Sources of Fats

Few foods are composed solely of fat. Usually fat is combined with other nutrients—protein, fat-soluble vitamins, and carbohydrate, for example. Foods that supply fat have traditionally been divided into two main groups: animal fat and vegetable fat. Animal fats refer to those found in such foods as meat, fish, poultry, milk and milk products, and egg yolk. The vegetable fats include margarines, seed and vegetable oils (corn oil, cottonseed oil), and vegetables or fruits (avocado and olives).

The fat content of these foods can vary considerably. In meat, for example, one species may contain more fat than another; for example, pork contains more fat than beef. Also, different cuts of the same kind of meat may vary—a rib roast of beef may have more fat than a chuck roast.

A study concerning the nutritive value of cooked meat by Leverton and Odell[8] set forth some interesting data on the differences in the fat content of meat. The report stated that cooked lean meat without marbling and with all separable fat trimmed away is no more than 5 to 10 per cent fat. When the lean cut marbled with fat was added and averaged with the cooked lean meat without marbling, the average fat content of the cooked meat was increased from 10 to 21 per cent. This figure illustrates to what degree "hidden fat" exists in meats.

The fat content of fish also varies. Haddock and cod are relatively low in fat, whereas mackerel is higher. Some fish, tuna for example, are frequently canned in oil, which supplies additional fat. Egg yolk is another source of fat; egg white is fat-free.

Milk and milk products contribute considerable amounts of fat to the diet. Milk itself is approximately 4 per cent fat; however, skim milk contains only a negligible amount. Buttermilk is usually low in fat content, but in some areas of the country buttermilk is cultured whole milk. Consequently, the fat content is similar to that of regular milk. "Light" cream is 20 per cent fat, while "heavy" cream is usually 35 to 40 per cent fat; other combinations of cream that range in fat content are also available.

Hydrogenated fats are generally made from the oils of cottonseed, corn, and, occasionally, soybean and peanut. These are the popular "shortenings," which are primarily used in pastries, cakes, and for deep-fat frying. The hydrogenation of fats has been discussed under

Health and Disease, Lea & Febiger, Philadelphia, 1973, pp. 135–137.

[6] Callie Mae Coons, "Fatty Acids in Foods," *Journal of the American Dietetic Association*, Vol. 34, No. 3 (March 1958), pp. 242–245.

[7] Food and Nutrition Board, National Research Council, *Recommended Dietary Allowances*, 8th ed., National Academy of Sciences, Washington, D.C., 1974, pp. 34–35, 49–50.

[8] Ruth Leverton and George V. Odell, *The Nutritive Value of Cooked Meat*, Miscellaneous Publication MP-49, Oklahoma Agricultural Experiment Station, Oklahoma State University, Stillwater, Okla., March 1958.

"The Chemistry of Fats" in relation to the difference between saturated and unsaturated fatty acids.

Another source of fats is nuts. The popular peanut contains approximately 50 per cent fat, Brazil nuts 65 per cent, and pecans as much as 73 per cent. Chocolate and cocoa are also vegetable foods that are fairly high in fat content. Chocolate has more than twice as much fat as cocoa. The amount of fat varies considerably among cocoa powders.

Margarine consumption has been increasing steadily in this country. Margarine is used as a spread and in seasoning foods. Although originally derived from animal fat, today it is primarily made from vegetable oils, such as cottonseed, corn, sunflower, safflower, and soybean oil.

Yogurt is a form of milk that may vary in its fat contribution to the diet. Generally it is simply cultured whole milk. However, many companies market a type made from skim milk, and other types are made from either skim or whole milk with additional skim milk powder.

Cheese supplies considerable milk fat, depending on the type of milk used. For example, cottage cheese is a skimmed milk product and therefore contains approximately 1 per cent fat. However, cream is often added to many varieties of cottage cheese, and this will, of course, increase the fat content. Cream cheese, cheddar cheese, or Swiss cheese may have as much fat as 30 to 35 per cent.

Another source of animal fat is lard and suet, the fats of pork and beef. These are frequently used in cooking, the former in pastry and the latter in a food dish like suet pudding. Bacon fat is a popular ingredient in cooking because of its well-liked flavor.

Vegetable fats are taken in either a liquid or solid form. Salad dressings contain oil pressed from seeds, such as olive, corn, or cottonseed. Some of these oils are used in many households for cooking purposes as well.

Besides the two major groupings of animal fats and vegetable fats, there are often references to "visible" or "invisible" fats, the latter sometimes called "hidden" fat. Most people are aware of eating visible fats, for instance, butter, cream, salad dressing, and lard. But many are not aware of the amount of fat consumed when eating meats, cheeses, olives, avocadoes, cake, pastries, and nuts.

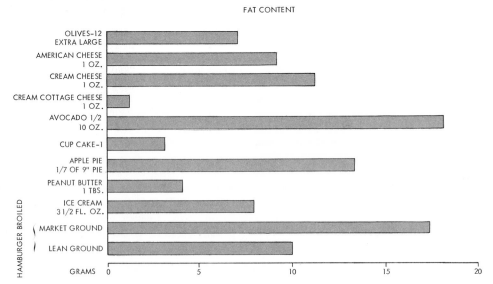

FIGURE 6–1. *Most persons are unaware of the amount of "hidden fat" in many foods. (Adapted from* Nutritive Value of Foods, *Home and Garden Bulletin No. 72, U.S. Department of Agriculture, 1971)*

The individual may control the amount of fat he consumes by what he eats and by the size of portion chosen. Some people use butter on many foods, others use it sparingly. Again an individual may choose the "extra" foods, such as gravies and sauces, that are high in fat, or he may refuse them. Consequently, there is a wide range in the amount and the kind of fat from one person's diet to another's.

Consumption

Preliminary figures for 1974 indicate the consumption of 158 g of nutrient fat available per capita per day, according to Friend and Marston,[9] 2 g less than 1973, which was the highest consumption since 1910. Since the 1947–1949 period, total nutrient fat has increased almost 11 per cent. Foods from three groups—fats and oils; meat, poultry, and fish; and dairy products—contribute 90 per cent of the total fat in the food supply.

Fats and oils are the largest contributors of fats and the share they contribute is increasing. In 1974 this group contributed 42.6 per cent of the total consumption. Use of salad and cooking oils doubled between the 1947–1949 period and 1967 and increased an additional third since that time. Nutrient fat provided by butter and lard declined to a record low, 9.5 per cent, because these food fats were replaced by margarine and shortening. In 1973, the quantity of fat provided daily by butter was 5 g, and by margarine, 11 g. The meat, fish, and poultry group is the next largest contributor of nutrient fat in the food supply. In 1973, 34 per cent of the total fat was provided by this group. The contribution of this group to the total fat supply has fluctuated little over the years. The share is higher in 1974 because of the rise in meat consumption. Pork provides a larger share of fat than beef. Dairy products, excluding butter, is a smaller contributor than the other two groups—12.4 per cent of the total fat contribution in 1974. Lower consumption of fluid whole milk and cream have resulted in de-

clines in the share of nutrient provided. The use of low-fat milks has more than doubled. The use of evaporated and condensed milks declined about 60 per cent from the 1947–1949 period. The consumption of cheese provides about 26 per cent of the total dairy-products contribution to the total fat consumption.

The increased amount of nutrient fat as well as shifts in sources of fat have influenced the fatty acid content of the diet. The levels of fatty acids have increased, but not equally. The net change in saturated fatty acids has been slight. The current level is 55 g per capita per day. Unsaturated fatty acid levels have increased with a marked change in linoleic acid consumption, an essential fatty acid; the level has steadily risen from 15 to 24 g per capita per day in 25 years. This change can be explained by the greater use of salad and cooking oils and greater use of margarine and shortening. A small gain in oleic acid, from 58 to 62 g per capita per day, can be accounted for by the same reasons, plus increased use of beef.

Pekkarinen[10] has studied world consumption of fats and oils with an emphasis on total consumption and the quality of the fats consumed. Highest consumption is in Europe and North America and the lowest is in Africa, the Far East, and in several countries in the Near East and Latin America. Dividing the parts of the world according to quantity of fat consumed results in three groups: Finland, West Germany, and Ireland are the users of large quantities of butter fat; Norway, Netherlands, Denmark, and Sweden use large quantities of margarine; Greece, Italy, Spain, and Bulgaria use large quantities of oil. Both butter and margarine are used in many countries. In North America, the United States is the largest user of shortenings in addition to margarine, butter, and lard. The main food fat in Canada is butter, besides margarine and shortenings. In Latin America the highest fat consumption is in Argentina. Several kinds of

[9] Berta Friend and Ruth Marston, "Nutrient Fat," *National Food Situation,* Economic Research Service, U.S. Department of Agriculture, Washington, D.C., November 1974, pp. 26–29.

[10] Maija Pekkarinen, "World Food Consumption Patterns," in Miloslav Rechcigl, Jr. (ed.), *Man, Food, and Nutrition,* CRC Press, Cleveland, 1973, pp. 30–31.

oil are most used in this region, plus small amounts of butter and margarine. In the rest of the world, with the exception of Israel and Libya, the consumption of fat is small. In many countries the predominant oil is olive oil. In Africa the use of palm oil is dominant. Groundnut and cottonseed oil are common in some areas.

Dietary Fat and Human Health

The relation of fat to coronary heart disease and other manifestations of atherosclerosis has gained considerable attention. Studies of the populations of many parts of the world have indicated an association of high intake of "saturated fats" and the prevalence of coronary heart disease, and a relatively low occurrence of this disease among populations having diets low in fats. In the "high-risk" populations, individuals tend to have higher plasma concentrations of cholesterol and triglycerides, whereas the "low-risk" populations tend to have low-plasma lipid levels. It must be recognized that populations have many variables, such as dietary characteristics, physical activity, smoking habits, and other influencing factors.[11] Research studies in the United States do indicate that genetics, body composition, sugar intake, personality, elevated plasma levels of cholesterol and possibly triglycerides are associated with greater susceptibility to coronary heart disease.[12] One is cautioned, however, against conceptualizing any atherosclerotic disease, especially coronary heart disease, with a single cause, although blood lipid levels can be used as a one predictor of clinical coronary events.

One explanation for the role of saturated fats in these conditions is that fatty substances, such as cholesterol, are deposited as fatty streaks on the lining of arteries. Gradually the lining of the arteries becomes heavy and irregular and displays heavy deposits called

"plaques." The whole process restricts the blood flow through the artery, and the roughened spots can break loose, weaken the walls of the blood vessel, and cause blood clots that interfere with blood flow. Although this may happen in any artery, the aorta and a number of arteries, middle-sized and large, situated in the brain, legs, and kidney appear to be more vulnerable. The most serious point of attack is in the three coronary arteries wrapped like a crown atop the heart. The process of atherosclerosis is slow—about 20 to 40 years. Early evidences have been found in children and young men.[13]

Christakis[14] gives an excellent review of the research that demonstrated the role of cholesterol and saturated fats and of the effect of nutritional factors in alleviating high serum cholesterol levels. Anderson and others[15] point out that diet has a powerful effect on serum cholesterol concentration in man, as demonstrated not only by epidemiological studies comparing large population groups who habitually subsisted on different diets, but also by experimental studies in which subjects were exposed to dietary changes under well-controlled conditions. In a study involving 14 groups of men with a sample of 500 or more men in each, living in seven different countries, Keys and others[16] demonstrated that 80 per cent of the serum cholesterol variability among these groups could be explained by the different proportions of saturated fat in the diet of these 40- to 59-year-old men.

A number of factors must be considered in planning cholesterol-lowering diets. Saturated fatty acid triglycerides, for example, have a

[11] Rosylin B. Alfin-Slater, "Fats, Essential Fatty Acids, and Ascorbic Acid," *Journal of the American Dietetic Association*, Vol. 64, No. 2 (February 1974), pp. 168–169.

[12] William B. Kannel, "Lipid Profile and the Potential Coronary Victim," *American Journal of Clinical Nutrition*, Vol. 24, No. 9 (September 1971), pp. 1074–1081.

[13] C. P. Gilmore, "The Real Villain in Heart Disease," *The New York Times*, March 25, 1973, pp. 31, 68, 72–80, 84–85, 92, 99.

[14] George Christakis, "The Case for Balanced Moderation or How to Design a New American Nutritional Pattern Without Really Trying," *Preventive Medicine*, Vol. 2, No. 3 (November 1973), pp. 329–336.

[15] Joseph T. Anderson, Francisco Grande, and Ancel Keys, "Cholesterol-Lowering Diets," *Journal of the American Dietetic Association*, Vol. 62, No. 2 (February 1973), pp. 133–142.

[16] Ancel Keys, "Coronary Heart Disease in Seven Countries," *Circulation*, Vol. 41, Supplement 1 (April 1970).

TABLE 6–1

Fat Content and Saturated and Unsaturated Fatty Acid Content of Some Common Foods

FOOD (APPROXIMATELY 1 CUP) AND WEIGHT (G)		FAT (g)	Saturated (total) (g)	FATTY ACIDS	
				Unsaturated	
				Oleic (g)	Linoleic (g)
Butter	226	184	102	60	6
Cooking vegetable fat	200	200	50	100	44
Corn oil	220	220	22	62	117
Cottonseed oil	220	220	55	46	110
Lard	205	205	78	94	20
Mayonnaise	240	96	16	16	48
Peanut oil	220	220	40	103	64
Olive oil	220	220	24	167	15
Safflower oil	220	220	18	37	165
Soybean oil	220	220	33	114	0

SOURCE: *Nutritive Value of Foods*, Home and Garden Bulletin No. 72, U.S. Department of Agriculture, Washington, D.C., 1971, pp. 32–34.

TABLE 6–2

Cholesterol Content in Milligrams of Portions of Some Common Foods

FOOD	PORTION	CHOLESTEROL (mg.)
Egg yolk, fresh	1 (17g)	255
Egg, whole	1 (50g)	275
Liver, raw	3½ oz (100g)	300
Butter	1 tbs (9g)	23
Sweetbreads	3½ oz (100g)	250
Lobster meat	3½ oz (100g)	200
Oyster	3½ oz (100g)	200
Crab, meat only	3½ oz (100g)	125
Cheese, cheddar	1 oz (28g)	28
Lard and other animal fat	1 tbs (13g)	12
Beef, without bone	3½ oz (100g)	70
Pork, without bone	3½ oz (100g)	70
Chicken, raw, flesh only	3½ oz (100g)	60
Ice cream	3 fl. oz (50g)	23
Cheese, cottage, creamed	½ cup (123g)	18
Milk, fluid, whole	1 cup (244g)	27
Milk, fluid, skim	1 cup (245g)	7

SOURCE: Bernice K. Watt and Annabel L. Merrill, *Composition of Foods*, Agriculture Handbook No. 8, U.S. Department of Agriculture, Washington, D.C., 1963, p. 146.

cholesterol-raising effect that is approximately twice the cholesterol-lowering effect of poly-unsaturated fatty acid triglycerides. The cholesterol content of the diet is another factor. Anderson and co-workers list the dietary alternatives that have a cholesterol-lowering effect (based on research) in approximate order of influence: decrease in saturated fatty acids such as lauric, myristic, and palmitic acids, especially those with a chain length of 12 to 16 carbons; increase in the proportion of polyunsaturated fatty acids; reduction of dietary cholesterol to less than the recommended 350 mg daily; addition of pectin; increase in the proportion of certain vegetables; and addition of plant sterols. In the planning of modification of the diet to decrease coronary heart disease risk, concern must be directed to appropriate kcaloric content and adequate intake of recommended nutrients. If polyunsaturated fatty acids dominate a diet, for example, there may be metabolic abnormalities related to vitamin E.

The role of fat in the problems of overweight and obesity are discussed in Chapter 10. See Table 6–1 for a listing of the fatty acids in common food and Table 6–2 for the cholesterol content of some common foods.

SELECTED REFERENCES

Alfin-Slater, Roslyn B., and Lilla Aftergood, "Fats and Other Lipids," in Robert S. Goodhart and Maurice E. Shils (eds.), *Modern Diet in Health and Disease*, Lea & Febiger, Philadelphia, 1973, Chapter 4.

Altschul, Aaron M., and G. E. Livingston (chairman, symposium), "Developing Foods for the Cardiac-Concerned," *Food Technology*, Vol. 28, No. 1 (January 1974), pp. 16–32.

Balart, L., M. C. Moore, L. Gremillion, and A. Lopez, "Serum Lipids, Dietary Intakes, and Physical Exercise in Medical Students," *Journal of the American Dietetic Association*, Vol. 64, No. 1 (January 1974), pp. 42–46.

Brown, Helen B., "Food Patterns That Lower Blood Lipids in Man," *Journal of the American Dietetic Association*, Vol. 58, No. 4 (April 1971), pp. 303–311.

Candau, M. G. "Your Health Is Your Heart," *The UNESCO Courier*, 25th Year (April 1972), entire issue.

Dietary Fat and Human Health, Publication 1147, Food and Nutrition Board, National Academy of Sciences–National Research Council, Washington, D.C., 1969.

"Exercise and Cholesterol Catabolism," *Nutrition Reviews*, Vol. 28, No. 8 (August 1970), pp. 211–212.

Feeley, Ruth M., Patricia E. Criner, and Hal T. Slover, "Major Fatty Acids and Proximate Composition of Dairy Products," *Journal of the American Dietetic Association*, Vol. 66, No. 2 (February 1975), pp. 140–146.·

Holt, Peter R., "Fats and Bile Salts," *Journal of the American Dietetic Association*, Vol. 60, No. 6 (June 1972), pp. 491–498.

McGandy, Robert G., and Jean Mayer, "Atherosclerotic Disease, Diabetes, and Hypertension: Background Considerations," and Mayer, Jean, "Heart Disease: Plans for Action," in Jean Mayer (ed.), *U.S. Nutrition Policies in the Seventies*, W. H. Freeman and Company, San Francisco, 1973, Chapters 4 and 5.

Strong, Jack P., Douglas A. Eggen, Margaret C. Oalman, Myra L. Richards, and Richard E. Tracy, "Pathology and Epidemiology of Atherosclerosis," *Journal of the American Dietetic Association*, Vol. 62, No. 3 (March 1973), pp. 262–268.

7

Protein and Amino Acids

From the days of the discovery of the "albuminous substances" to the present problem of kwashiorkor, a disease found in many nations throughout the world, investigations into the study of protein have brought about a greater appreciation of its importance to human nutrition. A historical review of the interesting research in this area includes the names of numerous well-known scientists.

Mulder is credited with recognizing that a certain substance that was essential to life existed in every cell. In his report in 1838 he named that substance *protein*, from the Greek word meaning "first." As protein was studied during the nineteenth century, the "building blocks" were identified one by one.

. In 1906 Wilcox and Hopkins demonstrated the nutritive indispensability of a single amino acid, tryptophan. Osborne and Mendel at Yale extended this concept by a series of classic experiments that elaborated the role of amino acids. Thus they were able to show the "limiting factors" of two amino acids, tryptophan and lysine. In 1915 they issued the report of their study: gliadin, a protein in wheat, would maintain life but would not promote growth in rats unless the amino acid lysine was added. They further demonstrated in their laboratory experiments that zein, a protein in corn, must be complemented with the amino acids tryptophan and lysine for both life and growth.

W. C. Rose, a pupil of Osborne and Mendel, continued to work with amino acids. Following years of painstaking, patient work, he and his associates at Illinois identified the last known amino acid in 1935. Through extensive detailed study, Rose established data that led to the current thinking about the nutritional role of protein and the amino acids.

Chemistry of Proteins

Proteins differ from carbohydrates and fats in that they contain nitrogen in addition to carbon, hydrogen, and oxygen. Some proteins also have sulfur, phosphorus, and iron. When extreme heat is applied, proteins will become coagulated. They may be precipitated out of solution by heavy metal salts. Plants can synthesize their own protein by combining the nitrogen from nitrogen-containing materials in the soil, such as nitrates and ammonia, with carbon dioxide and water. The energy for this process is provided by the sun. Legumes, such as beans, peas, and peanuts, have the capacity

71

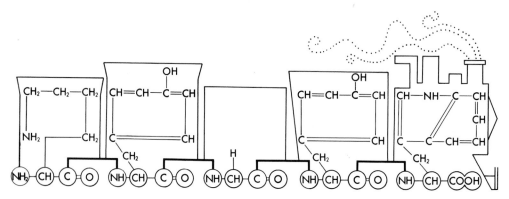

FIGURE 7–1. *A protein molecule is assembled from various kinds of amino acids, as a freight train is assembled from various kinds of cars. Whatever the differences, all the amino acids, like all the cars, have identical coupling devices. (Adapted from R. W. Gerard, ed.,* Food for Life, *University of Chicago Press, 1952)*

to utilize directly the nitrogen of the air with the aid of bacteria and to combine it with other necessary substances to make protein. Human beings cannot use such raw materials and are limited to securing their protein from plants and animals.

The protein that is found in foods and the protein that is synthesized are composed of giant molecules. Regardless of the size of the protein molecule, the percentage of nitrogen is approximately the same—16 per cent. The amount of protein in a given food can be obtained by first determining the nitrogen content by chemical analysis and then multiplying this result by 6.25.

This complex protein molecule is made up of the smaller structures called *amino acids.* There are approximately 22 known amino acids of varying nutritive value. The kind and structure of each protein depend on the amino acids involved. A molecule of protein may contain as many as several hundred or even thousands of amino acids. Apparently there are limitless possibilities for the formation of unique proteins, not only in the number of times amino acids are repeated, but in the order in which they are joined and in the arrangement of linkages into coiled, straight, or folded formations, which also influences the properties of the protein and further indicates the complexity of proteins.

These combinations of amino acids are connected together in a unique fashion, known as the *peptide linkage.* When the protein is broken down during digestion, the amino acids are split at this connecting link by the addition of water. And, conversely, when protein is synthesized, amino acids are combined by the elimination of water.

Only amino acids and, in rare instances, a few intact proteins are absorbed, according to Brown.[1] This absorption occurs at different rates and has little bearing on the quality of the amino acids. The premise is that the slow process provides for a more uniform and efficient rate of release, according to Griffith.[2]

Insulin, growth hormone, testosterone, adrenal corticoids, thyroid, and other hormones have a significant role in the absorption process. The amino acids are available to the individual body cells for such functions as the formation of new tissue and the synthesis of enzymes, hormones, and antibodies. Other nutrients, calories, vitamins, and minerals, as well as water, participate in this synthesis. The

[1] W. Duane Brown, "Present Knowledge of Protein Nutrition," in *Present Knowledge in Nutrition,* 3rd ed., Nutrition Foundation, New York, 1967, Chap. 2.

[2] W. H. Griffith, "Foods as a Regulator of Metabolism," *American Journal of Clinical Nutrition,* Vol. 17, 1965, p. 391.

digestion and metabolism of protein are discussed in Chapter 8.

Classification of Proteins

Protein sources of essential and nonessential amino acids are often classified as follows:

Complete proteins are those foods that contain all the essential amino acids in significant amounts and in the proportions to maintain life and support growth when used as the sole source of protein food. These foods are referred to as having a "high biological value."

Partially incomplete proteins are those foods that contain amino acids in amounts and in the proportions that may maintain life but not support growth. They may contain essential amino acids, but the proportionate amount of one may be low or a food may not contain one or more essential amino acids.

Incomplete proteins are those foods whose amino acid content is such that it is incapable either of maintaining life or of supporting growth.

Amino acids themselves may be divided into two groups: the essential and the nonessential (Table 7–1). Essential amino acids are those that cannot be synthesized by the body in sufficient quantities for growth and maintenance and therefore must be supplied in the daily diet. Histidine is considered essential for infants and small children, but its essentiality for adults has not been determined.

Each cell is responsible for building the type of protein that is typical of that cell and its function. The mechanism for this rather precise biosynthesis was the subject of dramatic research by scientists for a number of years. The discovery of deoxyribonucleic acid (DNA) and ribonucleic acid (RNA) helped to enlighten this riddle.[3] DNA is found in the nucleus of every cell. The biosynthesis of the needed protein takes place, however, in the cytoplasm of the cell. RNA acts as the messenger to transmit the appropriate protein synthesizing information. Another form of RNA, transfer RNA, collects the amino acid "packages" that match the code to the site of the synthesis or ribosomes in the cytoplasm, and the desired protein is formed according to the DNA pattern. Upon completion of the synthesis, the protein is released to perform its responsibilities in the cell and the cycle of biosynthesis is repeated again and again as necessary under the guidance of DNA. The importance of this code cannot be overestimated because it contains the information to duplicate the cells, tissues, and organs of an individual.

The dividing line between essential and nonessential amino acids is not sharply defined, according to Albanese and Orto.[4] Arginine is not essential for the adult but cannot be formed with necessary speed for infants, so it might be considered essential for early infancy. Tyrosine can be formed from the essential amino acid phenylalanine, and actually about 50 per cent of the phenylalanine need can be met by tyrosine. Cystine present in proteins may be substituted for approximately 30 per cent of the methionine requirement, if the dietary supply is low. Nonessential amino acids must be produced in intermediary metabolism so that essential amino acids will be optimally utilized. This has been demonstrated

TABLE 7–1

The Two Major Groups of Amino Acids

ESSENTIAL	NONESSENTIAL
Valine	Glycine
Lysine	Tyrosine
Threonine	Cystine
Leucine	Alanine
Isoleucine	Serine
Tryptophan	Glutamic acid
Phenylalanine	Aspartic acid
Methionine	Arginine
	Histidine
	Proline
	Hydroxyproline
	Citrulline

[3] Marion Thompson Arlin, *The Science of Nutrition*, Macmillan, New York, 1972, p. 68.

[4] Anthony A. Albanese and Louise A. Orto, "The Proteins and Amino Acids," in Robert S. Goodhart and Maurice E. Shils (eds.), *Modern Nutrition in Health and Disease*, Lea & Febiger, Philadelphia, 1973, Chap. 2A.

in feeding experiments in which a mixture of essential and nonessential amino acids was more effective than feeding only essential amino acids.

Protein Evaluation

The efficiency with which a protein is used for growth or maintenance is a measure of its quality, according to a Report of a Joint FAO/WHO Ad Hoc Expert Committee on energy and protein requirements.[5] The quality of a protein is determined first by its amino acid composition, but other factors bear consideration in a discussion of utilization. The amount of food consumed as well as the protein content of that food is important. For example, foods of low protein content can make a useful contribution to the diet if amounts are adequate. Unfortunately, the amount of food consumed is frequently considered in terms of energy requirements, and protein inadequacy may result. If the protein content of a food consumed by a child is low, such as in cassava, it may be impossible to consume the large quantity of food necessary to meet protein requirements.

Digestibility and metabolism may reduce the availability of the protein in the food consumed. Excessive heat processing, as in the production of milk powder, oil-seed meals, and protein-rich biscuits may reduce availability of protein content. In a carbohydrate-rich food, lysine and sulfur-containing amino acids may be affected. Home cooking and commercial canning methods cause little or no losses. Heat, on the other hand, is required to release the protein in soybeans so that it will be available in the body. Imbalance of amino acids may reduce food intake, or in the case of the high leucine content of corn and sorghum there is an apparent need for an increase of tryptophan and isoleucine.

Certain methods have been devised to evaluate protein quality. FAO recommends that the protein quality of any food be compared with the protein quality of egg or milk. Corrections are necessary when a food of lesser quality is included in the diet. In practice, persons, except young infants, consume diets that are less well utilized, at least by children, than are egg or milk protein. The FAO/WHO Committee recognized that this adjustment must be made in light of the quality of protein consumed by most age and sex categories. A 30 per cent increase in adjusted nitrogen requirements in accordance with balance and growth data was determined as necessary to meet physiological nitrogen requirements for all healthy people except for infants less than 6 months of age. From this adjustment another 30 per cent was added to allow for individual variability. This is cited in the report as "safe levels of intake of egg or milk protein." This implies that consideration has been given to proteins in a food or diet as compared with the quality of egg or milk protein, sometimes called the "biological value of protein."

Sometimes a correction must be arbitrary, as in studies of national diets. In rich countries, the diets are considered to have an 80 per cent relative quality protein and diets in poor countries are about 70 per cent. If 70 to 80 per cent of the protein is coming from foods like cassava or corn and there is little animal food consumed, the relative quality of protein in the diet may be as low as 60 per cent. It is recommended that a subpopulation be studied to determine the degree of relativity of protein quality.

Another method for determining protein quality is the *protein efficiency ratio* (PER). This ratio is defined as the weight gain of a growing animal divided by the protein intake. Feeding experiments are required that use small animals. This procedure has been valuable in studies with human infants. No chemical measurements are involved but standard dietary conditions are essential if protein quality is to be adequately measured. For example, inadequate kcalories or excessive protein may skew the data.

Nitrogen protein utilization (NPU) is the proportion of ingested nitrogen retained in the body, allowing for the degree of digestibility and the efficiency of utilization. This

[5] Report of a Joint FAO/WHO Ad Hoc Expert Committee, *Energy and Protein Requirements*, World Health Organization Report Series, No. 522, World Health Organization, Geneva, 1973, pp. 61–73.

method is time consuming and expensive, and because the procedure usually uses animals, ther may be an underestimate of the quality of the protein being tested.

Albanese and Orto[6] suggest that these methods of evaluation, although valuable, must be used with discretion because of the limitations of the procedures and the marked differences in the indicated nutritive value of samples of the same protein and in proteins with similar amino acid content.

Functions of Protein

Approximately 15 to 20 per cent of the human body is protein, and that protein exists in many forms. About one third of it is in muscle and one fifth in bone cartilage. Not only is protein present in every cell, but it is also an essential component of enzymes, hormones, and body secretions.

It is an important constituent of the blood. Among the forms of blood protein are hemoglobin, which transports oxygen from the lungs to the tissues and brings carbon dioxide from the tissues back to the lungs. Proteins also exist in the blood in the form of antibodies, our defense against disease. Still another function of blood protein is its role in helping to maintain the fluid balance within the body. Closely allied to this is the assistance protein gives in the exchange of nutrients between the blood and lymph cells and the cells and the fluid that surround them in supplying nutrients for cell metabolism. Protein is required for the growth of infants and children and for the maintenance of all tissues at all ages.

Protein is important in regulatory functions, acting as biocatalysts in every biological process at the biochemical stage. Proteins are enzymes or components of enzymes and structural elements in intracellular and extracellular materials; they comprise a large portion of the more solid matter of organs. The regulation of osmotic pressure is another function. The proteins in the important nucleic acids, DNA and RNA, are the bearers of inheritance characteristics. Hormones such as thyroxine and insulin are of a protein nature as well as

the antibodies that enhance immunity to disease. Body proteins are constantly being degraded and resynthesized. Proteins are amphoteric as a result of their basic amino acid groups and organic acid radicals. These characteristics enable proteins to assist in the mechanism that maintains an acid–base balance in the blood and tissues by uniting with either acidic or alkaline substances as the need arises.

Energy value is also supplied by protein— 4 kcalories per gram, the same amount provided by carbohydrate. The body's need for energy is of primary importance; thus if the diet does not supply sufficient kcalories from carbohydrate, tissue protein will be metabolized to provide the needed energy. On the other hand, adequate amounts of carbohydrate allow protein to participate in body functions that are specific only for protein. This relationship is referred to as the *protein-sparing action* of carbohydrate, for it avoids "dipping into" or breaking down tissue protein as a source of energy.

Protein Needs

Historically, wide variations in protein recommendations have been made throughout the years. In 1881 Voit,[7] on the basis of the analysis of diets of German men, suggested that 118 g of protein were needed in the diet each day. This diet also included 500 g of carbohydrate and 56 g of fat, and provided 3055 kcalories.

At the turn of the century, Atwater[8] in the United States made a similar recommendation of 125 g per day. He also studied the diets of American men and used them as his criterion of protein need. When both Voit and Atwater examined the diets of workingmen in their respective countries, the former suggested that protein be increased to 145 g and the latter to 150 g per day.

---

[6] Albanese and Orto, op. cit., pp. 41–53.

[7] E. V. McCollum, A *History of Nutrition*, Houghton Mifflin, Boston, 1957, p. 192.

[8] W. O. Atwater and A. P. Bryant, *The Chemical Compositions of American Food Materials*, Bulletin No. 28, U.S. Department of Agriculture, Washington, D.C., 1902.

Chittenden, after extensive studies on the nitrogen balance of athletes, professional men, and soldiers, suggested in 1904 that nitrogen equilibrium could be obtained on an intake of 44 to 53 g of protein per day. For many years Chittenden[9] maintained his own health on a diet of approximately 35 g of protein.

White[10] pointed out that, although not everyone is in agreement with Chittenden's suggestions for a low intake of protein, it is generally accepted that Voit's recommendation of 118 g of protein is too high. The answer lies somewhere in between.

The body's need for protein remains fairly constant, yet it can vary as a result of certain stresses or demands. When the diet supplies an adequate amount of amino acids for daily protein metabolism, the nitrogen intake (from food protein) equals the nitrogen output (in urine, sweat, and feces, in skin, nails, and hair, gas, saliva and sputum expectorated, nasal secretions, and blood lost from trivial wounds). Such a situation is known as being in nitrogen balance or nitrogen equilibrium. This balance, or lack of it, is used to determine protein needs.

When the nitrogen outgo exceeds the intake, indicating a loss of body nitrogen, the balance is said to be negative. Conversely, if intake exceeds outgo, indicating a deposition of protein tissue, the balance is said to be positive.

A negative nitrogen balance can be brought on by fever, surgery, toxemia, burns, or shock such as that following an accident. This negative balance is undesirable because body protein is being used to meet the emergency.

A positive balance exists during periods of growth—for example, during the growth stages of infancy, childhood, and adolescence; during pregnancy when the fetus is growing; and during lactation when the mother is storing protein for breast feeding. Other times when an adult may be in positive nitrogen balance would be when he is recovering from a debili-

tating illness or when he is increasing the amount of muscle tissues, for example, during a training period for sports events.

It is desirable for the adult to maintain nitrogen equilibrium. However, for the child it is highly important that enough protein be supplied in the diet so that the maximum nitrogen retention, with resultant growth of body tissue, occurs.

Additional information plus a recognition of certain errors led the FAO/WHO Committee[11] to change their method of estimating the nitrogen requirement for maintenance of nitrogen equilibrium. When individual male subjects weighing about 70 kg and consuming proteins of high quality were studied, the nitrogen losses were in a range of 4g/day to approximately 7g/day or an average value of about 5.2g/day. This is equivalent to a protein loss of 33 g per day for a 70-kg man, or 0.47 g per kg of body weight, according to *Recommended Daily Allowances*.[12] Energy intakes in these studies were adequate for maintenance of body weight. The results of these nitrogen-balance studies show that when nitrogen intake approaches the requirement even the highest quality proteins are not used with maximum efficiency, and the view that the measurement of nitrogen underestimates the minimum nitrogen requirement for maintenance is upheld. These results are the basis for establishing the recommended dietary allowance for protein.

Individuals do vary in their protein requirements according to their genetic backgrounds, but these differences cannot be documented in a highly heterogeneous human population. The figure of 30 per cent to be added to the average requirement will take individual variations into account based upon FAO/WHO suggestions.

During the first year of life, the body weight increases about 7 kg; concurrently, the protein content of the body increases from 11 to 14.6 per cent. Translated more specifically, there is

[9] Russell H. Chittenden, *Physiological Economy in Nutrition*, Stokes, New York, 1904.

[10] Abraham White, "Protein Metabolism," in Garfield G. Duncan (ed.), *Diseases of Metabolism*, Saunders, Philadelphia, 1964, Chap. 3.

[11] Report of a Joint FAO/WHO Ad Hoc Expert Committee, *Energy and Protein Requirements*, op. cit., pp. 40–44.

[12] Food and Nutrition Board, *Recommended Dietary Allowances*, 8th ed., National Academy of Sciences—National Research Council, Washington, D.C., 1974, pp. 40–43.

an average increase of body protein of about 3.5 g per day during the first 4 months of life and 3.1 g per day during the next 8 months, according to Fomon.[13] An allowance for maintenance must be added to ensure a satisfactory rate of growth.

Allowances for infants are based on the amount of protein provided in the quantity of milk required to ensure adequate growth in the infant. Estimates are 2 to 2.4 g per kg per day during the first month of life, falling gradually to about 1.5 g per kg per day by the sixth month, as suggested by the FAO/ WHO Committee. Allowances for children are calculated on information provided on growth rates and body composition. An assumption is made that protein will be used as efficiently for growth as for maintenance in adults.

---

[13] Samuel J. Fomon, *Infant Nutrition*, Saunders, Philadelphia, 1967, Chap. 5.

Protein is deposited in the fetus and accessory tissues of the mother for a total of 925 g and at a suggested rate of 0.6, 1.8, 4.8, and 6.1 g per day during the successive quarters of gestation. Some question has been raised about the protein allowances for pregnant women because some nitrogen-balance studies imply that protein utilization is lower than generally considered. The allowance for a pregnant woman must include needs for fetus and maternal accessory tissues as well as maintenance. Adjustments must be made for the efficiency of the utilization of protein. There is uncertainty about the amount of protein stored during gestation and to cover the needs previously stated, so a generous protein allowance is recommended for the pregnant woman or an additional 30 g per day. In determining the allowance for the lactating woman an adjustment has to be made for the conversion of dietary protein to human milk protein. Information is inade-

TABLE 7–2

Recommended Daily Dietary Allowances for Protein, Revised 1974

Designed for the maintenance of good nutrition of practically all healthy people in the United States.

	AGE (years)	WEIGHT (kg)	WEIGHT (lb)	HEIGHT (cm)	HEIGHT (in.)	ENERGY (kcal)	PROTEIN (g)
Infants	0.0–0.5	6	14	60	24	kg × 117	kg × 2.2
	0.5–1.0	9	20	71	28	kg × 108	kg × 2.0
Children	1–3	13	28	86	34	1300	23
	4–6	20	44	110	44	1800	30
	7–10	30	66	135	54	2400	36
Males	11–14	44	97	158	63	2800	44
	15–18	61	134	172	69	3000	54
	19–22	67	147	172	69	3000	54
	23–50	70	154	172	69	2700	56
	51+	70	154	172	69	2400	56
Females	11–14	44	97	155	62	2400	44
	15–18	54	119	162	65	2100	48
	19–22	58	128	162	65	2100	46
	23–50	58	128	162	65	2000	46
	51+	58	128	162	65	1800	46
Pregnant						+300	+30
Lactating						+500	+20

SOURCE: Food and Nutrition Board, *Recommended Dietary Allowances*, 8th ed., National Academy of Sciences—National Research Council, Washington, D.C., 1974, p. 129.

quate about the efficiency of this process. Twenty additional grams per day are suggested for the lactating woman.

The protein allowances for various ages, both sexes, and for pregnancy and lactation are indicated in Table 7–2.

There are other influences on protein requirement, according to the Report of a Joint FAO/WHO Expert Group. Extreme climatic variations, such as Arctic conditions, mean a kcaloric increase and hence a protein increase. If the extreme cold becomes a stress, it may result in increased nitrogen excretion. Exposure to high humidity conditions can result in losses of 3 g of nitrogen per day or more. It has not been investigated how much loss of nitrogen occurs through perspiration of populations living in hot climates.

Although kcalories are increased for persons doing heavy work, whether there is a need for additional protein is inconclusive. For persons who are increasing their muscle mass, extra protein intake is indicated.

Parasitic and other types of infections are quite common in developing countries and may result in severe protein deficiency, especially in children. The increased nitrogen loss due to dietary restriction, plus losses from infection, can be critical.

There is some evidence that psychological stress, such as anxiety and pain, may increase the excretion of nitrogen. If the situation is extreme, the loss may be as high as one third. In addition, psychological stress may impair the absorption of amino acids. Some recognition of the effect of stress is given in estimating recommended allowances.

Amino Acid Needs

Information about the precise quantitative amino acid requirements of man is less complete than for nitrogen requirements. The pattern of amino acids in foods is a critical factor that influences the total amount of protein required by man. The FAO/WHO Committee offers some tentative recommendations based on quite incomplete information, which must be used accordingly. The proportion of dietary protein that must be supplied as essential amino acids apparently changes with age. The

ratio appears to fall with age, but the rate and the magnitude have not been established.

There is some doubt about the adequacy of the protein requirements for women; they probably should be higher. The table of requirements for children was based on studies of amino acid requirements for boys, which are considered adequate for girls. A number of studies have been done with infants and there was considerable agreement among them about the amino acid requirements.

Harper and Benevenga[14] discuss the effects of disproportionate amounts of amino acids. It is important to recognize that organisms tolerate a measure of disproportion among the amino acids in a diet without adverse effects. The degree of tolerance for this condition depends upon the physiological and nutritional state. A continuous gradation of effects of disproportionate amounts of amino acids takes place depending upon the degree of disproportion.

Amino acid deficiency is the most obvious type, in which the inadequacy of one or more amino acids results in retarded growth and food intake. The content of the limiting amino acid will be reflected in the high correlation between amino acid content of the diet and both food intake and growth.

Amino acid imbalance is related to a dietary surplus of amino acids other than the one that is growth-limiting. Effects are depressed food intake and growth rate. An excess of individual amino acids has somewhat the same effect.

Protein Status

In the *Ten-State Nutrition Survey*[15] the findings indicated that a relatively large number of pregnant and lactating women demonstrated low serum albumin levels, which suggested marginal protein nutriture although

[14] A. E. Harper and N. J. Benevenga, "Effects of Disportionate Amounts of Amino Acids," in R. A. Lawrie (ed.), *Proteins as Food*, Avi Publishing, Westport, Conn., 1970, pp. 417–445.

[15] *Highlights, Ten-State Nutrition Survey 1968–1970*, DHEW Publication No. (HSM) 72–8134, Center for Disease Control, Health Services and Mental Health Administration, U.S. Department of Health, Education, and Welfare, Atlanta, Ga., 1972.

dietary intakes were above levels considered adequate. The recommendation of the survey is that dietary standards for this group should be reviewed, particularly in light of the relatively unsatisfactory outcome of pregnancy among low-income groups due to an excess of low-birth-weight babies.

In low-income-ratio states among both sexes of the black 6- to 9-year-olds, the 10- to 59-year-old females, and the over-60-year-olds in both sexes, there was a low prevalence of deficient values in protein. Among the Spanish-American, 10- to 16-year-old females and for both sexes from 17 to over 60 years of age, there was a low prevalence of deficient values in protein. Minimal deficiencies existed in all groups for both sexes in the high-income-ratio states and for whites, black and Spanish-American children of both sexes from 0–9 years of age, black males from 10–59 years of age, and Spanish-American males from 10–16 years of age in the low-income-ratio states. (See Table 2–2.)

In the preliminary findings of the *First Health and Nutrition Examination Survey*,[16] white persons under 45 years of age in both income groups had higher mean protein intakes (approximately 80.19 g with a range of 58.19 to 112.62 g) than blacks in similar age and income groups (approximately 69.54 g with a range from 52.30 to 99.31 g).

In the group 45 to 59 years of age, white adults had the lowest mean protein intake (62.83 g). This was considerably lower than for both racial groups in the income group above poverty level (white 83.45 g; black 80.33 g). Income was related to protein intake in the 60-years-and-over group. Both racial groups in the income group above poverty level had higher mean protein intakes than those in the lower income group.

Protein consumption is closely related to total kcaloric intake. Mean protein intakes per

1000 kcalories showed little or no variation by income or race within age groups with the exception of the 18- to 44-year-old group in which white males in the lower-income group had the highest mean intake, 42.22 g per 1000 kcalories. Another exception was in the 45 to 59 age group in which white persons of both income groups reported less protein intake per 1000 kcalories, 38.48 and 42.30 g, respectively, than did blacks of both income levels, 44.73 and 46.60 g, respectively.

In the biochemical evaluation, the mean protein level was higher for blacks than for whites for all age groups, regardless of income. In general, whites and blacks in the lower-income levels had higher serum protein levels than did whites and blacks in the income group above poverty level.

There was no prevalence of low serum albumin levels in the 1 to 5, 6 to 11, and 12 to 17 age groups. In the 18 to 44, 45 to 59, and 60-years-and-over age groups, whites had a higher percentage of low serum protein albumin values than did blacks, regardless of income. Females in the 18 to 44 age group had a higher percentage of low serum albumin values than did males of the same age for both incomes and races.

These findings indicate that, on the whole, the protein intake of the participants of this national survey met the 1974 recommended dietary allowances and in many instances surpassed the recommendation.

Sources of Protein

Which foods offer the best combinations of amino acids for the American diet? This question has been a consideration for many years. Animal sources, such as milk, eggs, cheese, meat, poultry, and fish, supply proteins of high biological value. Gelatin, because of its small amounts of threonine, methionine, and isoleucine and its lack of tryptophan cannot be classified with other animal sources as a complete protein. Rather, it is an example of an incomplete protein.

Cereals and vegetables provide a second source of proteins in the diet. These are "the partially incomplete proteins." Grains such as wheat and corn and rice as well as vegetable

---

[16] National Center for Health Statistics, *Preliminary Findings, First Health and Nutrition Examination Survey, United States, 1971–1972*, Dietary Intake and Biochemical Findings, DHEW Publication No. (HRA) 74-1219-1, Health Resources Administration, Public Health Service, U.S. Department of Health, Education, and Welfare, Rockville, Md., 1974.

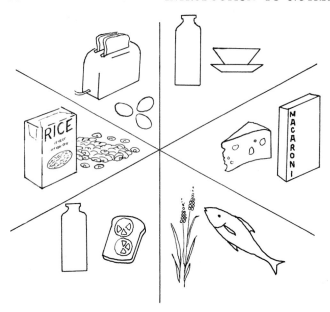

FIGURE 7–2. *Examples of mutual
supplementation of dietary protein.
These combinations of foods will
enhance the protein value of the
diet.*

proteins—for instance, legumes (peas, beans, lentils, peanuts)—and other vegetables are examples of this type of protein. Nuts are also included in this group.

There is a wide variation in the biological value of specific food sources of incomplete proteins; for example, such foods as nuts, grains, and legumes contain more amino acids than fruits and vegetables. The legumes are sometimes called "poor man's meat" because the protein of these foods are valuable when taken with animal protein.

Some of these legumes deserve additional attention. Soybeans, the first legume of which a written record was made when Emperor Shen Nung included soybeans among the principal and sacred crops of China, according to Altschul,[17] are rich in protein (40 per cent —more than any legume), fat, and other nutrients. The crops yield a great many "calories per acre." A method for preparing palatable soybeans was elusive for many years except among the Chinese who sprouted, fermented, and used other processes such as cheesemaking. The soybean is always cooked or toasted. Certain antinutritional factors identified as *tyrosine inhibitors* and others are

found in this legume. When treated to the right amount of heat as judged by research these factors are destroyed and the flavor enhanced, so that suitability for human consumption results. Another advantage of soybeans is that there is no evidence of allergenic properties.

A wide range of food products are made from soybeans, such as flours and grits that contain 40 to 60 per cent protein; soaked, blanched, and toasted beans used as nuts; soybean oil used for cooking and salad dressings; and meat, poultry, and fish analogs made from textured protein that simulates these products. Another textured vegetable protein product (often soybean, but it may be cottonseed or peanut) is added to meat patties, loaves, stews, or other dishes as an extender that reduces the cost. This product may be incorporated into ground meat by supermarkets and sold at the meat counter, labeled as such. Fibrous protein may be made into pieces to resemble bacon, ham, chicken, or beef.

The supplementation of vegetables, legumes, cereals, and nuts with limiting amino acid content has exciting possibilities. Keys and Keys[18] suggest that dishes of rice and

[17] Aaron M. Altschul, "The Revered Legume," *Nutrition Today,* Vol. 8, No. 2 (March–April 1973), pp. 22–29.

[18] Margaret Keys and Ancel Keys, *The Benevolent Bean,* Noonday Press, New York, 1972, p. 28.

beans, popular in Latin America and other regions, provide high-quality protein. Rice is deficient in the amino acids lysine and isoleucine but beans are rich in these amino acids. Wheat and legume meals are frequently used in Southern and Western Europe and in India; the proteins of these foods supplement each other. The beans and pasta of Italy and the chick-peas and chupatties (like *tortilla* but made from wheat instead of corn) used in India are other examples. The Japanese diet of rice and *tofu*, a concentrate of soybeans that resembles cheese, is highly nutritious. Other possibilities of supplementation are sesame seeds or Brazil nuts added to green vegetables. Nuts have supplemental potential, but nuts high in fat, such as pecans, almonds, English walnuts, or filberts, have their protein content diluted by the fat and are high in kcalories, so they are not as effective as other nuts. Peanuts are considered botanically a legume.

There are several problems associated with supplementation of proteins. The large quantities of food required to meet the protein requirements may be difficult to consume, especially for children. Limited information is available about the amino acid content of foods. To match two or more foods for the purpose of supplementation without causing an amino acid imbalance or deficiency may be difficult. From a practical standpoint the proportion of the foods used and their variety must be considered. For example, what proportion of beans and rice and which variety of these foods will provide the best supplementation of proteins? Supplementation must not be oversimplified or misinterpreted. For instance, it must be understood that the foods are to be eaten at the same time. Rice for breakfast and beans for dinner is not the answer. Another consideration is the contribution to amino acid content of any other foods that may be consumed at the same time. Supplementation is a challenging area for research.

Another form of supplementation is combining animal sources of protein with vegetable and cereal sources of this nutrient. A protein food from an animal source, such as milk, meat, or cheese, in combination with cereal protein will ensure that all essential components are present simultaneously so that protein synthesis will ensue. This practice is referred to as *mutual supplementation of dietary proteins.*

Many popular food habits reflect the practical approach and application of supplementation. For example, cereal with the addition of milk provides maximum effective use of the amino acids present in these foods. Other examples are such combinations as macaroni and cheese, casserole dishes containing the legumes with small amounts of meat, and sandwiches that are combinations of cereal grains, vegetables, and milk or cheese.

The Effect of Cooking on Protein

Modern methods of food processing and food preparation can influence the protein value of some foods. These techniques may either enhance or reduce the digestibility of protein foods. The digestibility of all foods, and in this instance protein, refers to the ability of the digestive enzymes to liberate the amino acids from the protein molecule.

Overheating or cooking by dry heat may reduce the nutritive value by destroying essential amino acids, especially those that are heat-labile, such as lysine and threonine. On the other hand, cooking in water or steaming increases the digestibility of some proteins and thereby enhances the nutritive value of a food. Furthermore, amino acids may be liberated by proper preparation. The importance of this function is illustrated by the fact that proteins in soybeans and wheat have a higher biological value when cooked. Moderately cooked meat is also better digested than raw or overcooked meat.

A comparison of the amounts of food that must be consumed to yield 20 g of protein can be of interest. A 2- to 3-oz serving of cooked lean meat from beef, pork, lamb, veal, chicken, or turkey will yield 20 g of high-quality protein, according to Peterkin.[19] To provide this same amount of protein would require about 10 slices of bacon, 14 slices of 3-

[19] Betty Peterkin, "The Cost of Meats and Meat Alternates," *Family Economics Review* (September 1970), p. 11.

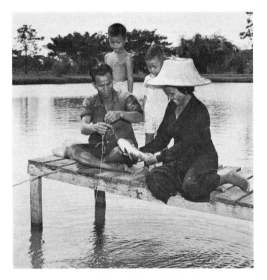

FIGURE 7–3. *This fish caught by a Thai family represents a healthful protein supplement to a primarily rice diet.* (FAO)

inch-diameter bologna, 3 frankfurters, 5 fish sticks, 3 oz of cheddar cheese, or ⅔ cup of cottage cheese.

Although vegetable proteins make a valuable contribution, it must be pointed out that many have serious amino acid limitations and the quantity of food to be consumed for even 20 g of protein can be forbidding. For example, 1½ cups of dried cooked or canned beans or peas, 5 tbs of peanut butter, ½ cup of roasted peanuts, ½ loaf of enriched white bread, 4 cups of cooked macaroni, or 4 cups of cooked oatmeal will yield 20 g of protein. In view of possible future protein shortages in this country, vegetable proteins will become more and more prominent in our diet. Amino acid fortification, the use of the least expensive animal protein sources that can be produced, supplementation, and other innovative approaches will need to be considered.

Protein Consumption

The American diet is rich in protein. In 1974 it was estimated that the mean per capita consumption was 101 g of protein per day. Over 69 per cent of the protein contribution comes from animal sources, which reflects

a high economic standard but also possible overconcentration.

According to preliminary data for 1974,[20] the source of protein in the food supply for civilians in the United States was distributed as follows: meat, including pork fat cuts, poultry, and fish, 41.5 per cent; eggs, 5.1 per cent; dairy products, excluding butter, 22.5 per cent; fats and oils, including butter, 0.1 per cent; citrus fruits, 0.5 per cent; other fruits, 0.6 per cent; potatoes and sweet potatoes, 2.4 per cent; dark-green and deep-yellow vegetables, 0.5 per cent; other vegetables, including tomatoes, 3.3 per cent; dry beans and peas, nuts, and soya flour, 5.4 per cent; flour and cereal products, 19.2 per cent; sugars and other sweeteners, less than 0.05 per cent; and miscellaneous, 0.4 per cent.

Meeting the Protein Requirement

Evidently meeting the protein need is not too great a problem in the United States. However, no aspect of the diet, from a nutritional standpoint, can be met by haphazard arrangement. Planning is necessary to ensure optimum nutrition.

The upsurge in inflation and possible recession in the world and especially in the United States are reflected in the consumption of food. Expensive cuts of meat have been substituted for, in part or on the whole, by less expensive cuts. Servings of meat have been reduced or eliminated for some meals. For instance, meat consumption has been curtailed for breakfasts and more cereal is being consumed. Unfortunately, foods such as rice, beans, and pasta that can be combined with meat for nutritious meals have risen dramatically in price.

Although there is no protein shortage for the country at large, it cannot be assumed that consumption is equally distributed. According to Bird,[21] within certain ethnic groups, among elderly people, teen-agers, and pregnant and lactating women, some individuals are lack-

[20] *National Food Situation*, Economics Research Service, U.S. Department of Agriculture, Washington, D.C., November 1974, p. 28.

[21] Kermit M. Bird, "Plant Proteins," *Food Technology*, Vol. 28, No. 3 (March 1974), pp. 31–39.

ing protein. The poor find it difficult to buy protein foods within their limited and somewhat static incomes.

Although the protein needs seem amply provided by the diet, the spacing of these foods must not be ignored. The fact was emphasized during the discussion of essential amino acids. Usually the suggestion is made that a complete protein be served at each meal so that through mutual supplementation the amino acids found in plant protein may be completely utilized. In fact, the combinations often improve the total biological value.

Protein Undernutrition

The most widespread nutritional condition of our time, according to McLaren,[22] is protein-kcalorie malnutrition. This disease has a broad spectrum from subclinical manifestations (which are more widely prevalent than severe forms) of retarded growth and development to more serious forms of marasmus, marasmic kwashiorkor, and kwashiorkor. Marasmus is generally considered to emerge from a restriction in the total food supply; kwashiorkor results from a diet specifically limiting in protein. Many consider these descriptions as oversimplified. Nutrition is generally only one of the major factors. These conditions reflect poverty, tradition, lack of parental understanding of child care, and inadequate medical care; the quality and quantity of the available food is either marginal or limiting, according to Hegsted.[23]

In addition, the physical environment may be unsatisfactory; many may suffer from repeated bouts with infection. All of these possible causes further accentuate a precarious nutritional state. In McLaren's opinion, conditions in urban areas that contribute to nutritional disaster are pressures for mothers to work; overcrowded, unhygienic living conditions; strong salesmanship to buy proprietary

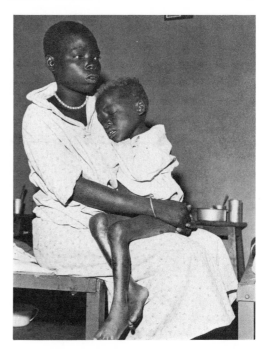

FIGURE 7–4. *A woman in the Congo holding a child suffering from kwashiorkor. Note change in hair color.* (*United Nations*)

milks that are expensive; or that may be diluted by the mother or improperly used (directions not followed); and low economic status. Unfortunately, because of these associated social problems, protein-kcalorie malnutrition cannot be solved solely by administering foods rich in protein or protein-fortified foods.

Protein malnutrition in children and adults may show its effects by stunted growth, mental retardation, and lack of muscle development. A lowered resistance to disease may also occur. Early signs of protein lack are fatigue and lassitude. In cases of a severe protein deficiency in the adult, such as occurred in World War II in many prison camps, muscle protein decreased as tissue protein was broken down to provide necessary amino acids for body metabolism.

Other evidences of protein deficiency include edema. This disturbance of the water balance is one of the symptoms of a protein lack. Continued physical restraint, such as being bedridden, may lead to nitrogen losses.

[22] Donald S. McLaren, "Undernutrition," in Miloslav Rechcigl, Jr. (ed.), *Food, Nutrition and Health*, Vol. 16, S. Karger, Basel, 1973, pp. 141–178.

[23] D. M. Hegsted, "Deprivation Syndrome of Protein-Calorie-Malnutrition," *Nutrition Reviews*, Vol. 30, No. 3 (March 1972), pp. 51–54.

Skin changes generally occur in the lower extremities of the body when there is inadequate protein or when the quality is poor. Loss of appetite is another indication.

In marasmus there is more severe growth retardation and wasting of subcutaneous fat and of muscles. Weight is more critically affected than skeletal measurements. Edema is absent, but enlarged liver and mild skin and hair changes are occasionally present. Precipitating factors are repeated attacks of gastroenteritis, respiratory infections, measles, and whooping cough. In reality, marasmus of a strictly nutritional nature does not exist. Marasmic kwashiorkor has mixed features of both conditions.

In kwashiorkor, a characteristic dermatitis and pigmentation change of the hair take place in many cases. Retardation of growth, weight loss, muscular wasting, apathy, and enlargement of the liver as a result of fatty infiltration are other symptoms found frequently. Kwashiorkor usually develops soon after a child is weaned. The child is susceptible if he does not receive a good supply of animal protein foods and subsists on a diet low in essential amino acids. The food intake may be adequate in kcalories, but because most of the food is supplied by cereals, there may be only a small supply of complete protein. Kwashiorkor is usually precipitated by some stress, such as an infectious disease.

Protein Overnutrition

If the diet contains protein foods far beyond the recommended allowance, there is a danger that other important nutrients may be lacking. The excess amino acids are used for purposes of energy. Because most protein foods of high quality are more expensive than other foods in the diet, the cost of the diet may be increased appreciably.

Protein and World Nutrition

If the protein gap in the world food crisis is to be met, considerable effort and resources must be brought to bear on the problem, according to the United Nations. Pulses, nuts, and seeds contribute to the protein content in countries where it is difficult to secure animal protein, and consumption has increased in many areas of the world. Lowest consumption of pulses is in North America and Oceania and in most European and Near East countries. Consumption of pulses, seeds, and nuts is highest in Africa, the Far East, and Latin America. The types of pulses vary from one part of the world to another. Although a large variety of nuts are available, few people in the Far East use them for food except for the countries that use coconut. More nuts are used for food in Africa than any other part of the world. The regions of highest meat consumption are Europe, North America, Oceania, and parts of South America. Consumption is highest in Argentina, the United States, New Zealand, and Australia. In developing regions of Africa, the Far East, and the Near East, the use of meat is moderate.

More milk is consumed in Europe, North America, and Oceania than any other part of the world. Of the Latin American countries, Uruguay is the only important consumer of milk. The Near East resembles Latin America, with Israel being the leading country in consumption. Milk is little used in the Far East and Africa. In addition to cow's milk, goat, sheep, and buffalo milks are used. France is the leading cheese consumer of the world; Bulgaria, Greece, Switzerland, and the Scandinavian countries, except Finland, are other users of cheese in Europe. North America and some countries in the Far East and in Latin America use cheese. Although the consumption of eggs is common, the quantity used in the world is small. Fish is consumed in quantity only in those countries where fishing is an important livelihood.[24]

Six avenues of investigation for solving the world's food problems are suggested by May.[25] They are the fortification of cereal grains, development of protein-rich types of rice, corn, and other grains, development of new

[24] Maija Pekkarienen, "World Food Consumption Patterns," in Miloslav Rechcigl, Jr. (ed.), Man, Food, and Nutrition, CRC Press, Cleveland, 1973, pp. 16–33.

[25] Jacques M. May, "Nutrition Science and Man's Food," in Food, Science and Society, Nutrition Foundation, New York, 1969.

foods based on oil seeds and the proteins of leaves and grasses, further development of fish protein concentrate, development of the animal husbandry industry, and development of single-cell protein foods. (See Chapter 34 for additional discussion.)

Although the importance of protein to man was recognized many years ago, studies since that time have reinforced and increased our knowledge. The critical shortage of protein in most of the world requires that attention be focused on the fact that world food production is falling behind population growth. Supplying adequate kcalories is not sufficient; adequate protein must be provided for the welfare of man and the development of nations.

SELECTED REFERENCES

Bird, Kermit M., "Plant Proteins: Progress and Problems," *Food Technology,* Vol. 28, No. 3 (March 1974), pp. 31–39.

Calvins, J. F., G. E. Inglett, and J. S. Wall, "Linear Programming Controls Amino Acid Balance in Food Formulation," *Food Technology,* Vol. 26, No. 6 (June 1972), pp. 46–49.

Food Policy and Food Science Service, Nutrition Division, *Amino Acid Content of Foods and Biological Data on Proteins,* Food and Agriculture Organization of the United Nations, Rome, 1970.

Harper, A. E., "Assessment of Human Protein Needs," *American Journal of Clinical Nutrition,* Vol. 26, No. 11 (November 1973), pp. 1168–1169.

Heiser, Charles B., Jr., *Seed to Civilization,* W. H. Freeman and Company, San Francisco, 1973.

Lipinsky, E. S., and J. H. Litchfield, "Single-Cell Protein in Perspective," *Food Technology,* Vol. 28, No. 5 (May 1974), pp. 16–24, 40.

Protein Advisory Group of the United Nations System, "International Review of Action to Improve World Protein Nutrition," *PAG Bulletin,* Vol. 2, No. 3 (Summer 1972), entire issue.

Rechcigl, Miloslav, Jr. (ed.), *Man, Food and Nutrition,* CRC Press, Cleveland, 1973.

Report of a Joint FAO/WHO Ad Hoc Expert Committee, *Energy and Protein Requirements,* World Health Organization Technical Report Series, No. 522, World Health Organization, Geneva, 1973.

Report of Joint FAO/WHO Committee on Nutrition, *Food Fortification and Protein–Calorie Malnutrition,* World Health Organization Technical Report Series, No. 477, World Health Organization, Geneva, 1971.

Scrimshaw, Nevin, and Aaron M. Altschul, *Amino Acid Fortification of Protein Foods,* The MIT Press, Cambridge, Mass., 1971.

"Some Aspects of Protein Nutrition," *Dairy Council Digest,* Vol. 43, No. 6 (November–December 1972), pp. 31–34.

8

The Release
and Utilization
of Nutrients

Man has long been intrigued by the mystery of what happens to food after it is eaten. Until the eighteenth century, many suggestions were made that had little bearing on the question. Then a French scientist, René de Réaumur, became the first man to use constructive thought and sound experimental procedures to determine the answer, in part at least, to what changes took place in food within the body.

Réaumur[1] noticed that his pet, a kite (a bird similar to an owl), would eat rather large pieces of food and later would spit up pellets of bone and other substances. He recognized that part of the food, which the animal could use, had been treated and retained in some manner and that the rejected part was indigestible. He then devised experiments that enabled him to obtain bits of partially digested foods from the kite by forcing the bird to swallow a metal tube open on both ends and containing meat. After the kite returned the indigestible tube, Réaumur studied the partially digested meat and noted for the first time the existence of digestive fluid. He then

forced the bird to swallow sponges attached to strings; he later removed the saturated sponges, thereby obtaining digestive fluid itself. He established the fact that gastric juice had greater solvent powers than water and that certain constituents of meat were dissolved by it.

Others followed Réaumur and studied digestion in many animals by various experiments. Different foods were tried and, in some cases, the digestive tract of a laboratory animal was examined periodically after eating.

One of the foremost contributors to the understanding of gastric digestion of man was William Beaumont.[2] He was an Army physician attached to the post on Mackinac Island in Michigan. In 1822 a trapper, Alexis St. Martin, was shot accidentally in the abdomen; this resulted in a large permanent hole in the abdominal wall. In the years that followed, Beaumont used St. Martin as a "human guinea pig" and conducted 116 experiments, which he recorded with painstaking thoroughness. He studied many aspects of gastric diges-

---

[1] E. V. McCollum, A History of Nutrition, Houghton Mifflin, Boston, 1957, p. 63.

[2] Dorothy Callahan and Alma Smith Payne, The Great Nutrition Puzzle, Scribners, New York, 1956, p. 82.

tion. He noted that gastric juice was secreted when food was swallowed normally, but not when food was placed into the stomach through its unnatural opening. He also found out the length of time each food remained in the stomach and which foods were digested there. He recognized the various motions that occurred within the stomach during the digestive process and speculated about the result of each. His research confirmed the surmises of earlier workers and prepared the way for later study.

As the science of chemistry advanced, various foods and the substances derived from them after their breakdown throughout the gastrointestinal tract were identified. The experiments of C. Bernard in 1856 (reported by McCollum[3]) contributed to the appreciation of fat and carbohydrate digestion. Bernard also added considerable knowledge about necessary enzymes and their reactions. Others too numerous to mention have provided additional information, so that today a fairly clear understanding of the digestive process exists.

Food is recognized as the sole source of nutrients. However, a food must undergo many changes before the nutrients are made available to the cell for utilization. The nutrients are bound in large molecules that cannot be absorbed because of their size and many are not water soluble. These changes progress in an intricate step-by-step pattern. Although there are still many gaps in the information on these reactions, each reaction is believed to be specific for a given nutrient at a given time at a given place; seldom can there be changes or substitutions. In addition, there are a considerable number of interrelationships among nutrients in their utilization.

This discussion is primarily concerned with the nutrients, protein, fat, and carbohydrate. Vitamins and minerals undergo little, if any, change in the process of digestion.

Basically, four steps are involved in the release and utilization of nutrients: (1) *ingestion*, the actual taking of food into the body; (2) *digestion*, the release of nutrients from food; (3) *absorption*, the process whereby the end products of digestion pass through the

[3] McCollum, op. cit., pp. 17, 18, 23, 35, 40.

wall of the gastrointestinal tract; and (4) *utilization*, the transport of these nutrients by the blood to all cells of the body and the ways in which the nutrients serve the body when needed. The total process is exceedingly complicated, yet orderly. Many factors, both internal and external, exert a marked influence upon digestion and utilization of nutrients.

Physiology of the Gastrointestinal Tract

The gastrointestinal tract, or, as it is commonly called, the digestive tract, is a muscular, mucosa-lined tube, approximately 30 feet long, that is subdivided into several sections. Each section has a particular shape suited to its specific function. The interrelationship of the muscles of the gastrointestinal tract with the special senses, smell and taste, along with the instinct thirst, needs to be fully appreciated. Through the nerve supply, the reactions of the gastrointestinal tract are both stimulated and inhibited.

The mouth, which is the first segment of the digestive tract, receives food, masticates it, and begins the digestive process. The food then goes to the esophagus, a long tube leading to the stomach. The function of the esophagus is merely that of a connective tube. The stomach, the next organ, serves a dual purpose: (1) that of a reservoir that holds food until the digestive process continues and (2) a phase of digestion itself. Next is the small intestine. This is subdivided into three areas—the duodenum, the jejunum, and the ileum—and is the longest part of the digestive tract, being approximately 12 to 15 feet in length. Secretions from the pancreas and the gall bladder are emptied into the duodenum, the upper portion of the small intestine. The major and final stages of the digestion of foods take place in the small intestine. The large intestine, which follows the ileum, serves as a reservoir. Residues from the digestive process are collected and stored before evacuation.

The nutrients are absorbed, for the most part, through the villi of the small intestine. After absorption, they are circulated either by the blood alone, or, as in the case of fats, by the lymph and then the blood. Utilization is

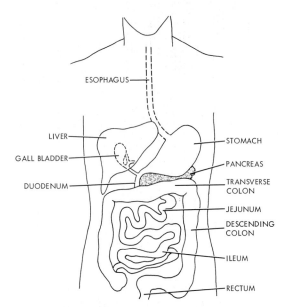

FIGURE 8–1. *Diagram of the gastrointestinal tract and those organs and glands concerned with digestion.*

facilitated by additional changes or reactions with other substances. These may take place at many sites: the individual cell, the liver, or the kidney. Some nutrients may be stored for future use. Others, if they are not needed and there is no provision for storage, are excreted.

Throughout all processes, the roles of respiration and of water metabolism play an important part. Electrolytes, secretions of hormones, and the complex enzyme systems with their component vitamin relationships are necessary for the effective preparation and ultimate utilization of nutrients.

Ingestion

Besides the cultural, economical, and emotional factors that determine the kind and amount of food that the individual eats, hunger and appetite play a dominant role. Though often referred to interchangeably, they have entirely different meanings, and, significantly, there is no agreement on an acceptable definition of either.

Hunger is an intrinsic desire for food that is accompanied with objective sensations.[4] Hunger has been described as a series of intermittent contractions of the stomach, or

at least a sensation of pressure and tension in this region. These hunger pangs are not continuous in an empty stomach. A hungry baby often cries loudly as if the hunger contractions were painful. The sensation of hunger may be inhibited by smoking or drinking cold water, or by strong emotions like anger. On the other hand, outdoor exercise and physical activity seem to increase hunger. Once an individual has begun eating a meal, the hunger sensation subsides. Thus hunger alone cannot determine the total food intake, although it probably exerts a great influence on one's desire to eat.

Appetite was defined by Newburgh[5] as "a sensation produced by happy memories." Appetite, as a desire to eat, is thus strongly governed by psychological factors like happy memories of previous experiences with certain foods. The smell and taste of these foods are reminders of those pleasant sensations. Often an individual will continue eating a meal or enjoy a dessert long after his hunger has been satisfied. Some believe that an appetite for a food may be acquired.

Recent experiments with laboratory animals and further observations in man have confirmed the belief held by many that there is an

---

[4] Arthur C. Guyton, *Textbook of Medical Physiology*, Saunders, Philadelphia, 1970, p. 1005.

[5] L. H. Newburgh, "Obesity," *Archives of Internal Medicine*, Vol. 70, No. 6 (December 1942), pp. 1033–1096.

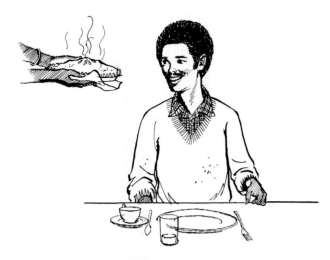

FIGURE 8–2. *Frequently an individual will have an appetite for dessert even though his hunger has been appeased by a hearty dinner.*

automatic regulating mechanism that determines the urge to eat. This mechanism is located in the hypothalamus. Reports have suggested that two distinct centers are involved, one governing appetite (the urge to eat) and a second one inhibiting the appetite center and determining the satiety level. The exact role of this hypothalamic regulation in relation to our total food intake remains to be seen.

Reports in the literature indicate the complexities of trying to define both hunger and appetite in a clear-cut fashion. Hoelzel[6] spoke of the many discussions that he and Carlson had had during their 40 years' association concerning hunger and its relationship to appetite. He stated that Carlson did not seem to consider hunger to be a simple gastric pain; rather, it was Hoelzel's impression, he regarded the essential element in hunger to be a keen desire, urge, or impulse to eat. This suggests that Carlson, who has been largely responsible for the consideration of hunger as a physiological reaction, also thought there were emotional influences.

Richter's[7] introductory remarks at a symposium on hunger and appetite enumerated three different points of view regarding the attention that should be paid to the sensation of hunger and appetite in feeding animals and man. Opinions were so divergent as to include those who considered that man could depend on his sensations to choose an adequate diet to those who believe that diets must be prescribed and not left to choice alone. Thus a statement of one of the speakers[8] at the symposium might serve as a summary: "The view that the quantity of food consumed measures a unitary 'appetite' must be abandoned for the reason that intake does not depend upon a single factor."

It is often believed that hunger and appetite if given free range will be a reliable guide to the correct foods to eat. This has been shown to be true under certain specific conditions.

Davis,[9] in describing her experiments in self-selection, reported that when a variety of simple nourishing foods—all the desirable foods that should be included in a child's diet—was presented for choice, children over a period of time chose foods that provided a good nutritional diet. At some meals it was

[6] Frederick Hoelzel, "Dr A. J. Carlson and the Concept of Hunger," *American Journal of Clinical Nutrition*, Vol. 5, No. 6 (March–April 1957), pp. 659–662.

[7] Curt P. Richter, "Hunger and Appetite," *American Journal of Clinical Nutrition*, Vol. 5, No. 6 (March–April 1957), pp. 141–153.

[8] Paul Thomas Young "Psychological Factors Regulating the Feeding Process," *American Journal of Clinical Nutrition*, Vol. 5 No. 6 (March–April 1957), pp. 154–161.

[9] C. M. Davis, "Self-selection of Diet by Newly Weaned Infants," *American Journal of Diseases of Children*, Vol. 36, No. 4 (October 1928), pp. 651–679.

found that the combinations were rather odd; children exhibited "food jags" and wanted varying amounts of food at different times. However, over a long span their diet proved to be nutritionally adequate. It must be noted that only simple nourishing foods were offered. The child did not have to make a choice between vegetables and potato chips, for example.

Furthermore, other studies have shown that an individual chooses not necessarily what is good but what he likes best.When popular, less-nourishing, and foods of low nutrient density are offered in competition with the "good foods," the nutritious foods are frequently slighted. So there is no basis for the generally accepted belief that a child, or an adult for that matter, "needs" the food that he chooses. Thus he cannot depend on hunger and appetite alone to guide him in the proper selection of nutrients necessary for health.

Digestion

Digestion is essentially a hydrolytic process; that is, insoluble foods are "broken down" into smaller particles suitable for absorption by the addition of water and the action of enzymes. An enzyme has protein in its makeup and may have minerals or vitamins in addition. Enzymes act as catalysts. When mixed with foods, they cause chemical changes without entering into the reaction themselves. Enzymes are specific; that is, each one acts upon a certain segment of food and it can act only under certain conditions. Digestive enzymes exist in an inactive state, and several factors influence secretion when needed. The sight and smell of food, or hormonal or other chemical influence, will stimulate secretion of enzymes.

Several important factors involved in digestion are interdependent. One is mechanical action. The most obvious example is the chewing of food. Another example is the contractions, the peristaltic waves and other motions, of the gastrointestinal tract. The mechanical influence on digestion is also illustrated by the stimulation of the secretion of enzymes by the mass of food, or *bolus* as it is known, as it is propelled along.

A second factor in digestion is the chemical influence. This may be illustrated in several ways. The activity of enzymes and other secretions may be considered as chemical reactions. Certain foods, like gravy, meat extracts, or spices, are chemical stimulants. The pH (the extent of acidity or alkalinity) of the digestive medium either inhibits or enhances the rate of digestion.

The term pH is an expression of the chemical characteristics of a solution; hence it is an important concept in appreciating why certain reactions take place. The pH of a solution is usually expressed numerically, with the neutral point at 7, the pH of water. If a solution is acid, then its numerical value is less than 7; the lower the number, the greater the concentration of acidity. If a solution is above 7, then it is alkaline (basic); the higher the number, the greater the degree of alkalinity. The pH of the body fluids varies, yet each fluctu-

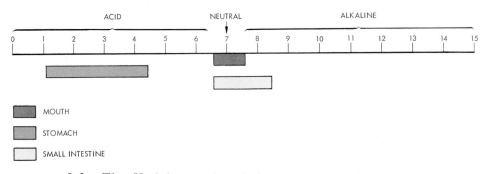

FIGURE 8–3. *The pH of the gastrointestinal tract varies according to the site and secretions as food is digested. There is a range of pH in each segment as the food is passed along.*

ates within very narrow limits. The pH of the solutions along the gastrointestinal tract are quite different.

The third factor in digestion is the regulatory influence of hormones and inorganic materials. Each of these exerts a specific influence upon certain phases of the breakdown of foods.

Digestion in the Mouth

Digestion starts in the mouth. Here two major reactions take place. By mastication, or chewing, food is broken down into small particles, thus making it more available to digestive enzymes. It is also well moistened with saliva, the digestive secretion of the mouth.

Saliva contains one principal enzyme, ptyalin. Ptyalin acts upon the starches, if they have been properly cooked, and begins to change them to maltose. Cooking does not "predigest" starch. However, it does make it more available to digestive enzymes by rupturing the starch granules. The pH of the mouth varies from 6.4 to 7.3, but ptyalin is able to react over a range of pH 4 to 9. The secretion of saliva is regulated by psychological factors. The taste, sight, odor, or even the thought of food, especially if one is hungry, can result in "mouth-watering." As much as 1000 to 1500 cc.—1 to 1½ quarts—of saliva, may be secreted in 24 hours. Saliva might also contain traces of an enzyme, maltase, which may convert some maltose to glucose.

Food remains in the mouth for a short time, and is pushed along by swallowing. The time spent in passage through the esophagus is approximately 5 seconds, the food being moved along as a result of wavelike motions known as *peristalsis*. A contracted band called the *cardiac sphincter* at the entrance to the stomach is released by the oncoming wave so food can pass into the stomach.

Digestion in the Stomach

The stomach is an elastic organ that can adjust its size to the volume of food eaten. Consequently, it serves more as a reservoir than as a digestive organ of food. This reservoir is primarily in the fundus, the large, rounded main portion of the stomach. The food entering the stomach first spreads out along its edge, subsequent amounts of food enter and are pressed out against the first mass, and the last food to enter then remains toward the center.

The action of saliva, which was begun in the mouth, continues in the stomach until the gastric juice, which is acid, permeates the food and stops the action of ptyalin. Saliva is not far from neutral in reaction, and its activity is inhibited by either highly acidic or basic conditions. This "carry-over" digestion may last for 30 minutes or more.

The secretion of gastric juices is stimulated by the hormone gastrin, which is secreted in the pyloric region of the stomach (the end nearest the small intestine) and then absorbed into the bloodstream and carried to the cells that secrete the gastric juices. When the factors that stimulate gastrin are no longer present, it ceases to be produced. When this action is depressed, the secreting cells will then have periods of rest.

The secretion of gastrin is stimulated in three ways: psychologically, mechanically, and chemically. The smell and taste of food, or even seeing or thinking about it, will stimulate secretion of the hormone gastrin. Conversely, such emotions as anger, excitement, fear, or unpleasant sights and odors may inhibit its secretion. The extension of the stomach musculature serves as a mechanical stimulant. The chemical stimulation may be meat extracts, broth, and seasonings of foods. As each of these stimuli diminishes, its effect upon gastrin secretion also diminishes.

Digestion begins in the outer layers of the stored food. The mechanical actions of the stomach, gastric contractions, gradually mix the food so that the gastric guices are worked in toward the food mass. A second type of muscular contraction, peristaltic waves, carries the food in wavelike motions to the pyloric end of the stomach. This pyloric section is connected to the small intestine by the plyoric sphincter.

The gastric juice contains several components: hydrochloric acid, mucin, water, and two enzymes. The secretion of hydrochloric acid causes the pH of the stomach to be highly acidic, thus providing the necessary medium for enzyme action. The pH of the gastric juice ranges from 1 to 4.

Pepsin, which digests protein, is the most important enzyme of the gastric juice. It acts upon proteins and reduces them to proteoses and peptones. Protein digestion is then completed in the small intestine. Pepsin requires an acid medium, an optimum pH of 1.5, which is brought about by the secretion of hydrochloric acid.

Another enzyme, gastric lipase, acts on fats. The value and extent of this enzyme are questionable. The gastric lipase may be able to split some fats into fatty acids and glycerol. However, if effective at all, it appears to be most active against emulsified fats such as milk, cream, and egg yolk. The optimum pH for its activity is approximately 7.8, and usually the pH of the stomach is far below this value. However, it may be important when the gastric juice is near neutral.

The gastric mucin serves as a lubricant to help the food mass move through the gastrointestinal tract. It may also protect the lining of the gastrointestinal tract against the acid digestive juice.

Generally food remains in the stomach from 3 to 5 hours; however, it may be there as little as 1 hour or as long as 7. The length of time depends primarily upon the kinds of foods eaten, psychological factors, or individual variation in gastric motility. Carbohydrates such as a sweet roll and orange juice leave the stomach rapidly. A meal that is high in protein leaves more quickly than a meal that is high in fat. Foods that are a combination of protein and fat remain in the stomach longest. This is why an individual is satisfied after a meal of protein and fat foods. They have satiety value. Large quantities of food can depress the flow of gastric juice and thereby slow the emptying time.

As a rule, foods are not absorbed from the stomach. Exceptions may be alcohol and, in some instances, small amounts of sugar. Since protein, fat, and carbohydrate digestion takes place primarily in the small intestine, these nutrients are not ready for absorption at this time. Waste passes through the stomach and is absorbed from the small intestine.

An important function of the highly acid gastric juice, apart from its role in preparing foods for eventual absorption, is its protective action. The gastric juice may either destroy or inhibit the activity of microorganisms that are part of a normal food intake. This reaction is the body's first defense against food-borne infection.

Digestion in the Small Intestine

As the highly acid *chyme* (liquefied mass of food) passes through the pyloric sphincter into the small intestine, a number of reactions take place. Most digestion occurs in the upper portion of the small intestine. Here there is an important interaction with hormonal, chemical, and mechanical factors. Pancreatic juice, bile, and intestinal juice are secreted almost simultaneously about 3 to 4 inches below the pyloric sphincter.

The pancreatic juice is believed to contain five enzymes: three that act upon protein substances, one that acts upon starches, and one that digests fats. One of the first group is trypsin, which splits proteins into polypeptides. Its secretion is activated by secretin, a component of the intestinal juice. A second enzyme is chymotrypsin, which is activated by trypsin. It brings about further breakdown of the protein products, for it attacks only specific linkages in a peptide chain. Carboxypolypeptidase, which is the third enzyme, influences peptides that contain a free carboxyl group. This results in free amino acid groups being split off. The fourth enzyme, amylase, is sometimes known as amylopsin. It is similar in action to ptyalin of saliva, since it is capable of splitting starch to maltose. The fifth enzyme, lipase, or steapsin as it is sometimes called, breaks down the emulsized fats into fatty acids and glycerol.

The intestinal juice contains seven enzymes in addition to secretin, which serves as an activator for trypsin of the pancreatic juice, and enterocrinin, which stimulates intestinal glands. The pH of the intestinal tract at this point is approximately 8.3. Two of these seven intestinal enzymes are for protein digestion, one for fat, and four for carbohydrate.

The first enzyme, aminopolypeptidase, specifically attacks the peptide next to a terminal amino acid with a free amino group, thereby splitting off a single amino acid from the chain. This complements the carboxypoly-peptidase of the pancreatic juice. The second enzyme, which is also concerned with protein digestion, is dipeptidase, which hydrolizes polypeptides into amino acids. The third enzyme, lipase, has the same effect as pancreatic lipase on fats, but it is of little importance.

The four enzymes concerned with carbohydrate digestion are amylase, sucrase, lactase, and maltase. Amylase acts upon starches, changing them to maltose. Sucrase acts upon sucrose, liberating one molecule of glucose and one molecule of fructose. Lactase acts upon lactose, yielding one molecule of glucose and one molecule of galactose. And maltase attacks maltose with the result of two molecules of glucose.

Bile is prepared by the liver, and concentrated and stored by the gall bladder. Technically it is not a digestive enzyme; however, it is extremely important to the digestion and absorption of fats. Approximately 1 pint of bile and its components, such as bile salts, pigments, lecithin, and cholesterol, is secreted each day.

The primary function of the bile salts is to facilitate the emulsification of fats, thereby rendering them more accessible to digestive enzymes. Other functions are to bring about a solution that will hold the fatty acids so they can be easily absorbed. Bile salts also aid in the absorption of fat-soluble vitamins and carotene.

Three types of mechanical action of digestion take place in the small intestine. One is the peristaltic actions, which are wavelike motions propelling food throughout the length of the gastrointestinal tract. However, there is an antiperistaltic wave that pushes back, at given intervals, some of the food mass, which is then carried forward again by the peristaltic wave. The third type of motion is a rhythmical movement of local constrictions that further mixes the food. All factors—the mechanical action, the chemical activity (enzymes), and the hormonal control—are interdependent and all are necessary for proper digestion.

Thus, in summary, protein digestion commences in the stomach and is completed in the small intestine where it is acted upon by enzymes from both the pancreatic juice and intestinal juice. Carbohydrate digestion begins in the mouth and is completed in the small intestine with enzymes from the pancreas and the small intestine. Fat digestion occurs in the small intestine, by action from a pancreatic enzyme aided by bile secreted by the gall bladder.

The end products of digestion of foods are amino acids, glucose, fructose, galactose, fatty acids, and glycerol. Table 8–1 illustrates the digestive process.

The term *digestibility* merits attention since so many meanings are associated with it. Table 8–2 shows the digestibility of foods by man when consumed in mixed diets. A distinction must be made between the ease of digestion and the length of time for food to digest. Approximately 95 per cent of all edible foodstuffs are digested and absorbed. Overeating may give a sense of "fullness." Sugars, for example, are rather quickly absorbed, whereas fats remain in the digestive tract for many hours, yet in a healthy person they are handled very efficiently. Complex proteins and carbohydrates are digested at a different pace, usually between the time necessary for sugars and fats.

Foods that ferment or cause gas, such as legumes, often result in discomfort. Inadequate mastication of food may cause disturbance because the digestive tract has difficulty in handling large pieces of food. Foods such as nuts must be masticated well so that digestive juices can penetrate.

The Large Intestine

One of the primary functions of the large intestine is to absorb water from the residual matter and to form the feces. Neither digestive action nor absorption of nutrients takes place. The mechanical motions are slower and may be described as sluggish.

The fecal matter contains numerous products. One portion is the unabsorbed food residue containing indigestible fiber, primarily cellulose that comes from fruits and vegetables. This fiber is an important part of the diet since it is necessary to maintain healthy muscle tone of the large intestine. Approxi-

TABLE 8–1

A Summary of Digestion

SITE	ENZYME	REACTION	ADDITIONAL COMMENTS
Mouth	Ptyalin (in saliva)	Starch ⟶ soluble starch ⟶ dextrin	Breakdown of food into small particles through process of mastication. Mucin in saliva lubricates foods. pH ranges from 6.4 to 7.3.
Stomach	Pepsin (in gastric juice)	Proteins ⟶ proteoses + peptones ⟶ polypeptides	Gastrin stimulates secretion of gastric juice. Salivary digestion continues until food mass is acidified. Hydrochloric acid (HCl) provides favorable pH for pepsin; swells proteins. pH ranges from 1.5 to 4. Fats depress gastric secretion. No general agreement that gastric lipase is secreted. Mechanical mixing of juices with food by means of muscular contraction.
	Rennin (abundant in babies)	Casein ⟶ paracasein	
Small intestine	*In pancreatic juice*		Secretin from pancreatic juice activates trypsin.
	(1) Trypsin	Proteoses ⟶ peptones ⟶ polypeptides	Chymotrypsin is activated by trypsin.
	(2) Chymotrypsin	Catalyzes hydrolysis of (breakdown of) polypeptides ⟶ amino acids	Mechanical mixing by means of rhythmic contractions, peristalsis and antiperistalsis.
	(3) Carboxypolypeptidase	Splits off amino acid from peptide end having free carboxyl	pH ranges from 8 to 9. No general agreement that pancreatic lactase and sucrase are secreted.
	(4) Lipase (steapsin)	Fats ⟶ fatty acids + glycerol	Bile salts activate pancreatic lipase.
	(5) Amylopsin (amylase)	Starch ⟶ soluble starches ⟶ dextrins ⟶ maltose	
	In intestinal juice		
	(1) Peptidases	Polypeptides ⟶ amino acids	Intestinal secretion stimulated by enterocrinin.
	(2) Amylase (Small amount)	Starches ⟶ dextrins ⟶ maltose	
	(3) Maltase	Maltose ⟶ glucose + glucose	
	(4) Sucrase	Sucrose ⟶ glucose + fructose	
	(5) Lactase	Lactose ⟶ glucose + galactose	
	(6) Lipase	Fats ⟶ fatty acids + glycerol	
	Gall bladder bile	Accelerates actions of pancreatic lipase	Gall bladder secretion stimulated by cholecystokinin. Neutralizes acid chyme.
	Bile salts	Lower surface tension and therefor aid in emulsification of fats.	Bile salts aid in absorption of fatty acids and fat-soluble vitamins.

Note: Digestive enzymes are not present in the large intestine.

TABLE 8–2

Average Percentage of Digestibility of Foods by Man When Consumed in Mixed Diets

FOODS	PROTEIN	FAT	CARBOHYDRATE[a]
Animal foods	97	95	98
Cereals and breads	85	90	98
Dried legumes (beans, etc.)	78	90	97
Vegetables	83	90	95
Fruits	85	90	90
Total food of average diet	92	95	98

SOURCE: Ralph W. Gerard (ed.), *Food for Life*, University of Chicago Press, Chicago, 1952, p. 99.

[a] Excepting fibrous carbohydrates.

mately one third of the feces is composed of bacteria, which originate in the large intestine itself. The remainder of the feces consists of intestinal secretion, some epithelial cells, and products of bacterial decomposition.

Eighteen to 24 hours may elapse from the time food is ingested until the final elimination of the indigestible or unabsorbed residue takes place. Reports of a longer period than this have been considered to be within a normal range of time. Bacterial action within the large intestine performs several important functions. It may reduce materials that were resistant to the process of digestion.

In addition, the intestinal flora are a factor in the digestive process. In infants, until a more solid diet is introduced, *Lactobacillus bifidus* predominates in the intestine of the breastfed infant and *L. acidophilus* in infants who are fed cow's milk. The bulk of the organisms found among the intestinal flora belong to the genera *Streptococcus*, *Lactobacillus*, and *Diplococcus*, according to Burton.[10]

When the diet is predominately carbohydrate, gram-positive fermentative organisms are encouraged. With a high protein intake, gram-negative putrefactive flora increase.

It is conjectured that the microbial population of the large intestine and cecum are more important than formerly assumed. When the intestinal flora of experimental animals has been significantly altered or inhibited, defi-

ciency syndromes appear. It seems that certain nutritional factors are synthesized here. Evidence points to the possibility of vitamin K, vitamin B12 thiamin, biotin, folic acid, and perhaps niacin being developed in the large intestine.

Absorption

Most of the absorption of nutrients takes place in the small intestine, by active transport and diffusion, particularly in the lower part of duodendum and the upper part of the jejunum; the stomach is considered a poor absorptive area of the gastrointestinal tract.[11] There is diffusion, however, of water and electrolytes in both directions. As the end products of digestion are liberated, they are absorbed, so that too great a concentration at any one place is avoided.

The lining of the small intestine consists of literally millions of villi, tiny finger-like projections similar to the nap on velvet that are highly specialized for this function. The villi increase the surface area for absorption to approximately 11 square yards. The epithelial cells of the villi are characterized by a brush border that increases the absorptive surface even more. Near the brush border area of these cells are mitochrondria that supply the cell with oxidative energy for the transportation of nutrients through or between the epithelial cells.

---

[10] Benjamin T. Burton, *The Heinz Handbook of Nutrition*, McGraw-Hill, New York, 1965.

[11] Guyton, op. cit., pp. 909–916.

Monosaccharides, monoglycerides, and amino acids are absorbed selectively and diffused into the blood of the capillaries of the cells and then into the portal vein. Short-chain fatty acids are absorbed from the endoplasmic membrane rather than the brush border of the epithelial cells. Some are absorbed directly into the portal vein, whereas longer-chain fatty acids are absorbed into the lymphatics. Calcium, sodium, perhaps some chloride, iron, hydrogen, magnesium, and phosphate ions are absorbed through the small intestinal mucosa. Vitamin D is required for calcium absorption. Vitamins C and E favor the absorption of iron.

Utilization

After absorption, the nutrients enter into a phase called *intermediary metabolism* in which they lose their identity as far as their food origin is concerned. Prior to this stage, it is convenient to speak of *protein metabolism, carbohydrate metabolism,* and *fat metabolism.* But a wide range of eventual pathways are available to all nutrients, and the needs of the body tissue at the time can determine how these nutrients will be utilized. For example, amino acids, glucose, and fatty acids can all contribute to the body's need for energy. Or segments of any of these molecules may be withdrawn from the metabolic pool and used to synthesize nonessential amino acids, glycogen, nonessential fatty acids, or compounds such as enzymes and hormones. In these reactions, various members of the B complex vitamins are important factors in the complex enzyme system that accompanies them. These functions are described in Chapter 13.

When amino acids are absorbed, they are circulated in the blood for a short time. An amino acid that is required by a particular cell will be selected. This need may be for synthesis of new tissue, for either maintenance or repair of body proteins, or for the manufacture of hormones or enzymes. The liver itself has a great demand for amino acids because it controls most of the human plasma proteins.

If amino acids are in excess of the immediate need, they enter into a catabolic, or break-down, process. This is believed to take place primarily in the liver. The amino group containing the nitrogen is detached from the nonnitrogenous fraction of the amino acid. This process is known as *deamination.* The nonnitrogenous fraction that contains the carbon–hydrogen–oxygen fraction then may enter a subsequent number of possible reactions. It may serve as a source of fuel, being converted into glucose. It may be stored as body fat by becoming adipose tissue or it may participate in the nonnitrogenous part of the synthesized nonessential amino acids.

The amino group may be utilized in the formation of nonessential amino acids. The synthesis is called *transamination.* Or, if it is not used in this way, it is eventually excreted by the kidney as a constituent of urine.

The glucose level of the circulating blood provides a continuous supply of energy to the tissues of the body. This level fluctuates within a given range, reflecting the immediate results of digestion and absorption of carbohydrate foods. For example, the blood glucose level rises considerably after a meal rich in carbohydrates, whereas it is low upon arising, when the long fast through the night has depleted the body''s glucose reserves. The monosaccharides galactose and fructose are believed to be converted to glucose by the liver following their absorption.

The glucose content of the blood that is in excess of the immediate needs is then converted to glycogen, the temporary fuel reserve. This conversion occurs primarily in the liver; however, the skeletal, cardiac, and smooth muscles can also synthesize glycogen and maintain their own stores. This conversion is thought to be a phosphorylation process (combination with phosphoric acid). Glycogen reserves are depleted during continuous or violent exercise. Glucose in excess of that needed for glycogen will be changed to adipose tissue, which serves as a more concentrated fuel reserve.

Still another function in which excess glucose might participate is the synthesis of nonessential amino acids. This would be the process of transamination in which the amino group would be supplied from another amino acid and the glucose participation would be

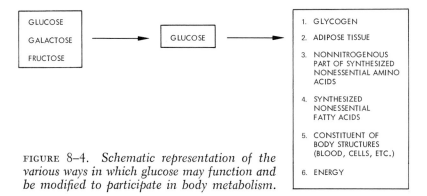

FIGURE 8–4. *Schematic representation of the various ways in which glucose may function and be modified to participate in body metabolism.*

limited to the carbon–oxygen–hydrogen fraction. Closely allied to this is the possible formulation of nonessential fatty acids. Thus, even though the primary function of glucose is to provide fuel, it may enter into other important reactions.

The two end products of fat digestion, fatty acids and glycerol, proceed along separate ways in metabolism. Glycerol follows a path similar to that of glucose. It is phosphorylated in the liver and converted into glucose. From this point on, its metabolism is merged with that of glucose itself.

In a manner similar to the immediate utilization of amino acids, the fatty acids may be picked up by the cells from the circulating blood and built into the structure of the cell if needed. But if this does not occur, fatty acid metabolism, which takes place primarily in the liver, will follow a considerably different pathway from that of other nutrients. First it is converted into phospholipids. This conversion must take place in the presence of choline (a member of the B complex) or methionine (one of the essential amino acids). These are known as lipotropic factors, for they promote the transport and utilization of fats. Fatty acids are oxidized in both liver

and muscle tissue with the release of energy accompanying this reaction. The oxidation of fatty acids refers to the breakdown of a long carbon chain into a shorter carbon chain. For example, an eighteen-carbon chain may be broken down to a four-carbon one.

There are several theories about the process of oxidation, but the essential point is that this does not take place all at once, but is rather a step-by-step reaction. Oxidation in the liver ends with the four-carbon chain fatty acid. These fatty acids, or ketone bodies, are then carried in the bloodstream to other tissues and further oxidized to supply energy. It is at this point that the oxidation of fatty acids becomes interrelated with that of glucose.

Fatty acids that are not needed, as well as glucose and amino acids that represent excess calories, are then converted into adipose tissue. This synthesis may take place in the liver, in the mammary gland, or in adipose tissue itself. If necessary, the fatty acid molecule may become part of a nonessential amino acid. The theory of formation of glucose from fatty acids is accepted by some and questioned by others.

Thus it is clear that there is no single role

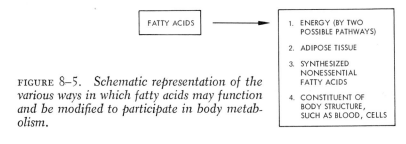

FIGURE 8–5. *Schematic representation of the various ways in which fatty acids may function and be modified to participate in body metabolism.*

for glucose, amino acids, or fatty acids once they have been absorbed. The utilization of these nutrients is complex, consisting of many interwoven reactions. None of these reactions takes place simply or singly; most seem to require a complicated enzyme system, plus vitamin and mineral catalysts. Consequently, it is especially true that the total diet must be considered when speaking of the metabolism and utilization of nutrients. No single food can begin to meet our bodies' needs; rather, they all seem to work together, yet depend upon one another for effective utilization of nutrients.

It is evident that the reduction of food for absorption and its consequent utilization is a step-by-step, interrelated, complex reaction. There are many gaps in the understanding of this process and much remains to be learned about the interrelationships of vitamins and minerals and their role in digestion and metabolism. The very important role of an individual's emotional health needs to be investigated further. What we do know about the roles of these many factors indicates that this is a fascinating, never-ending, changing part of the study of nutrition.

SELECTED REFERENCES

Beck, I. T., "The Role of Pancreatic Enzymes in Digestion," *American Journal of Clinical Nutrition*, Vol. 26, No. 3 (March 1973), pp. 311–325.

Guyton, Arthur C., *Textbook of Medical Physiology*, W. B. Saunders Company, Philadelphia, 1970, Chapters 60, 61, and 62.

Ingelfinger, Franz J., "Gastric Function," *Nutrition Today*, Vol. 6, No. 5 (September–October 1971), pp. 2–10.

———, "The Esophagus," *Nutrition Today*, Vol. 8, No. 1 (January–February 1973), pp. 3–8.

Lamanna, Carl, "Needs for Illuminating the Microbiology of the Lumen," *American Journal of Clinical Nutrition*, Vol. 25, No. 12 (December 1972), pp. 1488–1494.

Robinson, Corrine H., *Fundamentals of Normal Nutrition*, Macmillan Publishing Co., Inc., New York, 1973, Chapter 2.

9

Energy Metabolism

The word *energy* has many connotations. To some energy implies vitality; to others the specter of the energy crisis around the world spells an unpleasant way of life. The biologist classifies energy as solar, chemical, mechanical, or electrical. All energy comes from the sun, but animals cannot use this source directly. They rely on plants to convert water, carbon dioxide, and nitrogen and sulfur compounds with the aid of solar energy through a process called *photosynthesis* into carbohydrates, fats, and proteins—all sources of energy to man. Food, thus, becomes the source of the energy required for work and the many functions of the human body. Energy, for example, is needed for forming new cells, muscular activity, breathing, and all the countless vital life processes.

The availability of energy foods has a direct bearing on health. When foods for energy are readily procured there may be a surplus of kcalories and obesity may be a problem. When there is a lack of kcalories, the work capacity of individuals is impaired, and in children growth may be retarded or even cease in dire circumstances. Many peoples of the world do not have adequate kcalories. Energy needs must have high priority if optimal nutrition is to be attained.

Labor-saving devices, sophisticated means of transportation, inactive forms of leisure-time activities, higher standards of living, and other influences have led to decreased physical activity among adults and children in most industrialized countries, according to Montoye.[1] Although a relationship between physical activity and sedentary living has not been conclusively established, there is substantial evidence of an indirect nature to support the hypothesis that routine exercise has an essential role in preventive medicine, particularly for coronary heart disease.[2]

Historical

The history of nutrition in the United States begins with studies in energy metabolism. W. O. Atwater[3] conducted fundamental

---

[1] Henry J. Montoye, "Estimation of Habitual Physical Activity by Questionnaire and Interview," *American Journal of Clinical Nutrition*, Vol. 24, No. 9 (September 1971), p. 1113.

[2] Jack H. Wilmore and William L. Haskell, "Use of the Heart Rate–Energy Expenditure Relationship in the Individual Prescription of Exercise," *American Journal of Clinical Nutrition*, Vol. 24, No. 9 (September 1971), p. 1186.

[3] Henry C. Sherman, *Nutritional Improvement of Life*, Columbia University Press, New York, 1950, p. 10.

research that is basic to our knowledge and work today when he was at Wesleyan University in Middletown, Connecticut. Later, when the first Agricultural Experiment Station in the United States was established in Connecticut (1887), he was appointed its director.

However, the study about man's need for energy, the identification of kcalories, and, even more basic, how the individual utilizes food began many years before Atwater's work in the United States. Lavoisier,[4] a French chemist, is credited with making the first discovery that subsequently led to a study of energy metabolism, and he provided many new concepts about body needs. Among his investigations were studies of the consumption of oxygen and the output of carbon dioxide and of the factors that influenced these reactions. He also noted that oxygen consumption and carbon dioxide production were increased by body activity. Another basic discovery was the increase in heat production during the digestion of a meal. He also devised a calorimeter, a device whereby the amount of heat given off by an animal or a human being may be measured. It is fascinating to read of Lavoisier's studies, for they are masterpieces in scientific investigation. When one realizes the complete lack of information about the metabolism of either the human or the animal at this time, the importance of his contribution to modern science can be recognized.

Many others added to the knowledge of energy expenditure. Among them were von Liebig, Voit, Boussingault, Pettenkofer, Regnault, and Reiset. France, and later Germany, and then the United States, were centers for learning.

One of the greatest advances came in 1892 when Rubner,[5] the German physiologist, developed an accurate calorimeter, the forerunner of our calorimeters today. In this chamber it was possible to measure simultaneously the heat production, oxygen intake, and carbon dioxide output of the subject. Then when food intake was recorded and its energy value determined, and later when urine and feces were collected and their energy value measured, the complete balance procedure was established. As a result of developing this technique, Rubner demonstrated that the law of conservation of energy existed in animals and man as well as in other matter.[6] Briefly stated this law is: "energy is neither created nor destroyed, it is changed from one form to another in the animal body, it is neither lost nor gained." Rubner demonstrated that the energy liberated as heat or for activity was "the energy value of the food intake of the individual."

At the turn of the century Atwater, along with Benedict, began measuring the energy production of human beings in the United States. They devised a large calorimeter so that the subject could be studied for as long as 2 weeks. These studies were carefully controlled. The individual lived in the calorimeter chamber, which contained equipment for muscular activity and furniture for sleeping and eating. Arrangements were made whereby his food was placed in the chamber and the excreta removed without disturbing the measurement of oxygen consumption and carbon dioxide and water output. These experiments were so carefully conducted that, even though they were carried out over 60 years ago, the results are valid today.

From Atwater and Benedict's studies, research has progressed in the United States. Others who have contributed to our knowledge about energy metabolism are Sherman, Mitchell, McCollum, Armsby, Maynard, DuBois, Swift, and Mary Swartz Rose. Research conducted by these investigators uncovered fundamental facts currently used in professional application of energy metabolism.

Energy Measurement

Kcalories in food are a measure of the amount of energy supplied to the individual by his diet. The energy requirement of an in-

[4] E. V. McCollum, A *History of Nutrition*, Houghton Mifflin, Boston, 1957, p. 115.

[5] Raymond W. Swift and Cyrus E. French, *Energy Metabolism and Nutrition*, Scarecrow Press, New Brunswick, N.J., 1954, Part 1, p. 11.

[6] McCollum, op. cit.

dividual, also expressed in kcalories, refers to the amount of energy he needs to live and to work. In human nutrition, a kilocalorie (kcalorie is defined as the amount of heat necessary to raise 1 kg (2.2 pounds) of water 1 degree Centigrade (or 4 pounds of water 1 degree Fahrenheit). The oxidation of foods within the body results in the liberation of heat.

In an effort to standardize measurement units, some discussion has been given to the use of the kilojoule (kJ) in preference to the kcalorie. The kilojoule as a measure for both mechanical heat and energy has some advantages.[7] Nutritionists have not met this suggestion with enthusiasm. All the present food composition tables would have to be revised, considerable confusion might result, and the kilojoule seems to be less appropriate for nutrition problems of everyday life. In situations where it is important to use kilojoules, the kcalorie may be defined as a unit of food rather than of heat, and kilojoules may be determined by the following formula: kcalories × 4.2 = kilojoules.

There are two methods of determining the total energy expenditure of an individual as measured by a calorimeter. When only the heat that is dissipated is measured, the technique is known as *direct calorimetry*. Although there are a few variations in construction methods that alter the procedure somewhat, the basic principle remains the same. The heat the subject gives off is removed by a stream of cold water flowing through copper tubing. The heat eliminated by evaporation of water from the lungs is calculated and the temperature of the water entering and leaving the calorimeter is recorded at frequent intervals. Air or oxygen is usually supplied under carefully controlled conditions so that water determinations may be made when leaving the chamber. Thus the total energy expended is reflected in the amount of heat given off.

In contrast, the method of determining energy expenditure known as *indirect calorim-*

etry is more practical and lends itself to a greater flexibility in devising experiments. In this indirect method, three things are determined: the volume of oxygen consumed, the volume of carbon dioxide exhaled, and the urinary nitrogen. From these data, the amount of carbohydrate, fat, and protein that was utilized to provide energy for a given task can be determined.

Much of our data concerning the number of kcalories needed to perform certain tasks have been determined by variations on this principle. Needless to say, the same experiment has been conducted using both the direct and indirect methods of calorimetry, and the results have been comparable.

Components of Energy Expenditure

The human body requires sufficient energy from food for basal metabolism or, for practical purposes, resting metabolism; for the synthesis of body tissues as occurs in growth and maintenance; for physical activity; heat regulation; excretory processes; special needs during pregnancy and lactation; and for physiological and psychological stress. The specific dynamic action of food is included in the need for resting metabolism.

Basal Metabolism

Basal metabolism is the energy metabolism of the body at complete rest, in a comfortable position and comfortably warm and relaxed, both mentally and physically. The patient must also be in a postabsorptive state; that is, the last meal must have been eaten 12 to 18 hours previously. Since voluntary activity can be eliminated and since such activity is extremely variable, metabolism is generally measured under basal conditions.

Basal metabolism as measured is not, however, the lowest level of heat production. Sleep can produce a further lowering of from 10 to 13 per cent in the rate. The determination upon a sleeping individual is not practical, and, therefore, the minimum heat production under previously described conditions is considered basal.

The number of kcalories expended in basal metabolism represents the energy required to

[7] Thomas Moore, "The Calorie Versus the Joule," *Journal of the American Dietetic Association*, Vol. 59, No. 4 (October 1971), pp. 327–330.

perform normal body functions apart from any voluntary activity. This includes such activity as respiration, circulation, tissue maintenance, cellular metabolism, glandular activity, maintenance of muscle tonus, regulation of body temperature, and other body processes.

Several techniques are used to measure basal metabolism. One of the most common is a clinical machine designed for office and bedside use which measures the oxygen consumption over a given period of time. The metabolic rate is calculated from the volume of oxygen consumed in a given time period under *basal* conditions. The heat value is obtained indirectly—the oxygen consumption represents the extent of oxidation that has taken place within the body during the test period.

In making basal determinations, it was found that for the same age, sex, and size, individuals produce fairly constant amounts of heat over the same period of time if this heat is expressed on a basis of their surface area. As a result of many determinations under controlled conditions on individuals who were free from any medical condition that might affect their metabolism, tables were developed that can serve as a standard to compare the results of single basal metabolism determinations. An individual's metabolic rate is expressed in percent of deviation from this established standard. Each individual basal metabolic rate is expressed as either a + or − the percent deviation. Healthy individuals fall within ±15 per cent of the standards established for their body size, age, and sex. A minus represents a lower metabolic rate than the established norm; conversely, a plus indicates a higher metabolic rate.

Resting Metabolism

Durnin[8] describes resting metabolism as the metabolism of a person while at rest, in a life situation that is normal and under conditions of thermal neutrality. Resting metabolism is an average minimal metabolism for those periods of the day and night when there is no exercise, no exposure to cold, and with the inclusion of specific dynamic action of food.

There is considerable practical interest in resting metabolism.

Specific Dynamic Action

The effect of food to increase metabolism over the basal level was called "specific dynamic action" (sometimes spoken of as S.D.A.) by Rubner. Any food ingested in excess of that needed for immediate energy or structural purposes exerts this effect. The feeding of pure foodstuffs indicates, that the increase from each is not identical. Roughly, the increase from protein is 30 to 40 per cent, from fat 4 to 14 per cent, and from carbohydrate 5 to 7 per cent. On the average, food that is mixed in terms of proteins, fats, and carbohydrates causes an increase of some 5 to 6 per cent above the basal level. The explanation of this dynamic action is complicated and not clear. It is thought to be not the cost of digestion as was formely believed, but the total energy required for the utilization of foodstuffs within the body. It is a relatively small energy expenditure for the complex biological process involved.

Considerable emphasis has been given in popular literature to the "specific dynamic effect of protein" as a decisive factor in weight

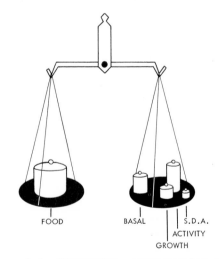

FIGURE 9–1. *Energy balance occurs when the energy intake (food) equals the energy expenditure: basal metabolism, muscle activity, growth, and specific dynamic action (S.D.A.) of food.*

[8] J. v. G. A. Durnin, *Energy, Work and Leisure,* Heinemann Educational Books, London, 1967.

loss diets of rather high protein content. The American diet consists of mixed foodstuffs, not pure protein. A pure protein diet would include only such foods as gelatin and egg white.

Swift[9] reports the results of extensive studies that he and his associates conducted at Pennsylvania State University in which they studied the dynamic effects of two diets that had the same energy content but differed in protein content. He concluded that if any difference exists for human beings in the overall energy utilization of equal-kcalorie diets of widely different protein contents, such differences must be very small.

He suggested that the dynamic effect may ordinarily amount to 5 or 6 per cent of the total food energy. If this were included in the calculations for total energy expenditure, an individual ingesting a diet of approximately 2000 kcalories would need about 100 kcalories for the specific dynamic effect. Thus it is clear that the energy expended each day in this manner is not considered a major factor; consequently, it is seldom calculated except in precise research experiments.

Garrow and Hawes[10] suggest that the term "specific dynamic action" as related to protein foods is misleading because the specific effect is not due to the protein in the diet, amino acid oxidation, or urea formation. The theory is advanced that the additional energy cost is related to protein synthesis.

Surface Area

The relationship of surface area to kcaloric expenditure was demonstrated first by Voit and later by Rubner. The metabolic rate may be expressed as kcalories per square meter of surface area per hour, or per 24 hours, which is the usual method in clinical and experimental studies. It is difficult to estimate the surface area, but from research studies a table

such as that of Du Bois,[11] and "nomograms" of Boothby[12] and Benedict have been worked out so that the surface area may be estimated from the height and weight of an individual.

Age

In addition to surface area, the basal metabolic rate is influenced by age. The rapidly growing child and the young adult have a higher metabolic rate than the older person or the aged. The highest basal metabolic rate per unit of surface area occurs at the age of approximately 2 years when it is estimated to be 55 kcalories per square meter per hour. It declines until the rise at puberty.

After early adulthood, energy requirements decrease progressively because of lessened physical activity and a lowering of the resting metabolism, according to the 1974 *Recommended Dietary Allowances*.[13] The approximate rate of decline in the resting metabolism is 2 per cent per decade with adults, according to Durnin. It is difficult to estimate the reduction of physical activity with age. It is proposed in the *Recommended Dietary Allowances* that kcalorie allowances above 50 years of age be reduced to 90 per cent of the amount required by a mature adult. If an individual is physically active, kcalories are reduced less. Special allowances must be made for men in the armed services or in active physical training.

Body Size

The total energy per unit of time for activities, such as walking, that involves moving mass over distance, will vary proportionately among individuals according to body size, larger body size requiring more energy and

[9] Raymond W. Swift, "Food Energy," *Food, The Yearbook of Agriculture, 1959*, U.S. Department of Agriculture, Washington, D.C., 1959, p. 39.

[10] J. S. Garrow and S. T. Hawes, "The Role of Amino Acid Oxidation in Causing 'Specific Dynamic Action' in Man," *British Journal of Nutrition*, Vol. 27, No. 4 (April 1972), pp. 211–219.

[11] E. F. Du Bois, *Basal Metabolism in Health and Disease*, Lea & Febiger, Philadelphia, 1936.

[12] W. M. Boothby, J. Berkson, and H. L. Dunn, "A Standard for Basal Metabolism with a Monogram for Clinical Application," *American Journal of Physiology*, Vol. 116, No. 2 (March–April 1936), pp. 468–484.

[13] Food and Nutrition Board, *Recommended Dietary Allowances*, 8th ed., National Academy of Sciences—National Research Council, Washington, D.C., 1974, pp. 29–30.

small body size less. Hourly resting metabolism rate may be lower or higher depending upon body size smaller or larger than average. True energy requirements of the underweight are best estimated on ideal weight or the kcalories may be inadequate, according to *Recommended Dietary Allowances.*

Energy needs of about 97 per cent of the population, according to occupation, fall within a variation of 300 kcalories. Special attention to energy requirements must be directed to individuals who are both large and active.

In making adjustments for the factor of

TABLE 9–1

Suggested Weight[a] and Basal Metabolic Rates (BMR)[b] of Adults[c]

HEIGHT		MEN			WOMEN		
		Median weight		BMR	Median weight		BMR
(in.)	(cm)	(lb)	(kg)	(kcal/day)	(lb)	(kg)	(kcal/day)
60	152				109 ± 9	50 ± 4	1399
62	158				115 ± 9	52 ± 4	1429
64	163	133 ± 11	60 ± 5	1630	122 ± 10	56 ± 5	1487
66	168	142 ± 12	64 ± 5	1690	129 ± 10	59 ± 5	1530
68	173	151 ± 14	69 ± 6	1775	136 ± 10	62 ± 5	1572
70	178	159 ± 14	72 ± 6	1815	144 ± 11	66 ± 5	1626
72	183	167 ± 15	76 ± 7	1870	152 ± 12	69 ± 5	1666
74	188	175 ± 15	80 ± 7	1933			
76	193	182 ± 16	83 ± 7	1983			

[a] Modified from Table 80, Hathaway and Foard, "Heights and Weights of Adults in the U.S." Home Economics Research Report No. 10, Agricultural Research Service, U.S. Department of Agriculture, 1960. Weights were based on those of college men and women. Measurements were made without shoes or other clothing. The ± refers to the weight range between the 25th and 75th percentile of each height category.

[b] Adapted from Talbot, FAO/WHO, 1973.

[c] To determine the daily energy need of an individual, allow for hours of sleep at 90 per cent of BMR and for time periods engaged in various activities as indicated below. Data are expressed as kilocalories per kilogram per hour.

ACTIVITY	MEN	WOMEN
Very light	1.5	1.3
Light	2.9	2.6
Moderate	4.3	4.1
Heavy	8.4	8.0

For example, a 50-kg woman employed as an agricultural worker and who maintains a home might have the following needs:

ACTIVITY	TIME (hr)	ENERGY NEED (kcal)
Sleep	8	420 (1399 × 0.9 ÷ 3)
Very light	6	390 (1.3 × 6 × 50)
Moderate	10	2050 (4.1 × 10 × 50)
Total	24	2860

SOURCE: Food and Nutrition Board, *Recommended Dietary Allowances*, 8th ed., National Academy of Sciences—National Research Council, Washington, D.C., 1974, p. 29.

size, weight may be used as a basis for individuals who are not appreciably underweight or overweight. With the obese, the lessened activity generally compensates for the increased energy allowance for carrying extra weight.

Linear growth is usually completed for females by the age of 17 and for males by 21, but most individuals in the United States continue to gain weight until the age of 60 years. The increase of muscle mass may continue into the third decade of life, especially if active physical training is taking place. Kcaloric allowances for adults are based on a desirable weight of given sex and height. Table 9–1 may be used as a guide.

Body Temperature

The body temperature of a healthy human remains constant regardless of variations in temperature in the surrounding atmosphere. This remarkable ability is due to a balance between two factors, heat production and heat elimination.

The heat production of the body results almost entirely from the oxidation of food. The amount of heat generated varies considerably with the extent of such factors as the intake of food, the environment, and exercise. Whenever the temperature of the surrounding atmosphere is lower than the body temperature, reflexes in the skin bring about an increase in the oxidative process, which results in a higher production of heat. If the temperature is still lower, an involuntary movement of muscles occurs (known as shivering) and even more oxidation takes place and still more heat is produced.

Heat is dissipated in a number of ways and by both voluntary and involuntary action. Most of the heat loss from the body takes place through the skin. It occurs by such routes as radiation, convection, conduction, evaporation of water from the skin and lungs, and loss of heat in the excreta. Several factors influence heat dissipation; among the most significant are environmental temperature, humidity, the presence or absence of fever, existing air currents, and the kind of clothing worn.

Usually the regulation of body temperature is easily maintained by the internal production of heat as the oxidation of food takes place and the regulation of heat loss by the wearing of clothing and maintenance of a favorable atmospheric temperature by modern methods of heating and air conditioning. As Newburgh[14] pointed out, the "mammalian organism rids itself of the heat at approximately the rate at which it is produced." The maintenance of this efficient heat regulation is a part of energy metabolism.

Climate

Few adjustments have to be made for climate. Most Americans live in comfortable temperatures that range from 66 to 77°F. Central heating, air conditioning, heated or cooled transportation, including automobiles, and the development of light, warm, and cool clothes are all considerations for a desirable temperature. If there is a prolonged exposure to either cold or heat, then some adjustment of kcalories is in order.

Kcalories must be increased approximately 5 per cent if work takes place in a temperature below 14°C., according to Johnson.[15] To this must be added 2 to 5 per cent to account for energy expenditure because of the weight of clothing and footwear for this climate and its impediment to activity. Similarly, energy requirement is increased for men working in a high temperature of 37.8°C. The explanation is that body temperature and metabolic rate increase, and more energy is required to maintain heat regulation. The desirable kcaloric increase, according to *Recommended Dietary Allowances*, for physically active men is 0.5 per cent for every degree of temperature rise between 30 and 40°C.

There is a tendency for activity to increase, both voluntary and involuntary (such as shiv-

[14] L. H. Newburgh, N. W. Johnson, and J. D. Newburgh, *Some Fundamental Principles of Metabolism*, J. W. Edwards, Ann Arbor, Mich., 1948, pp. 1–70.

[15] R. E. Johnson, "Caloric Requirements Under Adverse Environmental Conditions," *Federation Proceedings*, Vol. 22, No. 6 (November–December 1963), pp. 1439–1446.

ering), if the body becomes cold and additional kcalories are needed. Heat, on the other hand, appears to discourage activity. No adjustment, however, seems to be needed for climate, but for the exceptions noted.

Body Composition

The firm-muscled athlete uses more fuel than the individual with flabby, underdeveloped muscles. A man, probably because he has more active tissue and less fat than a woman in proportion to his actual weight, has a higher metabolic rate. The metabolic rate for women is about 8 per cent less than that of men and it also decreases with passing years. In view of her research findings and those of other research workers, Fulton[16] recommends that serious consideration be given to the adoption of changes in the standards for basal metabolism rates for women. The group mean basal of −10.53 for 499 tests on 60 women agrees with similar studies. This change is important in light of the use of the basal heat production of women for nutritional and physiological studies and by clinicans to determine BMR as an indicator of thyroid activity. Muscle tissue requires more oxygen and hence calories than adipose tissue. Individuals with large muscular development have a basal metabolic rate 5 to 6 per cent greater than persons of the same height and weight, according to Johnson.[17]

Although body composition has some effect on metabolic rate, there is considerable difficulty in securing accurate measurements of body composition, granted that this method is more exact than measuring body surface.

Growth

Growth itself may be defined as "a net increase in tissue substance." Whenever tissues

have been developed, an increased energy requirement has resulted. Growth is considered to occur when new tissue formation takes place. Thus such processes as pregnancy, lactation, convalescence with repair of injured tissue, as well as growth during childhood, would require additional energy expenditure.

The energy requirement for growth will vary directly with the rate of growth. It is difficult to make accurate predictions about the growth rate because it varies with individuals. The fourteenth year in boys and the twelfth year in girls, on the average, are periods of rapid growth. It must be emphasized that growth cannot take place until basal energy requirements are met, plus kcalories for activity and for environmental, nutritional, and other influences.

Pregnancy and Lactation

Kcalories for pregnancy are calculated by adding the increase demanded by the growth of the placenta, mammary glands, and the fetus to the usual requirements. A daily increase not exceeding 200 kcalories is suggested. It is estimated that 40,000 kcalories are required for the additional energy requirements during gestation.

The energy needs for lactation are much greater. The increase depends of course on the amount of milk that the mother secretes. *Recommended Dietary Allowances* recommends an increase of 500 kcalories. The production of milk is a costly energy process. The physical and mental health of the mother are other factors to be considered.

Stress

Physical, physiological, and emotional disturbances impose a stress on the body. The nutritional status of the person prior to the onset of stress has an important influence.[18] Stress of almost any origin will result in an effect on nutritional status if intense enough and of sufficient duration. No exact allowances have been predicted for stress, but it probably has some impact on energy requirement.

---

[16] Doris Elliot Fulton, "Basal Metabolic Rate of Women," *Journal of the American Dietetic Association*, Vol. 61, No. 5 (November 1972), p. 520.

[17] Ogden C. Johnson, "Present Knowledge of Calories," in *Present Knowledge in Nutrition*, 3d ed., Nutrition Foundation, New York, 1967, Chap. 1.

[18] "Nutrition and Common Stress," *Dairy Council Digest*, Vol. 37 (May–June 1966), pp. 14–16.

Activity

The amount of energy expended by the individual for the performance of work is the largest single variable factor in calculating his total energy needs. There are two primary reasons for this: (1) a person engages in many activities during the 24-hour period, and each one may require a different number of kcalories, and (2) the amount of time spent in activities can vary considerably.

Contrary to popular belief, *mental work* does not effectively increase the total metabolism. Investigators have found that mental work adds only 3 to 4 per cent to the total expenditure and for all practical purposes can be ignored.

If one wanted to estimate the energy a person needs to perform certain tasks or to speculate about the relative kcaloric cost of two activities, such as tennis and swimming, the usual procedure would be to consult tables of energy expenditure. However, the information included in these tables could only be regarded as an approximation of energy expenditure. The data found there are derived from a number of sources, and, at present, they are being revised extensively.

All tables of energy expenditures for specified activities must be used with caution. Individuals vary in size, age, and efficiency in accomplishing the task. Many other factors must be considered as well. Calculations can give only a relative answer.

Five categories of activities according to degree of physical exertion are indicated in

TABLE 9–2

TYPE OF ACTIVITY	KCALORIES PER HOUR
Sedentary activities, such as reading, writing, eating, watching television or movies, listening to the radio, sewing, playing cards, and typing. Miscellaneous officework and other activities done while sitting that require little or no arm movement.	80 to 100
Light activities, such as preparing and cooking food, doing dishes, dusting, handwashing small articles of clothing, ironing, walking slowly, and personal care. Miscellaneous officework and other activities done while standing that require some arm movement, and rapid typing and other more strenuous activities done while sitting.	110 to 160
Moderate activities, such as making beds, mopping and scrubbing, sweeping, light polishing and waxing, laundering by machine, light gardening and carpentry work, and walking moderately fast. Other activities done while standing that require moderate arm movement, and activities done while sitting that require more vigorous arm movement.	170 to 240
Vigorous activities, such as heavy scrubbing and waxing, handwashing large articles of clothing, hanging out clothes, stripping beds, and other heavy work. Walking fast, bowling, golfing, and gardening.	250 to 350
Strenuous activities, such as swimming, playing tennis, running, bicycling, dancing, skiing, and playing football.	350 and more

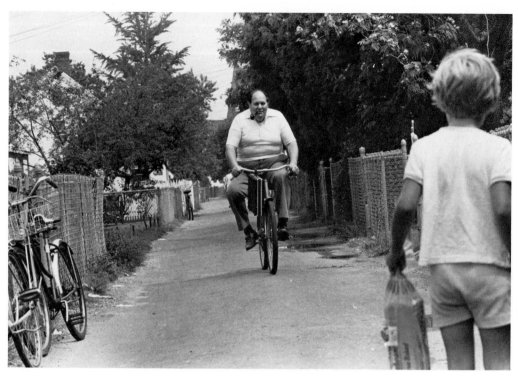

FIGURE 9–2. *Bicycling is an example of a strenuous activity.* (*Courtesy of Vandercook*)

Table 9–2 with appropriate examples.[19] The figures indicate the minimum kcalories needed per hour. The range is given for each type to allow for differences in activities and in persons. In the sedentary activities, for example, typing will require more kcalories than listening to the radio. One reason for difference is that some individuals are more efficient in their body action than others. Values at the upper limits of a range are probably more indicative of kcalorie needs for men and lower limits for women.

One of the most active areas of nutrition research in recent years has been that of energy expenditure. The development of newer techniques has allowed greater flexibility in collecting information. Earlier determinations of

energy expenditure were chiefly made by two methods, the respiration chamber mentioned earlier, which measured directly the heat produced, and, second, the indirect method, which consisted of collecting the total sample of expired air in a Douglas bag and having the air sample subsequently analyzed.

Just prior to World War II, the Max Planck Institut für Arbeitsphysiologie[20] in Dortmund, Germany, introduced the Kofranyi–Michaelis (KM) respirometer, which eliminated some of the difficulties inherent in other techniques. Even though there are many limitations to using this respirometer, it is possible to obtain data that were difficult to get by other means. The KM apparatus consists of a light (approximately 12 pounds) respirometer, which the subject wears on his back in a knapsack-like fashion. He needs to wear a nose clip and

[19] Louise Page and Lillian J. Fincer, *Food and Your Weight*, Consumer and Food Economic Research Division, Agricultural Research Service, U.S. Department of Agriculture, Washington, D.C., 1969, pp. 3–5.

[20] E. Kofranyi and H. F. Michaelis, *Arbeitsphysiologie*, Vol. 11, 1940, p. 148.

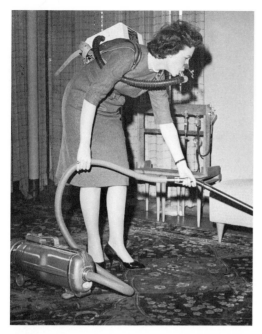

FIGURE 9–3. *Determining the energy expenditure in vacuuming a living room. Note the freedom of movement allowed by using the Kofranyi-Michaelis apparatus. (Home Economics Department, New York University)*

the amount of energy expended at various household tasks.

Energy Value of Foods

The energy of the combustion heat value of a food may be determined by burning it (or any other substance desired) in a "bomb" calorimeter in an atmosphere of pure oxygen. This represents a direct calorimetric method. The heat evolved is measured as a change in temperature of the water surrounding the "bomb." Such determinations indicate that

> 1 g of pure fat yields 9.3 kcalories
> 1 g of pure carbohydrate yields 4.1 kcalories
> 1 g of pure protein yields 4.1 kcalories

Fat and carbohydrate, consisting of C(arbon), H(ydrogen), O(xygen), are burned completely to carbon dioxide and water. Protein, with the elements C H O N(itrogen), P(hosphorus), S(ulfur), yields, in addition to carbon dioxide and water, a residue, and when correction is made for this incomplete combustion, the average value for proteins becomes 4.1 kcalories per gram.

There are slight variations in kcalorie values obtained for different foods within a given group as they are oxidized within the body for energy. But through the years, the rounded figures for the following came into common usage:

> 1 g fat, 9 kcalories
> 1 g carbohydrate, 4 kcalories
> 1 g protein, 4 kcalories

The development of food composition tables is described in Chapter 28. These tables of composition are merely approximations of the actual values of all such foods. There is considerable variation in composition, especially in the vitamin and mineral content. These differences may be due to such factors as the weather, the variety of food, the maturity, and the period of storage. In addition, some differences may be related to the method of analysis itself.

The table of food values in Appendix B is a U.S. Department of Agriculture contribution

mouthpiece or a mask that covers the nose and mouth. They are quite uncomfortable, but most subjects become accustomed to them. The respirometer is connected in such a way that a 3 or 6 per cent sample of expired air is collected in a small football-like bladder. This allows for an extended activity period since the bladder is filled in approximately 20 minutes and can be replaced to collect additional samples. An analysis of this sample, as well as that of atmospheric air, needs to be made. Figure 9–3 shows a KM respirometer in use.

The important contribution of the KM respirometer, and other recently developed portable methods, is that the subject has physical freedom which enables him to perform all aspects of a given activity. McCracken[21] and his associates have determined

[21] *Energy Expenditure of Women Performing Selected Activities*, Home Economics Research Report No. 11, Agricultural Research Service, U.S. Department of Agriculture, Washington, D.C., 1960.

TABLE 9–3

Approximate Kcalorie Content of Selected Foods

		KCALORIES				KCALORIES
BEVERAGES			**FATS, OILS, AND RELATED PRODUCE**			
Carbonated beverages:			Butter or margarine,	1 pat		50
Cola type	12-oz can or	145	16 per ¼-lb stick			
	bottle		Peanut butter	1 tbs		100
	8-oz glass	95	Mayonnaise	1 tbs		100
Fruit flavors	12-oz can or	170	Blue cheese	1 tbs		75
(10–13% sugar)	bottle		salad dressing			
	8-oz glass	115	Salad dressing, plain	1 tbs		65
Alcoholic beverages:			Salad oil	1 tbs		125
Wines:			**MEAT GROUP**			
Table wines	3-oz glass	75	Hamburger, broiled	3 oz		245
Beer 3–6%	12-oz can or	150	Steak, broiled, without	3 oz		175
alcohol	bottle		bone, lean			
	8-oz glass	100	Frankfurter, cooked	1		155
Whiskey, gin, rum,	1⅛ jigger	105	Sardines, canned in oil	3 oz		175
vodka (86 proof)			Egg, boiled	1 large		80
BREAD AND FLOUR-BASED FOODS			Omelet, plain, milk and	1 large egg		110
1-lb loaf, 16 slices:			fat for cooking			
Cracked wheat, raisin,	slice	75	Baked beans in tomato	½ cup		160
white			sauce with pork			
Whole wheat,	slice	70	**MILK GROUP**			
rye			Skim, fresh or dry	1 cup		90
Hamburger of	1 roll	120	Reconstituted whole	1 cup		160
frankfurter roll	(18 oz per		Sour cream	1 tbs		30
	dozen)		Yoghurt made from	1 cup		120
Doughnuts:			partially skim milk			
Cake-type, plain	1 average	125	Chocolate milk shake	12 oz		520
yeast-leavened, "raised"	2½–2¾ in.	175	Cheese, American	1 oz		105
	diameter		process			
Pancakes (griddle cakes),	4-in cake	60	Cottage cheese,	2 tbs		30
wheat			creamed			
Pizza, plain cheese	5½-in sector	185	**SNACKS**			
	of 14-in. pie		Corn chips	1 cup		230
Pretzels	5 small sticks	20	French fries	10, 2 x 2 x ½-in.		155
Waffle	1 average	210		diameter		
DESSERTS AND OTHER SWEETS			Hamburger with roll	2-oz patty		265
Cakes:			Hotdog with roll	1 average		245
Angel cake	2-in. sector of	105	Tomato catsup	1 tbs		15
	8½-in tube		**VEGETABLES AND FRUITS**			
	cake		Cabbage	½ cup shredded		10
Chocolate cake	2-in. sector of	345	Celery	Two 8-in. stalk		10
with chocolate icing	10-in. round		Lettuce	2 large leaves		10
	layer cake		Beans, snap, green or	½ cup		15
Pound cake	2¾ x 3 x ⅝-in.	140	yellow, cooked			
	slice		Peas, green	½ cup		60
Caramels	3 medium	115	Apple	2½-in. diameter		70
Chocolate cream	2 or 3 small	110	Avocado			
Milk chocolate	1-oz bar	150	California variety	½ of 10 oz		185
sweetened			Florida variety	½ of 13 oz		160
Plain and assorted cookie	3-in.	120	Strawberries	½ cup		30
Apple pie	⅟₇ of 9-in. pie	345	Banana	one 6 x 1½ in.		80
Gelatin with fruit	½ cup	80	Cantaloupe	½ of 5-in. melon		60
Ice cream, plain	½ cup	145	Grapefruit juice, fresh	½ cup		40
Ice milk	½ cup	110	Orange juice,	½ cup		55
Sherbet	½ cup	130	frozen, ready to serve			

to the long series of food composition tables. The kcaloric value of some common foods is given in Table 9–3.

Energy Needs of the Individual

The recommendations for kcalories of the Food and Nutrition Board of the National Research Council are included in Table 9–4. The energy allowance, in contrast to recommendations for other nutrients, is established at the lowest value believed to be compatible with good health for average individuals in each age group.

The kcaloric allowance for infants during the first year is based on an intake reflected by thriving infants. Allowances for the first 5 months are 117 kcalories per kilogram of body weight; from 5 months to 1 year the allowance is 108 kcalories per kilogram of body weight.

Energy allowances for children of both sexes decline gradually to about 80 kcalories per kilogram through ten years of age. After age 10, the energy allowance gradually declines further to 45 kcalories per kilogram for adolescent males and 38 kcalories for adolescent females. Energy allowances at the adolescent level must be individually adjusted because of the marked variation in energy output exhibited at this age.

Recommended allowances for energy for infants and adults are identical to international standards (FAO/WHO, 1973). Allowances for children are less because American children, on the whole, are less active.

Allowances for average adults are divided into two age categories, those aged 23 to 50 years and those over 50. Factors assumed in the determination of the allowances are (1) the practice of a light occupation, (2) an average temperature of 20°C, and (3) the

TABLE 9–4

Recommended Daily Dietary Allowances for Kcalories, Revised 1974

Designed for maintenance of good nutrition of practically all healthy people in the United States

	YEARS (From–To)	WEIGHT (kg)	WEIGHT (lb)	HEIGHT (cm)	HEIGHT (in.)	ENERGY (kcal)
Infants	0.0–0.5	6	14	60	24	kg × 117
	0.5–1.0	9	20	71	28	kg × 108
Children	1–3	13	28	86	34	1300
	4–6	20	44	110	44	1800
	7–10	30	66	135	54	2400
Males	11–14	44	97	158	63	2800
	15–18	61	134	172	69	3000
	19–22	67	147	172	69	3000
	23–50	70	154	172	69	2700
	51+	70	154	172	69	2400
Females	11–14	44	97	155	62	2400
	15–18	54	119	162	65	2100
	19–22	58	128	162	65	2100
	23–50	58	128	162	65	2000
	51+	58	128	162	65	1800
Pregnant						+300
Lactating						+500

SOURCE: Food and Nutrition Board, *Recommended Dietary Allowances*, 8th ed., National Academy of Sciences—National Research Council, Washington, D.C., 1974, p. 129.

wearing of clothes for thermal comfort. Adjustments must be made for increased physical activity, body size, and only rarely for climate.

Adjustments must be made for pregnancy and lactation. During pregnancy, additional energy is required to build new tissues in the placenta and fetus, for the increased work load associated with the movement of the mother, and to support the increase in the resting metabolic rate. Weight should be gained at a steady rate of 0.25 to 0.45 kg per week. An extra allowance of 300 kcalories throughout pregnancy is considered adequate for most women. The additional energy requirements of lactation are proportional to the quantity of milk produced, which varies from woman to woman. Energy allowances are increased by 500 kcalories per day but should be increased if necessary, such as if the mother begins to lose weight. If more than one baby is being suckled, allowances will have to be increased.[22]

According to Bradfield,[23] there are five methods for the assessment of energy expenditure: (1) assessment of kcaloric intake required to maintain body weight over a period of time; (2) an activity questionnaire–interview; (3) a diary of time activities maintained every minute or 5 minutes by the subject or an observer, accompanied by the determination of oxygen consumption for certain activities; (4) continuous indirect calorimetry with respirometers; and (5) the establishment of individual oxygen consumption–heart regression lines with subsequent continuous monitoring of the heart rate. Each method has advantages and limitations depending upon sample size, precision required, and the amount of tolerance a subject has physically for the equipment carried and psychologically for the maintenance of diaries by the subject or for the continual presence of an observer.

Generally speaking, an individual's weight can be taken as a reflection of whether or not he is eating enough kcalories to support his activities. If he gains weight, he is eating more kcalories than he needs and is, therefore, in a state of *positive energy balance*, since he is retaining more kcalories than he uses. Conversely, if he loses weight, he is consuming fewer kcalories than he needs and is in a state of *negative energy balance*. A person who maintains his weight is in a state of *energy balance*.

In determining the kcaloric needs of the individual, one must consider many points. First, the need for basal expenditure is determined. Then a critical look at the whole 24-hour activity must be taken. How many hours does a person spend in sleep, how many in riding in a train, car, or bus? Is his work really heavy, or are there short periods of heavy labor, with longer periods of "standing around"? Many jobs have changed radically and become mechanized. For example, carpenters use electric saws, cement is mixed by machine, children ride to school instead of walk, and many household appliances have reduced the number of kcalories spent per day. The reduction of the work week has made the number of hours that the individual spends in recreation vitally important to his total energy expenditure. Does he watch television, or does he play volleyball or swim? Does she garden or does she play bridge? Has the energy crisis increased activity, such as more walking or using a bicycle? All of these are important influences on the total energy expenditure of individuals. A constant check on body weight is the best way of knowing whether one is getting enough kcalories.

Adequate energy intake should be allowed to provide for efficient utilization of dietary protein for growth and maintenance. The type of foods selected for the daily diet must reflect high nutrient density so that not only will kcalories be sufficient but other nutrients as well, especially minerals that are widely distributed but are sometimes low in concentration. Americans may need to examine their diet for high concentrations of fats, sugars, and alcohol, which are low in nutrient density but high in kcalories. In other words, it is careless to look at only the number of kcalories in the daily diet. What other nutrients are being conveyed?

[22] *Recommended Dietary Allowances*, op. cit., pp. 25–33.

[23] Robert B. Bradfield, "Introduction, Symposium, Assessment of Typical Daily Energy Expenditure," *American Journal of Clinical Nutrition*, Vol. 24, No. 9 (September 1971), p. 1111.

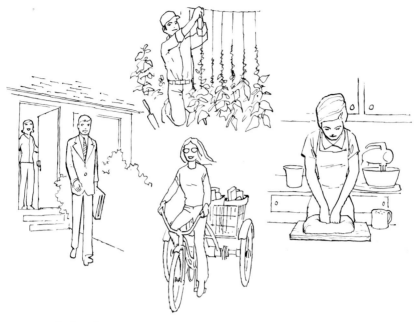

FIGURE 9–4. *An economic and energy crisis can encourage more physical activities, such as walking to work, using adult tricycles, gardening, and baking bread.*

Sedentary living, including low levels of work output, may present a problem in the maintenance of a balance between weight and dietary intake. A sedentary lifestyle for young or old can contribute to obesity and to degenerative arterial disease and complications, notably diabetes mellitus. Any tendency to gain excessive weight at any age may be counteracted by increased physical activity. Kcaloric undernutrition, in contrast, can be as serious as overnutrition. The problem continues to exist among the poor in America and in developing countries in the world.

Kcaloric Undernutrition

Cases of undernutrition exist in the economically underdeveloped countries and among the poor in the United States. In the United States, many cases of undernutrition may be due to physical factors that interfere with food consumption, absorption, or storage of nutrients, as well as factors that are economic in origin.

There is a very high correlation between the average body weight of a people and their estimated average kcalorie supply in both Latin American countries and the Asian countries, according to the U.S. Department of Agriculture.[24] Men and women in the Asian countries do not differ significantly in mean height from Latin Americans, but they weigh significantly less even though both groups consume about the same mean of kcalories. Possible explanations are that the estimates of kcalorie supplies are incorrect or that environmental differences, such as a larger incidence of intestinal parasites, prevail, interfering with food absorption. Yet within each country the boys and girls with the fastest rates of growth, and the ones having the heaviest body at maturity generally, have the highest daily supply of kcalories.

[24] Rose Frisch and Roger Revelle, "Variations in Body Weights Among Different Populations," in *The World Food Problem*, vol. III, Report of the Panel on World Food Supply, The President's Science Advisory Committee, Washington, D.C., September 1967, Chap. 1.

Odum[25] believes that the design of a system

[25] Howard T. Odum, "Energetics of World Food Production," in *The World Food Problem*, vol. III, Report of the Panel on World Food Supply, The President's Science Advisory Committee, Washington, D. C., September 1967, Chap. 3.

of world food production and consumption can be aided by a study of energy-flow networks that show the basis for man's progress. The ability of a nation to hold leadership will depend upon its ability to control flows of food and fuel.

SELECTED REFERENCES

Bradfield, R. B. (ed.), "Assessment of Typical Energy Expenditure," *American Journal of Clinical Nutrition*, Part I, Vol. 24, No. 9 (September 1971), pp. 1111–1192; Part II, Vol. 24, No. 12 (December 1971), pp. 1403–1493.

Davidson, Stanley, R. Passmore, and J. F. Brock, *Human Nutrition and Dietetics*, The Williams & Wilkins Company, Baltimore, 1972, Chapter 2.

Durnin, J. v. G. A., *Energy, Work and Leisure*, Heinemann Educational Books, Ltd., London, 1967.

Food and Nutrition Board, *Recommended Dietary Allowances*, 8th ed., National Academy of Sciences—National Research Council, Washington, D.C., 1974.

Konishi, Frank, "Exercise Equivalents of Foods," Southern Illinois University Press, Carbondale, Ill., 1973.

Report of a Joint FAO/WHO Ad Hoc Expert Committee, *Energy and Protein Requirements*, World Health Organization Technical Report Series, No. 522, World Health Organization, Geneva, 1973.

Robinson, Corrine H., *Fundamentals of Normal Nutrition*, Macmillan Publishing Co., Inc., New York, 1973, Chapter 7.

10

Nutrition and Weight

A preoccupation of the twentieth century is a concern about overweight. There are many evidences of this high interest. Newspapers and magazine articles about easy ways to lose weight have high readership. Supermarkets and other stores have shelves of low kcaloric foods. Drugstores offer pills and potions for reducing. Health stores, reducing salons, and stores with an array of home-exercise gadgets lure the public with an image of svelte fitness. Commercials on television bombard viewers with information about the low kcaloric value of many foods. The before-and-after pictures induce many gullible persons to part with money for products that bring little or no results.

The peddling of special foods, remedies, and devices for losing weight has become big business—so large that several congressional subcommittees have investigated this serious trend. They were concerned that Americans were being bilked of large sums for phony reducing preparations.

The mention of obesity in the literature is interesting. Garrison in his *History of Medicine* cites evidence of obese women in the sculpture and carvings of prehistoric caves as far back as the Stone Age. This implies that

overweight is not a new condition. Prior to the twentieth century, however, moderate overweight was often considered an indication of wealth, beauty, and health. In fact, the entire matter of weight appears to have strong overtones of cultural approval or disapproval even today in many parts of the world.

Incidence of Overweight in the United States

The Public Health Service acknowledges that statistics on prevalence and incidence of overweight and obesity in the United States are inadequate.[1] Crude statistical data indicate that obesity is a problem at all ages and in both sexes. There is a greater frequency of excessive weight gain at certain ages and physiological periods. In women, weight problems are more likely to occur after the completion of growth (around 20), during pregnancies, and after the menopause. There are no similar periods during which men tend to

---

[1] *Obesity and Health*, PHS Publication No. 1485, National Center for Chronic Disease Control, Public Health Service, U.S. Department of Health, Education, and Welfare, Arlington, Va., 1966.

become obese, but they are inclined to gain weight between 25 and 40 years of age, with some acceleration after the age of 40.

Few statistics are available about the prevalence of obesity[2] in infants and small children. Studies on elementary and high school students give estimates of from 10 to 39 per cent for obesity. There is general agreement that prevalence increases with age and that more girls are obese than boys.

There are some indications that there is less overweight among the high socioeconomic class and that there may be an inverse correlation between socioeconomic classes and the prevalence of obesity—more true of women than of men.

Some data about obesity were secured in the *Ten-State Nutrition Survey*.[3] Black females in the age group 15 to 19 in low- and high-income-ratio states had a high prevalence of obesity. White females from ages 17 to over 60 in both income levels had a medium prevalence of obesity. Black females over 60 years of age in both income levels were also in the medium prevalence value. A minimal prevalence of obesity was present among black males from 17 to over 60 years in both income levels and among white males over 60 years of age and in both income levels. No data were available in the Spanish-American sample. (See Table 2–2.)

In a study[4] of a large representative sample of adults in midtown Manhattan, New York City, almost one third of the women in the lower socioeconomic bracket were overweight by the standard used. A weaker correlation between men and weight levels was evident. In this same study, correlation between prevalence of obesity and national background was found. For example, a larger proportion of women of Italian than British backgrounds was overweight.

Racial differences[5] have been studied. Black women tended to be heavier in all age groups than white women of corresponding heights. Similar differences between men were not so marked. Attitudes of black and white persons toward obesity have suggested that white women are more concerned with excess weight than black women or men of either race.

Herman[6] found that education was the best indicator of social or economic level in her study of individuals who attended a Health Maintenance Clinic at Thomas Jefferson University in Philadelphia. Significant differences in the prevalence of overweight as related to education was found among women 40 to 59 years of age. Women with less than 12 years of education were more likely to be overweight than the women. Among women at the higher educational level there were almost no differences among ethnic groups in the proportion overweight. The percentage of overweight men increased up to 60 years of age and then declined.

More evidence is needed concerning the differences in obesity due to education, race, and similar factors. *Obesity and Health* emphasizes that insufficient data exist to make statements with assurance concerning obesity in the total population or for any particular group.

Definition of Obesity

A distinction must be made between overweight and obesity.[7] Overweight implies excessive weight as related to an arbitrary standard, such as a table. These standards are of two types: average weights, and desirable, best,

[2] "Natural History of Obesity: Infancy Through Adolescence," *Dairy Council Digest*, Vol. 39, No. 1 (January–February 1968), p. 1.

[3] *Highlights, Ten-State Nutrition Survey, 1968–1970*, DHEW Publication No. (HSM) 72–8134, Center for Disease Control, Health Services and Mental Health Administration, U.S. Department of Health, Education, and Welfare, Atlanta, Ga., 1972, pp. 4–5.

[4] P. B. Goldblatt, M. E. Moore, and A. J. Stunkard, "Social Factors in Obesity," *Journal of the American Medical Association*, Vol. 192, No. 12 (June 21, 1965), pp. 1039–1044.

[5] *Obesity and Health*, op. cit., p. 21.

[6] Mary W. Herman, "Excess Weight and Sociocultural Characteristics," *Journal of the American Dietetic Association*, Vol. 63, No. 2 (August 1973), pp. 161–164.

[7] Charlotte M. Young, "Overnutrition," in Miloslav Rechcigl, Jr. (ed.), *Food, Nutrition and Health*, Vol. 16, S. Karger, Basel, 1973, pp. 179–186.

or ideal weights. The average-weight tables are based on average weight, height, and age found in various populations of individuals that met certain criteria and from national surveys. Average weights usually increase with age. Ideal-weight tables have been designed for all individuals over 25 years of age based on the concept that growth in height has been attained and there is no biological need for further gain. These ideal-weight tables do not allow for increase in weight with age.

These weight–height–age tables have serious limitations. Most tables are not representative cross sections of the population. No agreement has been reached as to the level of excess weight that connotes overweight or obesity. Consideration is not always given to the size of bones or amount of muscle of an average person.

Obesity, according to Bray,[8] exists when fat makes up a greater than normal fraction of total body weight. Obese persons are usually overweight but overweight persons may not be obese, such as certain athletes, like heavyweight boxers or football defensive players. However, it is easy to measure weight but much more difficult to measure fatness.

Identification of Obesity

A determination of obesity may be ascertained by practical methods or by scientific procedures. A fairly realistic but gross evaluation for determining evidence of obesity is the "look"—an examination of the nude body in a mirror for excessive fat deposits. Another method is the "pinch test." In young individuals and adults under 50, at least half the body fat is found directly under the skin. A fold of skin and subcutaneous fat can be lifted between the thumb and forefinger at several locations on the body, such as back of upper arm and side of lower chest. Care must be taken so that the skin is held free from soft tissue or bony structure. Persons with normal amounts of fat beneath the skin have folds

that vary from ¼ to ½ inch thick. Skinfolds thicker than 1 inch of double thickness indicate excessive body fatness. The thin fold measuring less than ½ inch may indicate underweight. To pinch and measure the body in several places is recommended.

Another test is a comparison of the circumference of the chest at the level of the nipples with the circumference of the abdomen at the level of the navel. If the abdominal measurement is near, the same, or exceeds the girth of the chest, it generally indicates excess fat. Scientific techniques to determine body fatness, according to Young,[9] include data from studies in body density,[10] total body water, body electrolyte estimation or body potassium 40 content,[11] and anthropometry.[12] These techniques are complex, time-consuming, expensive, and require considerable professional preparation. Their use is confined largely to researchers.

The skinfold measurement with the use of calipers in the triceps or subscapular areas of the body is recommended by the Committee on Nutritional Anthropometry as a fairly precise, simple, and good method for determining the fat content of an individual's body and for judging the degree of his obesity. It is not necessary to measure both areas, but a more definitive quantification will result if both are used. Of the two methods, the triceps measurement alone is satisfactory. There is agreement that skinfold tests are of proved value in measuring total adiposity although valid

---

[8] George A. Bray, "The Myth of Diet in the Management of Obesity," *American Journal of Clinical Nutrition*, Vol. 23, No. 9 (September 1970), pp. 1141–1148.

[9] Young, op. cit., p. 181.

[10] Charlotte M. Young, M. Elizabeth Kerr Martin, Rosalinda Tensuan, and Joan Blondin, "Predicting Gravity and Body Fatness in Young Women," *Journal of the American Dietetic Association*, Vol. 40, No. 2 (February 1962), pp. 102–107.

[11] G. B. Forbes, J. Gallup, and J. B. Hirsh, "Estimation of Body Fat from Potassium 40 Content," *Science*, Vol. 133, No. 3446 (January 1961), pp. 101–102.

[12] Committee on Nutritional Anthropometry, Food and Nutrition Board, National Research Council (Ancel Keys, chm.), "Recommendations Concerning Body Measurements for Characterization of Nutritional Status," in J. Brozek (ed.), *Body Measurements for Human Nutrition*, Wayne University Press, Detroit, 1956, p. 10.

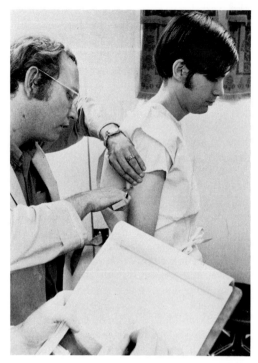

FIGURE 10–1. *Skinfold measurement of triceps area to determine the degree of fatness.* (HANES)

standards are arbitrary at the moment. Table 10–1 gives obesity standards using skinfold thickness. Norms for population groups throughout the world are needed.

Obesity is characterized by a positive energy balance. In other words, obese individuals consume more calories than are utilized in the energy requirements of their bodies. Nutrition experts are becoming increasingly aware that, although this explanation appears very simple, the causes for this overconsumption are varied and multiple. For that reason, *Obesity and Health* states that some investigators refer to "obesities" rather than obesity. Naturally, many concepts have been advanced and some of them have considerable evidence to substantiate them. Some of the more important ones will be examined here.

Physiological Concepts About Obesity

One of the most recent concepts about obesity, the relation of the condition to the

TABLE 10–1

Obesity Standards for Caucasian Americans

Minimum Triceps Skinfold Thickness Indicating Obesity (Millimeters)

AGE (years)	SKINFOLD MEASUREMENTS Males	Females
5	12	14
6	12	15
7	13	16
8	14	17
9	15	18
10	16	20
11	17	21
12	18	22
13	18	23
14	17	23
15	16	24
16	15	25
17	14	26
18	15	27
19	15	27
20	16	28
21	17	28
22	18	28
23	18	28
24	19	28
25	20	29
26	20	29
27	21	29
28	22	29
29	23	29
30–50	23	30

SOURCE: *Obesity and Health*, PHS Publication No. 1485, National Center for Chronic Disease Control, Public Health Service, U.S. Department of Health, Education, and Welfare, Arlington, Va., 1966, p. 13.

number and size of adipose cells, was the major thrust of a paper given by Professor of Experimental Medicine Jules Hirsch at Rockefeller University. This paper and others presented at a Conference on Childhood Obesity in New York City on November 15 and 16, 1973, were reviewed by the chairman of the conference, Myron Winick,[13] Director of the

[13] Myron Winick, "Childhood Obesity," *Nutrition Today*, Vol. 9, No. 3 (May–June 1974), pp. 6–12.

Institute of Human Nutrition, Columbia University. Early in his research, Hirsch noted that nonobese individuals averaged 0.6 to 0.7 mg of fat per cell, whereas obese persons averaged about 20 per cent more. The nonobese individual had about 300 billion fat cells, but obese individuals had about twice that number. In very obese adults, the spectacular cellular difference was in the number of fat cells. When these adults lost weight, the effect was almost entirely on cell size; cell number changed very little, if at all.

Additional studies by Hirsch suggested two types of obesity. Too many fat cells is characteristic of one type and is known as *hyperplastic obesity*. The other type occurs when an individual has fat cells that are too large and is identified as *hypertrophic obesity*. The obesity that occurs in childhood is primarily hyperplastic, whereas the late onset of obesity at the adult age is hypertrophic. Hirsch cautions that the two types are not clear-cut and some overlapping may occur. Critical periods for the onset of obesity in life are the first three years, adolescence, and the last trimester of pregnancy.

One obesity theory resulting from research on experimental animals is that the hypothalamus does not function properly.[14] The hypothalamus is a part of the brain which is situated at the base of the larger brain mass. It is responsible for the control of many of the body functions.

There is considerable evidence from animal experimentation that the hypothalamus contains a mechanism that initiates eating and another mechanism that deters overeating. If even small lesions are induced in those areas of the hypothalamus, the changes in eating are quite dramatic. Depending upon which mechanism is disturbed, the experimental animal might either starve or increase his food intake markedly.

Other animal experimentation, which involved the digestive tract, had some interesting results. If a digestive organ such as the stomach was removed or injured, there was no consequent change in the feeding mechanism. The conclusion suggested by investigators is that food intake is controlled by the nervous system with the hypothalamus playing a major role, and that the digestive system has no regulatory function on feeding. This work on experimental animals can only be postulated for human beings. More research is needed in this area.

Stunkard[15] produced evidence that the obese were less responsive to internal physiological cues indicative of hunger or satiety. There was a smaller correlation among the obese than in normal persons, for example, between gastric motility and verbal reports of hunger.

There is insufficient evidence to determine the influence of heredity on obesity. Studies of human populations give rise to speculation of a hereditary factor.[16] According to a study,[17] when one parent was obese, the prevalence among the children increased 40 per cent; and when both parents were obese, it rose to 80 per cent. This finding was corroborated by similar studies. The impact of family food patterns must not be overlooked.

It is well known that animal breeders for centuries have selected cattle or hogs, or even poultry, which are either inclined to be lean or to be fat, depending on the type which the market was demanding. Studies by human geneticists and anthropologists, such as Angel, Bauer, Rony, and Siemens, have indicated that certain genes may determine obesity as is indicated in certain human populations. Mayer, at Harvard, found that certain breeds of mice possessed a peculiar gene which resulted in overweight. These genetic factors apparently are responsible for causing alterations in metabolism.

Many obese individuals are under the il-

---

[14] Jean Mayer, "Physiology of Hunger and Satiety; Regulation of Food Intake," in Robert S. Goodhart and Maurice E. Shils (eds.), *Modern Nutrition in Health and Disease*, Lea & Febiger, Philadelphia, 1973, Chap. 4.

[15] Albert J. Stunkard, "The Relationship of Gastric Motility and Hunger, a Summary of Evidence," *Psychosomatic Medicine*, Vol. 33, No. 2 (March–April 1971), pp. 123–134.

[16] H. H. Newman, F. N. Freeman, and J. J. Holzinger, *A Study of Heredity and Environment*, University of Chicago Press, Chicago, 1937.

[17] R. F. J. Withers, "Problems in the Genetics of Human Obesity," *Eugenics Reviews*, Vol. 56, No. 2 (February 1964), p. 81.

lusion that their endocrine glands are responsible. Research reveals, however, that very few obese individuals show any clinical or laboratory evidence of difficulty with the endocrine glands. Hypothyroidism, for example, is grossly overrated as a possible cause of obesity, according to Lawrence.[18]

The amount of exercise in the life of the individual is considered of increasing importance. In a study done by Dorris and Stunkard,[19] the activities of 15 women of normal weight were matched to the activities of 15 obese women. The obese women walked less than half as much as their nonobese controls. This aversion to activity appears to develop after the onset of obesity. Oddly enough, the obese women in estimating their activites, however, indicated that they were as active as or even more active than the nonobese women.

The body types that are most conducive to obesity have been studied. Seltzer and Mayer[20] did research based on the somatotype classification of body-build differentiations (used widely in medical research); their research indicated that obesity does not occur in all varieties of physical types and is found more frequently in some types than others. Conclusions were that obese adolescent girls tended to be more endomorphic (softness and roundness), somewhat less mesomorphic (a combination of bone and muscle development), and considerably less ectomorphic (linearity, fragility, thinness, and slenderliness). These same somatotypic traits were found among women.

These are some of the major physiological considerations that have been advanced in relation to obesity. Some of these studies are still in a hypothetical stage. No doubt other physiological reasons are yet to be unearthed in current and future research projects.

Psychological Theories

There is considerable evidence that psychological factors may play a role in obesity. It has been found that many obese persons eat food to derive certain types of satisfactions or to compensate for certain personality lacks. The overweight girl who is not socially acceptable may appease her discomfiture and ego by indulging in rich desserts or some other type of unwise eating. Persons who are undergoing tensions, such as fear, boredom, or frustration, may find that eating seems to relieve the situation. The individual who lacks affection, recognition, or the fulfillment of other emotional needs may turn to food as a solace.

Other psychological aspects of eating can lead to overweight. Eating itself may satisfy a simple need for pleasure. For individuals who have been hungry at one time or another, food represents a change of fortune and consequently is indulged in to the hilt. To many, elaborate meals or a good family table are the symbols of financial security and social status. Naturally, these attitudes can lead to the consumption of more food than is needed.

Bruch[21] categorizes psychological influences related to obesity as (1) factors that played a role in the development of obesity, (2) problems created by the obese state, and (3) tension and conflicts precipitated by efforts to reduce weight. Traumatic or less dramatic events in the lives of individuals may lead to the onset of obesity. The loss of a loved one, subjection to war, crises, or crime are examples. Loneliness, separation from family, failures in school or in personal relationships, or family conflicts may be contributing factors. Failure of the family to recognize a child's individual needs or to respect the urge for self-expression can facilitate the onset of excess weight.

Problems of the obese state lead to an un-

[18] Ann M. Lawrence, "Obesity—New Happening," *Food and Nutrition News*, Vol. 43, Nos. 8–9 (May–June 1972), pp. 1, 4.

[19] R. J. Dorris and A. J. Stunkard, "Physical Activity: Performance and Attitudes of a Group of Obese Women," *American Journal of Medical Science*, Vol. 233, No. 6 (June 1957), pp. 622–628.

[20] Carl C. Seltzer and Jean Mayer, "Body Build (Somatotype) Distinctiveness in Obese Women," *Journal of the American Dietetic Association*, Vol. 55, No. 5 (November 1969), pp. 454–458.

[21] Hilde Bruch, "Psychological Implications of Obesity," *Nutrition News*, Vol. 35, No. 3 (October 1972), pp. 9, 12.

wholesome self-concept and poor body image. Many of these individuals are quite dependent upon others. Obese adolescents and adults whose excess weight emerged in childhood are especially vulnerable to rejection. Reduction of weight may bring even greater unhappiness and emptiness. Individuals who became obese as adults are inclined to be more objective and less self-derogatory.

However, individuals do vary and inflexible categories are not advisable. Bruch cites a study, for example, of a follow-up of development into adulthood of a large group of fat children from a pediatric clinic. There was a wide variation in self-concept and overall adjustment. An accepting and encouraging attitude from their families helped to develop a good self-concept and a positive body image. This healthy adaptation included an ability to maintain control over their weight, but often at a level above average. Those adults who had shown signs of emotional disturbances in childhood or who had been associated with serious problems and conflicts among family members did poorly in regard to weight and adjustment. They suffered excessively from the cultural attitude of rejection. Many in this group became psychiatric patients. Bruch emphasizes the importance of assessing the functional significance of abnormal weight to each individual in relation to his total development.

Stunkard and Mendelson[22] maintain that only two forms of neurotic behavior seem specifically related to obesity—overeating and disturbance of the body image. Individuals may overeat because they react more strongly to visual, taste, or food-related cues.[23] Some obese persons are quite disturbed about their body image. This concept, according to Stunkard and Mendelson, is indicated in descriptions of feelings when they look at themselves. Typical comments are related to hatred of self or avoidance of looking at self in a store window or mirror. Others can take an objective view of their appearance. Factors that contribute to a predisposition for disturbed body image are the age of onset of obesity, presence of neurosis, and how the individual's parents evaluated the child's obesity. Disturbed body images do not remain stable but fluctuate widely in intensity even for short periods of time. Body image disturbances may linger even after successful weight reduction.

Spark[24] reviewed some of the studies that explored possible reasons for the increased hunger experienced by many obese individuals. In one experiment,[25] lean and obese subjects were instructed to come to the laboratory without lunch or dinner, depending upon the time of the experiment. On arrival, one half of the group were fed sandwiches. All participants were told that the purpose of the study was to evaluate several types of crackers and to rate them appropriately as to taste qualities. Subjects were told to help themselves to as many crackers as they wanted. The rating of crackers was only a device to secure information about the number of crackers consumed by the lean and by the obese subjects. Results indicated that the lean subjects who had not been served sandwiches ate more crackers than the lean participants who had previously consumed sandwiches. However, the obese subjects who had and who did not have sandwiches ate the same number of crackers. Spark concluded that "the obese do not know when they are hungry or when they are full."

In this same study by Schachter the effect of a fear stimulus on eating was studied. Generally, fear inhibits eating behavior. When the lean and obese subjects were subjected to a fear-provoking stimulus, the lean subjects decreased food consumption while the obese subjects ate the same amount or slightly more food than in a neutral emotional situation.

Until these emotional problems can be alleviated, there is considerable evidence that little permanent progress can be made in

[22] Albert Stunkard and Myer Mendelson, "Disturbances of Body Image in Some Obese Persons," *Journal of the American Dietetic Association*, Vol. 38, No. 4 (April 1961), pp. 328–331.

[23] "Cues Affecting Eating Behavior and Obesity," *Nutrition Reviews*, Vol. 27, No. 1 (January 1969), pp. 11–14.

[24] Richard F. Spark, "Fat Americans," *The New York Times Magazine*, January 6, 1974, pp. 10, 41–43, 50–51.

[25] S. Schacter, "Obesity and Eating," *Science*, Vol. 161, No. 8 (August 1968), pp. 751–756.

weight reduction. The intensity of the problem will bear a direct relationship here. Authorities indicate that obesity originating in childhood, with an emotional problem as at least one of its bases, is more difficult to handle than obesity occurring later in life. For that reason, an early diagnosis and treatment of emotional problems to prevent this situation are important.

Environmental Theories About Obesity

Modern living has a conspicuous influence on weight. The fact that food is freely available to many people in America has a direct bearing on the development of obesity. When food is sufficient, people can become fat from eating large amounts of porterhouse steaks as easily as by consuming fatback and corn bread.

The environment abounds with inducements to buy and to eat food. Television and radio commercials have many lures. Magazines and newspapers offer pages of advertisements as well as pages of recipes, and, in the case of magazines, many articles and advertisements with four-color pictures of tempting dishes.

Food is very important to most Americans.

Thus there is great probability of becoming obese. Our food markets provide many incentives. All too often a homemaker or other member of the family with a shopping list will emerge from the store with many extras that he or she could not resist. There is no question but that many families today are buying much more food than they need for energy purposes.

The conditions under which people have to eat meals away from home sometimes makes it difficult for them to control their weight. The choice of fruits and vegetables on many restaurant and cafeteria menus is usually limited. Corn, which is actually a cereal, is frequently served in addition to potatoes as the extra vegetable, for example. When lunch has to be eaten away from home, sometimes the only foods available are desserts and sandwiches. Also the person who works odd hours may add extra meals in order to eat with his family or may make other adjustments, and consequently consume more food.

The spectator role in sports and general disinclination to participate in physical activity contribute to the obesity syndrome. The concentration of the population in cities that afford little opportunity for exercise is another contributing factor.

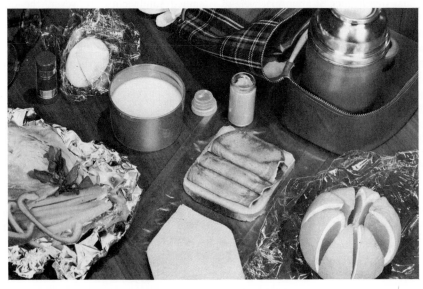

FIGURE 10–2. *A low kcalorie lunch can be appetizing.* (Everywoman's Family Circle Magazine)

Certain ethnic groups take pride in setting a lavish table. Sociability, with the concomitant high kcaloric refreshments and alcoholic beverages that contribute considerable kcalories, can be a hazard.

If the family diet tends to stress foods that are high in kcalories, it is logical to assume that the intake may exceed the need for energy purposes. Sometimes a father urges members of his family to eat well so that his role of a good provider will be reflected. Sometimes a mother's reputation for being a good cook is reflected in extra poundage in her family members.

Sheer ignorance of food values is often the cause of overeating. Again and again individuals will comment that their diet has not varied, yet suddenly they have gained a great deal of weight. Actually, upon examination, it proves that they have indulged in malted milks, candy, rich desserts, or some other food that they did not realize was high in kcalories.

People are not only unaware of food values, but they may also be addicted to food fads or fallacies. The eat-all-you-want kind of reducing diets certainly leaves much to be desired and gives false impressions. Some persons, for example, will eat the food that they regularly consume, plus certain foods that are advertised as having reducing qualities.

The frequency of eating or the consumption of one half of the day's kcalories at one meal has no correlation to the degree of body fatness.[26] However, the habit of overeating in the evening[27] appears more frequently among the obese than among the nonobese.

Obesity in Childhood and Adolescence

Obesity in childhood and adolescence is particularly important. A significant percentage of obese youngsters become obese adults— one of the most difficult groups to treat. The damaging physiological and psychological effects are equally deserving of attention.

The interest in childhood and adolescent obesity has been accelerated with the realization that increased numbers of fat cells can occur in the first 3 years of life and during early adolescence, according to Hirsch,[28] as discussed at the Conference on Childhood Obesity. Mayer[29] of Harvard University emphasized that certain body types are inherited, so a genetic component to obesity must be considered. If neither parent is obese, there is only a 7 per cent chance of a child being obese. If one parent is obese, the chance is 40 per cent; if both parents are obese, the chance increases to 80 per cent. Mayer grants that environmental factors are also important, but as physical activity is not highly prized in our society, the genetic potential for obesity has greater opportunity to be expressed. Physical activity is the most important environmental variable affecting obesity, according to this authority. This concept about physical activity has been reenforced in the 1974 dietary recommendations for energy[30] for children, which are less than United Nations Food and Agriculture/World Health Organization recommendations for children, because American children are on the whole less active than children in other parts of the world.

Mayer also discussed the psychological consequences of being a fat child. Such a child often suffers from social rejection. These social pressures have been reflected in psychological testing in which obese children had a profile similar to other children who suffer from prejudice and discrimination.

Felix P. Heald,[31] Professor of Pediatrics at the University of Maryland School of Medicine, in his discussion at the conference of child and adolescent obesity, noted peak

---

[26] E. J. Hutson et al., "Measures of Body Fat and Related Factors in Normal Adults. III. Diet and Physical Activity." *Journal of the American Dietetic Association*, Vol. 47, No. 2 (February 1965), pp. 179–186.

[27] Albert J. Stunkard, W. J. Grace, and H. G. Wolff, "The Night-Eating Syndrome: Pattern of Food Intake Among Obese Patients," *American Journal of Medicine*, Vol. 19, No. 1 (July 1955), pp. 55–86.

[28] Winick, op. cit., p. 8.

[29] Winick, op. cit., p. 9.

[30] Food and Nutrition Board, *Recommended Dietary Allowances*, 8th ed. National Academy of Sciences—National Research Council, Washington, D.C., 1974, p. 33.

[31] Winick, op. cit., p. 9.

periods of obesity in children—infancy, early childhood around 6 years of age, and adolescence. Upon entering adolescence, two patterns are noted in obesity. One is a distinct family history of obesity among girls that begins in infancy. The other is no family history but the occurrence of a specific stressful experience.

While obese adolescents are usually taller than their peers and their skeletal age is beyond their body age, they grow up to be less tall adults. Puberty comes earlier, and there is a question of the psychological effect of shortening childhood by 1 year. Weight reduction must occur slowly to prevent interference with growth. Treatment then becomes difficult. Prevention is preferred to weight reduction later.

A further concern is the relation of the fat content of a child's diet and the hyperlipidemias (excessive amount of lipids in the blood) found so commonly in adult populations and also among children and adolescents. The family and individual lifestyles, including diet, are a critical factor. A. K. Khachadurian,[32] Professor of Medicine at Rutgers Medical School, in his discussion noted that the most common type of hyperlipidemia found in children was hypercholesterolemia, with plasma cholesterol in the children he treated approximately four times above normal. As these children grow older, dietary treatment becomes less effective.

Glen Friedman,[33] a practicing pediatrician on the faculty of the University of Arizona, contended that reducing risk factors related to coronary heart disease should begin during childhood because patterns of living that lead to risk factors emerge at that time. Parents may reduce risk factors, too. Atherosclerosis can develop in the pediatric age and may be "irreversible" in this age group.

Jerome Knittle,[34] Professor of Pediatrics at Mount Sinai School of Medicine in New York City, indicated at the conference that only when dietary treatment is begun early can the number of fat cells be altered. Children who have too many fat cells for their age, but still fewer than a normal number for adults, have a better chance to avoid obesity. The goal is to slow down the rate of fat cell division while attempting to maintain normal growth. If children have already acquired the adult number of fat cells, the situation is serious.

Huenemann[35] identified the child environmental factors associated with the development of obesity. Factors found for 6-month-old infants in comparison with leanness were more rapid weight gain since birth, lower birth weight, primary birth order, a trend to greater kcalorie consumption (but not statistically significant), obesity of the mother, less nutrition knowledge on the part of the mother, and a less conventional lifestyle.

A follow-up study of these 6-month-old infants at the age of three years provided a number of conclusions. The first 6 months of life may be a vulnerable period for the development of obesity. Lifestyle is significantly associated with obesity. Many mothers had become aware of obesity prevention and control and of the desirability of implementing practices to prevent excessive weight, such as appreciation of food and physical activity control, a trend toward breast feeding, and a generally good nutrient intake among the young children.

Peckos[36] has described the potentials of a summer camp for assisting teen-agers to lose weight and to develop sound nutritional habits. The campers were 11- to 18-year-old overweight teen-agers. A wide variety of commonly available foods was served. Portion control of all foods was taught in preference to "forbidden foods." In this way campers learned how to handle high kcaloric foods and still lose or maintain their weight. Parental involvement was encouraged. Physical activity was included, but campers were helped to face the actual

[32] Winick, op. cit., p. 20.

[33] Winick, op. cit., p. 11.

[34] Winick, op. cit., p. 12.

[35] Ruth L. Huenemann, "Environmental Factors Associated with Preschool Obesity, I. Obesity in Six-Month-Old Children and II. Obesity and Food Practices of Children at Successive Age Levels," *Journal of the American Dietetic Association*, Vol. 64, No. 5 (May 1974), pp. 480–491.

[36] Penelope S. Peckos, "The Teenage Obesity Problem—Why," *Food and Nutrition News*, Vol. 42, Nos. 5–6 (February–March 1971), pp. 1, 4.

potential for activity in their lives and to adjust their diet accordingly.

Problems of Overweight

Often the image of a fat person is a jolly, easy-going, and very friendly individual. Occasionally such derogatory attributes as being lazy and slow or dull and uninteresting are conceived. Actually, it is questionable whether obese individuals are contented with their physical state.

Women on the whole are much more sensitive to obesity than men are.

The reason for women having a greater concern about their weight is that physical appearance is much more important to a woman than to a man. Women's clothes reveal figure defects, such as overweight, much more readily than men's attire. In other words, fashion designers have sometimes motivated a desirable weight pattern to a greater degree than have health educators.

Health and Obesity

The idea that excess weight has a deleterious effect on health was noted as early as 400 B.C. by Hippocrates. Shakespeare commented on it also in his play *Henry IV*. Present-day information about the relation of overweight to health has come largely from life insurance statistics. The Metropolitan Life Insurance Company[37] made an extensive analysis of 250,000 life histories of persons insured by their company. They demonstrated that length of life and the incidence of a number of degenerative diseases were associated with overweight. The length of life had an inverse ratio to the degree of overweight. This fact has led to the statement, "The longer the belt line, the shorter the life line." Actual statistics reveal that individuals who are 10 to 25 pounds overweight showed a 5 per cent increase in mortality; those 25 to 40 pounds overweight showed a 31 per cent increase in mortality; those 45 to 60 pounds overweight showed a 44 per cent in-

crease; 60 to 80 pounds, a 65 per cent increase; and 80 pounds and over, a 123 per cent increase.

Four types of health hazards are associated with obesity, according to *Obesity and Health*. They are

1. Changes in various normal bodily functions.
2. Increased risk of developing certain diseases.
3. Detrimental effects on diseases already established.
4. Adverse psychological reactions.

Changes, at least transitory, have been reported of practically every body function in obese individuals. Obesity may not only be a causal factor but also a coexisting one. Certain disorders appear frequently in the obese, such as respiratory disorders and difficulty in breathing. The more excess adipose tissue present, the greater the problem of adequately oxygenating the blood that has to supply this extra tissue. Obese individuals apparently experience more respiratory infections than the nonobese.

Another disturbance in body function is that carbon dioxide accumulates in the blood more readily, causing lethargy. Red blood cells tend to be produced in greater numbers, causing a ruddy complexion. Problems of blood clotting and a predilection to thrombosis are associated with obesity.

Obesity does not have a direct effect on the normal functioning of the heart, yet there is incidence of cardiac enlargement and congestive heart failure. Elevated blood pressure is associated with increased body weight, but the nature of this situation is not clear. Studies do show that more hypertension exists among the obese than among the nonobese.[38] Obese hypertensive patients experience a greater risk of coronary heart disease than the nonobese hypertensive patient. Mortality rates for obese hypertensive individuals are higher than for persons with obesity alone or hypertension

[37] *Statistical Bulletin, Metropolitan Life Insurance Company*, Vol. 41 (February–March 1960), pp. 5–8.

[38] J. Stamler, "The Early Detection of Heart Disease," *Heart Disease Control*, Continuing Educational Series No. 97, University of Michigan School of Public Health, Ann Arbor, Mich., 1962.

alone. An alarming increase in other degenerative diseases, such as diabetes, coronary artery disease, and cancer, is indicated. There appears to be a particularly strong relationship between diabetes and overweight. Joslin termed diabetes "the fat man's folly." In addition, Olson in his work at the University of Pittsburgh found a high rate of chronic illness among patients who were 25 per cent or more overweight, particularly in the middle-age years 40 to 60.

Other conditions, such as toxemias of pregnancy, chronic neuritis, and conditions of the liver, are known to be aggravated by obesity. It is also recognized that a surgeon is always apprehensive in operating upon an obese person, for operative risk and the rate of mortality increase. Arthritis has been found to be much more severe in the case of obese persons. There is an earlier appearance of varicose veins in some individuals and an increased incidence of gall bladder disease.

Overweight persons appear to be much more prone to accident. Dublin and Marks found that accidents increase at least 12 per cent. It is possible that obese individuals are clumsy and incur accidents much more frequently.

Most of these conditions increase with age. The death rate is higher, too. Someone has aptly stated that it is possible for individuals to dig their graves with their teeth. When health problems are added to psychological problems, it is easily conceived that an obese individual may have a very difficult time in life.

Symptoms of many established diseases are greatly improved by the reduction of adipose tissue. This is especially true of conditions associated with the circulatory and locomotive systems. In general, obesity is accompanied by alterations in blood pressure, serum lipids, and carbohydrate tolerance, according to Kannel.[39] Risk for coronary heart disease, atherosclerosis, and other conditions is in proportion to the degree of alteration in the above metabolic processes. The risk of developing major illness appears higher in fat persons in good health than in persons of normal weight. Psychological problems may occur at various stages in the life of an obese individual. The degree of risk cannot be accurately predicted. In all instances, the person's total health assessment is a vital factor. The complexity of obesity is obvious.

Loss of Weight

Losing weight is not easy. One has only to look around among one's friends or acquaintances and even family members to realize how many of them have tried to lose weight, have been successful for a time, and then have regained their weight. The more obese an individual is, the more difficult it generally is to lose that weight. The lesson here is that one should begin to lose weight as soon as one is aware of being obese. This is much more easily said than done. Also, some persons refuse to recognize their problem. Considering all the handicaps that confront an obese person, however, it would seem sensible to remove these excess pounds.

To lose weight, the energy intake must be less than the energy output. A pound of fat averages about 3500 kcalories. This means that an individual must oxidize 3500 kcalories of his own fat, more or less, for every pound that he wishes to lose. Through the reduction of kcalories in his diet or by increasing his energy output, this loss becomes possible.

The loss of weight is a medical problem and no individual should place himself or herself upon a reducing regimen without the advice of his doctor. Most physicians agree that the weight loss of an individual should not exceed 2 pounds per week. This means that he will have to have a diet that will allow for this energy deficiency. Since losing weight involves certain metabolic processes, it is possible that there will be fluctuations in this rate of weight loss owing primarily to changes in water balance. As the fatty tissue is used for energy, it is frequently replaced by water. Until that water can be eliminated, there may be little if any weight loss. Fatty tissue within a person varies somewhat in composition, some containing more fat and less water. This factor will influence rate of weight loss.

---

[39] William B. Kannel, "Obesity and Coronary Heart Disease," The Framingham Heart Study, *Nutrah* (American Heart Association), Vol. 1, No. 3 (March 1973), pp. 1-4.

Nutritional Needs During Weight Loss

A diet for weight loss should be adequate in all areas of nutrition except kcalories. The number of kcalories prescribed on such a diet will depend on the physician's advice. Many self-prescribed reducing diets are too low in kcalories. If the kcaloric intake becomes extremely low, then it is difficult to include an adequate amount of other nutrients.

The following foods should be included every day[40]:

MILK AND MILK PRODUCTS One pint, 600 cc or more, of skim milk is important. If the kcalories are to be only slightly reduced, then it is possible to have a pint of whole milk. Cream should be avoided. Pot, skim milk, or farmer cottage cheese is an excellent source of protein. Other cheeses that are high in fat should be omitted or substituted for meat. For children under 9 years, 2 to 3 cups (600 to 900 cc) of milk are required; for children 9 to 12 years, 3 or more cups (900 cc or more); and for teen-agers, 4 or more cups (1200 cc or more). For young children, the physician will determine if the milk should be whole or skim.

BREADS AND CEREALS At least four servings a day should be included. They may be chosen from ½ cup of cold or cooked cereal, a slice of whole-grain or enriched bread, ½ cup of enriched macaroni, spaghetti, or rice, or two or three crackers, depending on the size. Weight varies with the type of cereal; cold cereal is about 13 to 15 g and cooked cereal around 120 g for ½ cup. If this amount is not included, there is grave danger of a lack of thiamin, other B vitamins, and iron.

FRUITS AND VEGETABLES At least two to three servings of fruit should be included every day. Emphasis should be on at least one serving of a citrus fruit or tomato juice. Fruit should be fresh, frozen, or canned without the addition of sugar. Water-packed canned fruits can be easily obtained and will add variety to the diet. At least one serving of the fruit should be uncooked. Vegetables will add fiber and give a filling aspect to a reducing diet. Two or three generous servings of vegetables or salad greens are suggested. Watery or green vegetables such as asparagus, broccoli, Brussels sprouts, cabbage, cauliflower, celery, cucumber, escarole, eggplant, all types of greens, radishes, sauerkraut, Swiss chard, spinach, summer squash, young tender green beans, tomatoes, and vegetable juices are the best choices. Some vegetables are much higher in kcalories and the amount should be limited to ½ cup per day; these include beets, carrots, onions, winter squash, turnips, and parsnips. Vegetables that should be eaten in very small quantities are beans (except string beans), corn, peas, and lentils. Potatoes should be small and not covered with gravy or fat.

MEAT, FISH, POULTRY, AND EGGS At least one to two servings a day. Five to six ounces of meat, fish, or poultry should be allowed. Dark-colored flesh, such as in mackerel or blue fish, should be avoided. Emphasis should be placed on light-colored flesh, such as in haddock, cod, halibut, or perch. Salt pork and bacon should be omitted. Meats should be broiled, braised, or boiled, but not fried. Three or four eggs each week are suggested. They may be prepared in any way except fried. In the case of poultry, allowances should be made for the bones. Canned fish such as salmon or sardines may be used if most of the oil is poured off. If meat is not eaten, cheese, additional milk, and eggs may be substituted. Dry beans, dry peas, and nuts, including peanut butter, may be used as alternates occasionally. On a strict vegetarian diet there is a problem of reconciling fewer kcalories and adequate protein because of the large servings of legumes and nuts required. Meat dripping should be omitted.

A diet that supplies nutrients similar to those of the normal diet but that is lower in total kcalories can accomplish satisfactory weight loss, is acceptable over a long period of time, and serves as a basis for establishing good food habits for weight maintenance. Other advantages to using the four food groups are the utilization of common foods, flexible allow-

---

[40] Louise Page and Lillian J. Fincher, *Food and Your Weight*, Home and Garden Bulletin No. 74, U.S. Department of Agriculture, Washington, D.C., 1971.

ances in planning, and the possibility for recognizing personal food preferences. Moreover, cost may be controlled in food selection and adjustments can be easily made in size of servings for persons of different ages, sizes, and activities. Recognition of familial patterns, economic status, usual eating patterns, and the intelligence of the person responsible for the preparation of the meals are other considerations. Educating the obese person so that he understands the nature of his condition and learns the kcaloric content of various foods according to portion is imperative. For example, ½ cup of fresh cherries has 58 kcalories, a scant ½ cup of canned cherries in heavy syrup has 89 kcalories, and a piece of cherry pie has 418 kcalories. These differences highlight the effect of food preparation on caloric value.

Although bizarre plans for the reduction of weight that underemphasize certain nutrients and overemphasize other nutrients as well as promote specific foods may have appeal, they are of dubious value and may be dangerous. It is extremely important that there be adequate carbohydrate in a diet for the loss of weight. It is essential for the metabolism of fat. When insufficient carbohydrate is not available, then certain bodies that are remnants of the unburned fat known as acetone bodies accumulate in the blood. This can result in a very serious condition. Large amounts of fat in a reducing diet must also be avoided, for the body is using its own fat for additional energy purposes. If the body has to metabolize large amounts of fat in the diet as well as body fat, then the possibility for acetone bodies in the blood, which may result in ketosis, is naturally much greater.

For individuals who are fond of food, a reducing diet may appear to be sheer punishment. However, there are many ways of making the food in such a diet palatable and interesting.

The use of liquid formula diets that provide exact amounts of kcalories and nutrients has the advantage of requiring no knowledge of foods and their nutritive content; still, there are serious shortcomings. There is no opportunity to develop desirable food habits and

the diet can become highly monotonous. Such side effects as constipation, due to lack of bulk, or diarrhea have been indicated.[41]

Starvation has been used as therapy for grossly obese patients. Because of the potential of a health hazard, this treatment is extremely limited and undertaken only in a hospital under the close supervision of a physician. Safeguards must be observed for prevention of ketosis, loss of lean body tissue, loss of nitrogen, phosphorus, calcium, potassium, sodium, B vitamins, and water. These undesirable losses accompany the loss of fat. The cost is questionable. Should a person who is still growing undertake fasting? What are the possible psychological effects? What are the long-term consequences? These and other questions have not been answered. Although there may be such discomforts as headaches, weakness, or nausea during starvation, hunger sensations subside quickly, according to Swendseid.

Salt restriction is not recommended unless advised by the physician. Haphazard omission of salt in the diet may lead to disturbed water balance in the body.

Exercise and Weight Reduction

Mayer[42] believes that too little attention has been given to the role of exercise in the reduction of weight as well as in weight maintenance. Violent exercise for a person who has had sedentary habits is questionable. And it is true that considerable exercise is required to remove a substantial number of pounds.

However, Mayer suggests that consideration be given to forms of exercise that a person might do with little inconvenience. Individuals who have tried to belittle exercise in weight reduction have commented that it is necessary to walk for 36 miles to remove 1 pound of fat or to split wood for 7 hours or

---

[41] Marian E. Swendseid, "The Metabolic Response to Starvation in Obesity," *Nutrition News*, Vol. 29, No. 2 (April, 1966), pp. 1, 4.

[42] Jean Mayer, *Human Nutrition*, Charles C Thomas, Springfield, Ill., 1972, pp. 393–394, 397–398.

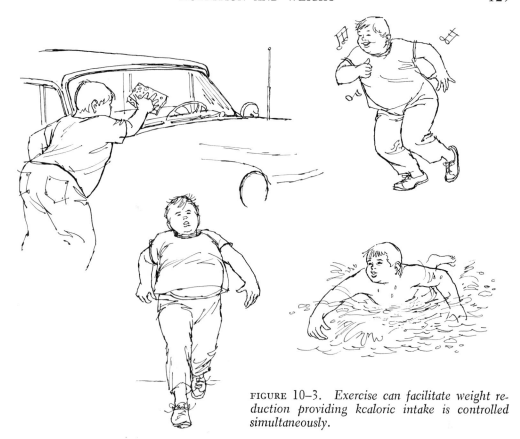

FIGURE 10–3. *Exercise can facilitate weight reduction providing kcaloric intake is controlled simultaneously.*

to play volley ball for 11 hours. One does not need to perform these physical activities at one time. To walk for 36 miles is unreasonable. To walk for 1 mile, however, would mean that 1/36 of a pound of fat would be needed for energy purposes.

Mayer is also very quick to dispel the commonly held misconception that exercise whets the appetite so that individuals will actually eat more. An accumulation of considerable evidence indicates that this is not true. The relation of appetite to exercise is somewhat questionable. Certainly, inactivity does not reduce appetite. Individuals who have taken a long sea voyage can vouch for the fact that although they may be comparatively inactive they are ready to eat whenever food is served.

A definite plan for some form of daily exercise is worthy of consideration. Not only would it aid in the reducing process, but it

would do much to aid in the maintenance of weight, and help to maintain or develop firm muscle tone and skin as weight loss progresses.

Planning the Weight-Loss Regimen

To lose weight cannot be a casual matter. A definite plan for action subject to a physician's advice and approval is necessary. Sufficient time to accomplish goals is important. All too often a woman will decide to follow a "crash" diet and lose all excess weight within a week in order to wear a particular dress to some social function or for some other personal reason. Hundreds of articles, pamphlets, and books have been directed to this purpose and yet the overall results are somewhat discouraging.

People must realize that the outcome is in their own hands and success cannot depend on others. Adjustments have to be made. Vegetables may be removed from the pan before sauces, butter, or other ingredients are added. A portion of the salad bowl may be removed before the salad dressing is added. Some families keep a fruit bowl on the table, and the dieter may take fruit instead of the high-kcaloric dessert that may be offered.

If the family feels strongly that the individual should partake of the food served, then it might be well to reduce the size of the servings and to compensate by low-kcaloric foods at other meals eaten away from home. In addition, snacks and other ways of adding kcalories should be limited. It is certainly possible to avoid extra amounts of bread and butter, some sauces, and rich desserts. If possible, the cooperation of the family should be encouraged.

Maintenance of Weight

One of the problems that has been of great concern to physicians and researchers in the area of obesity is that individuals frequently do not maintain their weight after they have reduced. This fact is not easily explained and is generally due to complex reasons. If a psychological problem has not been remedied, then an individual may return to overeating as a form of compensation. Many people believe that once they have lost the desired number of pounds they can eat anything they wish. Anyone who was overweight cannot go back to former eating habits and expect to maintain a desirable weight. This fact is sometimes difficult to face. Individuals must learn that new food habits will have to be acquired and maintained. One must realize also that his smaller size demands fewer kcalories. For example, a man at 190 needs 2800 kcalories, but at 150 pounds he needs only 2300 kcalories. If an individual eats heavily at one meal, some compensation must be made for it at a later meal. Also, when an individual realizes he or she is gaining weight, food habits should be changed as soon as possible. The reduced person must allow himself only 2 to 3 pounds leeway to maintain new weight. There may be other important reasons why it is so difficult to maintain this desired weight.

A problem that is even more serious than maintaining a desirable weight is that of the individual who is an on–off dieter. Olson[43] has reported that the fitful dieter, particularly the one who tries to lose weight rapidly, can set off recurrences of rheumatic fever and asthma, precipitate attacks of gout, flare ups of thyroid disease, or even coronary attacks. "On and off" dieting has been known to lead to severe mental depression and even addiction to alcohol. Weakness, dizziness, and even reactivating latent tuberculosis are other results.

Bruch[44] makes a number of valuable suggestions about maintenance of weight. A well-established routine for weight reduction, such as regular weighings, a knowledge of nutrition that is applied to the planning of daily food intake, and a positive attitude are helpful in the achievement of acceptable food and living patterns in the maintenance of weight. Some who have difficulty in maintaining weight might well examine if they are attempting to lose weight that is not compatible with their body build or healthful living. Accepting a sensible weight may be part of the battle. Obesity can be a lifetime problem.

Individuals are often unaware of the continuous attraction of food around them and their seeming helplessness to avoid eating it. Behavior modification may be helpful,[45] such as confining all eating to a designated table. Keeping daily records of the amount, kind, time, and circumstances of eating may provide insights about one's patterns. One man, for example, found that many extra kcalories were consumed during his evening snacking because he was bored. Other techniques are counting each mouthful of food during a meal, placing utensils on the plate after every second or third mouthful, or planning short interruptions during mealtime—all of which may assist in

[43] Robert E. Olson, "Obesity as a Nutritional Disorder," Federation Proceedings, Vol. 18, No. 2, Part I (July 1959), pp. 58–67.

[44] Hilde Bruch, Eating Disorders, Basic Books, New York, 1973, Chap. 16.

[45] S. Penick, R. Filion, S. Fox, and Albert J. Stunkard, "Behavior Modification in the Treatment of Obesity," Psychosomatic Medicine, Vol. 33, No. 1 (January 1971), pp. 49–55.

developing control of food consumption. Further studies are needed, particularly on the long-range effects of these forms of behavioral modification.

Bruch cites that certain group methods tend to alleviate the dreariness of dieting alone. American-type spas, reducing salons, and programs, such as Weight Watchers and TOPS, have been a means of finding congenial company for losing weight. In the Weight Watchers program, the dietary advice seems sound and is given in interesting and sufficient detail. Stunkard[46] found TOPS to compare favorably with contrasting groups in medical clinics. Bruch believes that these programs are less helpful to the obese with complex psychological problems. Also, information about the effectiveness of these programs in the maintenance of weight would be valuable.

It is the hope of experts in the field that some help can be given to individuals who succumb to erratic reducing and regaining of weight, as well as to those who have difficulty in maintaining weight.

Underweight

Sometimes underweight individuals bemoan the fact that all the attention is given to overweight individuals and little information is available for them. Many of the ideas suggested here for obese individuals will operate for underweights in reverse.

One of the serious difficulties of underweight persons is that very often they lack an appetite and are not interested in food. Furthermore, they may have their strong likes among foods that are low in kcaloric value. An underweight individual should have a complete physical checkup and should be advised by the physician. Excessive fatigue, some type of infection, or other disturbances may be the real cause. If possible, underweight persons should concentrate on having an adequate diet, that is, all nutrients present in required amounts, and with emphasis on high-kcaloric foods.

Increasing the size of servings or adding sauces, salad dressings, and the like to foods will do much to add kcalories. In-between feedings of food that do not deter the appetite for the next meal are advisable. In some cases physicians recommend a number of small feedings since such a person may be reluctant to eat large amounts of food at one sitting. A rather large snack at bedtime has been successful in many cases. This should consist of foods that are high in kcalories but are easily digested so that sleep will not suffer interference. It might include such foods as malted milk shakes, crackers, or plain cookies. Crackers may be spread with peanut butter, jelly, or the like. Some individuals have managed to tolerate a simple sandwich with milk and perhaps a piece of fruit.

Fortifying foods may be another way of adding kcalories. For example, instead of drinking plain whole milk, it may be fortified with a considerable amount, say up to ¾ or 1 cup per quart, of dried skim milk. Drinking half cream and half milk may be another suggestion. Quick breads, mashed potatoes, milk desserts, and the like are other foods that may be fortified with extra dried skim milk. Since many high-kcaloric foods are lacking in texture, it is well that sufficient fruits and vegetables be added for variety in the diet as well as for important nutrients.

Care must be taken that foods are not drowned with heavy sauces or dressings. It is especially important that foods be attractive and palatable so that an underweight person will be interested in eating them. Those that are too sweet or too high in fat may discourage appetite and must be watched carefully.

Sometimes the mental health of such an individual needs to be improved. Having outside interests and doing everything to avoid an intense preoccupation with oneself may do a great deal to improve eating habits. A person who is underweight also needs to rest and to conserve energy in every possible way. This does not mean that exercise is to be avoided. A brisk walk may do a great deal to build morale and to add zest to eating. A certain amount of fat is necessary for the padding

46 Albert J. Stunkard, H. Levine, and S. Fox, "The Management of Obesity, Patient Self-help and Medical Treatment," *Archives of Internal Medicine*, Vol. 125, No. 6 (June 1970), pp. 1067–1072.

of vital organs. Individuals sometimes have a fallen stomach or fallen kidney because there is insufficient fat to hold them in place. An extremely thin person has the same difficulty with clothes that the overweight one does. These individuals may not be as attractive as they could be, and may encounter the same problems as the obese in finding a job or in gaining social approval.

Physicians, as a rule, are not so concerned about underweight if the person has a desirable food pattern, enjoys good health, and has a positive mental attitude toward life.

In regard to weight, Americans will probably always have a greater concern for excess pounds rather than too few pounds.

SELECTED REFERENCES

Bray, G. A., "The Myth of Diet in the Management of Diet," *American Journal of Clinical Nutrition*, Vol. 23, No. 9 (September 1970), pp. 1141–1148.

Bruch, Hilde, *Eating Disorders, Obesity, Anorexia Nervosa, and the Person Within*, Basic Books, Inc., New York, 1973.

Dwyer, Johanna, "Who Is Concerned About Weight?" *Journal of Nutrition Education*, Vol. 1, No. 4 (Spring 1970), p. 16.

———, and Jean Mayer, "Potential Dieters: Who Are They? Attitudes Toward Body Weight and Dieting Behavior," *Journal of the American Dietetics Association*, Vol. 56, No. 6 (June 1970), pp. 510–514.

———, Jacob J. Feldman, and Jean Mayer, "The Social Psychology of Dieting," *Mental Health Digest*, Vol. 3, No. 5 (May 1971), pp. 1–13.

"Effects of Meal Frequency During Weight Reduction," *Nutrition Reviews*, Vol. 30, No. 7 (July 1972), pp. 158–162.

Finkelstein, B., and B. A. Fryer, "Meal Frequency and Weight Reduction of Young Women," *American Journal of Clinical Nutrition*, Vol. 24, No. 4 (April 1971), pp. 465–468.

Jordan, Henry A., "In Defense of Body Weight," *Journal of the American Dietetics Association*, Vol. 62, No. 1 (January 1973), pp. 17–21.

Jourdan, Martin H., and Robert B. Bradfield, "Body Composition Changes During Weight Loss Estimated from Energy, Nitrogen, Sodium, and Potassium Balances," *American Journal of Clinical Nutrition*, Vol. 26, No. 2 (February 1973), pp. 144–149.

Lewis, Kathleen J., and Margaret D. Doyle, "Nutrient Intake and Weight Response of Women on Weight-Control Diets," *Journal of the American Dietetics Association*, Vol. 56, No. 2 (February 1970), pp. 119–125.

Linton, P. H., M. Conley, C. Kuechenmeister, and H. McClusky, "Satiety and Obesity," *American Journal of Clinical Nutrition*, Vol. 25, No. 4 (April 1972), pp. 368–370.

Mayer, Jean, "Obesity," in Robert S. Goodhart and Maurice E. Shils (eds.), *Modern Nutrition in Health and Disease*, Lea & Febiger, Philadelphia, 1973, Chapter 22.

Mead, Margaret, "Why Do We Overeat?" *Redbook*, Vol. 140, No. 9 (January 1971), pp. 28–30.

Schauf, George E., "All Calories Don't Count—Perhaps," *Nutrition Today*, Vol. 6, No. 5 (September–October 1971), pp. 16–24.

Seltzer, Carl C., and Jean Mayer, "An Effective Weight Control Program in a Public School System," *American Journal of Public Health*, Vol. 60, No. 4 (April 1970), pp. 679–689.

Sohar, Ezra, and Ephraim Sneh, "Follow-up of Obese Patients: 14 Years After a Successful Reducing Diet," *American Journal of Clinical Nutrition*, Vol. 26, No. 8 (August 1973), pp. 845–848.

Spark, Richard F., "Fat Americans," *The New York Times Magazine*, January 6, 1974, pp. 10, 42–43, 50–52.

Stunkard, Albert J., "The Obese: Background and Programs," in Jean Mayer (ed.), *U.S. Nutrition Policies in the Seventies*, W. H. Freeman and Company, San Francisco, 1973, Chapter 3.

Thomas, Donald W., and Jean Mayer, "The Search for the Secret of Fat," *Psychology Today*, Vol. 7, No. 4 (September 1973), pp. 74–79.

Van Itallie, Theodore B., and Robert G. Campbell, "Multidisciplinary Approach to the Problem of Obesity," *Journal of the American Dietetic Association*, Vol. 61, No. 4 (October 1972), pp. 385–390.

Winick, Myron, "Childhood Obesity," *Nutrition Today*, Vol. 9, No. 3 (May–June 1974), pp. 6–12.

Wooley, O. W., S. C. Wooley, and R. B. Dunham, "Can Calories Be Perceived and Do They Affect Hunger in Obese and Non-Obese Humans?" *Journal of Comparative and Physiological Psychology*, Vol. 80, No. 2 (February 1972), pp. 250–258.

Worthington, Bonnie S., and Lynda E. Taylor, "Balanced Low-Calorie vs. High-Protein–Low-Carbohydrate Reducing Diets," *Journal of the American Dietetic Association*, Vol. 64, No. 1 (January 1974), pp. 47–51.

Young, Charlotte M., Sonia S. Scanlan, Hae Sook Im, and Leo Lutwak, "Effect on Body Composition and Other Parameters in Obese Young Men of Carbohydrate Level of Reduction Diet," *American Journal of Clinical Nutrition*, Vol. 24, No. 3 (March 1971), pp. 290–296.

———, "Overnutrition," in Miloslav Rechcigl, Jr. (ed.), *Food, Nutrition, and Health*, Vol. 16, S. Karger, Basel, 1973, pp. 179–186.

11

An Overview of Vitamins

Nutrition has frequently been called a "twentieth-century science." This is especially true of the study of vitamins. At the turn of the century, interest was centered upon studies of energy requirements and protein needs. The discovery and identification of the many vitamins were to occur in a brief 40-year span that followed.

Credit for noting that there was some other factor essential to health is given to Lunin, who observed in experiments in 1881 that

> mice can live well under these conditions [his experimental ones] when receiving suitable foods (e.g., milk), but as the experiments show that since they cannot subsist on proteins, fats, and carbohydrates, salts and water, it follows that other substances indispensable for nutrition must be present in milk beside casein, fat, lactose, and salts.[1]

Lunin's comment seems to have been unnoticed, for in 1905 Pekelharing showed that there was "an unknown substance in milk which even in very small quantities is of para-

mount importance to nourishment." This conclusion was reached after he had fed small amounts of whey (from milk) to mice in addition to a diet made up of those substances which at the time were considered essential. The control mice, which did not receive the additional whey, died. Pekelharing's observations were published in Dutch and were not translated into English until 1926, so the significance of his discovery was not fully realized at the time.

Hopkins, a British scientist, found similar results, and coined the phrase "accessory food factors" in 1906 for those heretofore unnamed substances essential for growth. The British used this term for many years. Studies were being conducted that would lead to the identification of specific foods containing some of the accessory food factors.

In 1912 at the Lister Institute in London, Funk, a Polish scientist, was studying the extract of rice polishings, trying to find an antiberiberi factor. He was able to isolate a substance that would prevent beriberi; hence he concluded that this substance was vital to life. Further, his preparation was an amine (a chemical structure that contained nitrogen in a specific configuration), so he named the preparation "vitamine."

[1] E. V. McCollum, *A History of Nutrition,* Houghton Mifflin, Boston, 1957, p. 204.
1881 that

134

McCollum and Davis identified the first vitamin, vitamin A, in 1915, and later showed that it was not one vitamin but two and that the second one was water-soluble rather than fat-soluble like vitamin A. The water-soluble one was named vitamin B. As time passed, further research revealed that each group was a group of vitamins, one fat-soluble and the other water-soluble.

Finally, in 1920 Drummond suggested that the "e" be dropped from the name "vitamine" as the only vitamin by that time that contained an amine was thiamine; consequently, the original spelling was inappropriate. As they were identified, vitamins were given names along the alphabetic spectrum, so to speak. They were also referred to in terms of the conditions they prevented, such as "anti-beriberi," "antiscorbutic," and "antirachitic." These latter designations were dropped gradually as it became apparent that each vitamin did much more than just prevent disease. Thus today a vitamin is called by the name that most clearly reflects its chemical structure.

General Characteristics of Vitamins

What is a vitamin? How does it differ from the other food substances?

The vitamins are a group of organic compounds that are essential in small quantities for the normal metabolism of other nutrients. The body is unable to synthesize most vitamins; hence they must be obtained from some other source. As indicated in Chapter 4, vitamins function as catalysts; that is, they do not enter into a reaction but they must be present in order for a specific reaction to take place. In this way they regulate body processes.

One of the characteristics of vitamins is that they are required in such minute quantities, usually as small as milligrams, and in some instances micrograms, yet these minute quantities are absolutely necessary. They are easily obtainable from foods, although the content varies from food to food and no one food can supply all of them in sufficient amounts for health. The vitamins vary in chemical construction and in their reaction in body metabolism. There is very little that all of them have in common, except the way that they act within the body, and even this varies somewhat.

The vitamins are all soluble however, some in fat and some in water. This distinction was among the earliest discoveries and served as a basis for research during their identification. Currently, it is helpful in regard to sources and also to subsequent care in food preparation and storage for maximum retention of the vitamin value of food.

Table 11–1 includes the contemporary vitamins known to be essential to the nutrition of man. The way in which they function will be discussed in Chapters 12–14.

Once the vitamins were identified, their specific activity in human nutrition was determined.

Vitamin research has followed a general pattern. After a vitamin was identified, the need to establish its structural formula followed. This accomplished, it became necessary to develop a process whereby the vitamin could be synthesized simply and inexpensively. With this knowledge behind him, the scientist could embark upon long and sometimes tortuous research to determine how much of each vitamin was needed. First, the minimum amount that was necessary to prevent recognized symptoms of a disease or condition was established. Next was determined the amount that would provide the best possible state of health in the human being, from the standpoint of existing knowledge of nutrition. The philosophy and differentiation between minimum and recommended allowances have been discussed elsewhere.

Once the quantitative requirement of a vitamin has been determined, research is then directed toward investigation of the ways in which vitamins function within the human body. Many insights have been obtained concerning interrelationships among vitamins and the action of vitamins in the utilization of other foodstuffs, such as amino acids, fats, and carbohydrates.

Functions of Vitamins

The role of vitamins in human nutrition may be divided into two broad categories: pre-

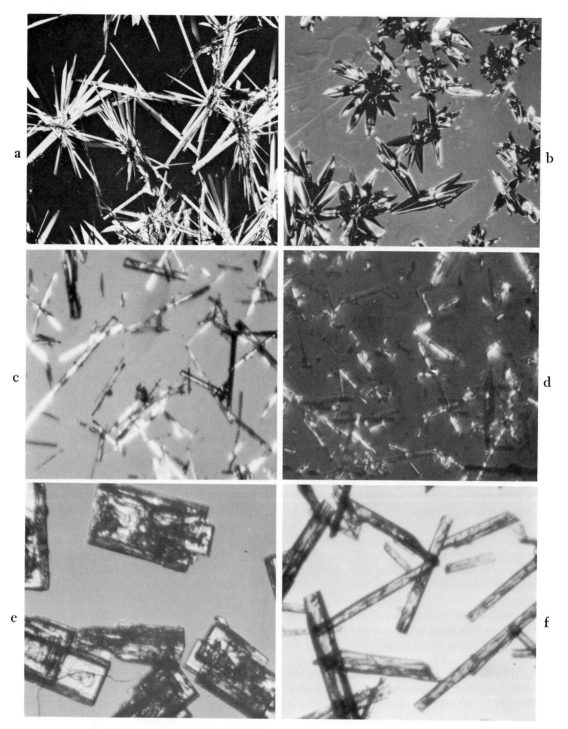

FIGURE 11–1. Variations in crystal formation furnish one technique whereby a vitamin may be identified in the laboratory: (a) vitamin A, (b) beta-carotene, (c) vitamin B_1, (d) riboflavin, (e) vitamin B_6 (f) biotin. (Hoffman-LaRoche, Inc., Nutley, N.J.)

136

TABLE 11-1

Vitamins Essential to Man

CONTEMPORARY NAME	OTHER DESIGNATION	CONTEMPORARY NAME	OTHER DESIGNATION
Vitamin A	Fat-soluble vitamin A, antixerophthalmia factor, retinol, retinal, retinoic acid, carotenes, carotenoids.	Pantothenic acid	Pantothen, liver filtrate factor, chick antidermatitis factor, chick antipellagra factor, factor II, antichromotrichia factor (antigray hair factor), vitamin B_3, Vitamin Bx.
Vitamin D	Ergocalciferol, cholecalciferol.		
Vitamin E	The tocopherols, antisterility factor.	Folacin	Folic acid, pteroylglutamic acid, folinic acid, vitamin M, vitamin B factor U, *L. casei* factor, citrovorum factor
Vitamin K	The antihemorrhagic factor, Koagulations vitamine (Danish), menadione (K_1 and K_2).		
Thiamin	Vitamin B, antineuritic factor, antiberiberi factor.	Vitamin B_{12}	Cyanocobalamin, antipernicious anemia factor, animal protein factor, extrinsic factor, includes vitamin B_{12} group (cobalamin) of B_{12a}, B_{12b}, B_{12c}.
Riboflavin	Vitamin B_2, vitamin G, lactoflavin, ovoflavin, hepatoflavin, yellow enzyme.		
Niacin	Nicotine acid, nicotinamide (niacin amide), pellagra preventive (PP) factor, antiblack tongue factor.	Biotin	Antiegg white injury factor, vitamin H, biotinic acid, coenzyme R, bios II, factor S, factor W, factor X.
Vitamin B_6	Pyridoxine, includes pyridoxal, pyridoxamine, pyridoximers, the eluate factor, rat acrodynia factor, adermine, vitamin Y.	Choline	Bilineaurine.
		Ascorbic acid	Vitamin C, antiscorbutic factor, cevitamic acid.

vention of disease and participation in the regulation of body processes. The impetus that led to the discovery of specific vitamins grew out of the need to determine the causative factors of certain diseases which at that time were not recognized as deficiency diseases so much as scourges upon humanity. Beriberi, scurvy, and pellagra are examples. It was while studying the conditions themselves to determine the causes that investigators established the concept of deficiency diseases. This awareness redirected research and thereby led to the identification of certain vitamins.

A deficiency disease is one that is caused by a lack of a specific nutrient in the diet. In the case of a vitamin deficiency, the disease can be cured or prevented by giving only the missing vitamin. Thus one has a "controlled" con-

dition in which only one variable exists—the vitamin in question.

Each deficiency disease has its own syndrome (series of symptoms), which manifests itself in different ways in different species. For example, a deficiency of pantothenic acid may exhibit a different kind of dermatitis in the chick than in man. In one species, a disease may result from a deficiency of a given vitamin, whereas when a different laboratory animal is used, data may show an entirely different reaction. Also, it is unwise to transfer knowledge obtained from animal experimentation to human nutrition. A vitamin may be an essential item in the diet of man, whereas the laboratory animal may be able to synthesize it. However, experiments with laboratory animals do give an insight into what might be found in man and direction for further investigations.

Seldom does one individual suffer a deficiency of only a single nutrient. Usually if the diet is inadequate in one respect, it is poor in another. Many deficiencies are multiple; consequently, it is difficult to find signs that will distinguish one from another. This may not be true, however, in parts of the world where a large percentage of the diet comes from one food alone, and one nutrient might be lacking. This can explain why a condition like beriberi might arise in a country that depended upon refined rice as practically its sole source of thiamin. Deficiencies may occur not only from a lack of vitamins but if there is a failure in the body to properly metabolize or absorb the vitamins.

Vitamins do not function entirely alone but are often interrelated with other vitamins in their nutrient group or with other nutrients. Cobalt, for example, is a part of vitamin B_{12}. Selenium is associated with vitamin E. Thiamin and biotin contain sulfur. Excessive amounts of vitamins E and C may interfere with the utilization of vitamin A.[2]

Recognition of deficiency diseases has been discussed in Chapter 4 when methods for evaluating nutritional status were considered. The specific deficiency diseases caused by a lack of each vitamin are covered in the following chapters.

How do vitamins function within the body? It has been shown for some of them, and suggested for the others, that they react as coenzymes. In other words, the vitamins become part of an enzyme system, acting as catalysts to facilitate the metabolism of other nutrients and biochemical processes in cells and tissues, by means of which nutrients are used for energy and for building cells or maintaining cells and tissues.

The Food and Nutrition Board of the National Research Council has recommended that specific amounts of nine vitamins, A, E, ascorbic acid, folacin, niacin, riboflavin, thiamin, B_6, and B_{12}, be included each day in the diet of the adult, with a tenth, vitamin D, added during periods of growth, which would include the diets of children from infancy through adolescence and of women during pregnancy and lactation. These recommendations appear in Chapters 21–27.

Vitamin Preparations

What is the role, then, of the vitamin preparation that is sold in drugstores and supermarkets across the country? The domestic sales of vitamin capsules, tablets, drops, and multivitamin and vitamin–mineral preparations run into many millions of dollars annually. Apart from those who include vitamin supplements as part of the medical care program outlined by the physician (primarily during pregnancy, childhood, and older age), a large number of persons routinely take a vitamin tablet or capsule each day. The question arises concerning this segment of the public, "Is this money spent wisely or foolishly?"

White,[3] as executive secretary of the Council of Foods and Nutrition of the American Medical Association, discussed the role of pharmaceutical vitamin preparations. He pointed out that the council had reviewed the indications for use and that a clear distinction should be made between vitamins as dietary supplements and vitamins as therapeutic agents.

In reviewing the recommended daily allowances and the plan to satisfy these through use of the U.S. Department of Agriculture's *Guide to Good Eating* (both discussed in Chapter 2), the council states: "If the diet contains the key food groups in sufficient amounts, nutritional supplementation should be unnecessary. The proper selection and preparation of foods are important to the achievement of an adequate diet."

However, White commented that the council felt that healthy persons whose diets were ordinarily considered adequate might benefit from dietary supplements at certain periods.

[2] John G. Bieri, "Effect of Excessive Vitamins C and E on Vitamin A Status," *American Journal of Clinical Nutrition*, Vol. 26, No. 4 (April 1973), p. 382.

[3] Philip L. White, "Vitamin Preparations as Dietary Supplements and as Therapeutic Agents," *Journal of the American Medical Association*, Vol. 169, 1959, p. 41.

These might be such times as during pregnancy or lactation when there is increased need for vitamins, during illness or a deranged mode of life that might result in an impairment of absorption, or perhaps when an individual, owing to ignorance, emotional illness, or many other reasons, does not eat an adequate diet.

Nutrition surveys, such as those cited elsewhere, have indicated that certain segments of the population are not receiving sufficient varieties of foods to supply vitamins in amounts necessary to meet the recommended dietary allowances. However, the council feels that generalizations of these findings as a basis for vitamin supplementation of healthy individuals are not rational.

The widespread use of vitamin preparations is highlighted in a national survey conducted by the Food and Drug Administration on health practices and opinions.[4] The belief that taking vitamin preparations will provide anyone with more pep and energy is so widespread as to be characteristic of the society as a whole. This is contrary to a consensus of qualified medical opinion that fatigue is seldom due to deficiencies of nutrients, especially in the absence of other pronounced symptoms. In addition, 20 per cent of the sample surveyed believed that arthritis and cancer are caused at least in part by vitamin and mineral deficiencies, in contradiction to scientific findings and opinions.

Over 25 per cent of the sample had reservations that eating a variety of available foods will supply essential vitamins. Ten per cent believed that it was beneficial to take more vitamins than needed. This means that over 20 million people hold this misconception. Women are more likely to use vitamin preparations than men. Vitamin pill usage clearly increases with higher socioeconomic status and higher levels of education. A greater tendency to worry about health was found among these users, about 60 per cent of the sample. Forty-five per cent of the population was influenced to use vitamin preparations by

sources other than physicians or health personnel, such as relatives, television and radio commercials, or friends.

The impact of these statistics is impressive when considering the effect of the cost of vitamin preparations and tonics on personal and family finances, the possible danger of an overload of certain vitamins, the tenacity of the misconceptions of the benefits to be derived from vitamin preparations, and the widespread use of unreliable resources as influences for the use of vitamins.

The notion that organic or natural vitamins provide special benefits over synthetic vitamins is debatable, according to Kamil.[5] The substances are molecularly identical but the natural vitamins are more costly. Many of the preparations labeled organic or natural are without qualification. For example, a vitamin C preparation containing rose hips was made with natural rose hips combined with chemical ascorbic acid, but the label may give the impression that the tablet is made entirely from rose hips. Other vitamins have been found to have some natural base, such as yeast, but with synthetic chemicals added. Consumers are advised to read the labels carefully if they insist upon natural vitamins.

Megavitamin therapy appears to have a strong hold on consumers, according to Halberstam.[6] The popularity of certain vitamins rise and then wane according to the fad of the times. Linus Pauling's enthusiasm for vitamin C for colds set loose a high usage of this vitamin. Vitamin E is especially popular with older people because they believe that it is good for circulation and sex. Vitamin A is purchased by some of the young because it is considered helpful in cases of acne. Some of these claims are dubious. Another concern is that consumers are using high-potency vitamins that may be triggering another danger, that of overload.

Another question under consideration is if vitamins should be a food supplement or a

---

[4] Final Report, A *Study of Health Practices and Opinions*, Food and Drug Administration, Department of Health, Education, and Welfare, Washington, D.C., 1972, Chap. 1, pp. 68–69; Chapter 2.

[5] Adolph Kamil, "How Natural Are Those Natural Vitamins?" *Journal of Nutrition Education*, Vol. 4, No. 3 (Summer 1972), p. 92.

[6] Michael Halberstam, "The A, B-12, C, D, and E of Vitamins," *The New York Times Magazine*, March 17, 1974, p. 68.

drug. The Food and Drug Administration considers all mineral and vitamin preparations that contain over 150 per cent of the U.S. RDA (recommended daily allowances) in most cases as drugs. The FDA regulation limiting dosages of vitamin A to 10,000 IU and vitamin D to 400 IU went into effect October 1, 1973.[7]

People have a much stronger concern about the vitamins in their diet than any other nutrient. This is unjustified because vitamins cannot compensate for the lack of protein, minerals, or other nutrients.

Vitamin Enrichment

Enrichment of foods with vitamins has come to be commonplace to the consumer, yet it took considerable effort on the part of influential and farsighted nutritionists to initiate a sound beginning for this important phase of nutrition. Although potassium iodide was added to table salt in 1924 to prevent goiter, and milk was fortified with vitamin D in the early 1930's, the enrichment program did not get fully under way until the early 1940's.

It was in August of 1940 that the Subcommittee on Medical Nutrition of the National Research Council[8] pointed out the generally accepted view that the American diet was minimal in its provision of vitamin B₁. The subcommittee felt that in case of war the deleterious effect of an inadequate supply of vitamin B₁ was likely to manifest itself unfavorably.

The bread and flour enrichment program was inaugurated by the National Nutrition Conference for Defense,[9] May 1941. State legislation followed federal action, and it is estimated that 90 per cent of all white bread

and white family flour produced is enriched. Exact figures are not available.

What is the difference between the terms enrichment, fortification, and restored? The term *enriched* legally means that thiamin, riboflavin, niacin, and iron are required ingredients and all four must be included if the product is labeled "enriched." (See Table 11-2.) The position of the Food and Nutrition Board has been to discourage the addition of vitamin D to bread.

Fortification, on the other hand, is applied to the addition of nutrients other than those found in natural amounts, or if not found at all, to foods that are suitable vehicles for such nutrients. Fortification may be advisable when a widespread nutritional deficiency exists or when natural sources of nutrients are not acceptable or available. Examples of fortification would be the addition of 15,000 IU of vitamin A per pound to margarine. Evaporated milk is fortified to include 400 IU of vitamin D per quart of reconstituted milk.

Restoration is the addition of a nutritive ingredient to a processed food in amount sufficient to restore to the normal level what was unavoidably lost during the processing. This term is not as broad in application as enrichment and fortification. Many foods on the market today are both enriched and fortified.

State enrichment laws have ensured the enrichment of such products as corn and rice when they are considered staples in the diet. Although there is no legal provision requiring the enrichment of any cereal or macaroni products, standards have been issued by the Food and Drug Administration that govern enrichment if it is done. About half the total production of macaroni, spaghetti, and other alimentary pastes is systematically enriched and half is not. Standards for the enrichment of rice became effective in 1958.

The Food and Nutrition Board[10] has stated the following policies in regard to the improvement of the nutritive quality of food. The following conditions must be met: (1) the intake of the nutrient(s) is below the

[7] Helen Ullrich, "Vitamins as Food or Drug," *Journal of Nutrition Education*, Vol. 6, No. 1 (January–March 1974), p. 6.

[8] *Cereal Enrichment in Perspective, 1958*, The Committee on Cereals, Food and Nutrition Board, National Academy of Sciences—National Research Council, Washington, D.C., 1958.

[9] *Enrichment of Flour and Bread, A History of the Movement*, Bulletin No. 110, National Academy of Sciences—National Research Council, Washington, D.C., 1944.

[10] Food and Nutrition Board, "General Policies in Regard to Improvement of Nutritive Quality of Foods," National Academy of Sciences—National Research Council, Washington, D.C., 1973.

TABLE 11–2

Standards for Vitamin Enrichment of Cereal Products in the United States (milligrams per pound)

FOODS	THIAMIN		RIBOFLAVIN		NIACIN	
	Min.	Max.	Min.	Max.	Min.	Max.
Breads and other baked goods		1.8		1.1		15
Flour, white		1.8		1.1		15
Macaroni and noodle products	4.0	5.0	1.7	2.2	27	34
Cornmeal, white or yellow, and grits	2.0	3.0	1.2	1.8	16	24
Rice and related products	2.0	4.0	1.2	2.4	16	32

SOURCE: *Federal Register*, October 15, 1973, p. 28558.

desirable level in the diets of a significant number of people; (2) the food(s) used to supply the nutrient(s) is likely to be consumed in quantities that will make a significant contribution to the diet of the population in need; (3) the addition of the nutrient(s) is not likely to create a dietary imbalance; (4) the nutrient(s) added is stable under customary conditions of storage and use; (5) the nutrient(s) is physiologically available from the food; (6) the enhanced levels attained in the total diet will not be harmfully excessive for those who may employ the foods in varying patterns of use; and (7) the additional cost is reasonable for the intended customers.

Enrichment has been a major public health measure in other countries. The importance of rice enrichment is discussed in Chapter 13. Benefits have been described in various areas such as Puerto Rico, Cuba, Scandinavia, Canada, and Latin America. One of the most outstanding nutritional surveys has been the Newfoundland Survey, which showed improvement in the health of individuals following the enrichment of all bread and flour for 4 years.

Some have raised the point that, instead of enriching staple products, the public should be educated to select foods that provide nutrients in the natural form. However, individuals are loath to modify their food habits, and previous educational efforts have sometimes proved fruitless. When it became clear that the public would not abandon its preference for refined breads, it seemed in the best public interest to enrich the accepted product.

Underload and Overload

Vitamin deficiency diseases are seldom found in the United States. In the *Ten-State Nutrition Survey*,[11] Spanish-Americans in the low-income-ratio states had a major problem of a lack of vitamin A in their diets and young people in the entire population had a high prevalence of low vitamin A levels. Vitamin C was not a major problem, but males generally had a lower vitamin C intake than females. Riboflavin status was poor among blacks and among young people of all ethnic groups.

Vitamins, according to Young,[12] have be-

[11] *Highlights, Ten-State Nutrition Survey, 1968–1970*, DHEW Publication No. (HSM) 72–8134, Center for Disease Control, Health Services and Mental Health Administration, U.S. Department of Health, Education, and Welfare, Atlanta, Ga., 1972, p. 12.

[12] Charlotte M. Young, "Overnutrition," in Miloslav, Rechcigl, Jr. (ed.), *Food, Nutrition and Health*, Vol. 16, S. Karger, Basel, 1973, p. 187.

come almost universal placebos. It is quite common for individuals to take a vitamin pill for a cold, skin disorders, fatigue, chronic infections, and other conditions. When a physician prescribes vitamins for a rational purpose, the patient may continue to take the vitamins after the prescribed period. Furthermore, some individuals are inclined to increase the dose, believing that more will be better.

Hypervitaminosis, or overload, may result from accidental overdosage, especially in young children or in the aged. Metabolic disease or disturbance may cause an intolerance for the vitamin. Food faddism may encourage an overload. The medical literature gives increasing evidence of hypervitaminosis and other cases may not have come to the attention of a physician. An overload of vitamins A and D has received the greatest attention. There is concern for vitamin K toxicity in infants, hypercarotenemia, often caused by a high consumption of carrot juice, and niacin and folacin overdosage.

Criteria for Food Sources

Nutritional labeling will assist the consumer in selecting foods according to their vitamin contribution to the diet. The consumer can usually find better buys among common food sources rather than from equivalents or substitutes. The purchase of convenience foods may present problems because the exact measure of individual nutrients in the product are difficult to determine. In the case of fresh fruit and vegetables, the degree of ripeness, wilting, and length of time from field or orchard to the counter may affect the vitamin content.

The losses in processing and preserving of foods are especially important in considering vitamin content. Lund[13] states that ascorbic acid, thiamin, vitamin D, and pantothenic acid in foods are the most heat labile. Significant losses of water-soluble vitamins occur in the washing and blanching steps for canning. Fat-soluble vitamins are less heat labile but are susceptible to degradation at high temperatures in the presence of oxygen.

During the dehydration and storage of dried foods there may be considerable destruction of water-soluble and fat-soluble vitamins, according to Labuza.[14] Ascorbic acid is probably the most labile of all vitamins contained in foods. Losses vary from 10 to 50 per cent during preparation of the food for drying because of washing, leaching, and blanching. Rate of loss of ascorbic acid during storage increases significantly if the water content of the food is high. The B vitamins are more stable than vitamin C in processing. Thiamin is probably the most heat sensitive of the B vitamins, especially in nonacid foods. During storage the amount of water in the food is a determining factor; the greater the water content the greater the loss of thiamin. The major loss of fat-soluble vitamins in dehydration and storage is also related to the amount of water and the presence of oxidants.

To be assured of an adequate vitamin component in the daily diet, it is necessary for planners to become informed of superior sources of the various vitamins, to include a wide variety of food, and to guard against vitamin losses during food preparation.

---

[13] D. B. Lund, "Effects of Heat Processing," *Food Technology*, Vol. 27, No. 1 (January 1973), p. 16.

[14] T. P. Labuza, "Effects of Dehydration and Storage," *Food Technology*, Vol. 27, No. 1 (January 1973), pp. 23–25.

SELECTED REFERENCES

Davidson, Stanley, R. Passmore, and J. F. Brock, *Human Nutrition and Dietetics*, The Williams & Wilkins Company, Baltimore, 1972, Chapters 11 and 12.

Gifft, Helen H., Marjorie Washbon, and Gail G. Harrison, *Nutrition, Behavior, and Change*, Prentice-Hall, Inc., Englewood Cliffs, N.J., 1972, pp. 91, 126.

Goodhart, Robert S., and Maurice E. Shils, *Modern Nutrition in Health and Disease*, Lea & Febiger, Philadelphia, 1973, Chapter 5.

Margolius, Sidney, *Health Foods, Facts and Fakes*, Walker & Company, New York, 1973, Chapter 7.

McCollum, Elmer V., A *History of Nutrition*, Houghton Mifflin Company, Boston, 1957, Chapter 14.

Pike, Magnus, *Man and Food*, McGraw-Hill Book Company, New York, 1970, pp. 147, 231.

Rechcigl, Miloslav, Jr. (ed.), *Food, Nutrition and Health*, Vol. 16, S. Karger, Basel, 1973, pp. 142–198.

12

The Fat-Soluble Vitamins

Of the four known fat-soluble vitamins recognized as necessary to human nutrition, three—vitamins A, E, and D—are included in the table of the *Recommended Dietary Allowances* of the National Research Council.[1] The fourth, vitamin K, is necessary for health, but because of insufficient data related to the needs of man, an absolute allowance for it has not been established.

Although it is difficult to make generalizations that will be equally applicable to all the fat-soluble vitamins, some characteristics are common to all. These characteristics help to identify them as members of this group.

Since they are fat-soluble, they are found in foods that are in association with lipids. They are absorbed with food fats, and the same factors that influence fat absorption seem to influence the absorption of the fat-soluble vitamins. This is an important consideration when the diet needs to be modified for medical reasons. Absorption of fat may be reduced by inhibiting influences, such as mineral oil;

by rendering the absorption of fats ineffective, as by fat combining with calcium salts; or by bringing about a lowered or lesser absorption such as might occur in conditions that affect the health of the intestinal tract, like ileitis and diarrhea.

Once absorbed, vitamins from this group are stored in moderate quantities. Therefore, the individual is not absolutely dependent upon day-to-day dietary intake. Because these vitamins are fat-soluble, the segment that is unable to be absorbed is not excreted in the urine but in the feces.

The final characteristic that the fat-soluble vitamins share is that they are all fairly stable to heat. Thus the effect of cooking and food processing upon the subsequent vitamin content of food is negligible.

Vitamin A

Although Hopkins, as discussed by McCollum,[2] had recognized that there were "accessory food factors" and Funk had named these

---

[1] Food and Nutrition Board, *Recommended Dietary Allowances*, 8th ed., National Academy of Sciences—National Research Council, Washington, D.C., 1974, pp. 50–62.

[2] E. V. McCollum, A *History of Nutrition*, Houghton Mifflin, Boston, 1957, p. 209.

144

factors "vitamines," it was an exciting day in 1913 when McCollum and Davis announced from the University of Wisconsin the discovery of a fat-soluble substance, which they named fat-soluble A. This resulted from their studies of an artificial diet that promoted good growth in experimental rats. The diet consisted of protein, lactose, starch, and inorganic salt, further supplemented with butterfat. But they found that if they gave the same diet but substituted another fat, olive oil, or lard for the butterfat, the rats failed to grow and were not in good health.

At almost the same time, Osborne and Mendel (at Yale) who had earlier published their discoveries in protein metabolism, reported findings similar to those of McCollum and Davis.

Early investigations of vitamin A were complicated, for they included the study of other unknown factors, later identified as vitamin D and the provitamin A, beta-carotene. In 1917 McCollum[3] and his co-workers studied an eye disease, xerophthalmia, in which the eyeball becomes dry and lusterless. They noted that it was caused by a lack of a fat-soluble vitamin and indicated that it was the same one that caused rickets. However, in 1922 McCollum and his colleagues suggested that two separate factors might be involved. The following year Goldblatt provided evidence to support this theory.

Even though Steenbock and Gross observed in 1919 that yellow foods were good sources of vitamin A, further experiments over the ensuing years by other investigators as well as studies of his own enabled Moore in 1929 to announce that carotene was provitamin A (see Glossary). In 1937, Holmes and Corbet isolated and crystallized vitamin A from the liver oil of mackerel and other fishes. That same year, Kuhn and Morris synthesized the vitamin for the first time. In the years that followed, studies revealed the formulas, characteristics, and syntheses of various forms of vitamin A and its provitamins.

Hence, more than 20 years passed between the recognition of the first fat-soluble vitamin, later called vitamin A, and its isola-

tion and synthesis. These were two decades of exciting primary research, which also included many discoveries other than those concerned with vitamin A.

Chemical and Physical Properties of Vitamin A

Vitamin A occurs in nature in several forms, the most common being retinol (vitamin A_1), which is found in mammals and saltwater fish. Freshwater fish contain dehydroretinol (vitamin A_2), which is considered less important. It is also supplied in the form of a provitamin (or precursor) commonly known as the carotenes. Retinol is found only in the animal kingdom, whereas the carotenes and carotenoids are found in plants and are the original source of vitamin A for animals. For example, the carotenoid of vegetable marine plankton might well be the source of provitamin A for fish. The herbivorous land animals, such as the cow, probably synthesize vitamin A from the carotenoid of the grass that is used for grazing. Vitamin A_1 is usually the form that is referred to as vitamin A.

The provitamin A carotenes, alpha, beta, and gamma, and sometimes cryptoxanthin (of the carotenes, beta has the highest vitamin A activity), are converted by a chemical process into fragments, one being vitamin A. In the blood, retinol is transported in association with a specific protein, referred to as a retinol-binding protein by Kanai and others.[4] Carotenoids are associated with lipid-bearing proteins. Several forms of carotenes and carotenoids are closely related chemically; these occur in yellow and green plants. It is believed that the conversion of carotene to vitamin A takes place in the intestinal wall.

Vitamin A is not synthesized in the body and must be supplied by food or supplements. When vitamin A and precursors are consumed in amounts beyond daily needs, the excess is stored in the liver for future use. Carotene precursors are less efficiently utilized than true vitamin A. Dietary adequacy of

---

[3] Ibid., p. 232.

[4] M. Kanai, M. A. Raz, and D. S. Goodman, "Retinol-Binding Protein: The Transport Protein for Vitamin A in Human Plasma," *Journal of Clinical Investigation*, Vol. 47, No. 2 (July–December 1968), pp. 2025–2044.

protein[5] and vitamin E are necessary for maximum utilization of the vitamin by the body.

Vitamin A is almost colorless (having a pale yellow tinge). It is soluble in fat solvents and insoluble in water, acids and alkalies. It is relatively stable to heat, and ordinary cooking procedures exert little effect upon it. However, it is destroyed by oxidation, especially if heat is present. In addition, it is fairly unstable to light. Vitamin A is stored in the animal body in combination with fatty acids, palmitic acid being the preferred acid.

Functions of Vitamin A

One of the best-defined roles of vitamin A is its requirement for normal vision. The rods of the retina of the eye contain rhodopsin (also known as *visual purple*), which is composed of vitamin A, aldehyde, retinal, and a protein substance, opsin. As the eye is exposed to light, visual purple is converted to visual yellow and then to visual white. During these steps, retinal is converted to retinol, and, in order to complete the cycle of regeneration, the reconversion of retinol to retinal and then the recombination with opsin to form rhodopsin, vitamin A must be replaced. This replacement is provided by the circulating blood supply. The rods in the retina are responsible for vision in dim light. The retina also contains cones, which are responsible for vision in bright light. The cones contain a vitamin A–protein substance, iodopsin, which is believed to follow a cycle similar to that of rhodopsin.

When an inadequate supply of vitamin A exists, incomplete regeneration of visual purple occurs. This results in a condition known as night blindness, or lack of dark adaptation, characterized by an impairment of vision in subdued light after an exposure to bright light. Night blindness may be especially noted when driving a car during the evening. The driver may have difficulty adjusting to the subdued light of the highway after being subjected to

the headlight of an oncoming car. McCollum has pointed out that both night blindness and xerophthalmia were recognized by the Egyptians in 1900 B.C. They realized that diet was an etiological factor in these two conditions. Both Egyptian and early Greek physicians recommended raw liver as a treatment.

Vitamin A is necessary for the health of the epithelial cells. These are the cells that form the outer layer of skin; they also are part of the cells that line any part of the body having contact with the exterior air; and they are the cells that are specialized for secretion in organs, such as the liver and the gastrointestinal tract. The health and normal growth of these cells are vitally important to the individual. A deficiency in the vitamin A intake may result in the epithelial tissue cells becoming hard and dry, instead of being in a normal soft, moist condition. These changes are called *keratinization*.

Vitamin A has often been mentioned as important in the body's resistance to infection. This reaction may be explained by its relationship to the health of the epithelial cells. Because the mucous membrane serves as a barrier against many kinds of bacterial invasion, a lowered resistance to infection may result when the structure of epithelial cells is impaired because of a deficiency in vitamin A.

Vitamin A is also necessary in the formation of the teeth. The critical phase occurs when the tooth buds are ready for the formation of the enamel while they are embedded in the child's gum. Vitamin A seems to participate in the orderly development of the enamel-forming cells. If developed normally, the cells form prisms that are laid together so perfectly that they become a dense, thick, smooth enamel. If there is an inadequate supply of vitamin A during this period of development, the imperfectly formed enamel will contain small pits. After the teeth have erupted, these pits may become "catches" for food deposits and may eventually lead to decay.

It has been demonstrated that vitamin A is necessary for growth; however, the mechanism by which this occurs is unknown. Vitamin A appears to be essential in bone formation.

[5] L. K. Kothari, K. B. Lal, D. K. Srivastava, and Rameshwar Sharma, "Correlation Between Plasma Levels of Vitamin A and Proteins in Children," *American Journal of Clinical Nutrition*, Vol. 24, No. 5 (May 1971), pp. 510–512.

Thus the importance of vitamin A to the health of the individual cannot be minimized. The structural development and adequate maintenance of major portions of the body, the epithelial tissues, retina, and teeth, will be affected adversely if an adequate amount is not included in the diet.

Effects of a Deficiency of Vitamin A

An inadequate dietary intake of vitamin A can cause a primary deficiency. A secondary deficiency may follow whenever there is any disease condition that interferes with the absorption, storage, or metabolism of vitamin A. In addition, interference with the conversion of carotene to vitamin A can cause a deficiency. The effects of the deficiency can range from a relatively mild condition to a severe one, depending upon the extent and duration of inadequate dietary intake and the age and health of the individual.

Hypovitaminosis A is a term that applies to all manifestations of the deficiency state. However, the severe form of vitamin A deficiency disease is known as *xerophthalmia*. This condition has long been recognized as a disease associated with malnutrition, and the eye is seriously affected. In 1904 it was observed in infants in Japan whose diet was devoid of fat. Similar symptoms were noted in 1917 in children in Denmark who suffered from a lack of dairy products in their diets. *Keratomalacia* applies to advanced and largely irreversible corneal damage.[6]

Although xerophthalmia occurs infrequently in the United States and Western Europe, it is regarded as a serious health problem elsewhere. Individual studies have reported a high incidence in countries of South and East Asia and in many countries of the Middle East. It has also been recognized as a serious problem in areas in Africa and Latin America.

Hypovitaminosis A has been a nutritional problem common to tropical and subtropical regions of the world. The northeast section of Brazil is one of the most seriously affected areas, particularly among preschool children, according to Varela and co-workers,[7] of whom 18 per cent of the group studied had serum retinol levels of less than 20 g per 100 ml. One third of the malnourished population also had low serum retinol levels. Protein-calorie malnutrition is often accompanied by vitamin A deficiency. The diet of the area was predominantly vegetables with low carotene content and consequently low vitamin A activity.

Xerophthalmia seldom occurs in isolation; frequently it is associated with malnutrition, and in some countries, with marasmus and kwashiorkor.[8] When xerophthalmia was accompanied by protein-calorie malnutrition, the mortality has been as high as 80 per cent, contrasted with a mortality rate of only 15 per cent in a group that was equally malnourished yet not deficient in vitamin A.[9]

In xerophthalmia, there is a loss of the normal protective secretions of the eye, since there is a keratinization of the epithelial cells. The eye becomes dry; the cornea, which is the transparent outer covering of the eye, also becomes dry and loses its sensitivity. Later, roughness occurs, followed by ulcers. Xerophthalmia itself is due to a secondary infection of the cornea. There are clearly defined clinical symptoms for which public health personnel in areas where xerophthalmia might be a problem need to be alerted. Then detection of potential xerophthalmia can be made before irreversible damage occurs. The maximum incidence of the disease is in the second and third year of life, with the range being about 3 months to 4 years. The most serious concern is that tens of thousands of children go

---

[6] D. S. McLaren, "The Effects of Vitamin A Deficiency in Man," in W. H. Sebrell and Robert S. Harris (eds.), *The Vitamins*, Vol. 1, 2nd ed., Academic Press, New York, 1967, pp. 267–280.

[7] Ramanita Mayer Varela, Suzana Gomes Teixeria, and Malaquias Batista, "Hypovitaminosis A in the Sugarcane Zone of Southern Pernambuco State, Northeast Brazil," *American Journal of Clinical Nutrition*, Vol. 25, No. 9 (August 1972), pp. 800–804.

[8] Paul György, "Protein-Calorie and Vitamin A Malnutrition in Southeast Asia," *Federation Proceedings*, Vol. 27, No. 3 (March 1968), pp. 949–953.

[9] D. S. McLaren, "Xerophthalmia: A Neglected Problem," *Nutrition Reviews*, Vol. 22, No. 9 (September 1964), p. 289.

blind each year because of insufficient intake of vitamin A and its precursors, according to Bauernfeind and others.[10] Other symptoms of vitamin A deficiency are growth depression, suspected greater susceptibility to disease, and death.

Hypervitaminosis A

It is possible to provide an overdose of vitamin A that will result in a serious condition known as hypervitaminosis A. Characteristic symptoms include a drying and peeling of skin, nausea, headaches that may be severe, dizziness, and lack of vigor or apathy, according to Bauernfeind and others.[11] In children, the symptoms most often noted are drowsiness, vomiting, and bulging of the fontanelle. If hypervitaminosis A becomes chronic, other symptoms appear, such as itching, fissures at the corners of the mouth, swelling of the extremities, growth failure, loss of appetite, irritability, and loss of hair. In prolonged cases, skeletal changes occur. In many cases when excessive vitamin A intake is stopped, symptoms disappear. There are no known causes of death attributed to hypervitaminosis A.

Hypervitaminosis A occurs when a single dose is sufficiently high in relation to body weight or a chronic dose administered over a period of time is sufficient to produce symptoms. The previous vitamin A nutritional status would have some influence. For example, a child suffering from protein-calorie malnutrition may receive a dose of 100,000 IU of water-miscible vitamin A by intramuscular injection without producing symptoms of hypervitaminosis A, according to Pereira and others.[12] Chronic hypervitaminosis A in children results usually from overzealous parents who are uninformed or believe that high dosages will provide beneficial results. Teen-

agers and adults may suffer from excessive intakes for somewhat the same reasons, often self-medicated. A skin disorder such as acne, for which a remedy is sought, may lead to excessive dosage of vitamin A.

Various levels of excessive vitamin A daily intake have been reported from 10,000 to 75,000 IU. The symptoms gradually disappear following a cessation of vitamin A intake. However, some permanent effects have been noted in the bone development of children.

Absorption, Transport, and Storage of Vitamin A

The absorption of vitamin A takes place in a stepwise fashion: dietary vitamin A (as retinyl ester) is hydrolyzed in the intestinal tract to retinol before passing across the mucosal wall of the cell. Within the cell, retinol combines with a fatty acid, palmitic acid. Thus, in the form of retinyl palmitate, it passes from the intestinal wall into the lymph system via the thoracic duct, into the bloodstream, and then to the liver.

Carotene is absorbed into the intestinal wall and then it follows two possible pathways. Some is converted to vitamin A and the remainder is absorbed as carotene. Unabsorbed carotene appears in the feces. The conversion of carotene to vitamin A usually takes place in the intestinal wall, although it has been demonstrated that other tissues can also perform this process. Absorbed carotene enters the lymph and then the bloodstream. Some carotene is stored in adipose tissue, giving it its light yellow color. Carotene converted to vitamin A follows the same route as preformed vitamin A.

A number of factors influence the absorption of carotene from the intestine; one is the level of dietary fat. In parts of the world where diets are low in fat (such as diets reported from Central Africa with only 7 percent of the total calories coming from fat), a vitamin A deficiency appeared even though there was a sufficient supply of carotenoids. The presence of bile is also necessary for absorption of carotene. The absorption of both preformed vitamin A and carotene has been adversely affected by low-protein diets of poor biological value. Vitamin A is especially sensitive to

---

[10] J. C. Bauernfeind, H. Newmark, and M. Brin, "Vitamins A and E Nutrition via Intermuscular or Oral Route," *American Journal of Clinical Nutrition*, Vol. 27, No. 3 (March 1974), pp. 234–253.

[11] Ibid, pp. 235–236.

[12] S. M. Pereira, A. Begum, and M. E. Dumm, "Vitamin A Deficiency in Kwashiorkor," *American Journal of Clinical Nutrition*, Vol. 19, No. 2 (February 1966), pp. 182–187.

oxidation, and vitamin E may act as an anti-oxidant. Mineral oil interferes with the absorption of both vitamin A and carotene. And, finally, any disease that impairs the function of the intestinal tract or its secretions will interfere with the absorption of vitamin A and carotene. The absorption of both vitamin A and carotene is slow in the young and in the aged over 70.

Vitamin A is stored primarily in the liver. It has been estimated that roughly 95 per cent of the body's vitamin A reserves are found there. A normal supply of a healthy individual may be enough to last for as long as several months on a diet devoid of vitamin A and carotene.

Vitamin A is released from the liver into the bloodstream, where it is circulated in a lipoprotein form to supply tissue needs. Maintenance of a normal blood level of vitamin A is regulated by a liver enzyme and replenished from liver stores. Thus an individual on a vitamin A deficient diet can maintain adequate blood levels until his stores are exhausted.

Nutritive Needs for Vitamin A

Although data for establishing the minimum and optimum requirements of vitamin A are limited, the National Research Council has recommended the allowances set forth in Table 12–1.

The basis for determining recommended dietary allowances for vitamin A are two studies, one done in England by Hume and

TABLE 12–1

Recommended Daily Dietary Allowances for Vitamin A, Revised 1974

Designed for the mainteance of good nutrition of practically all healthy people in the United States

	AGE (years)	WEIGHT (kg)	WEIGHT (lb)	HEIGHT (cm)	HEIGHT (in.)	ENERGY (kcal)	VITAMIN A ACTIVITY (re)[a]	VITAMIN A ACTIVITY (iu)
Infants	0.0–0.5	6	14	60	24	kg × 117	420[b]	1400
	0.5–1.0	9	20	71	28	kg × 108	400	2000
Children	1–3	13	28	86	34	1300	400	2000
	4–6	20	44	110	44	1800	500	2500
	7–10	30	66	135	54	2400	700	3300
Males	11–14	44	97	158	63	2800	1000	5000
	15–18	61	134	172	69	3000	1000	5000
	19–22	67	147	172	69	3000	1000	5000
	23–50	70	154	172	69	2700	1000	5000
	51+	70	154	172	69	2400	1000	5000
Females	11–14	44	97	155	62	2400	800	4000
	15–18	54	119	162	65	2100	800	4000
	19–22	58	128	162	65	2100	800	4000
	23–50	58	128	162	65	2000	800	4000
	51+	58	128	162	65	1800	800	4000
Pregnant						+300	1000	5000
Lactating						+500	1200	6000

SOURCE: Food and Nutrition Board, *Recommended Dietary Allowances*, 8th ed., National Academy of Sciences—National Research Council, Washington, D.C., 1974.

[a] Retinol equivalents.

[b] Assumed to be all as retinol in milk during the first 6 months of life. All subsequent intakes are assumed to be half as retinol and half as beta-carotene when calculated from international units. As retinol equivalents, three fourths are as retinol and one fourth as beta-carotene.

Krebs[13] and a recent one by the University of Iowa and the U.S. Army by Hodges and Kolder.[14] The results of these two studies were in relative good agreement. Conclusions were that 500 to 600 μg of retinol or twice as much beta-carotene are a minimum requirement for adults to maintain adequate blood concentrations and to prevent deficiency symptoms.[15] Because significant sections of the population in the United States have low vitamin A reserves, an allowance must be made. The usual foods available to individuals provide about half the total vitamin A activity in the form of retinol and half as carotenoids, precursors of vitamin A. Presently, food tables provide little information about the amount or type of carotenoids to allow for possible discrepancies, so the adult male recommended allowance continues as 5000 IU or 1000 retinol equivalents, about 25 per cent higher than the FAO/WHO recommendations. Because of the smaller size of women, their allowance is 80 per cent, or 4000 IU or 800 retinol equivalents.

The recommended allowances for infants is based on the average retinol content of human milk, approximately 49 μg per 100 ml. The allowance for infants to 6 months of age is 420 retinol equivalents, and 400 retinol equivalents from 6 months to 1 year of age. Allowances for children and adolescents are interpolated largely from the recommended allowance for infants and for male adults. Consideration is given to body weight and some arbitrary allowance for growth. The increased allowance for children levels off at adolescence and remains at that intake for life.

Additional allowance is made during pregnancy to 5000 IU or 1000 retinol equivalents to allow for storage of vitamin A in the fetus. An even greater allowance is recommended during lactation, 6000 IU or 1200 retinol equivalents to provide for the vitamin A secreted in the milk.

The term, retinol equivalent, has been accepted by a number of countries in preference to the international unit, according to Bieri.[16] The Expert Committee of the Food and Agriculture Organization/World Health Organization (FAO/WHO) decided to abandon the use of international units. The primary advantage is that the variable absorption and intestinal conversion of provitamin A carotenoids is automatically included in the term "retinol equivalent." When using international units there could be considerable variation because allowances are not made for the variations in vitamin A activity in carotenoids. In the 1974 table of allowances, both the retinol equivalents and international units are identified, but it is hoped that the change to retinol equivalents can be accomplished by the time of the next edition of the allowances.[17]

To calculate the vitamin A value of diets, according to the Food and Nutrition Board, it is important to be familiar with the various equivalencies. Retinol equivalents can be computed by using the following information:

1 retinol equivalent = 1-μg retinol
= 6 μg beta-carotene
= 12 μg other provitamin A carotenoids, such as alpha- and gamma-carotene and cryptoxanthin
= 3.33 IU vitamin activity from retinol
= 10 IU vitamin A activity from beta-carotene
= 20 IU vitamin activity from other provitamin A carotenoids

[13] E. M. Hume and H. A. Krebs (compilers), *Vitamin A Requirement of Human Adults*, Report of the Vitamin A Sub-committee of the Accessory Food Factors Committee, Medical Research Council (Great Britain), Special Report Series, No. 264, His Majesty's Stationery Office, London, 1949.

[14] R. E. Hodges and H. Kolder, "Experimental Vitamin A Deficiency in Human Volunteers," in J. G. Bieri (chairman), *Summary of Proceedings, Workshop on Biochemical and Clinical Criteria for Determining Human Vitamin A Nutriture*, National Academy of Sciences, Washington, D.C., 1971, pp. 10–16.

[15] *Recommended Dietary Allowances*, op. cit., pp. 53–54.

[16] John G. Bieri, "Fat-Soluble Vitamins in the Eighth Revision of the Recommended Dietary Allowances," *Journal of the American Dietetic Association*, Vol. 64, No. 2 (February 1974), pp. 171–174.

[17] *Recommended Dietary Allowances*, op. cit., p. 52.

1 IU = 0.3 μg retinol

= 0.6 μg beta-carotene

= 1.2 μg other provitamin A carotenoids, such as other carotenes

Several formulas may be helpful in these calculations.

1. If retinol and beta-carotene are given in micrograms, then

$$\mu g \text{ retinol} + \frac{\mu g \text{ beta-carotene}}{6} = \text{retinol equivalents}$$

An example is a diet containing 400 μg retinol and 1200 μg of beta-carotene:

$$400 + \frac{1200}{6} = 600 \text{ retinol equivalents.}$$

2. If both retinol and beta-carotene are given in international units, then

$$\frac{\text{IU retinol}}{3.33} + \frac{\text{IU beta-carotene}}{10} = \text{retinol equivalents}$$

An example is a diet containing 999 IU of retinol and 2000 IU of beta-carotene:

$$\frac{999 \text{ retinol}}{3.33} + \frac{2000 \text{ IU beta-carotene}}{10} = 500 \text{ retinol equivalents}$$

3. If beta-carotene and other provitamin A carotenoids are given in micrograms, then

$$\frac{\mu g \text{ beta-carotene}}{6} + \frac{\mu g \text{ other carotenoids}}{12} = \text{retinol equivalents}$$

An example is a food containing 1800 IU beta-carotene and 600 IU of other provitamin A carotenoids:

$$\frac{1800}{6} + \frac{600}{12} = 350 \text{ retinol equivalents}$$

It will be necessary for food composition tables to provide information about the form in which vitamin A is found, such as retinol and the various provitamin A carotenoids, so that a more accurate calculation of vitamin A content of foods can be made.

Nutritional Vitamin A Status

The findings of the *Ten-State Nutrition Survey* indicate that black and Spanish-American children from 0 to 5 years of age in low-income-ratio states have a high prevalence of deficient values in vitamin A, as did Spanish-Americans at all age levels and both sexes in this income level. The white and black groups had a low prevalence of vitamin A deficient values from 0 to 16 years of age for both sexes in the low-income level. In the high-income-ratio states, black and white children from 0 to 16 years of age had a low prevalence of deficient values in vitamin A, while the Spanish-Americans had only minimal deficiencies at all age levels and both sexes, as did blacks and whites from the ages of 17 to over 60.[18] (See Table 2-2.)

In the preliminary findings of the *First Health and Nutrition Examination Survey* (HANES),[19] the mean vitamin A intakes for all ages, at income levels below or above poverty, for both sexes, and for both blacks and whites approached 90 to 100 per cent of the standard or above the standard in dietary intakes. White females in the 18 to 44-year-old group in the lower-income group had mean intakes below the standard and 12 to 17-year-old black boys and girls in the higher-income level were slightly below standard.

In the *biochemical tests* the mean serum vitamin A levels for whites was higher than for blacks for all income levels and age groups. With the exception of blacks in the 1- to 5-year-olds, whites and blacks in the income group above poverty levels had higher mean levels of serum vitamin A than did the lower-income group. In general, mean vitamin A

[18] *Highlights, Ten-State Nutrition Survey, 1968–1970,* DHEW Publication No. (HSM) 72–8134, Center for Disease Control, Health Services and Mental Health Administration, U.S. Department of Health, Education, and Welfare, Atlanta, Ga., 1972.

[19] National Center for Health Statistics, *Preliminary Findings, First Health and Nutrition Examination Survey, United States, 1971–1972,* DHEW Publication No. (HRA) 74–1219–1, Health Resources Administration, Public Health Service, U.S. Department of Health, Education, and Welfare, Rockville, Md., 1974.

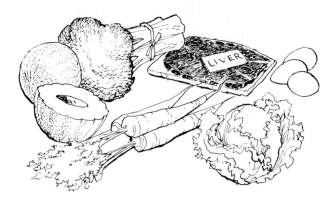

FIGURE 12–1. *Some foods that are rich in vitamin* A.

serum levels increased with age group regardless of race or income group. The percentage of low serum vitamin A values for blacks of 1 to 5 years of age was relatively more than four times that of whites 1 to 5 years of age for both income groups. The percentages with low serum vitamin values in the total population were whites, 2.36, and blacks, 10.20. In the low-income level, the percentages with low serum vitamin A levels were 1.61 for whites and 9.08 for blacks. In the income level above poverty, the percentages of low serum vitamin A values were 2.41 for whites and 10.34 for blacks. Although the population as a whole appears to be meeting vitamin A requirements, it must be borne in mind that among the various groups there is a substantial group of individuals that are below standard, as revealed by their intake range for vitamin A of from 37 to 74 per cent of the standard. These are preliminary findings and further analysis may provide additional data.

Sources of Vitamin A

The animal sources of vitamin A are liver, kidney, whole milk, eggs, and butter. Margarine is fortified with vitamin A and skimmed milk also. Fish-liver oils are the richest source of vitamin A; however, they appear in the diet as a supplement. There is considerable variation in the natural sources of vitamin A content, which reflects the feed of the animal.

The major sources of carotene are the yellow and green leafy vegetables and yellow fruits, such as salad greens (with the exception of iceberg lettuce), kale, collard greens, spinach, carrots, pumpkin, butternut or Hubbard squash, broccoli, beet, mustard, turnip or dandelion greens, red or green peppers, yellow sweet potatoes, apricots, and cantaloupe. The red palm oil used in West and Central Africa and some parts of the Far East has been shown to be an excellent source of carotene. It has been proved that the vitamin A value of fruits and vegetables is directly proportional to the intensity of color; that is, the deeper the green or yellow, the higher the vitamin A content. Table 12–3 shows the amounts of vitamin A that are supplied by some common foods.

Since both carotene and vitamin A are insoluble in water, there is no loss through solubility during cooking. However, vitamin A may be lost through oxidation especially in the presence of heat. This may occur if vegetables or eggs, for example, are preserved by drying, but vacuum drying can prevent its loss. By rupturing the cellular structure, cooking of vegetables, such as carrots, improves the availability of carotene.

It is difficult to determine the contribution to the diet of the formulated and processed foods used in America. De Ritter and others[20] studied the vitamin content of typical frozen heat-and-serve dinners and pot pies. Foods analyzed were chicken pie, fried chicken dinner, turkey dinner, beef pie, beef dinner, Salisbury steak dinner, fish dinner, fried shrimp dinner, and macaroni and cheese. The findings indicated that the available vitamin A varied

---

[20] Elmer De Ritter, Modest Osadca, Jacob Scheiner, and John Keating, "Vitamins in Frozen Convenience Dinners and Pot Pies," *Journal of the American Dietetic Association*, Vol. 64, No. 5 (April 1974), pp. 391–397.

TABLE 12–3

Vitamin A Contributions to Day's Diet of Some Common Foods

FOOD	AMOUNT	VITAMIN A VALUE (IU)
Liver, beef	4 oz	60,660
Egg	1	590
Mackerel, Atlantic	3 oz.	450
Milk, whole	8 oz.	390
Cream, heavy, whipped	1 tbs	240
Cheese, cheddar	1 oz	350
Carrot, raw	1 (5½ × 1 in.)	6,000
Kale, cooked	½ cup	4,610
Spinach, cooked	½ cup	10,600
Squash, winter, cooked	½ cup	1,270
Apricots, dried	½ cup (20 halves)	8,195
Cantaloupe	½ (5-in. diam.)	3,295

SOURCE: *Nutritive Value of Foods*, Home and Garden Buletin No. 72, U.S. Department of Agriculture, Washington, D.C., 1971.

considerably from product to product, ranging from 90 to 2430 IU in the prepared dinners. Most of the vitamin A activity, except for one turkey dinner and the macaroni and cheese combination, occurred in the form of carotene. Losses of vitamin A activity during the preparation of the dinners for eating were small. The minimum nutrient level established by the Food and Drug Administration for vitamin A is 150 IU per 100 kcalories or a minimum level of 520 IU for a total dinner. Only three dinners analyzed contained less than the FDA guideline and six were above the guideline.

Consumption

The contribution in percentages of major food groups to vitamin A nutrient supplies available for civilian consumption for 1974 were meat (including pork fat cuts), poultry, and fish, 21.5 per cent; eggs, 5.8 per cent; dairy products, excluding butter, 12.9 per cent; fats and oils, including butter, 8.1 per cent; citrus fruits, 1.5 per cent; other fruits, 5.5 per cent; potatoes and sweet potatoes, 5.3 per cent; dark-green and deep-yellow vegetables, 21.2 per cent; other vegetables, including tomatoes, 15.5 per cent; dry beans and peas, nuts, soya flour, less than 0.05 per cent; flour and cereal products, 0.4 per cent; sugars and other sweetners, 0 per cent; and miscellaneous, 2.3 per cent.[21]

Vitamin D

Although deformed bone conditions and varied quality among bones had been known for centuries, it was not until 1922[22] that the cause of rickets was discovered. Observations had been made in historical records concerning variation in bone density and quality of skulls of soldiers slain in battle. Then, in 1650, Francis Glisson was the first to describe the clinical manifestation of the bone disorder known as rickets. The historical background of the research leading to the ultimate discovery of vitamin D is primarily concerned with the study of the development of the bone and the factors that various investigators considered important in good or poor bone growth.

Many investigators noted that a poor environment, consisting of poor hygiene, a lack of sunshine and exercise, and often city dwelling was associated with the incidence of rickets. Thus for many years the concept of environment, especially of hygiene and sanitation, dominated the thinking of those who were investigating the cause of this disease. This opinion prevailed in spite of the fact that as early as 1824 cod-liver oil had been recommended as a remedy for rickets.

Using puppies as experimental animals, Sir Edward Mellanby[23] demonstrated that rickets was a dietary deficiency disease. He further showed that certain fats, and specifically cod-liver oil, could prevent and cure it. To Mellanby goes the credit for dispelling the belief

[21] "Contribution of Major Food Groups to Nutrient Supplies Available for Civilian Consumption, 1957–59 and 1974," *National Food Situation* Economic Research Service, U.S. Department of Agriculture, November 1974, p. 28.

[22] McCollum, op. cit., p. 20.

[23] E. Mellanby, *Proceedings of the Physiological Society*, 1918, pp. 1–26.

that environment was the sole cause of rickets.

In 1922 McCollum[24] reported that the vitamin A content of cod-liver oil could be destroyed by oxidation, leaving the antirachitic property of cod-liver oil intact. He had demonstrated that there existed a second fat-soluble vitamin, which was named vitamin D. McCollum and his associates at Johns Hopkins further investigated the importance of vitamin D and the strong influence exerted on the development of rickets by calcium and phosphorus. They also showed that the proportion between calcium and phosphorus is important for good bone development. This proportion has been referred to as the *calcium–phosphorus ratio*. Thus vitamin D, by virtue of its major function, is frequently called the antirachitic vitamin.

Chemistry of Vitamin D

Although there are many members of the vitamin D complex, two forms are equally effective in human nutrition, vitamin D_2 and D_3. Vitamin D_2 is formed by ultraviolet irradiation of ergosterol, found in yeast and fungi, and is identified as ergocalciferol. Vitamin D_3 occurs naturally in egg yolk, milk, and fish-liver oils, and is identified as cholecalciferol.

The human skin contains a sterol known as 7-dehydrocholesterol, which, when exposed to the ultraviolet light found in sunlight, is converted to vitamin D_3. Such things as clothing, clouds, dust, fog, and window glass absorb ultraviolet light. This makes it necessary for each person to examine his surrounding environment to be sure that conditions are favorable for sunlight to activate the provitamin.

Vitamin D_2 is produced commercially first by the irradiation of the sterol, ergosterol, of yeast and then by dissolving the resultant calciferol in oil; it is sold as viosterol. It has been shown to be effective in preventing development of rickets in infants and in a few experimental animals such as rats, pigs, and calves.

The importance of irradiation was discovered in 1924 by both Hess, who was in New York, and Steenbock from Wisconsin. Ergosterol was identified in 1929, and further experiments revelaed the existence and character of calciferol during the years 1930 to 1933.

The intensity of the ultraviolet rays from the sun can vary from one geographic area to another. For example, the sunlight in the tropics is rich in these rays, whereas the temperate areas are less fortunate. Also, there is a greater degree of exposure in the mountain areas than in the valleys or at sea level.

Both vitamins D_2 and D_3 are soluble in fat and fat solvents, and insoluble in water. They are stable to heat, acids, alkalis, and oxidation. For purposes of general discussion, these vitamins are referred to as vitamin D.

Functions of Vitamin D

Vitamin D is vital to a number of aspects of metabolism in the body, but the exact mechanism for these operations is not fully understood. Some of the most important functions are listed here:

1. Increases absorption of calcium and phosphorus from the intestinal tract, thus heightening their availability, and facilitates bone development by influencing mineral deposits.
2. Ensures an adequate supply of calcium and phosphorus in the extracellular fluids bathing growing points of the bones.
3. Maintains desirable levels of calcium and phosphorus in the blood.
4. Reduces excretion of phosphorus in the urine and calcium in the feces.
5. Facilitates eruption of teeth.
6. Increases the absorption of phosphate in kidney tubules.
7. Necessary for mobilization of calcium and phosphorus from bone through promoting physiologic concentrations of parathyroid hormone.
8. Prevention of rickets.

Vitamin D plays an important role in the optimal nutrition of human beings.

Metabolism and Storage of Vitamin D

Like vitamin A, vitamin D is absorbed in the intestine with other fats. Consequently,

---

[24] McCollum, op. cit., p. 276.

TABLE 12–4

Recommended Daily Dietary Allowances for Vitamin D, Revised 1974

Designed for the maintenance of good nutrition of practically all healthy people in the United States

	AGE (years)	WEIGHT (kg)	WEIGHT (lb)	HEIGHT (cm)	HEIGHT (in.)	ENERGY (kcal)	VITA-MIN D (iu)
Infants	0.0–0.5	6	14	60	24	kg × 117	400
	0.5–1.0	9	20	71	28	kg × 108	400
Children	1–3	13	28	86	34	1300	400
	4–6	20	44	110	44	1800	400
	7–10	30	66	135	54	2400	400
Males	11–14	44	97	158	63	2800	400
	15–18	61	134	172	69	3000	400
	19–22	67	147	172	69	3000	400
	23–50	70	154	172	69	2700	
	51+	70	154	172	69	2400	
Females	11–14	44	97	155	62	2400	400
	15–18	54	119	162	65	2100	400
	19–22	58	128	162	65	2100	400
	23–50	58	128	162	65	2000	
	51+	58	128	162	65	1800	
Pregnant						+300	400
Lactating						+500	400

SOURCE: Food and Nutrition Board, *Recommended Dietary Allowances*, 8th ed., National Academy of Sciences—National Research Council, Washington, D.C., 1974.

anything that interferes with the absorption of fats, such as mineral oil or certain disease conditions, will result in the decrease of the absorption of vitamin D. The individual is able to store large amounts of vitamin D, primarily in the liver, but other depots may be the spleen, brain, bones, and skin.

Nutritive Needs for Vitamin D

A minimum requirement for vitamin D has not been established, according to *Recommended Dietary Allowances*.[25] Although the need for vitamin D can be met through skin irradiation if there is sufficient exposure to ultraviolet light, there are many deterrents. Variables are length and intensity of exposure and the color of the skin. Heavily pigmented skin may prevent as much as 95 per cent

[25] *Recommended Dietary Allowances*, op. cit., pp. 54–56.

of the ultraviolet radiation from reaching the deeper layers of the skin, where vitamin D is synthesized.

The prevention of rickets, adequate absorption of calcium in the intestine, satisfactory growth rate, and normal mineralization of bone can occur in the infant on an intake of 2.5 μg or 100 IU of vitamin D. However, 7.5 to 10 μg promotes better calcium absorption and enhances some increase in growth. Infants should be provided with a vitamin D supplement and not risk sunlight as the source.

No information is available concerning the exact requirement of vitamin D for older children and adults. Persons who have limited access to sunlight should have a dietary source of vitamin D. Although no recommended allowance is indicated for adults, a dietary intake of 400 IU for healthy adults of all ages is not risk-producing. For the pregnant and lactating women, 400 IU are advised. See Table 12–4.

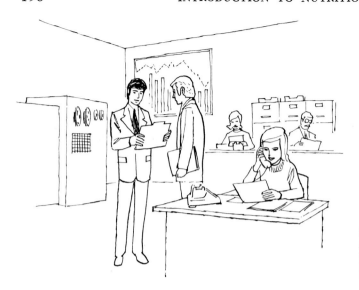

FIGURE 12-2. *Sunshine as a source of vitamin D is limited because of clothes and indoor living.*

Sources of Vitamin D

The ultraviolet light of sunshine, wherever and whenever it is available, is an inexpensive source but not dependable because of clothes, indoor living, and other influences. The use of mercury quartz window glass or similar products that permit ultraviolet light to penetrate is expensive but desirable for individuals who cannot be taken out of doors.

Vitamin D has a limited distribution among foods. Eggs, cream, milk, and liver have small amounts. Fortified foods, fish-liver oils, fatty fish or water-miscible preparations of the vitamin are the primary sources of vitamin D.

Milk was selected as the one food most suitable to be fortified by vitamin D by the Council of Foods and Nutrition of the American Medical Association.[26] Homogenized milk, skim milk, evaporated milk, and nonfat milk solids are fortified by using the standard of 400 IU per quart of liquid milk, an amount that provides the recommended daily allowance. Indiscriminate fortification of other foods is not desirable or necessary. Vitamin D is very stable in foods during storage, marketing, and food preparation and cooking.

Toxicity of Excess Vitamin D

Excessive amounts of vitamin D are dangerous, according to the *Recommended Dietary Allowances*. The dosage that is toxic is considerably beyond the requirement for the vitamin. No extra benefits are gained from higher intakes than those required; 2000 IU per day or five times the recommended allowance for prolonged periods can produce high levels of blood calcium and other evidences of hypercalcemia. Irreversible kidney damage from prolonged hypercalcemia has been reported, according to Omdahl and DeLuca.[27] Some individuals may have a hypersensitivity to vitamin D.

Vitamin E

In 1922 Evans and others[28] observed that experiments with rats raised on certain diets resulted in growth but low fertility in the first generation and complete sterility in the second. These experiments led to the discovery of a third fat-soluble vitamin called vita-

[26] Council on Foods and Nutrition, American Medical Association, "Decision," *Journal of the American Medical Association*, Vol. 159, 1955, p. 1018.

[27] J. L. Omdahl and H. F. DeLuca, "Vitamin D," in Robert S. Goodhart and Maurice E. Shils (eds.), *Modern Nutrition in Health and Disease*, Lea & Febiger, Philadelphia, 1973, Chapter 5.

[28] McCollum, op. cit., Chapter 23.

min E. By giving supplements of lettuce, yeast, and other foods, this sterility condition was corrected. In 1924 vitamin E was named by Sure. Finally, in 1936, the tocopherols were isolated and shown to be the vitamin E. Later, in 1938, alpha-tocopherol was synthesized and thus further experimentation was possible. Vitamin E was available in both the natural and synthetic forms so that its biological activity could be studied further.

Chemical and Physical Properties of Vitamin E

Vitamin E is identified as a series of compounds of plant and animal origin called tocopherols and tocotrienols. There are four naturally occurring tocopherols, but alpha-tocopherol is given primary consideration because it is the most active biologically and has a relatively higher potency than other forms. Vitamin E is soluble in fat solvents and insoluble in water. It is stable to heat and acids and visible light; however, it is unstable to alkali, ultraviolet light, and oxygen. All tocopherols are antioxidant, meaning that they unite with oxygen both within and outside the body.

Functions of Vitamin E

Definite biochemical mechanisms by which vitamin E functions in the body are unknown.[29] The vitamin has been found in all body tissues. The pituitary and adrenal glands have especially high concentrations, but body storage is mainly in the muscle and adipose tissue.

This vitamin plays a role as a nonenzymatic antioxidant that inhibits the oxidation of unsaturated fatty acids and vitamin A. It helps to maintain normal resistance of the red blood cells to rupture by oxidizing agents. Partial substitutes for vitamin E may be selenium and certain antioxidants found in food. Some evidence has been found of very low tocopherol blood levels in the blood serum of premature infants. Vitamin E therapy appeared to have a positive effect on capillary fragility. Majaj[30] and others have shown that infants with severe kwashiorkor, macrocytic anemia, and creatinuria showed positive improvement with vitamin E therapy. This vitamin has an apparent role in the maintenance of stability and integrity of biological membranes.

Nutritive Needs for Vitamin E

There is a correlation of the amount of vitamin E required and the intake of fat and polyunsaturated fatty acids. As the intake of fat and polyunsaturated fatty acids increases, there is a corresponding increase in need for vitamin E. The vitamin E content of diets consumed in the United States is another consideration in determining the recommended allowances. Although there is no evidence that there is a vitamin E deficiency in the "normal" American population, certain medical populations may develop deficiences, such as premature infants on formulas that may lack vitamin E and individuals with impaired fat absorption, according to Bieri.[31] For these reasons, the vitamin E recommended allowances for 1974 are lower. See Table 12–5.

There is some discussion that in future editions of Recommended Dietary Allowances, international units as a measurement will be eliminated and replaced by alpha-tocopherol equivalents. One reason is that in the past alpha-tocopherol was the major source of vitamin E, but the large consumption of soybean oil in American diets has increased the amount of gamma-tocopherol to approximately 20 per cent of the total vitamin E activity in foods, in spite of the fact that the biologic activity of gamma-tocopherol is only 10 per cent of alpha-tocopherol. Confusion between the milligrams of various forms of alpha-tocopherol (natural, synthetic, or esterfied) and international units would be eliminated.

The minimum adult requirement for vitamin E is unknown but is probably from 3 to 6

[29] I. Molenaar, J. Vos, and F. A. Hommes, "Effect of Vitamin E Deficiency on Cellular Membranes," in Robert S. Harris et al. (eds.), Vitamins and Hormones, Academic Press, New York, 1972, p. 45.

[30] A. S. Majaj et al., "Vitamin E Responsive Megaloblastic Anemia in Infants with Protein-Calorie Malnutrition," American Journal of Clinical Nutrition, Vol. 12, No. 3 (March 1963), pp. 374–377.

[31] Bieri, op. cit., pp. 172–173.

TABLE 12–5

Recommended Daily Dietary Allowances for Vitamin E, Revised 1974

Designed for the maintenance of good nutrition of practically all healthy people in the United States

	AGE (years)	WEIGHT (kg)	WEIGHT (lb)	HEIGHT (cm)	HEIGHT (in.)	ENERGY (kcal)	VITA-MIN E ACTIVITY[a] (iu)
Infants	0.0–0.5	6	14	60	24	kg × 117	4
	0.5–1.0	9	20	71	28	kg × 108	5
Children	1–3	13	28	86	34	1300	7
	4–6	20	44	110	44	1800	9
	7–10	30	66	135	54	2400	10
Males	11–14	44	97	158	63	2800	12
	15–18	61	134	172	69	3000	15
	19–22	67	147	172	69	3000	15
	23–50	70	154	172	69	2700	15
	51+	70	154	172	69	2400	15
Females	11–14	44	97	155	62	2400	12
	15–18	54	119	162	65	2100	12
	19–22	58	128	162	65	2100	12
	23–50	58	128	162	65	2000	12
	51+	58	128	162	65	1800	12
Pregnant						+300	15
Lactating						+500	15

SOURCE: Food and Nutrition Board, *Recommended Dietary Allowances*, 8th ed., National Academy of Sciences—National Research Council, Washington, D.C., 1974.

[a] Total vitamin E activity, estimated to be 80 per cent as alpha-tocopherol and 20 per cent other tocopherols. See text for variation in allowances.

IU per day.[32] Allowances for low-birth-weight-infants on formulas are suggested as 3 mg or about 4.5 IU of alpha-tocopherol per liter of formula containing 3.5 per cent of fat in a mixture of saturated and unsaturated fats. Human milk is considered adequate in vitamin E activity. For normal infants, breast milk is adequate. A total of 4 IU of vitamin E should be provided to the infant during the first 5 months and 5 IU for the remainder of the first year on a mixed diet of solid foods and milk. The basis for allowances for growing children is to increase the intake of vitamin E from 5 IU at 9 kg of body weight to 12 IU at 40 kg of body weight, provided 4 to 7 per

[32] *Recommended Dietary Allowances*, op. cit., pp. 60–61.

cent of the calories are in linoleic acid. Seven IU is recommended for children 1 to 3; 9 IU for 4 to 6; 10 IU for 7 to 10; and 12 IU for both boys and girls 11 to 14 years.

For adults a dietary intake of vitamin E that maintains a blood concentration of 0.5 mg per 100 ml will ensure an adequate supply in all tissues. Adaquate in this context means a ratio of tocopherols to polyunsaturated fatty acids that encourages normal physiological functioning and also allows for potential stress situations. The ratio for this human tissue functioning is unknown. No reports have emerged of vitamin E deficiencies, so a range of 10 to 20 IU for balanced diets of 1800 to 3000 kcalories appears adequate for adults. For men, 15 IU is recommended daily and for women, 12 IU. During pregnancy and lactation the allowance is increased to 15 IU to compensate for amounts deposited in the fetus and secreted in human milk. International units in *Recommended Dietary Allowances* indicate total vitamin E activity and are not to be interpreted as milligrams of d-alpha-tocopherol tabulations.

Vitamin E, unfortunately, has caught the fancy of faddists, who recommend massive doses, in some instances, to relieve such conditions as acne, heart disease, sterility, muscular weakness, cancer, ulcers, burns, and shortness of breath.[33] The elderly, many of whom can ill afford to buy expensive vitamin preparations, take vitamin E to ward off the signs of old age and to increase sexual potency. These misconceptions have arisen from misinterpretations of animal experimental studies, such as antisterility studies. There is no scientific evidence that vitamin E will either cure or prevent any of these human ailments, according to a statement of the Food Nutrition Board, Division of Biology and Agriculture, of the National Research Council.

Sources of Vitamin E

The richest dietary sources are the cereal seed oils, such as wheat germ oil, but vitamin E is widely distributed among foods. Hence there is little possibility of a deficiency in the American diet unless there is limited choice and the individual's absorptive mechanisms are not normal. Food processing and storage including freezing of foods tend to destroy some of the tocopherol content. Ordinary cooking, except for deep-fat frying, has little effect.

American sources of this vitamin are provided by salad oils, shortening, and margarine, fruits and vegetables and cereal products. Table 12–6 gives the alpha-tocopherol content of some common foods. Food composition tables for vitamin E are somewhat limited. Indications of the types of tocopherols have not been accessible. The availability of this information will give more accurate data about the sources of vitamin E in the diet.

[33] "Supplementation of Human Diets with Vitamin E," *Nutrition Reviews*, Vol. 31, No. 10 (October 1973), pp. 327–328.

TABLE 12–6

Some Common Food Sources of Vitamin E in the Form of Alpha-Tocopherol

FOOD	ALPHA-TOCOPHEROL (mg/100 g)
Fats and oils	
Coconut oil	0.8
Corn oil	13.0
Cottonseed oil	50.0
Margarine	4.8
Olive oil	7.6
Soybean oil	4.8
Cereals	
Cornmeal, yellow	0.84
Oatmeal	1.94
Rice, polished	0.57
Wheat germ	12.9
Fruits	
Apple	1.0
Bananas	0.37
Grapefruit	0.25
Tomato	0.5
Vegetables	
Asparagus	2.5
Broccoli	3.5
Cabbage, white	0.6
Carrots	0.45
Dandelion greens	2.5
Green peas	0.1
Spinach	2.71
Nuts	
Brazil nuts	6.5
Peanuts	12.0
Pecans	1.5
Walnuts	20.5
Meats, fish, poultry, and eggs	
Egg	0.99
Beef liver	1.40
Chicken breast	0.15
Codfish	0.63
Haddock	0.35

SOURCE: Martha W. Dicks, *Vitamin E Content of Foods and Feeds for Human and Animal Consumption*, Bulletin 435, Agricultural Experiment Station, University of Wyoming, Laramine, Wyo., 1965.

Vitamin K

The discovery of the antihemorrhagic vitamin, last of the fat-soluble vitamins to be discovered, was accomplished by Damm[34] in 1934. This investigator recognized that there existed a factor that was causing a hemorrhagic disorder in chickens. It was not until 1939 that Damm, along with others, isolated vitamin K.

Chemical Properties of Vitamin K

Vitamin K is similar to the other vitamins in having a number of forms. The two principal natural sources are K_1 (phylloquinone), which is the form of vitamin K that is found in food in the normal diet, especially leafy vegetables, and vitamin K_2 (menaquinone) with about 75 per cent of the activity of K_1, which is synthesized by the bacterial flora of the human intestinal tract.

All the K vitamins are insoluble in water; therefore there is no loss in cooking. They are fat-soluble and stable to heat and reducing agents. They are labile to alcoholic alkali, oxidizing agents, strong acids, and light. Vitamin K_1 is found primarily in green leaves, and vitamin K_2 is synthesized by intestinal microorganisms. The synthetic water-soluble forms are those usually used for therapy.

Functions of Vitamin K

Vitamin K has one major function; it seems to be necessary for the synthesis of prothrombin, an enzyme synthesized by the liver. Prothrombin is required for normal clotting of blood. A deficiency of vitamin K is manifested by a prolonged clotting time. Other blood-clotting factors may be involved.

Vitamin K Deficiency

Infants, especially the premature or ones that have feeding problems, may develop vitamin K deficiency. Incidence of neonatal hemorrhage in newborn infants has been corrected by the administration of vitamin K promptly after birth. In adults a deficiency of this vitamin may occur with the intake of antibiotics or similar drugs that interfere with the synthesis of vitamin K in the intestine. Anticoagulants are antagnoistic to the activity of the vitamin.

Other conditions that may hinder the vitamin K content of the body may be associated with those that interfere with proper absorption of vitamins, such as chronic diarrhea or ingestion of mineral oil. Bile salts are essential for absorption and any illness that interferes with the production of bile may then result in a vitamin K deficiency.

The ability to store vitamin K seems limited, as evidenced by the fact that a mother is unable to provide a reserve in the fetus. What little storage exists seems to take place with the liver as the primary site.

Nutritive Needs for Vitamin K

An exact dietary allowance for vitamin K has not been established. The lack of adequate information about human intakes of vitamin K, factors noted in experimental animals but not evaluated in man, the role of synthesis in the intestinal tract, and the absorption of this vitamin from food sources complicate the determination of an allowance.

Sources of Vitamin K

As mentioned previously, there are two major sources of vitamin K: ingested foods and intestinal synthesis. The latter occurs in the small intestine, and vitamin K then follows the usual pathways in metabolism. Of the foods, green leafy vegetables and alfalfa are among the richest sources. In fact, alfalfa is one of the original known sources. Vitamin K is widely distributed in other foods, such as egg yolk, soybean oil, liver, cauliflower, and tomatoes. Cow's milk is somewhat richer in the vitamin than human milk.

[34] McCollum, op. cit., Chap. 25.

SELECTED REFERENCES

GENERAL

Bauernfeind, J. C., H. Newmark, and M. Brin, "Vitamins A and E Nutrition Via Intra-muscular or Oral Route," *American Journal of Clinical Nutrition*, Vol. 27, No. 3 (March 1974), pp. 234–253.

Bieri, John G., "Fat-Soluble Vitamins in the Eighth Revision of the Recommended Dietary Allowances," *Journal of the American Dietetic Association*, Vol. 64, No. 2 (February 1974), pp. 171–174.

Davidson, Stanley, R. Passmore, and J. F. Brock, *Human Nutrition and Dietetics*, The Williams & Wilkins Company, Baltimore, 1972, Chapter 11.

Food and Nutrition Board, *Recommended Dietary Allowances*, 8th ed., National Academy of Sciences—National Research Council, Washington, D.C., 1974, pp. 50–62.

Halberstam, Michael, "The A, B-12, C, D., and E of Vitamins," *The New York Times Magazine*, March 17, 1974, pp. 16, 68–72.

Kutsky, Roman J., *Handbook of Vitamins and Hormones*, Van Nostrand Reinhold Company, New York, 1973.

Robson, John R. K., et al., *Malnutrition, Its Causation and Control*, Volume 2, Gordon and Breach, New York, 1972, pp. 337–338, 340.

VITAMIN A

Brooke, Clinton L., and Winifred M. Cort, "Vitamin A Fortification of Tea," *Food Technology*, Vol. 26, No. 6 (June 1972), pp. 50–52, 58.

Roels, Oswald A., "Vitamin A Physiology," *Journal of the American Medical Association*, Vol. 214, No. 6 (November 9, 1970), pp. 1097–1102.

Sweeney, J. P., and A. C. March, "Effect of Processing on Provitamin A in Vegetables," *Journal of the American Dietetic Association*, Vol. 59, No. 3 (September 1971), pp. 238–243.

Zaklama, Mona S., Mamdouh K. Gabr, Safinaz El Maraghy, and Vinayak N. Patwarhan, "Serum Vitamin A in Protein-Calorie-Malnutrition," *American Journal of Clinical Nutrition*, Vol. 26, No. 11 (November 1973), pp. 1202–1206.

VITAMIN D

DeLuca, H. F. "Vitamin D: A New Look at an Old Vitamin," *Nutrition Reviews*, Vol. 29, No. 8 (August 1971), pp. 179–181.

Food and Nutrition Board, *Hazards of the Overuse of Vitamin D*, National Research Council, National Academy of Sciences, Washington, D.C., 1974.

"Recent Developments in Vitamin D," *Dairy Council Digest*, Vol. 41, No. 4 (July–August 1970), pp. 19–22.

Report of a Joint FAO/WHO Expert Group, *Requirements of Ascorbic Acid, Vitamin D, Vitamin B-12, Folate, and Iron*, World Health Organization Technical Report Series, No. 452, World Health Organization, Geneva, 1970

VITAMIN E

Bieri, John G., and Titva Poukka Evarts, "Tocopherols and Fatty Acids," *Journal of the American Dietetic Association*, Vol. 62, No. 2 (February 1973), pp. 147–151.

Bunnell, R. H., J. Keating, A. Quaresimo, and G. K. Parman, "Alpha-Tocopherol Content of Foods," *American Journal of Clinical Nutrition,* Vol. 17, No. 7 (July 1965), pp. 1–10; Addendum, pp. 1–6.

Christianson, M. M., and Ethelwyn B. Wilcox, "Dietary Polyunsaturates and Serum Alpha-Tocopherol in Adults," *Journal of the American Dietetic Association,* Vol. 63, No. 2 (August 1973), pp. 138–142.

Committee on Nutritional Misinformation, *Supplementation of Human Diets with Vitamin E,* Statement of Food and Nutrition Board, Division of Biology and Agriculture, National Academy of Sciences—National Research Council, Washington, D.C., 1973.

Hodges, Robert E., and Roslyn B. Alfin-Slater, "Vitamin E- -A Review," *Nutrah,* Vol. 1, No. 3 (January 1972), pp. 1–3.

Olson, Robert E., "Vitamin E and Heart Disease," *Food and Nutrition News,* Vol. 44, Nos. 5–6 (February–March 1973), pp. 1, 4.

"Pitfalls in Calculating the Vitamin E Content of Diets," *Nutrition Reviews,* Vol. 30, No. 3 (March 1972), pp. 55–57.

Tappel, A. L., "Vitamin E.," *Nutrition Today,* Vol. 8, No. 4 (July–August 1973), pp. 4–12.

"Vitamin E," *Consumer Reports,* Vol. 38, No. 1 (January 1973), pp. 60–66.

Witting, Lloyd A., "Recommended Dietary Allowance for Vitamin E., *American Journal of Clinical Nutrition,* Vol. 25, No. 3 (March 1972), pp. 257–261.

VITAMIN K

Suttie, J. W., "Vitamin K and Prothrombin Synthesis," *Nutrition Reviews,* Vol. 31, No. 4 (April 1973), pp. 105–109.

13

The B Vitamins— Water Soluble

The identity of the B vitamins emerged in a number of ways. Some were discovered as solutions to public health problems, such as pellagra and beriberi. Others were isolated during experimentation to secure a pure form of the vitamin when two or more forms were found. Still others emerged from laboratory and clinical experimentation. Although these vitamins have commonalities, they are distinctly different vitamins with unique functions and characteristics.

Thiamin

The disease beriberi has been recognized for centuries. However, it was Eijkman's[1] observations during the 1890's that led to the first clear concept of a deficiency disease. Eijkman was a Dutch physician who was in Java in the Dutch East Indies studying the problem of the high incidence of beriberi among the military. Accidentally, he noticed that chickens that ate the polishings from rice failed to develop a condition similar to beriberi, whereas those that ate polished rice

seemed to suffer from the disease. Eijkman then experimentally induced polyneuritis among the chickens. This study represents a milestone in nutrition history, since it was the first time that a deficiency disease was produced experimentally.

Prior to Eijkman's reports, Takaki had found in 1882 that beriberi among the sailors in the Japanese navy could be cured and prevented by providing extra meat. He concluded, erroneously, that the additional protein was the beneficial factor.

Eijkman thought that there was a toxic substance in the white rice that produced the beriberi. However, Grijns suggested in 1906 that beriberi was a deficiency disease due to the absence of an essential nutrient.

At the Lister Institute in London, Casimir Funk obtained a crystalline material from rice polishings, which he named "a vitamine" because of its chemical structure.

It was not until 1926 that Jansen and Donath in Holland isolated the antiberiberi vitamin. Later, in 1936, Robert R. Williams[2]

---

[1] E. V. McCollum, A History of Nutrition, Houghton Mifflin, Boston, 1957, p. 216.

[2] R. R. Williams, Toward the Conquest of Beriberi, Harvard University Press, Cambridge, Mass., 1961.

163

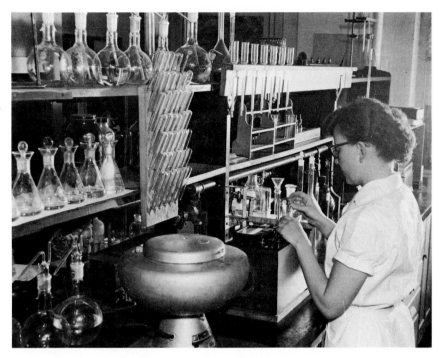

FIGURE 13–1.   *A laboratory technician analyzes a food for thiamine.* (*General Mills, Inc.*)

and his colleagues determined the structure of the antiberiberi factor, which they called *thiamine*. Once the structure was determined, they synthesized the vitamin. Williams coined the word *thiamine* to indicate its structure: the presence of both sulfur and an amine group.

Chemistry of Thiamin

The pure vitamin is identified as thiamin hydrochloride, a crystal compound. It is soluble in water and insoluble in fat. It has a characteristic odor described as "nutty and yeasty." Thiamin is stable in dry heat but destroyed rapidly in a neutral or alkaline solution. An acid solution enhances its stability.

Functions of Thiamin

The most important function of thiamin seems to be its role in the utilization of carbohydrate. Glucose is broken down (oxidized) in the tissue to supply energy. This breakdown occurs through a series of reactions,

each requiring specific enzymes. Thiamin is part of the coenzyme structure (small organic molecules, nonprotein in nature, which are essential to the activity of the particular enzyme). In this case, the reaction of the enzyme system brings about the oxidation of glucose. Thiamin, then, participates in reactions that, through the release of energy, result in the formation of carbon dioxide. This coenzyme, known as cocarboxylase, acts on pyruvic acid, an intermediate product in the oxidation of glucose. Cocarboxylase is required for the subsequent breakdown of pyruvate, and then further energy is released through this reaction. However, if a thiamin deficiency exists, the oxidation of glucose cannot proceed beyond this stage, and pyruvic acid levels of the blood increase.

Another function is that the enzyme transketolase requires thiamin as a coenzyme. This enzyme is present in red blood cells, the liver, kidney, and other tissue, except skeletal. Transketolase is essential for the synthesis within the body of certain sugars, such as ribose, found in nucleotides. A third role is in the metabolism of fat and carbohydrate in an intermediary stage in which a form of keto-glutaric acid is decarboxylated to succinic acid.

Other functions ascribed to thiamin are varied and seemingly unrelated. Thiamin seems to be necessary in maintaining a functionally normal nervous system. However, it has not been shown that nervous disorders are due to thiamin deficiencies. Thiamin also seems to be related to cardiac function, as evidenced by the characteristic "beriberi heart" that occurs in the thiamin deficiency disease.

Deficiency of Thiamin

A thiamin deficiency may occur in one of two ways: a primary deficiency is the result of an inadequate dietary supply, or a secondary deficiency may come about as a result of conditioning factors that interfere with the proper utilization of thiamin or that increase the demand for thiamin, such as pregnancy and lactation.

A mild deficiency can be produced by a moderately low intake of thiamin. It is characterized by such symptoms as loss of appetite, apathy, fatigue tendencies, nausea, and numbness in the legs. Certain mental disturbances occur: moodiness, irritability, and mild depression. An electrocardiogram may show variations from normal.

More advanced deficiences result in the disease beriberi. There are two types of beriberi. The dry or peripheral neuritis is characterized by severe muscular wasting, loss of sensation in the skin, loss of weight, and paralysis in the lower extremities. The wet form produces marked edema, which usually starts at the extremities and develops upward. When it reaches the trunk, the heart becomes involved, enlarged, and frequently the end result is heart failure. Beriberi in infants is characterized by edema, gastrointestinal difficulties, retarded growth, and often cardiac failure.

Beriberi seldom occurs in this country, although it is still quite prevalent in many areas of the world, particularly where people depend on rice for the major portion of their calorie needs. Some of these countries are the Philip-pines, Burma, Vietnam, Malaya, and Indonesia. Most incidences of beriberi in the United States appear in chronic alcoholics whose diet patterns are so poor that they have substituted alcohol in its various forms for food.

Metabolism and Storage of Thiamin

Thiamin is absorbed readily from the small intestine as it is released from foods. It is circulated by the bloodstream to various sections of the body where it can be utilized as the need arises. The total amount in the body will supply enough for only a few weeks of normal functioning. If the individual ingests more thiamin than he can use or store in the small amounts that are possible, the excess thiamin is excreted.

Thiamin Nutritive Needs

Allowances for thiamin have usually been related to energe intake.[3] Most of these experimental diets had a ratio of carbohydrate and fat similar to those consumed in the United States. Although there is some evidence that dietary fat spares thiamin to some extent, there is inadequate basis for making adjustments in the carbohydrate and fat ratios in the diet. Other studies about dietary thiamin intake have dealt with intakes that produce clinical signs of deficiency, intakes that are consistent with good health, the amount of thiamin excreted in the urine, or with red cell transketolase.

After reviewing the findings of research on thiamin intake, the Food and Nutrition Board decided on a thiamin allowance for adults of 0.5 mg per 1000 kcalories. Some data indicate that older persons may use thiamin less efficiently, so 1 mg per day is recommended even though less than 2000 kcalories are consumed. Thiamin allowances increase for pregnant and lactating women with the increase in kcalories, but the formula continues to be 0.5 mg per 1000 kcalories. Scarcity of information limits the basis for thiamin allowance for infants. From available research findings, the

---

[3] Food and Nutrition Board, *Recommended Dietary Allowances*, 8th ed., National Academy of Science—National Research Council, Washington, D.C., 1974, pp. 65–68.

TABLE 13–1

Recommended Daily Dietary Allowances for Thiamin, Revised 1974

Designed for the maintenance of good nutrition for practically all healthy people in the United States

	AGE (years)	WEIGHT (kg)	WEIGHT (lb)	HEIGHT (cm)	HEIGHT (in.)	ENERGY (kcal)	THIA-MIN (mg)
Infants	0.0–0.5	6	14	60	24	kg × 117	0.3
	0.5–1.0	9	20	71	28	kg × 108	0.5
Children	1–3	13	28	86	34	1300	0.7
	4–6	20	44	110	44	1800	0.9
	7–10	30	66	135	54	2400	1.2
Males	11–14	44	97	158	63	2800	1.4
	15–18	61	134	172	69	3000	1.5
	19–22	67	147	172	69	3000	1.5
	23–50	70	154	172	69	2700	1.4
	51+	70	154	172	69	2400	1.2
Females	11–14	44	97	155	62	2400	1.2
	15–18	54	119	162	65	2100	1.1
	19–22	58	128	162	65	2100	1.1
	23–50	58	128	162	65	2000	1.0
	51+	58	128	162	65	1800	1.0
Pregnant						+300	+0.3
Lactating						+500	+0.3

SOURCE: Food and Nutrition Board, *Recommended Dietary Allowances*, 8th ed., National Academy of Sciences—National Research Council, Washington, D.C., 1974.

recommended allowance is 0.5 mg per 1000 kcalories. Information on which to base allowances for children and teen-agers is equally limited. The recommended allowance is 0.5 mg per 1000 kcalories. See Table 13–1 for specific recommendations for all ages, sexes, and for pregnancy and lactation.

Thiamin Nutritional Status

According to the *Ten-State Nutrition Survey*,[4] the only groups of concern were 10- to 16-year-old black boys and girls in low- and high-income-ratio states and white boys and girls at this same age level in low-income-ratio states; these groups had a low prevalence of

[4] *Highlights, Ten-State Nutrition Survey 1968–1970*, DHEW Publication No. (HSM) 72–8134, Center for Disease Control, Health Services and Mental Health Administration, U.S. Department of Health, Education, and Welfare, Atlanta, Ga., 1972.

thiamin deficiencies. All other age levels, both sexes, and at both income levels had only minimal deficiencies. (See Table 2–2.)

Sources of Thiamin

Thiamin is present in many foods, but the amount supplied by any given one is relatively small. No single food in the American diet can be depended upon to supply a major portion of the individual's daily thiamin needs. Some foods contain more thiamin than others, and these primary sources include such items as lean pork, organ meats, liver, sausage, lean meats, eggs, whole-grain and enriched breads and cereals, green leafy vegetables, nuts, and legumes. Table 13–2 indicates the amount of thiamin found in an average portion of these foods.

In those parts of the world where as much as 70 per cent of the kcalories of the diet may be provided by rice, it is common practice in the milling of the cereal to remove the part

TABLE 13–2

Thiamin Content of Selected Foods

FOOD	PORTION	CONTENT THIAMIN (mg)
Milk, fluid whole	1 cup (8 oz)	0.08
Pork, roast	3 oz	0.78
Liver, beef, fried	3 oz	0.24
Beef, roast, round	3 oz	0.06
Egg, boiled	1	0.05
Peanuts, halves	¼ cup	0.12
Spinach	1 cup	0.14
Broccoli	1 cup	0.10
Dates	1 cup	0.16
Peas	1 cup	0.40
Orange, navel	1	0.12
Pineapple, raw	1 cup	0.12
Watermelon	1 wedge 4 × 8 in.	0.20
Oatmeal, cooked	1 cup	0.22
Enriched white bread	1 slice	0.06
Whole-wheat bread	1 slice	0.06
Rice, cooked, white	1 cup	0.02

SOURCE: *Nutritive Value of Foods*, Home and Garden Bulletin No. 72, U.S. Department of Agriculture, Washington, D.C., 1971.

of the grain that is richest in thiamin. This action has created conditions favorable to the development of beriberi in more than half the human race.

Effect of Food Preparation on Thiamin

Here in the United States thiamin is lost through some processing procedures, like the milling of cereals, the pasteurization of milk, and the canning of meat.

But thiamin can also be lost in cooking because it is water-soluble. And it can be lost through oxidation, a loss that is further increased by heat and that is accelerated in an alkaline medium.

The thiamin loss in cooking will depend on the amount of water used, the length of the cooking period, and the amount of surface area exposed. When meats are cooked, water-soluble thiamin often goes from the meat itself into the juices and is found in the drippings. The time-honored technique of searing meats also causes some loss of thiamin. As frozen meats thaw, the drippings also contain thiamin.

Bowers and Fryer[5] analyzed the effects of cooking and reheating (after 1 day of refrigeration and 5 weeks of freezer storage) in microwave and gas ovens on the thiamin content of turkey muscle. The turkey muscle held for 1 day at refrigerator temperature and reheated retained the highest amount of thiamin in comparison to reheating turkey muscle held in freezer storage for 5 weeks and reheated. Variation was much greater among birds than between methods.

Noble[6] analyzed thiamin retention in cooked variety meats such as frozen calf sweetbreads, fresh beef kidney, and fresh lamb and pork heart. Results differed among the meats analyzed. Sweetbreads, for example, retained the highest amount of thiamin (60 per cent), followed in descending order, by beef, veal, and pork hearts (lowest with 29 per cent). Braised meats on the average, lost 19 per cent of the thiamin.

DeRitter and others[7] analyzed the vitamin content of frozen convenience dinners and pot pies. The highest level of thiamin was found in one type of beef pot pie and in one Salisbury steak dinner, probably because the label indicated that thiamin had been added, and in macaroni and cheese, possibly because of the enriched macaroni. Losses during preparation varied considerably, ranging from 0 to 85 per cent. According to FDA guidelines for thiamin, only one frozen dinner exceeded the

[5] Jane A. Bowers and Beth A. Fryer, "Thiamin and Riboflavin in Cooked and Frozen, Reheated Turkey," *Journal of the American Dietetic Association*, Vol. 60, No. 5 (May 1972), pp. 399–401.

[6] Isabel Noble, "Thiamine and Riboflavin Retention in Cooked Variety Meats," *Journal of the American Dietetic Association*, Vol. 56, No. 3 (March 1970), pp. 225–228.

[7] Elmer DeRitter, Modest Osadca, Jacob Scheiner, and John Keating, "Vitamins in Frozen Convenience Dinners and Pot Pies," *Journal of the American Dietetic Association*, Vol. 64, No. 4 (April 1974), pp. 391–397.

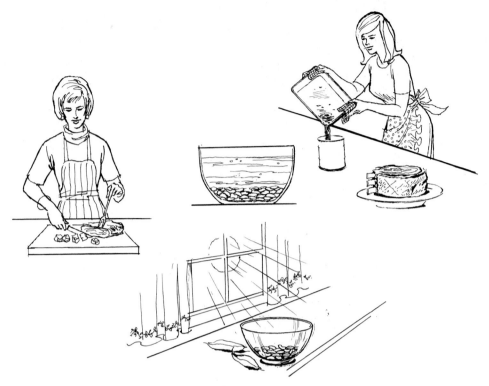

FIGURE 13–2.   *Thiamin losses in food preparation.*

minimum level of thiamin and two dinners were close.

Since the thiamin content of the diet may come from many sources, it seems wise for persons preparing food to become aware of the many ways in which they can minimize the loss of this essential nutrient.

Thiamin Consumption

Food groups contribute the following percentages of thiamin in the American diet according to preliminary 1974 data: eggs, 2.2 per cent; dairy products, excluding butter, 9.0 per cent; fats and oils, including butter, 0 per cent; citrus fruits, 2.8 per cent; other fruits, 1.8 per cent; potatoes and sweet potatoes, 6.2 per cent; dark-green and deep-yellow vegetables, 0.9 per cent; other vegetables, including tomatoes, 6.9 per cent; dry beans and peas, nuts, soya flour, 5.7 per cent; flour and cereal products, 36.3 per cent; meat (including pork fat cuts), poultry, and fish, 28.1 per

cent; and sugars and other sweeteners, less than 0.05 per cent.[8]

Riboflavin

The separation of the water-soluble group was often confusing. It was not until 1926 that it was shown that part of the B complex was heat-labile (thiamin) and part heat-stable. In the same year, Goldberger and Lilly[9] developed pellagra in the rat and cured the condition by the administration of a diet from which thiamin had been removed. They named the curative factor P-P (pellagra preventive). It was also called B_2 by the British Committee on Accessory Food Factors; American scientists referred to it as vitamin G in honor of Goldberger. Later this heat-stable

---

[8] *National Food Situation*, Economic Research Service, U.S. Department of Agriculture, Washington, D.C., November 1974, p. 28.

[9] McCollum, op. cit., p. 296.

fraction was shown to include other vitamins as well.

In 1932, Warburg and Christian[10] reported that they had separated a "yellow enzyme" that exhibited oxidative reactions. The next year riboflavin was identified and reported as isolated in pure form from natural materials by Kuhn and his associates. Later György[11] demonstrated the significance of riboflavin as an essential growth factor in both its synthesized and naturally occurring forms.

Chemical and Physical Properties of Riboflavin

Riboflavin crystals are in the form of orange-yellowish brown needles. Riboflavin has an intense yellow-green fluorescence in water. Since it is soluble in water, losses may occur in food preparation. This vitamin may be destroyed in the presence of alkali or if exposed to ultraviolet light. (Special attention must be given to milk so that it does not stand in a glass container in the sunlight.) Riboflavin is relatively stable to heat, especially in an acid solution, and to oxidizing agents.

Functions of Riboflavin

The primary function of riboflavin seems to be its activity in the oxidative process of the living cell. It participates in the respiration of tissue cells and seems to combine with protein to form a number of very important enzymes and coenzymes known as flavoproteins, sometimes called the yellow enzymes. These flavoproteins act closely with other enzymes containing niacin and are important in the metabolism of protein, fat, and carbohydrate. They are identified as flavin mononucleotide (FMN) and flavin adenine dinucleotide (FAD).

Riboflavin is an essential component of living cells. Cellular growth depends upon this vitamin. It is necessary for the release of energy in the cell. Riboflavin contributes to normal tissue maintenance, as of the skin, mucous membranes, and possibly the eye.

Riboflavin Deficiency

No clear-cut disease is associated with a deficiency of riboflavin intake, as beriberi is intimately associated with a deficiency of thiamin. A low dietary intake of riboflavin may result in fissures at the angle of the mouth, accompanied by a yellow crust. This characteristic condition is known as *cheilosis*. A local inflammation may also be associated with this condition. However, it is not necessarily specific for ariboflavinosis. Sometimes changes appear in the eye, such as a vascularization of the cornea, and the patient also may complain of a sensitivity to light. The tongue may exhibit a glossitis, turning a purplish red in color, accompanied by a painful, burning sensation. Dermatitis about the nose and scrotum in the male has been observed. Although there have been well-controlled experiments with human volunteers to try to bring about a deficiency syndrome, the subjects have hardly ever displayed an acute uniform manifestation of riboflavin deficiency that involved all these vague and somewhat isolated symptoms. However, it is necessary that we include adequate amounts of riboflavin in the diet each day, for its essential role in tissue respiration is extremely important.

Riboflavin Nutritive Needs

Riboflavin nutriture is generally evaluated by urinary excretion of the vitamin. Studies of clinical symptoms, such as cheilosis and changes in red blood cell riboflavin, and their relation to riboflavin dietary intake have been useful.[12] After reviewing this research, allowances for individuals of all ages were computed to be 0.6 mg per 1000 kcalories. Activity of all individuals is judged to be normal, neither sedentary nor heavy. Additional allowances are required for pregnancy; an additional 0.3 mg is recommended. To allow for the amount of riboflavin required for the production of milk in a lactating woman and for the amount of riboflavin secreted in the milk, an additional daily intake of 0.5 mg is recommended.

---

[10] Ibid., p. 297.

[11] Paul György, "Early Experiences with Riboflavin—A Retrospect," *Nutrition Reviews*, Vol. 12, No. 3 (March 1954), p. 97.

[12] *Recommended Dietary Allowances*, op. cit., pp. 68–69.

TABLE 13–3

Recommended Daily Dietary Allowances for Riboflavin, Revised 1974

Designed for the maintenance of good nutrition for practically all healthy people in the United States

	AGE (years)	WEIGHT (kg)	WEIGHT (lb)	HEIGHT (cm)	HEIGHT (in.)	ENERGY (kcal)	RIBO-FLAVIN (mg)
Infants	0.0–0.5	6	14	60	24	kg × 117	0.4
	0.5–1.0	9	20	71	28	kg × 108	0.6
Children	1–3	13	28	86	34	1300	0.8
	4–6	20	44	110	44	1800	1.1
	7–10	30	66	135	54	2400	1.2
Males	11–14	44	97	158	63	2800	1.5
	15–18	61	134	172	69	3000	1.8
	19–22	67	147	172	69	3000	1.8
	23–50	70	154	172	69	2700	1.6
	51+	70	154	172	69	2400	1.5
Females	11–14	44	97	155	62	2400	1.3
	15–18	54	119	162	65	2100	1.4
	19–22	58	128	162	65	2100	1.4
	23–50	58	128	162	65	2000	1.2
	51+	58	128	162	65	1800	1.1
Pregnant						+300	+0.3
Lactating						+500	+0.5

SOURCE: Food and Nutrition Board, *Recommended Dietary Allowances*, 8th ed., National Academy of Sciences—National Research Council, Washington, D.C., 1974.

Table 13–3 includes the riboflavin allowances recommended by the Food and Nutrition Board.

Riboflavin Nutritional Status

In the *Ten-State Nutrition Survey*[13] there was evidence of a riboflavin deficiency among certain groups. In the low-income-ratio states, there was a medium prevalence of deficient values of riboflavin among blacks of all ages and both sexes and among Spanish-Americans from ages 0 to 16 and of both sexes. There was a low prevalence of deficient values among whites from 0 to 16 years of both sexes and among Spanish-Americans from 17 to over 60 years of age. All other groups had only minimal deficiencies.

In the high-income-ratio states there was a low prevalence of deficient values of riboflavin among blacks of all ages and both sexes and for whites from 0 to 5 years of age. All other groups had only minimal deficiencies of riboflavin. (See Table 2–2.)

Sources of Riboflavin

Chief among the sources that supply considerable amounts of riboflavin are the organ meats such as liver, heart, and kidney. Milk and its by-product, cheese, are also excellent sources. Other foods that supply a considerable amount of riboflavin are eggs, lean meat, leafy green vegetables, and whole-grain and enriched cereals. These are all easily available and common in the American diet. Table 13–4 indicates the riboflavin content of some common foods in the diet.

Riboflavin Consumption

In the United States, riboflavin is among those nutrients that are added to bread and

---

[13] *Ten-State Survey,* op. cit., pp. 4–5.

TABLE 13–4

Riboflavin Content of Selected Foods

FOOD	PORTION	RIBOFLAVIN CONTENT (mg)
Beef liver	3 oz	3.55
Almonds	½ cup	0.65
Milk, nonfat, skim	1 cup	0.44
Milk, whole	1 cup	0.41
Yeast, brewer's, dry	1 tbs	0.34
Avocado, 3⅛-in. diameter	½	0.22
Oysters, raw	½ cup	0.22
Collards, cooked	½ cup	0.18
Chicken, broiled, flesh only	3 oz	0.16
Winter squash, baked, mashed	½ cup	0.14
Cheese, cheddar	1 oz	0.13
Cream of mushroom soup, commercial	1 cup	0.12
Asparagus spears, cooked, ½-in. diameter	4	0.11
Beet greens, cooked, drained	½ cup	0.11
Frankfurter	1	0.11
Peanuts, roasted	½ cup	0.10
Bread, white	1 slice	0.05
Potato, baked, peeled	1 medium	0.04
Grapefruit juice	½ cup	0.02

SOURCE: *Nutritive Value of Foods*, Home and Garden Bulletin No. 72, U.S. Department of Agriculture, Washington, D.C., 1970.

cereal products through the enrichment program. However, in the rice-eating countries of the world, riboflavin is often omitted in the enrichment.

According to a preliminary 1974 estimate,[14] the percentages of riboflavin present in major food groups available to civilian consumption is as follows: meat (including pork fat cuts), poultry, and fish, 24.5 per cent; eggs, 5.1 per cent; dairy products, excluding butter, 41.0 per cent; fats and oils, including butter, 0 per cent; citrus fruits, 0.5 per cent; other fruits, 1.5 per cent; potatoes and sweet potatoes, 1.7 per cent; dark-green and deep-yellow vegetables, 1.1 per cent; other vegetables, including tomatoes, 4.5 per cent; dry beans and peas, nuts, and soya flour, 2.0 per cent; flour and cereal products, 17.4 per cent; sugars and other sweeteners, less than 0.05 per cent; and miscellaneous, 0.7 per cent.

Effect of Food Preparation on Riboflavin

Because riboflavin is stable to heat, little is lost in cooking. The question is often raised about the possibility of a loss of riboflavin when milk is pasteurized and subjected to such a high temperature. However, it has been shown that neither pasteurizing nor drying milk lowers its riboflavin content appreciably. Light destroys the vitamin.

As much as 70 to 80 per cent of the riboflavin in meat is retained after either roasting or broiling. The riboflavin loss, or at least a small portion of it, can be recovered from the meat drippings.

Niacin

Elvehjem's announcement in 1937, according to McCollum,[15] that nicotinic acid (later

[14] *National Food Situation*, op. cit., p. 28.

[15] McCollum, op. cit., p. 311.

known as niacin) was the elusive factor in curing black tongue in dogs, a condition similar to pellagra in human beings, concluded 200 years of study devoted to this deficiency disease.

The condition received its name from two Italian words, *pella* and *agra*, which mean "rough skin." The first description of pellagra was clearly set forth in 1735 by Casal, a physician in northern Spain. At that time pellagra was commonly seen in Italy, France, the Balkans, Egypt, and Rumania. The condition has been called a sickness of the four D's—dermatitis, diarrhea, dementia, and death.

McCollum describes the incidence of pellagra in the United States as an "explosive outbreak" that appeared between 1905 and 1910 and was principally confined to the Southern states. Medical opinion of the day was about equally divided between the "corn poison" and "infection" theories as to the cause of pellagra. The "corn poison" theory sprang from a long association of the disease with people of relatively poor background who seemed to exist on a diet composed mostly of corn. It was generally accepted that pellagra was probably due to a toxic or infectious substance in spoiled corn.

The earliest study to prove that human pellagra was caused by a dietary deficiency was reported by Voegtlin in 1914. He tested the effects on pellagra patients of two contrasting diets in a hospital in Spartanburg, South Carolina.

Goldberger[16] has perhaps contributed the most to our background knowledge of the conditions that prevailed in this country. In 1915 he began investigations on pellagra among inmates of all kinds of institutions in the areas where the disease was endemic to determine whether a faulty diet could be the cause. He became convinced that it could. In Mississippi, where pellagra was rampant among 6- to 12-year-olds, he was able to eradicate pellagra by providing liberal amounts of eggs, milk, and meat in the diet.

Goldberger's most famous experiment was made in Mississippi in 1915, and is referred to as the "Rankin Farm" or "Prison Farm" experiment. He secured the cooperation of prisoners who volunteered to serve as subjects in return for a promise of a pardon from the governor. These prisoners were put on the kind of diet they had been used to before they entered prison. (Their regular prison diet before the experiment had been quite good; they had been given milk, fresh fruits and vegetables, and adequate amounts of meat. However, they missed the tasty, but less nutritious, foods they had consumed at home and were happy to have these familiar foods again.) It took 6 months of this familiar type of diet to bring about evidences of pellagra among these volunteer subjects. However, in spite of the evidence Goldberger obtained from this experiment, the symptoms that he was able to induce in these men were not accepted by everyone as evidence of pellagra.

Black tongue in dogs was discovered to be a condition similar to that of pellagra in the human being. Through studying the composition of diets that were effective in treatment of induced black tongue, it was hoped that the responsible factor could be determined. In 1925 Goldberger felt that he was able to list common foods in fairly stable classifications on the basis of their effectiveness in preventing and curing the deficiency disease of pellagra. He then created the term *pellagra preventive factor*. From that time on, scientists hunted for the unknown factor that could treat black tongue in dogs and also exist in the list of foods that were pellagra preventing. It was not until 1937 that the nutritive significance of nicotinic acid, or nicotinamide, was fully established. After Elvehjem[17] at Wisconsin had shown that niacin could cure black tongue in dogs, Krehl showed later, in 1945, that either niacin or tryptophan, an essential amino acid, could counteract a retarded growth in rats. This was the beginning of an appreciation of the relationship that existed between tryptophan and niacin.

[16] V. P. Sydenstricker, "The History of Pellagra, Its Recognition as a Disorder of Nutrition, and Its Conquest," *American Journal of Clinical Nutrition*, Vol. 6, No. 4 (July–August 1968), pp. 409–414.

[17] Conrad A. Elvehjem, "Early Experiences with Niacin—A Retrospect," *Nutrition Reviews*, Vol. 11, No. 10 (October 1953), pp. 289–292.

Chemical and Physical Properties of Niacin

Niacin (nicotinic acid) is a white compound that is soluble in water and fairly stable to heat. It is also stable to acids and alkalis. It is not destroyed in ordinary cooking procedures. Niacin is found in plant tissues, and the physiologically active niacinamide (the amide of nicotinic acid) is present in animal tissues. Man is able to change ingested niacin to niacinamide.

Perlzweig[18] demonstrated in 1946 that tryptophan could be converted to niacin in the human being. Krehl[19] investigated the amount of tryptophan needed for niacin synthesis. Thus the relationship between niacin and tryptophan has been established, and now the term "niacin equivalent" is used when the nutritive need is discussed. The bacterial synthesis of niacin from tryptophan must take place in the presence of pyridoxine.

Functions of Niacin

The primary function of niacin seems to be to serve as a component of two coenzymes, coenzyme I and coenzyme II, which participate in tissue respiration and oxidation of glucose for release of energy. They are identified as nicotinamide adenine dinucleotide (NAD) and nicotinamide adenine dinucleotide phosphate (NADP). Coenzymes are required for fat and cholesterol synthesis.

Niacin Deficiencies

Pellagra,[20] the deficiency disease of niacin, is characterized by a dermatitis, particularly in the areas of the skin that are exposed to light or injury. Diarrhea usually occurs, as well as inflammation of mucous membrane, including that of the entire gastrointestinal tract. The latter may be identified by a red swollen tongue and a mouth that is quite sore. One of the outstanding characteristics of niacin deficiency is its manifestations of mental disorders, including, in mild cases, irritability, depression, and anxiety. In the advanced state, conditions of such severity as delirium and hallucinations occur. In severe pellagra, hydrochloric acid may be lacking in the gastric juice.

Even though there is no evidence of how something like the simple lack of niacin in the diet induces these symptoms of pellagra, they do disappear remarkably upon the administration of an adequate amount of niacin. In fact, recovery is quite spectacular, especially the recovery from mental depression manifestations. Like other deficiency diseases, human pellagra seldom exists without deficiencies in thiamin and riboflavin.

Pellagra in the United States is practically nonexistent today. Of course, a few cases are reported among chronic alcoholics, cases resulting from a long-standing substitution of alcohol for food. Occasionally a patient appears who has long existed on a low-kcalorie diet of low protein and low vitamin and mineral content. Such a diet may be primarily high in carbohydrate and fat and minus such foods as fresh fruits and vegetables, meat, eggs, and milk. Also, there are those who might have pellagra in association with other conditions. This secondary type of deficiency could be due to illnesses that would interfere with the appetite or the absorption and utilization of foods. Examples would be chronic diarrhea, cirrhosis, and tuberculosis.

Roe[21] points out that pellagra was a disease of the poor who lived on the land and had to eat a diet that was cheap and lacked variety. Over the years there was association of pellagra with "corn eaters." One example related to the Italian peasants of past centuries, many of whom were pellagrins subsisting on polenta, a cornmeal porridge. In other parts of the

[18] W. A. Perlzweig et al., "The Excretion of Nicotinic Acid Derivatives After Ingestion of Tryptophane by Man," *Journal of Biological Chemistry*, Vol. 167, No. 1 (January 1947), pp. 511–514.

[19] W. A. Krehl, L. J. Teply, P. S. Sarma, and C. A. Elvehjem, "Growth-Retarding Effect of Corn in Nicotinic Acid-Low Rations and Its Counteraction by Tryptophane," *Science*, Vol. 101, No. 2628 (May 1945), pp. 489–490.

[20] M. K. Horwitt, "Niacin," in Robert S. Goodhart and Maurice E. Shils (eds.), *Modern Nutrition in Health and Disease*, Lea & Febiger, Philadelphia, 1973, Chapter 5.

[21] Daphne A. Roe, A *Plague of Corn, the Social History of Pellagra*, Cornell University Press, Ithaca, N.Y., 1973.

world where pellagra existed, corn was often an important part of the diet, such as other parts of Europe and in Africa.

The question has arisen as to how the inhabitants of Central America, for whom corn was the basis of the diet, managed to remain healthy. The corn consumed was treated with lime, which improved the nutritional qualities, including niacin. Also, corn was eaten with beans, and sometimes toasted corn pests or locusts that enchanced the protein values and such foods as squashes, chili peppers, and other fruits and vegetables were included. Roe emphasizes that the total diet must be scrutinized, not just the inclusion of corn, when analyzing the diet of the pellagrin.

Nutritive Needs for Niacin

Both Goldsmith[22] and co-workers at Tulane and Horwitt and his associates at the University of Illinois College of Medicine produced experimental pellagra in human subjects. From these data it was shown that the minimal niacin requirement, including niacin derived from its precursor tryptophan, for the prevention of pellagra appeared to be about 9 mg daily. The requirement for niacin is in relation to body weight. Goldsmith showed that the minimal need was slightly greater than 0.1 mg per kilogram of body weight daily when the diet also furnished 250 mg of tryptophan. Horwitt,[23] after both he and Goldsmith noticed a relationship to kcaloric intake, suggested that the minimal amount of niacin which would prevent pellagra was 4.4 mg per 1000 kcalories, except with diets that provided less than 2000 kcalories. In this case 8.8 mg was required.

The human being may depend upon the conversion of tryptophan to niacin for part of his niacin supply. The problem, therefore, is to determine approximately how much trypto-

phan can produce a given amount of niacin. Although there is wide variation among individuals, on the basis of studies conducted by Goldsmith[24] and by Horwitt,[25] it was determined that approximately 60 mg of dietary tryptophan would furnish 1 mg of niacin.

The interpretation here is not that 60 mg of tryptophan are oxidized to form 1 mg of niacin, but rather that when 60 mg of tryptophan are ingested a sufficient amount of tryptophan is oxidized to provide about 1 mg of niacin. Also, this formula can be used to determine the amount of niacin in foods if the tryptophan content is known. Most animal protein sources contain 1.4 per cent tryptophan, and proteins of vegetable origin contain about 1 per cent tryptophan. This information is helpful in estimating the tryptophan and niacin content of foods. In the 1974 *Recommended Dietary Allowances*, the term *niacin equivalents* is not used, but recommendations for niacin allowances are presented in milligrams of niacin.

The niacin allowance recommended for adults is 6.6 mg per 1000 kcalories and not less than 13 mg at kcaloric intakes of less than 2000 kcalories.

No data are available as a basis for niacin requirements of children from infancy to adolescence. There is a possibility that the efficiency of tryptophan conversion to niacin during these ages differs from the adult. Based on the niacin and tryptophan content of human milk, the niacin allowance for infants up to 6 months of age is 8 mg per 1000 kcalories, about two thirds of which comes from tryptophan. For children over 6 months and adolescents, 6.6 mg per 1000 kcalories is recommended but not less than 8 mg daily.

Pertinent information is limited for use as a basis for determining the niacin requirements

---

[22] Grace Goldsmith et al., "Studies of Niacin Requirement in Man," *American Journal of Clinical Nutrition*, Vol. 4, No. 2 (March–April 1956), pp. 151–160.

[23] M. K. Horwitt, "Niacin–Tryptophan Requirements of Man," *Journal of the American Dietetic Association*, Vol. 34, No. 9 (September–October 1958), pp. 914–919.

---

[24] Grace Goldsmith, "Niacin-Tryptophan Relationships in Man and Niacin Requirements," *American Journal of Clinical Nutrition*, Vol. 6, No. 5 (September—October 1958), pp. 479–460.

[25] M. K. Horwitt et al., "Tryptophan–Niacin Relationships in Man: Studies with Diets Deficient in Riboflavin and Niacin, Together with Observations on the Excretion of Nitrogen and Niacin Metabolites," *Journal of Nutrition*, Vol. 60, Supplement 1 (October 1956), pp. 3–63.

TABLE 13–5

Recommended Daily Dietary Allowances for Niacin, Revised 1974

Designed for the maintenance of good nutrition for practically all healthy people in the United States

	AGE (years)	WEIGHT (kg)	WEIGHT (lb)	HEIGHT (cm)	HEIGHT (in.)	ENERGY (kcal)	NIACIN[a] (mg)
Infants	0.0–0.5	6	14	60	24	kg × 117	5
	0.5–1.0	9	20	71	28	kg × 108	8
Children	1–3	13	28	86	34	1300	9
	4–6	20	44	110	44	1800	12
	7–10	30	66	135	54	2400	16
Males	11–14	44	97	158	63	2800	18
	15–18	61	134	172	69	3000	20
	19–22	67	147	172	69	3000	20
	23–50	70	154	172	69	2700	18
	51+	70	154	172	69	2400	16
Females	11–14	44	97	155	62	2400	16
	15–18	54	119	162	65	2100	14
	19–22	58	128	162	65	2100	14
	23–50	58	128	162	65	2000	13
	51+	58	128	162	65	1800	12
Pregnant						+300	+2
Lactating						+500	+4

SOURCE: Food and Nutrition Board, *Recommended Dietary Allowances*, 8th ed., National Academy of Sciences—National Research Council, Washington, D.C., 1974.

[a] Although allowances are expressed as niacin, it is recognized that on the average 1 mg of niacin is derived from each 60 mg of dietary tryptophan.

of pregnant and lactating women. There is some evidence that the conversion of tryptophan to niacin is more efficient in the pregnant than the nonpregnant state. The recommended allowance provides an increase of 2 mg of niacin daily during pregnancy based on the recommended increased energy intake. On the same basis, the recommendation for lactating women is an additional daily allowance of 4 mg of niacin for the extra 500 kcalories suggested. See Table 13–5.

Sources of Niacin

The sources of niacin can also be considered in relation to their tryptophan content, for tryptophan is a precursor of this essential vitamin. The chief sources of niacin that are also rich in tryptophan are such foods as liver, lean meat, fish, and poultry. Plant sources include peanuts, which are very rich in both niacin and tryptophan, and peanut butter, beans and

peas, other legumes, and most nuts. Several whole-grain or enriched cereal products should also be included in this list. Milk is a poor source of niacin, but is rich in tryptophan. Foods that are low in tryptophan are gelatin, which has none, and corn and rice, which are also quite low in niacin in contrast to other grains, which are relatively high.

Table 13–6 includes a list of common foods in the normal diet that contain niacin. The contribution from each food can be easily compared.

Horwitt noted that even though it has been shown that pellagra can be prevented by tryptophan alone, with niacin excluded from the diet, it must be recognized that niacin is more efficiently converted to coenzyme I and coenzyme II than tryptophan. Therefore, an enrichment program should include niacin rather than depend upon tryptophan to supply the niacin needed.

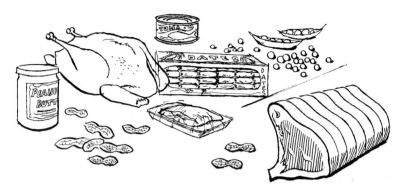

FIGURE 13–3. *Some food sources of niacin: peanut butter, peanuts, dates, peas, pork, liver, chicken, and tuna.*

TABLE 13–6

Niacin Content of Selected Foods

FOOD	PORTION	NIACIN (mg)
Milk	1 cup	0.2
Cheese, cheddar	1 oz	Trace
Liver, beef, fried	3 oz	12.6
Beef, round, roast	3 oz	3.8
Pork, roast	3 oz	4.7
Chicken	3 oz without bone	7.1
Fish, tuna, drained	3 oz	10.9
Egg	1	0.05
Peanuts	¼ cup	6.2
Peanut butter	2 tbs	3.0
Peas, cooked	1 cup	3.7
Collards, cooked	1 cup	3.2
Kale, cooked	1 cup	1.9
Potato, baked	1 medium	1.7
Spinach	1 cup	1.1
Tomato juice	1 cup	1.8
Dates, fresh and dried	1 cup	3.9
Prune juice	1 cup	1.1
Macaroni, enriched, cooked	1 cup	1.9
Enriched white bread	1 slice	0.5
Whole-wheat bread	1 slice	0.7
Oatmeal	1 cup	0.4

SOURCE: *Nutritive Value of Foods*, Home and Garden Bulletin No. 72, U.S. Department of Agriculture, Washington, D.C., 1971.

Effect of Food Preparation on Niacin

Since niacin is stable to air, light, and heat and is not destroyed in ordinary cooking processes, it is generally unaffected by most cooking. However, it is a water-soluble vitamin, and, as such, part of the niacin content of meat may be lost in the meat drippings and juices. Studies have shown that niacin losses from cooking meat may range from 10 to 40 per cent. Another food in which preparation might affect the niacin value is cooked cereals. The niacin in cereals is often in "bound" forms. Enrichment alleviates this problem. The treatment of corn with lime may release some niacin.

Cereal and bread and cereal products are enriched with niacin, as well as with thiamin and riboflavin. This point was discussed in Chapter 11.

Niacin Consumption

Food groups contribute the following percentages of the total niacin consumption, according to preliminary 1974 data:[26] meat (including pork fat cuts), poultry, and fish, 45.6 per cent; eggs, 0.1 per cent; dairy products, excluding butter, 1.6 per cent; fats and oils, including butter, 0 per cent; citrus fruits, 0.9 per cent; other fruits, 1.7 per cent; potatoes and sweet potatoes, 7.1 per cent; dark-green and deep-yellow vegetables, 0.7 per cent; other vegetables, including tomatoes, 6.1 per cent; dry beans and peas, nuts, soya flour, 7.6 per cent; flour and cereal products, 24.0 per cent; sugars and sweeteners, less than 0.05 per cent; and miscellaneous, 4.8 per cent.

Vitamin B₆ (Pyridoxine)

Vitamin B₆ might be better termed the B₆ complex, for it exists as a group of three closely related (functionally and metabolically) chemical compounds: pyridoxine, pyridoxal, and pyridoxamine. Usually the complex is referred to by the name *pyridoxine.*

It was about 1934 that György, according to McCollum,[27] demonstrated that B₆ was a distinct vitamin. Later, in 1938, it was isolated almost simultaneously in several different laboratories. And the following year it was synthesized in two independent laboratories. Through laboratory studies on the rat, György was able to identify B₆ as a substance that would prevent and cure the syndrome known as acrodynia. This was characterized by severe cutaneous lesions accompanied by edema, redness, and scaliness of the paws, snout, nose, and ears.

[26] *National Food Situation,* op. cit., p. 28.

[27] McCollum, op. cit., p. 413.

These initial studies by György have been followed by many others. Their aim has been to determine the metabolic activity and specific needs, if possible, of several species of animals and, ultimately, the human need for vitamin B₆.

Chemical and Physical Properties of Vitamin B₆

Pyridoxine, or the B₆ complex, a white solid, is water soluble, fairly stable to heat, sensitive to ultraviolet light, and also sensitive to oxidation. The three forms that comprise the complex have approximately equal metabolic activity for animals, but they show a different activity for different microorganisms. This difference provides a technique for the assay of various forms of vitamin B₆. Pyridoxal and pyridoxamine are the forms of B₆ found in animal food, whereas pyridoxine is present in plant foods. Of the three forms of the vitamin, pyridoxine is most resistant to destruction by heat or chemical action. As all three are interconverted to the biologically active form pyridoxol within the body, there is no difference in their function for man.

Functions of Vitamin B₆

Considerable interest has centered upon vitamin B₆, and many investigations have been made in an effort to determine its function in human nutrition. Vitamin B₆ is related to a large number and wide variety of enzyme systems, as the coenzyme pyridoxal phosphate, which is associated with nitrogen metabolism, including the synthesis of proteins, according to Sauberlich.[28] Studies in brain metabolism indicate that the B₆ vitamin participates in the metabolism of the nervous system, possibly in the regulation of the central nervous system. The conversion of trytophan to niacin requires B₆. Many studies indicate that this vitamin has a role in erthrocyte formation, so a deficiency may lead to anemia. Other studies report that B₆ has an effect on various endocrine activities, such as growth hormone, insulin,

[28] H. E. Sauberlich, "Biochemical Systems and Biochemical Detection of Deficiency," in W. H. Sebrell, Jr., and Robert S. Harris (eds.) *The Vitamins,* Vol. 2, Academic Press, New York, 1968, pp. 44–80.

thyroid, adrenal, pituitary gonadal hormones, and neurohormones. But only in the case of neurohormones has a definite relationship been established. Although the mechanisms are not understood, this vitamin appears to be involved in stress, electrolyte balance, energy production, and water metabolism.

For some time it has been recognized that B_6 participates in lipid metabolism, but the mechanism has not been established. Vitamin B_6 supplements have reduced dental caries in man, but the process has not been identified. The absorption of the amino acid methionine requires the presence of this vitamin, and if the diet has extra amounts of methionine, more B_6 is required.

Vitamin B_6 Deficiencies

Although pyridoxine deficiency has been induced in experimental animals of several different species, there has been little in the literature concerning deficiencies in man. Vitamin B_6 is recognized as necessary, but there is no evidence that a diet can be so deficient in pyridoxine content that a deficiency state will occur.

Wachstein[29] and his associates noted that a higher than normal excretion of xanthurenic acid occurred during toxemia and pre-eclampsia in pregnancy. The administration of relatively small doses of pyridoxine resulted in a statistically significant decrease in the incidence of toxemia as compared with a control group. These results were not repeated in studies of liver disease, cancer, muscular dystrophy, febrile infections, heart failure, problems of geriatric patients, and other pathological conditions.

Vitamin B_6 may be associated with immunity to disease because a partial depression of the immunologic response occurred with a B_6 vitamin deficiency, according to Axelrod and Traketellis.[30] This effect may be attributed to the ability of vitamin B_6 to catalyze the biosynthesis of the nucleic acids—essential in cellular proliferation and the building of specific immune proteins.

Vitamin B_6 Nutritive Needs

The fact that in no area in the world has a vitamin B_6 deficiency been sharply defined hampers the establishment of allowances for this vitamin. Many unrelated conditions have implicated vitamin B_6. Information on the vitamin B_6 content of foods is limited and knowledge about the availability of it is scanty, although a number of methods have been employed for determination of the forms of vitamin B_6. In general, estimates of vitamin B_6 nutritional status have been based on excretion of tryptophan metabolites after tryptophan load tests, measurement of the activity of serum and red blood transaminases, urinary excretion of the vitamin or its metabolite, pyridoxic acid, and the amount or lack of the vitamin required to produce cures or clinical signs of deficiency.

For healthy babies, the allowance is based on general experience with proprietary formulas and is 0.015 mg per g of protein or 0.05 mg per 100 kcalories, an amount that should satisfy metabolic requirements. The allowance for adult men and women is 2 mg daily. Additional allowances for pregnancy and lactation are suggested as 0.5 mg per day, making a total of 2.5 mg per day.

Table 13–7 indicates the recommended allowances for both sexes and all ages, as well as for pregnancy and lactation, as reported by the Food and Nutrition Board.

Women using estrogen-containing oral contraceptives may require additional vitamin B_6 above the recommended allowance to correct increased urinary excretion of tryptophan metabolites and symptoms of a vitamin B_6 deficiency, according to Rose and co-workers[31]

[29] M. Wachstein, "Related Deficiency of Vitamin B_6 in Pregnancy and Some Diseases," *Vitamins Hormones*, Vol. 22, 1964, p. 705.

[30] A. E. Axelrod and A. C. Traketellis, "Vitamin B_6 and Immunological Phenomena," *Vitamins Hormones*, Vol. 22, 1964, p. 581.

[31] D P. Rose, R. Strong, Janet Folkard, and P. W. Adams, "Erthrocyte Aminotransferase Activities in Women Using Oral Contraceptives and the Effect of Vitamin B_6 Supplementation," *American Journal of Clinical Nutrition*, Vol. 26, No. 1 (January 1973), pp. 48–52.

TABLE 13–7

Recommended Daily Dietary Allowances for Vitamin B$_6$, Revised 1974

Designed for the maintenance of good nutrition for practically all healthy people in the United States

	AGE (years)	WEIGHT (kg)	WEIGHT (lb)	HEIGHT (cm)	HEIGHT (in.)	ENERGY (kcal)	VITAMIN B$_6$ (mg)
Infants	0.0–0.5	6	14	60	24	kg × 117	0.3
	0.5–1.0	9	20	71	28	kg × 108	0.4
Children	1–3	13	28	86	34	1300	0.6
	4–6	20	44	110	44	1800	0.9
	7–10	30	66	135	54	2400	1.2
Males	11–14	44	97	158	63	2800	1.6
	15–18	61	134	172	69	3000	2.0
	19–22	67	147	172	69	3000	2.0
	23–50	70	154	172	69	2700	2.0
	51+	70	154	172	69	2400	2.0
Females	11–14	44	97	155	62	2400	1.6
	15–18	54	119	162	65	2100	2.0
	19–22	58	128	162	65	2100	2.0
	23–50	58	128	162	65	2000	2.0
	51+	58	128	162	65	1800	2.0
Pregnant						+300	2.5
Lactating						+500	2.5

SOURCE: Food and Nutrition Board, *Recommended Dietary Allowances*, 8th ed., National Academy of Sciences—National Research Council, Washington, D.C., 1974.

and Lumeng and others.[32] Drenick and others[33] found a vitamin B$_6$ deficiency developing among obese males who were fasting to lose weight. The common premenstrual edema and late massive edema of pregnancy are prevented or therapeutically influenced by high doses of vitamin B$_6$ without the use of pharmaceutical antidiuretics, according to György.[34] There is

[32] Lawrence Lumeng, Robert E. Cleary, and Ting-Kai Li, "Effect of Oral Contraceptives on the Plasma Concentration of Pyridoxal Phosphate," *American Journal of Clinical Nutrition*, Vol. 27, No. 5 (April 1974), pp. 326–333.

[33] Ernest J. Drenick, Elizabeth Vinyard, and Marian E. Swendseid, "Vitamin B$_6$ Requirements in Starving Obese Males," *American Journal of Clinical Nutrition*, Vol. 22, No. 1 (January 1969), pp. 10–13.

[34] Paul György, "Developments Leading to the Metabolic Role of Vitamin B$_6$," *American Journal of Clinical Nutrition*, Vol. 24, No. 10 (October 1971), pp. 1250–1256.

evidence, according to this researcher, that physiological disturbances of B$_6$–enzyme activity increase with age, and doses of pyridoxine have been helpful in the early stages of acute rheumatism and osteoarthritis among the aged.

Sources of Vitamin B$_6$ in Foods

Although vitamin B$_6$ activity can be measured in foods by a number of methods, these methods have not been compared adequately or used widely to provide for an acceptable table of B$_6$ values for the variety of foods consumed in the American diet. Table 13–8 gives a listing of the vitamin B$_6$ content of a few common foods.

Although there is limited information on the vitamin B$_6$ content of foods, organ meats, especially liver, are a rich source. Meat, fish, and poultry (especially light meat) are excellent sources. Dried beans, peanuts, and nuts

TABLE 13-8

Vitamin B₆ Content of Some Common Foods

FOOD	VITAMIN B₆ (μg/100 g)
Banana	320
Barley	320–560
Beef	230–320
Cabbage	120–290
Carrot, raw	120–220
Corn, yellow	360–570
Egg	22–48
Heart, beef	200–290
Kidney, beef	350–990
Lamb	250–370
Liver, beef	600–710
Milk, whole	54–110
Orange juice, fresh	18–56
Peanuts	300
Peas, dry	160–330
Pork	330–680
Potato	160–250
Rice, white	340–450
Soybeans	710–1200
Tomatoes, canned	710
Wheat bran	1380–1570
White flour	380–600

SOURCE: W. H. Sebrell and R. S. Harris, *The Vitamins*, Vol. 2, Academic Press, New York, 1968, pp. 222–228.

are good sources. Among the fruits, bananas and avocadoes are excellent sources. Cereals vary in their contribution with whole-grain cereals being much richer than milled products. Egg yolk makes a good contribution. Raw cabbage and cauliflower, potatoes, canned yellow corn, leaf spinach, and ripe tomatoes are noted for the amount of vitamin B₆ provided.

Vitamin B₆ Consumption

According to preliminary 1974 data,[35] meat (including pork fat cuts), poultry, and fish contributed 45.8 per cent of the vitamin B₆ consumption from major food groups; eggs, 1.9 per cent; dairy products, excluding butter, 10.2 per cent; fats and oils, including butter,

[35] *National Food Situation,* op. cit., p. 28.

0 per cent; citrus fruits, 1.2 per cent; other fruits, 5.5 per cent; potatoes and sweet potatoes, 11.2 per cent; dark-green and deep-yellow vegetables, 1.7 per cent; other vegetables, including tomatoes, 9.2 per cent; dry beans and peas, nuts, soya flour, 4.3 per cent; flour and cereal products, 8.9 per cent; sugar and sweeteners, 0 per cent; and miscellaneous, 0.1 per cent.

Vitamin B₁₂ (Cyanocobalamin)

For many years it was recognized that patients with pernicious anemia would respond to "heroic" amounts of liver in the diet. This followed Minot and Murphy's[36] announcement in 1927 that the feeding of whole liver brought about remission in pernicious anemia patients. Through the years, investigators searched for the elusive factor that was present in liver that brought about this desired change.

It was not until 1948 that the isolation of vitamin B₁₂ was announced at almost the same time by two separate investigators. Rickes and his associates are credited with isolating B₁₂ in 1948, but Smith, in England, isolated the same material at almost the same time by an entirely different method. He observed the red color of the compound and set out to determine exactly what it was.

Chemical and Physical Properties of Vitamin B₁₂

Vitamin B₁₂ is water soluble and has a characteristic red color. It is labile to acids, alkalis, and light. One of its most interesting characteristics is that it is the first cobalt-containing substance that has been found essential for life, and, in addition, it is the only vitamin known for man that contains an essential mineral element. Vitamin B₁₂ is a very potent and active biological substance. Its molecule is unusually large and intricate so that problems of absorption may arise, complicated by the fact that the *intrinsic factor,* also a complex molecule, must be present in gastric secretions to facilitate the transfer of B₁₂ into the ileal epithelium. This transfer takes much more

[36] *Present Knowledge in Nutrition,* 2nd ed., Nutrition Foundation, New York, 1956, Chap. 25, p. 119.

time than that of other water-soluble substances. Calcium is necessary for this process. Vitamin B_{12} is stored in the body tissues, especially the liver.

Functions of Vitamin B_{12}

Vitamin B_{12} is present and essential for the adequate functioning of all mammalian cells. As a component of various coenzymes, it plays an important role in nucleic acid formation and in fat and carbohydrate metabolism. With folic acid, this vitamin is involved in the synthesis of DNA. Vitamin B_{12} appears to take part in the synthesis of myelin because a lack of the vitamin results in neurological damage.[37]

Vitamin B_{12} Deficiencies

A deficiency of vitamin B_{12} results in defective synthesis of deoxyribonucleic acid (DNA). The specific defect with a lack of vitamin B_{12} is due to a failure to utilize 5-methyltetrahydrofolate, which requires B_{12} for its conversion back into the folate pool.[38] Vitamin B_{12}, in addition to its function in folate metabolism, is involved in certain isomerization reactions and possibly in unknown reactions in carbohydrate, fat, and protein metabolism. Infertility or even complete sterility may be linked with severe vitamin B_{12} deficiency. Neural cell dysfunction may result from a lack of this vitamin, but the biochemical mechanism is unknown. Epithelial cell alterations occur when there is an inadequate amount of vitamin B_{12} available.

The lack of vitamin B_{12} is seldom found in the United States, owing to the high protein diet consumed. Food faddists or individuals on a deficient diet may show indications of a lack of this vitamin. In countries where nutritious food is at borderline levels, a dietary B_{12} deficiency is not uncommon. Inadequate gastric absorption accounts for many of the cases of B_{12} deficiency.

A lack of vitamin B_{12} may be found among individuals who consume a diet consisting largely of vegetables. Evidences of sore tongue; signs of degeneration of the spinal cord; prickling, itching, or abnormal sensations; and low serum levels of vitamin B_{12} are common, according to Mehta and associates[39] and Hines.[40] A low serum level of folic acid is often found among vegetarians, strengthening the possible relationship of folic acid with B_{12}.

The commonest deficiency of vitamin B_{12} is pernicious anemia facilitated by an absence of the intrinsic factor (IF). This anemia is characterized by abnormally large red blood cells with half the normal lifespan, somewhat oval in shape, with an adequate supply of hemoglobin. The disease primarily affects older persons, with a definite predilection found among northern European peoples. It is rare among children.

Vitamin B_{12} Nutritive Needs

On the basis of findings by the Joint FAO/WHO Expert Group on vitamin B_{12} and of Herbert,[41] the recommended allowance for this vitamin was placed at 3 μg per day for adolescents and normal adults. Overt vitamin B_{12} deficiency does not occur in a breast-fed baby, but for artificially fed infants the recommended allowance is 3 μg per day. Reasonal extrapolations suggest an allowance of 3 μg daily for children up to adolescence.

Little evidence is available for a basis for allowances for pregnancy. Estimates made on fetal demands would suggest 4 μg daily for the pregnant woman and the same will suffice

---

[37] Victor Herbert, "Folic Acid and Vitamin B_{12}" in Robert S. Goodhart and Maurice E. Shils (eds.), *Modern Nutrition in Health and Disease*, Lea & Febiger, Philadelphia, 1973, Chap. 5.

[38] Report of a Joint FAC/WHO Expert Group, *Requirements of Ascorbic Acid, Vitamin D, Vitamin B_{12}, Folate, and Iron*, World Health Organization Technical Report Series, No. 452, World Health Organization, Geneva, 1970.

[39] B. M. Mehta, D. V. Rege, and R. S. Satoskar, "Serum Vitamin B_{12} and Folic Acid Activity in Lactovegetarian and Non Vegetarian Healthy Adult Indians," *American Journal of Clinical Nutrition*, Vol. 15, No. 2 (August 1964) pp. 77–84.

[40] J. D. Hines, "Megaloblastic Anemia in an Adult Vegan," *American Journal of Clinical Nutrition*, Vol. 19, No. 4 (October 1966) pp. 260–268.

[41] Victor Herbert, "Nutritional Requirements for Vitamin B_{12} and Folic Acid," *American Journal of Clinical Nutrition*, Vol. 21, No. 8 (August 1968), pp. 743–752.

TABLE 13–9

Recommended Daily Dietary Allowances for Vitamin B$_{12}$, Revised 1974

Designed for the maintenance of good nutrition for practically all healthy people in the United States

	AGE (years)	WEIGHT (kg)	WEIGHT (lb)	HEIGHT (cm)	HEIGHT (in.)	ENERGY (kcal)	VITA-MIN B$_{12}$ (μg)
Infants	0.0–0.5	6	14	60	24	kg × 117	0.3
	0.5–1.0	9	20	71	28	kg × 108	0.3
Children	1–3	13	28	86	34	1300	1.0
	4–6	20	44	110	44	1800	1.5
	7–10	30	66	135	54	2400	2.0
Males	11–14	44	97	158	63	2800	3.0
	15–18	61	134	172	69	3000	3.0
	19–22	67	147	172	69	3000	3.0
	23–50	70	154	172	69	2700	3.0
	51+	70	154	172	69	2400	3.0
Females	11–14	44	97	155	62	2400	3.0
	15–18	54	119	162	65	2100	3.0
	19–22	58	128	162	65	2100	3.0
	23–50	58	128	162	65	2000	3.0
	51+	58	128	162	65	1800	3.0
Pregnant						+300	4.0
Lactating						+500	4.0

SOURCE: Food and Nutrition Board, *Recommended Dietary Allowances*, 8th ed., National Academy of Sciences—National Research Council, Washington, D.C., 1974.

for the lactating woman. Requirements are increased if the body metabolic rate is raised in fever or hyperthyroidism.

Table 13–9 presents the recommended dietary allowances of the Food and Nutrition Board for all ages and for both sexes, and includes pregnancy and lactation.

Sources of Vitamin B$_{12}$ in Foods

Vitamin B$_{12}$ is found only in foods of animal origin, although a diet that is entirely from plant sources might provide traces of it. There is the possibility of intestinal synthesis, but this does not seem to be sufficient, so it is important to obtain it from the diet.

The best sources are liver and kidney, closely followed by muscle meats, milk, cheese, fish, and eggs. The Food and Nutrition Board has pointed out that 1 cup of milk, 4 oz of meat, and one egg per day would provide 2 to 4 μg

of vitamin B$_{12}$. Rosenthal[42] summarizes the sources of vitamin B$_{12}$ in foods as follows:

BEST SOURCES	INTERMEDIATE SOURCES	POOR SOURCES
Liver	Steaks	Green vegetables
Kidney	Muscle meats	Potatoes
Brain	Dairy products	Egg white
Heart	Fish	Cereals
Clams	Shrimp	
Oysters	Lobster	
Egg yolk		

See Table 13–10 for detailed information about the vitamin B$_{12}$ content in foods.

[42] Harold L. Rosenthal, "Occurrence in Foods," in W. H. Sebrell, Jr., and Robert S. Harris (eds.), *The Vitamins*, Vol. 2, Academic Press, New York, 1968, pp. 170–174.

TABLE 13–10

Vitamin B$_{12}$ Content of Some Common Foods in Milligrams

FOOD	EDIBLE PORTION OF 100 g	EDIBLE PORTION OF 1 POUND AS PURCHASED
Liver, lamb	0.10400	0.4717
beef	0.08000	0.3629
calf	0.06000	0.2722
hog	0.03200	0.1452
chicken	0.02500	0.1134
Clams, meat only	0.09800	0.4445
Kidneys, lamb	0.06300	0.2858
beef	0.03100	0.1406
calf	0.02500	0.1134
Oysters, meat only	0.01800	0.0816
Liverwurst	0.01390	0.0631
Mackerel, salted, smoked	0.01200	0.0544
Sardines, canned in oil or tomato sauce	0.01000	0.0454
Herring, whole	0.01000	0.0231
Crab, cooked	0.01000	0.0454
Beef and beef heart	0.00682	0.0309
Egg yolks	0.00600	0.0272
Eel, smoked	0.00560	0.0254
Brains	0.00400	0.0181
Cod, dried, salted	0.00310	0.0163
Chicken	0.00200	0.0081
Milk, whole	0.00040	0.0018
Yoghurt	0.00011	0.0005
Crackers, saltines	0.0	0.0
Grapefruit, raw	0.0	0.0
Kale	0.0	0.0
Lettuce, raw	0.0	0.0
Corn flakes	0.0	0.0
Cantaloupe	0.0	0.0
Strawberries	0.0	0.0

SOURCE: Martha Louise Orr, *Pantothenic Acid, Vitamin B$_6$ and Vitamin B$_{12}$ in Foods*, Home Economics Research Report No. 36, Agricultural Research Service, U.S. Department of Agriculture, Washington, D.C., 1969.

Vitamin B$_{12}$ Consumption

The major food groups contribute the following percentages of vitamin B$_{12}$ to the American diet, according to preliminary 1974 data.[43] Meat (including pork fat cuts), poultry, and fish contribute 69.7 per cent; eggs, 8.3 per cent; dairy products, excluding butter, 20.5 per cent; fats and oils, including butter, 0 per cent; citrus fruits, 0 per cent; other fruits, 0 per cent; potatoes and sweet potatoes, 0 per cent; dark-green and deep-yellow vegetables, 0 per cent; other vegetables, including tomatoes, 0 per cent; dry beans and peas, nuts, and soya flour, 0 per cent; flour and cereal products, 1.5 per cent; sugars and sweeteners, 0 per cent; and miscellaneous, 0 per cent.

[43] *National Food Situation*, op. cit., p. 28.

Folacin

The discovery of folacin stems from a number of research studies. Lucy Wills in Bombay in 1931 was concerned about the nutritional megaloblastic anemia found in pregnant women. This anemia was reproduced in monkeys by feeding them a diet similar to that eaten by her patients, a diet consisting of polished rice and white bread. The anemia did not respond to any of the known vitamins or to purified liver extract. A good response was secured with an autolyzed yeast preparation that had been found generally ineffective in cases of pernicious anemia. This was the beginning of a distinction between folacin and vitamin B_{12}.

Mitchell in 1941 obtained a preparation called folic acid from spinach that would cure a dietary anemia of chicks. The name folic acid was originally given because the substance came from foliage material. Spies used folacin clinically in 1945 in the treatment of the macrocytic anemias of pregnancy and of tropical sprue and found it effective.

The pure synthetic form of folacin is pteroylglutamic acid, and this group of vitamins is sometimes called by the general term *pterglutamates*. In 1949 the American Institute of Nutrition[44] suggested that the term *folacin* be adopted. *Folacin* and *folic acid* are used interchangeably.

Chemical and Physical Properties of Folacin

Folacin is a yellow crystalline substance that is sparingly soluble in water and stable in an acid medium. It is readily destroyed in a heated alkaline solution. The biologically active form of the vitamin is known as the *citrovorum factor* of folinic acid. Folacin is absorbed readily if there are no metabolic disturbances. The chief center for storage is the liver.

Functions of Folacin

Folacin is required for the synthesis of essential components of red blood corpuscles,

other cells, and enzymes. The utilization of the amino acid histidine is facilitated by folacin. The five known forms of folacin coenzymes, according to Vitale,[45] have as a primary function the transfer of one-carbon units to facilitate the synthesis of DNA, RNA, methionine, and serine. The major role of folacin is the prevention of megaloblastic anemia in man.

Folacin Deficiencies

The main evidences of a folacin deficiency are megaloblastic anemia (not pernicious anemia), diarrhea, and inflammation of the tongue. Individuals with scurvy and infants on goat's milk or nutritionally inadequate proprietary formulas may develop a megaloblastic anemia because of combined folacin and ascorbic acid deficiencies. These results have been reported by Vilter and associates.[46] In tropical sprue, combined deficiencies of folacin and vitamin B_{12} may exist, according to Rivera and co-workers.[47]

Megaloblastic anemia is a concern in pregnancy, especially during the last trimester, owing to increased demands of the fetus. Vomiting, metabolic derangements in the production of folacin coenzymes, as well as a dietary lack, are other causes that may lead to deficiencies of this vitamin. In the event of leukemia, Hodgkin's disease, cancer, and other diseases in which the demand for folacin may be greatly increased, a folacin deficiency may occur. Certain drugs, including oral contraceptives, may have a deleterious effect on folacin metabolism. Protein malnutrition deters the

---

[44] *Present Knowledge in Nutrition*, Nutrition Foundation, New York, 1950, p. 107.

[45] Joseph J. Vitale, "Present Knowledge of Folacin," in *Present Knowledge in Nutrition*, 3rd ed., Nutrition Foundation, New York, 1967, Chap. 25.

[46] R. W. Vilter et al., "Interrelationships of Vitamin B_{12}, Folic Acid, and Ascorbic Acid in Megaloblastic Anemias," *American Journal of Clinical Nutrition*, Vol. 12, No. 2 (February 1963), pp. 130–144.

[47] Julio V. Rivera, F. Rodriquez de la Obra, and M. M. Maldonaldo, "Anemia Due to Vitamin B_{12} Deficiency After Treatment with Folic Acid in Tropical Sprue," *American Journal of Clinical Nutrition*, Vol. 18, No. 2 (February 1966), pp. 110–115.

utilization and functioning of folacin, as indicated by Spector and associates.[48]

A deficiency of folic acid results directly in a defective synthesis of deoxyribonucleic acid (DNA).[49] Severe lack of the vitamin may cause infertility and even sterility. Fetal and placental abnormalities may be associated with a folate deficiency. Striking abnormalities in skin pigmentation may occur. A folate deficiency in the newborn may result in mental retardation.

Folacin Nutritive Needs

One influence on the determination of folacin dietary allowances is information about the availability of this vitamin in foods.[50] Folacin is present in a wide variety of foods but generally in the form of polyglutamates that require the action of conjugase to release the vitamin for metabolic activity. This action may occur within the proximal intestinal mucosal cells, although a minimal amount of conjugase activity can be demonstrated in intestinal juices and greater activity occurs in tissues and plasma.

The folic acid content of food is biologically assayed by demonstrating growth response of selected bacterial organisms. Results of such tests indicate that approximately 25 per cent of dietary folacin is in the free form. The extent of absorption of food folacin is uncertain. The amount of total folacin absorbed is unknown, but, assuming that mucosal conjugase is active in normal individuals, significant amounts of conjugated folic acid should be available for folic acid activity. No exact figures are available. Once folic acid is absorbed it must undergo further metabolism to convert this vitamin into its coenzymatic forms.

Allowing for the wide range of folacin availability on a mixed diet and for other uncertainties, the recommended dietary allowances for adolescents and normal adults is 400 μg. For infants under 1 year of age, the recommendation is 50 μg. Few studies have been done on children's needs for this vitamin, but sensible interpolations suggest allowances for children ranging from 100 μg for 1 year of age to 400 μg for preadolescents. For the pregnant woman, 800 μg is recommended to protect the fetus and maternal stores of the vitamin for subsequent pregnancies. For the lactating mother, 600 μg is recommended to allow for excretion of folacin in milk and for lack of efficiency in absorption of dietary folic acid. Table 13–11 gives the recommended allowances for both sexes and all ages, and for pregnancy and lactation.

Sources of Folacin in Food

The content of folacin has not been established for many foods. Losses in storage, processing, and cooking can be considerable. Good sources include green leafy vegetables, liver, kidney, asparagus, lima beans, whole-grain cereals, nuts, and legumes. Table 13–12 gives a list of the folacin content of some common foods.

Biotin

Biotin was named in 1936 by Kogl and Tonnis when it was recognized that it was a potent yeast growth factor. Later it was established that the vitamin H of György and the coenzyme R were also the same substance, biotin. During 1941–1942, the structural formula of biotin was discovered by du Vigneaud, and Harris and his associates announced its synthesis.[51]

Chemical and Physical Properties of Biotin

Biotin is a water soluble compound. In food and tissues, this vitamin is bound to protein and contains sulphur. It is very stable to light, heat, and acids. It is somewhat unstable in the presence of alkalis and oxidizing agents.

---

[48] I. Spector et al., "Observations on Urocanic Acid and Foriminglutamic Acid Excretion in Infants with Protein Malnutrition," American Journal of Clinical Nutrition, Vol. 18, No. 6 (June 1966), pp. 426–436.

[49] Report of a Joint FAO/WHO Expert Group, op. cit., pp. 35–36.

[50] Recommended Dietary Allowances, op. cit., pp. 71–74.

[51] McCollum, op. cit., pp. 408–412.

TABLE 13-11

Recommended Daily Dietary Allowances for Vitamin Folacin, Revised 1974

Designed for the maintenance of good nutrition for practically all healthy people in the United States

	AGE (years)	WEIGHT (kg)	WEIGHT (lb)	HEIGHT (cm)	HEIGHT (in.)	ENERGY (kcal)	FOLA-CIN[a] (µg)
Infants	0.0–0.5	6	14	60	24	kg × 117	50
	0.5–1.0	9	20	71	28	kg × 108	50
Children	1–3	13	28	86	34	1300	100
	4–6	20	44	110	44	1800	200
	7–10	30	66	135	54	2400	300
Males	11–14	44	97	158	63	2800	400
	15–18	61	134	172	69	3000	400
	19–22	67	147	172	69	3000	400
	23–50	70	154	172	69	2700	400
	51+	70	154	172	69	2400	400
Females	11–14	44	97	155	62	2400	400
	15–18	54	119	162	65	2100	400
	19–22	58	128	162	65	2100	400
	23–50	58	128	162	65	2000	400
	51+	58	128	162	65	1800	400
Pregnant						+300	800
Lactating						+500	600

SOURCE: Food and Nutrition Board, *Recommended Dietary Allowances*, 8th ed., National Academy of Sciences—National Research Council, Washington, D.C., 1974.

[a] The folacin allowances refer to dietary sources as determined by *Lactobacillus casei* assay. Pure forms of folacin may be effective in doses less than one fourth of the recommended dietary allowance.

It can be synthesized by many microorganisms. Small amounts have had a marked effect on the growth of yeast and certain bacteria. Avidin, found in egg white, appears to be antagonistic to biotin. Cooking the eggs destroys this action.

Functions of Biotin

Biotin is essential in many biochemical reactions in the body. Among the important functions, biotin acts as a coenzyme in the metabolism of fatty acids and amino acids and in reactions in which carbon dioxide is fixed into certain organic acid molecules. Biotin is a very active biological substance.

Biotin Deficiencies

A deficiency of biotin results in anemia, depression, dermatitis, loss of hair, muscle atrophy and pain, nausea, loss of appetite, high cholesterol levels, and changes in heart functioning.

The widespread occurrence of biotin in foods, as well as its synthesis by intestinal flora, reduces the possibility of a deficiency in man, except in cases where faddism occurs, large amounts of raw egg white are eaten, inadequate diets are consumed, or the presence of metabolic disturbances causes utilization interference.

Biotin Nutritive Needs

A recommended dietary allowance has not been established for biotin by the Food and Nutrition Board because of the uncertainty as to the level of contribution of intestinal microorganisms. Daily intake of biotin is estimated between 100 µg and 300 µg per day.

TABLE 13–12

Sources of Folacin in Foods

FOOD	FOLACIN (μg/100 g)
Beef liver	290
Kidney	58
Hamburger	5
Egg, whole	5.1
Filberts	67
Peanuts	57
Walnuts	77
Asparagus	110
Lima beans, dry	100
Escarole	26
Spinach	80
Turnip greens	83
Potatoes, peeled	8
Tomatoes	9
Apples	0.5
Apricots, dried	4.7
Avocado	30
Dates, dry	25
Orange juice	4.8
Bread, white	15
Breakfast cereal, corn, and soya	80
Wheat, shredded	58
Whole milk	1.5
Buttermilk	11
Cottage cheese	34

SOURCE: *Agricultural Handbook 29*, Bureau of Human Nutrition and Home Economics, U.S. Department of Agriculture, Washington, D.C., 1951.

Sources of Biotin in Foods

Biotin will be found in liver, kidney, other organ meats, egg yolk, nuts, cauliflower, legumes, and mushrooms. Dairy products are only a fair source. Cereals are a poor source.

Choline

Choline is one of the methyl groups in nutrition. Methionine is the ultimate methyl donor as choline is synthesized in the body. Folate and vitamin B_{12} appear to be important. The amount of choline required by the body is therefore influenced by the amount of methionine, folate, and vitamin B_{12} in the diet, as well as growth rate, energy intake and expenditure, fat intake, and the type of dietary fat.[52]

Choline is a component of all cell membranes and lipoproteins that are involved in the transport of fat-soluble substances in the body. This vitamin is an important constituent of the brain and of acetylcholine, which functions in the transmission of nerve impulses. Choline may also be the source of labile methyl groups.

The most prominent signs of choline deficiency in experimental studies in mammals are fatty infiltration of the liver and hemorrhagic kidney disease. Under similar experimental conditions, a choline deficiency has not been demonstrated in man; consequently, there is no basis for establishing requirements or dietary allowances.[53] The only possibility of deficiency contemplated is in protein-calorie malnutrition of infants and children on diets of highly refined products. Mixed diets are estimated to yield from 400 to 900 μg of choline daily. The most important sources in foods are the organ meats, liver and kidney, muscle meats, nuts, the legumes, and skim milk.

Pantothenic Acid

Williams originated his long period of investigation in 1918, and in 1933 he reported on an acidic substance that was required as a growth factor for yeast. He named this substance *panthothenic acid* from the Greek meaning "everywhere." The name is particularly appropriate, for it is found everywhere in nature. Foods are rich in pantothenic acid content. In 1940, Williams isolated a nearly pure sample, and later in 1940 Stiller and his colleagues determined its structure.[54]

[52] W. H. Griffith, J. F. Nye, W. S. Hartroft, and E. A. Porta, "Choline," in W. H. Sebrell and R. S. Harris (eds.), *The Vitamins*, Vol. III, 2nd ed., Academic Press, New York, 1971, pp. 1–154.

[53] *Recommended Dietary Allowances*, op. cit., pp. 64–65.

[54] R. J. Williams, "Early Experience with Pantothenic Acid—A Retrospect," *Nutrition Reviews*, Vol. 12, No. 3 (March 1954), pp. 65–68.

Chemical and Physical Properties of Pantothenic Acid

This vitamin is a pale, yellow, oily liquid that has not been crystallized, but its calcium salt—calcium pantothenate—crystallizes readily. Pantothenic acid is readily available in the form of its salt. It is water soluble, stable in neutral solutions, but deteriorates rapidly in acid or alkaline solutions. It is not stable in dry heat. If temperatures are kept at a normal level, little loss occurs in cooking. Chemically, pantothenic acid contains the simple amino acid alanine.

Functions of Pantothenic Acid

Pantothenic acid is an active component of coenzyme A and participates in intermediary metabolism of carbohydrates, fats, and proteins that lead to energy release, the synthesis of fatty acids and sterols, and many other important reactions. This vitamin appears to be necessary for all organisms.

Pantothenic Acid Deficiencies

Deficiency symptoms are fatigue, prickling in the hands and feet, abdominal distress, nausea, sleep disturbances, headaches, leg cramps, motor impairment, flatulence, and occasional vomiting. Major cellular aberrations have resulted in death. These evidences of deficiency of pantothenic acid have occurred in animals but not in man.

Pantothenic Acid Nutritive Needs

Insufficient evidence is available to develop dietary allowances. Marginal deficiencies may exist along with other vitamin B complex deficiencies. This vitamin is widely distributed in food so only individuals on extremely limited diets may be subject to a deficiency. A daily intake of 5 to 10 mg of pantothenic acid is probably adequate for all adults, with the upper limits suggested for pregnant and lactating women. Diets that meet all other nutritional needs of children contain from 4 to 5 mg per day. Human milk contains approximately 2 mg per liter and cow's milk about 3.5 mg per liter, which may be the basis for estimating amounts of pantothenic acid for infants.[55]

Sources of Pantothenic Acid

Pantothenic acid is widely distributed among foods. The best sources are liver, kidney, fresh vegetables, other organ meats, whole-grain cereals, yeast, and egg yolk.

---

[55] Recommended Dietary Allowances, op. cit., pp. 79–80.

SELECTED REFERENCES

GENERAL

Davidson, Stanley, R. Passmore, and J. F. Brock, *Human Nutrition and Dietetics*, The Williams & Wilkins Company, Baltimore, 1972, Chapter 12.

De Ritter, Elmer, Modest Osadca, Jacob Scheiner, and John Keating, "Vitamins in Frozen Convenience Dinners and Pot Pies," *Journal of the American Dietetic Association*, Vol. 64, No. 4 (April 1974), pp. 391–397.

Economic Research Service, *National Food Situation*, U.S. Department of Agriculture, Washington, D.C., November 1973.

Food and Nutrition Board, *Recommended Dietary Allowances*, 8th ed., National Academy of Sciences National Research Council—Washington, D.C., 1974.

Goodhart, Robert S., and Maurice Shils (eds.), *Modern Nutrition in Health and Disease*, Lea & Febiger, Philadelphia, 1973, Chapter 5, Sections E–J and L.

Kutsky, Roman J., *Handbook of Vitamins and Hormones*, Van Nostrand Reinhold Company, New York, 1973, Chapters 7–10 and 12–15.

Orr, Martha Louise, *Pantothenic Acid, Vitamin B₆, and Vitamin B₁₂ in Foods*, Home Economics Research Report No. 36, Consumer and Food Economics Research Division, Agricultural Research Service, U.S. Department of Agriculture, Washington, D.C., 1969.

THIAMIN

Bowers, Jane A., and Beth A. Fryer, "Thiamin and Riboflavin in Cooked and Frozen, Reheated Turkey," *Journal of the American Dietetic Association*, Vol. 60, No. 5 (May 1972), pp. 399–401.

Frey, Charles N., Alfred S. Schultz, and Lawrence Atkin, "Recent Developments in the Vitamin Technology of Bread," *Food Technology*, Vol. 26, No. 6 (June 1972), pp. 54–58.

Henshaw, J. L., G. Noakes, S. O. Morris, M. Bennion, and C. J. Gubler, "Method for Evaluating Thiamine Adequacy in College Women," *Journal of the American Dietetic Association*, Vol. 57, No. 5 (November 1970), pp. 436–441.

"Influence of Malnutrition and Alcohol on Thiamine Absorption," *Nutrition Reviews*, Vol. 29, No. 1 (January 1971), pp. 13–15.

Noble, Isabel, "Thiamine and Riboflavin Retention in Cooked Variety Meats," *Journal of American Dietetic Association*, Vol. 56, No. 3 (March 1970), pp. 225–228.

Sebrell, W. H., and Robert Harris (eds.), *The Vitamins*, Vol. 5, Academic Press, Inc., New York, 1972, Chapter 15.

RIBOFLAVIN

Sauerberlich, H. E., J. H. Judd, G. E. Nicholalds, H. B. Broquist, and W. J. Darby, "Application of the Erythrocyte Glutathione Reductase Assay in Evaluating Riboflavin Nutritional Status in a High School Student Population," *American Journal of Clinical Nutrition*, Vol. 25, No. 8 (August 1972), pp. 756–762.

Sebrell, W. H., and Robert S. Harris (eds.), Academic Press, Inc., *The Vitamins*, New York, 1972, Chapter 14.

NIACIN

"Conversion of Tryptophan," *Nutrition Reviews*, Vol. 32, No. 3 (March 1974), pp. 76–77.

Goldsmith, Grace A., "Niacin: Antipellagra Factor, Hypocholesterolemic Agent," *Journal of the American Medical Association*, Vol. 194, No. 2 (October 11, 1965), pp. 167–173.

VITAMIN B₆

Cinnamon, Dale A., and John R. Beaton, "Biochemical Assessment of Vitamin B₆ Status in Man," *American Journal of Clinical Nutrition*, Vol. 23, No. 6 (June 1970), pp. 696–702.

Donald, Elizabeth, Lois D. McBean, Mary H. W. Simpson, Mary F. Sun, and Hekmat E. Aly, "Vitamin B₆ Requirement of Young Adult Women," *American Journal of Clinical Nutrition*, Vol. 24, No. 9 (September 1971), pp. 1028–1041.

György, Paul, "Developments Leading to the Metabolic Role of Vitamin B₆,"

American Journal of Clinical Nutrition, Vol. 24, No. 10 (October 1971), pp. 1250–1256.

"Oral Contraceptives and Vitamin B_6," *Nutrition Reviews*, Vol. 31, No. 2 (February 1973), pp. 49–50.

Polansky, Marilyn M., and Elizabeth W. Murphy, "Vitamin B_6 Components in Fruits and Nuts," *Journal of the American Dietetic Association*, Vol. 48, No. 2 (February 1966), pp. 109–111.

Sauberlich, H. E., J. E. Canham, E. M. Baker, N. Raica, and Y. F. Herman, "Biochemical Assessment of the Nutritional Status of Vitamin B_6 in the Human," *American Journal of Clinical Nutrition*, Vol. 25, No. 6 (June 1972), pp. 629–642.

VITAMIN B_{12}

Alvarado, Jorge, William Vargas, Napoleon Diaz, and Fernando E. Viteri, "Vitamin B_{12} Absorption in Protein-Calorie Malnourished Children and During Recovery: Influence of Protein Depletion and of Diarrhea," *American Journal of Clinical Nutrition*, Vol. 26, No. 6 (June 1973), pp. 595–599.

A Staff Report, "Discovery and Synthesis of Vitamin B_{12} Celebrated," *Nutrition Today*, Vol. 8, No. 1 (January–February 1973), pp. 24–27.

FOLACIN

"Alcoholism and Folic Acid," *Nutrition Reviews*, Vol. 30, No. 3 (March 1972), pp. 57–60.

Butterfield, Susan, and Doris Howes Calloway, "Folacin in Wheat and Selected Foods," *Journal of the American Dietetic Association*, Vol. 60, No. 4 (April 1972), pp. 310–314.

Dong, Faye M., and Susan M. Oace, "Folate Distribution in Fruit Juices," *Journal of the American Dietetic Association*, Vol. 62, No. 2 (February 1973), pp. 162–166.

"Folic Acid Absorption, Anticonvulsant and Contraceptive Therapy," *Nutrition Reviews*, Vol. 32, No. 2 (February 1974), pp. 39–41.

Herbert, Victor, et al., "Symposium, Folic Acid Deficiency," *American Journal of Clinical Nutrition*, Vol. 23, No. 6 (June 1970), pp. 841–860.

Hoppner, B. Lampi, and D. E. Perrin, "Folacin Activity of Frozen Convenience Foods," *Journal of the American Dietetic Association*, Vol. 63, No. 5 (November 1973), pp. 536–539.

Santini, Rafael, Maj. Florence M. Berger, Gloria Berdasco, Capt. Thomas W. Sheey, Josefina Aviles, and Ivonne Davila, "Folic Acid Activity in Puerto Rican Foods," *Journal of the American Dietetic Association*, Vol. 41, No. 6 (December 1962), pp. 562–567.

Saraya, A. K., V. P. Choudhry, and T. P. Ghai. "Interrelationships of Vitamin B_{12}, Folic Acid, and Iron in Anemia of Infancy and Childhood: Effect of Vitamin B_{12} and Iron Therapy on Folate Metabolism," *American Journal of Clinical Nutrition*, Vol. 26, No. 6 (June 1973), pp. 640–646.

Streiff, Richard R., "Folate Levels in Citrus and Other Juices," *American Journal of Clinical Nutrition*, Vol. 24, No. 12 (December 1971), pp. 1390–1392.

———. "Folate Deficiency and Oral Concentrates," *Journal of the American Medical Association*, Vol. 214, No. 1 (October 5, 1970), pp. 40–43.

BIOTIN

Goodhart, Robert S., "Biotin," in Goodhart, Robert S., and Maurice E. Shils, (eds.), *Modern Nutrition in Health and Disease*, Lea & Febiger Company, Philadelphia, 1973, Chapter 5, Section L, pp. 256–258.

CHOLINE

Barak, Anthony J., Dean J. Tuma, and Michael F. Sorrell, "Relationship of Ethanol to Choline Metabolism in the Liver: A Review," *American Journal of Clinical Nutrition*, Vol. 26, No. 11 (November 1973), pp. 1234–1241.

PANTOTHENIC ACID

Cohenour, Sally Hansen, and Doris Howes Calloway, "Blood, Urine, and Dietary Pantothenic Acid Levels of Pregnant Teenagers," *American Journal of Clinical Nutrition*, Vol. 25, No. 5 (May 1972), pp. 512–517.

14

Ascorbic Acid

Vitamin C (Ascorbic Acid)

Comments in historical reports and diaries by famous men through the years give some indications of the seriousness of scurvy. One example is Sir Richard Hawkins' statement during the latter half of the sixteenth century that in his 20 years at sea he had seen about 10,000 mariners destroyed by this disease.

An even more dramatic report was given by Lord Anson as described by Tisdall and Jolliffe.[1] He had left England in November 1740, with six ships and crews totaling 961 men. When he reached the southwest coast of South America in June of the following year, he had lost two thirds of his crew as a result of scurvy, and he had to abandon three ships. By November 1741, 1 year later, scurvy had further reduced the number of his men to the point that he had to abandon two more ships. Finally returning to England in June 1744, 3½ years after he left, he reported that more than four fifths of his crew had succumbed to scurvy and he had lost five of his six ships.

James Lind's *Treatise on Scurvy*, published in 1753, as described in *A History of Nutrition*,[2] tells of men who were cured of the disease by an Indian remedy over two centuries earlier. They were part of the company that had joined Jacques Cartier in the early explorations of North America. During the winter of 1536, 110 of the men were afflicted with scurvy. The Indians, who were apparently familiar with the disease, effectively treated them with a medicine prepared from the needles of a certain pine tree.

Lind published a second edition of his *Treatise* in 1757 that told of the first experimental investigations into the value of various substances in treating scurvy. He reported that in May 1747 he had treated 12 scurvy patients, whose conditions were of a similar degree of severity. He divided the patients into pairs and experimented with six different diets. Among the diets he tried such things as vinegar, cider, and something that he called elixir vitriol (sulfuric acid, alcohol, and an extract of ginger and cinnamon). Lind found that the best effects were obtained when the diet was supplemented with oranges and

---

[1] Frederick F. Tisdall and Norman Jolliffe, "Water-Soluble Vitamins," in Norman Jolliffe (ed.), *Clinical Nutrition*, Hoeber, New York, 1950, p. 586.

[2] E. V. McCollum, *A History of Nutrition*, Houghton Mifflin, Boston, 1957, p. 252.

192

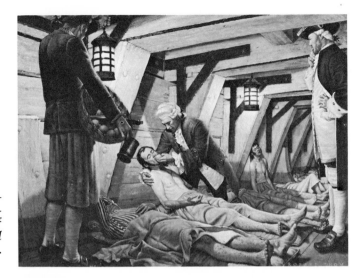

FIGURE 14–1. *Lind experimented with various substances in the treatment of scurvy and found oranges and lemons to be most effective. (Park-Davis; see page 12)*

lemons. This and subsequent experiments caused the British navy in 1795 to order all its ships to carry supplies of lemons or limes. Thus British sailors subsequently became known as "limeys." But they also became known as sailors who did not have scurvy!

In 1928, Szent-Györgi isolated hexuronic acid from adrenal glands, cabbage, and oranges. In 1931, King and Waugh obtained the crystalline form of this hexuronic acid and discovered that 0.5 mg could serve as a protective dose against scurvy for a guinea pig. This evidence established that the crystals were antiscorbutic vitamin C. Szent-Györgi and Svirbely in 1932 confirmed the biological effectiveness of their hexuronic acid crystals. Haworth and others established the molecular structure, and Reichstein· and associates synthesized ascorbic acid in 1933.

Chemical and Physical Properties of Vitamin C

Ascorbic acid, or vitamin C, is a water-soluble, crystalline compound. Although fairly stable in an acid or fatty solution, it is a strong reducing agent and, as such, is very sensitive to oxygen and can thus be called the least stable of vitamins. It can be lost through exposure to heat and air and to light, which stimulates the activity of oxidative enzymes. Furthermore, it is quite sensitive to alkalis.

Functions of Vitamin C

The primary contribution of vitamin C is to the normal functioning of all cells, including subcellular structures, according to King.[3] It is essential to the formation of normal collagen, sometimes referred to as "intercellular cement." This important constituent is necessary for the structural integrity of bones, teeth, connective tissue, skin, cartilage, and capillary walls.

Vitamin C has significant relationships with other nutrients. It converts the inactive form of folic acid to the active form, folinic acid. The metabolism of the amino acids phenylalanine and tyrosine is facilitated by ascorbic acid. The absorption of iron is enhanced by this vitamin, and it may have a role in calcium metabolism. There is a significant sparing action (utilized to better advantage) of vitamin C on thiamin, riboflavin, folic acid, pantothenic acid, and on vitamins A and E, according to Schwieter and Isler,[4] because of

[3] C. G. King, "Present Knowledge of Ascorbic Acid (Vitamin C)," in *Present Knowledge in Nutrition*, 3rd ed., Nutrition Foundation, New York, 1967, Chap. 18.

[4] U. Schwieter and O. Isler, "Chemistry," in W. H. Sebrell, Jr., and Robert S. Harris (eds.), *The Vitamins*, Vol. 1, Academic Press, New York, 1967, Chap. 2.

its antioxidant qualities. Extra doses of vitamin C appear to be beneficial to an individual exposed to extremely low environmental temperatures. Although the mechanism is not clear, Baker[5] believes that there is an increased requirement for all forms of stress, but the amount is not known. There is either an increased need or an increased destruction of vitamin C in fevers and infections.

A severe deficiency is necessary to interfere with wound healing, according to Schwartz.[6] Leroy and Schendel[7] suggest that oral contraceptives depress plasma ascorbic acid levels, so supplementation may be necessary to counteract this effect. Croft[8] evaluated ascorbic acid levels of the drug addict and 58 per cent of his patients revealed a deficiency. This is another area for fruitful research.

Some relationship exists between ascorbic acid and the adrenal glands, but its exact nature is unclear.

Vitamin C in prescribed amounts has a role in the healing of wounds because it facilitates the formation of strong connective tissue in the scar. Similarly, it is important in the healing of burns. Ascorbic acid is necessary in the synthesis of epinephrine and anti-inflammatory steroids, for example, hydrocortisone by the adrenal gland.

Glandular tissues, such as in the adrenal cortex, the pituitary, and glandular cells of the intestinal tract, as well as embryonic tissue and leucocytes, are especially high in ascorbic acid content, according to King. Intermediate

content is found in the pancreas, kidney, liver, thymus, spleen, brain tissue, and salivary glands. Muscle tissue is relatively low in ascorbic acid content.

Without doubt, vitamin C is essential to human beings. Although many important functions have been proposed for it, much remains to be discovered about this elusive vitamin.

Manifestations of Vitamin C Deficiency

Scurvy is seldom seen today, but when it does occur it appears in the infant and young child more frequently than in the adult. However, many clinical manifestations of suboptimal nutritional status have been correctly or incorrectly attributed to an ascorbic acid deficiency.

Some of the most obvious signs of scurvy are found in the growing bone. The essential nutrients for bone formation, the minerals and proteins, may be present, but they cannot be set down in the necessary orderly fashion unless an adequate amount of ascorbic acid is also present. Without it, the intercellular cementing substance is not available and the mineralization is incomplete. The bone, therefore, may be formed improperly. This condition can be detected by X ray.

A frequent sign of scurvy in the young child is "beaded" ribs. The front ends of the ribs are sore, and breathing may be uncomfortable and difficult. It is painful to the child even to turn in bed, and he will cry upon being handled because of the bone condition.

Another characteristic of scurvy in the young child is that the soft tissue around the joints is swollen and painful if touched. The area at the end of the bone shaft where normal development takes place is especially affected. After the child is given ascorbic acid, these symptoms are dramatically changed within a few days.

The symptoms of scurvy in an adult are somewhat different because he is not subjected to the stress of growth. However, the same fundamental manifestations occur. Changes in the soft tissues are usually the first and most evident symptom of a deficiency of vitamin C. Because the cementing substance is missing, cells tend to disintegrate and fall apart. Since

[5] Eugene M. Baker and W. H. Griffin, "Vitamin C Requirements in Stress," American Journal of Clinical Nutrition, Vol. 20, No. 5 (May 1967), pp. 583–586.

[6] Peter L. Schwartz, "Ascorbic Acid in Wound Healing—A Review," Journal of the American Dietetic Association, Vol. 56, No. 6 (June 1970), pp. 497–503.

[7] Vera Joyce McLeroy and Harold Eugene Schendel, "Influence of Oral Contraceptives on Ascorbic Acid Concentration in Healthy Sexually Mature Women," American Journal of Clinical Nutrition, Vol. 26, No. 2 (February 1973), pp. 191–196.

[8] Lloyd K. Croft, "Ascorbic Acid Status of the Drug Addict Patient," American Journal of Clinical Nutrition, Vol. 26, No. 10 (October 1973), p. 1042.

the mouth is so accessible to clinical observation, it is usually the first area that is examined when scurvy is suspected. In these cases, the gums become swollen, they bleed readily, and are spongy. The unhealthy condition results in a high susceptibility to infection; teeth may even loosen if the condition is of sufficient severity. This syndrome is usually called *gingivitis*.

In addition to the oral signs, the skin may be scaly and thickened. Small capillary hemorrhages have been observed, although this does not always occur in mild cases. If pressure is exerted, these small hemorrhages may result in large bluish-green or yellow patches. A patient may complain of lassitude and general ill health. Wounds do not heal easily and there seems to be a lessened ability to resist generalized infection.

Symptoms that might be ascribed to a mild case of ascorbic acid deficiency are quite vague —weakness, irritability, loss of weight, vague aches and pains in muscles or joints, and apathy. There may be an additional complaint of bleeding gums.

Infectious diseases are much more common among people with scurvy and animal experiments have supported these observations. Despite this evidence, the leucocyte count and the immune response to antigenic challenge have not altered when tested in men and animals with scurvy. Conflicting evidence appears in a number of experimental areas, indicating the need for further research.

There has been considerable discussion of and research into the relation of ascorbic acid to colds. Linus Pauling made the observation that after he and his wife took large doses of vitamin C daily for several years there was a striking decrease in the number of colds and their severity. Pauling's conclusions were based upon theoretical speculation; he discounted reports of controlled studies, which indicated that vitamin C had little or no value for the prevention or the treatment of colds, and the recommended dietary allowances of this vitamin.[9]

Some Canadian physicians in Toronto[10] have evaluated the effect of large doses upon the frequency and duration of colds. Approximately 1,000 volunteers participated in the study. Information was secured about a vast number of details. In the vitamin group (dosage of 1 g daily and during illness, 4 g), 26 per cent of the subjects remained free from illness; in the placebo group, 18 per cent remained free from illness. The difference was statistically significant. The greatest difference was found in the days confined to the house, a 21 per cent reduction for the vitamin group compared with the placebo group. The data apparently show an effect of vitamin C, primarily upon the severity of the cold as indicated by the number of days confined to house, and a modest but barely significant effect on the frequency of colds.

An earlier study was reported from Minnesota[11] in which supplements of 200 mg of vitamin C were provided to college students. The estimated reduction of colds was about 15 per cent. Students taking the placebo lost an average of 1.6 school days compared with 1.1 days in the group receiving the vitamin. These studies were in considerable agreement with later research.

Coulehan[12] and others did a double-blind study to evaluate vitamin C supplements for respiratory-infection prophylaxis among 641 children at a Navajo boarding school over a 14-week period. Supplements of 1 and 2 g of ascorbic acid or placebo were given daily. Although findings indicated no differences between treatment groups in the number of respiratory episodes, those given vitamin C had fewer days of morbidity than those re-

[9] Editorial, "Vitamin C for Colds," *American Journal of Public Health*, Vol. 61, No. 4 (April 1971), pp. 649–652.

[10] T. W. Anderson, R. B. W. Reid, and G. H. Beation, "Vitamin C and the Common Cold: A Double-Blind Trial," *Canadian Medical Association Journal*, Vol. 107, No. 6 (June 1972), pp. 503–508.

[11] D. W. Cowan, H. S. Diehl, and A. B. Baker, "Vitamins for the Prevention of Colds," *Journal of the American Medical Association*, Vol. 120, No. 16 (August 1942), pp. 1268–1271.

[12] John L. Coulehan, Keith S. Reisinger, Kenneth D. Rogers, and Daniel W. Bradley, "Vitamin C Prophylaxis in a Boarding School," *New England Journal of Medicine*, Vol. 290, No. 1 (January 3, 1974), pp. 6–9.

TABLE 14–1

Recommendations for Daily Dietary Allowances for Iodine, Revised 1974

Designed for the maintenance of good nutrition of practically all healthy people in the United States

	AGE (years)	WEIGHT (kg)	WEIGHT (lb)	HEIGHT (cm)	HEIGHT (in.)	ASCORBIC ACID (mg)
Infants	0.0–0.5	6	14	60	24	35
	0.5–1.0	9	20	71	28	35
Children	1–3	13	28	86	34	40
	4–6	20	44	110	44	40
	7–10	30	66	135	54	40
Males	11–14	44	97	158	63	45
	15–18	61	134	172	69	45
	19–22	67	147	172	69	45
	23–50	70	154	172	69	45
	51+	70	154	172	69	45
Females	11–14	44	97	155	62	45
	15–18	54	119	162	65	45
	19–22	58	128	162	65	45
	23–50	58	128	162	65	45
	51+	58	128	162	65	45
Pregnant						60
Lactating						80

SOURCE: Food and Nutrition Board, *Recommended Dietary Allowances*, 8th ed., National Academy of Sciences—National Research Council, Washington, D.C., 1974.

ceiving the placebo. The researchers state that the actual clinical meaning of this experiment remains unclear and recommend further clinical trials.

The cost of colds in the population are a matter of concern not only from the standpoint of health but of economics.[13] These data raise many points for future studies. The findings did not conclude that large doses of vitamin C are necessarily the most effective method for treating or preventing colds. The best dosage has not been evaluated. The possibility of fortified foods may be more practical. Other methods of treatment may be explored that are equally effective.

There have been many warnings about large dosages of vitamin C. Goldsmith[14] states that 1 g of ascorbic acid daily may cause diarrhea. Amounts of 4 to 12 g can lead to urate and cystine stones in the urinary tract. Large amounts of the vitamin will be excreted in the urine on large dosages. In animals excessive amounts can cause infertility and abortion. The main role for vitamin C is as an essential nutrient.

Nutritional Needs for Ascorbic Acid

Evidence is available that a daily intake of 10 mg of ascorbic acid will alleviate scurvy in

[13] "Vitamin C and the Common Cold," *Nutrition Reviews*, Vol. 31, No. 10 (October 1973), pp. 303–305.

[14] Grace A. Goldsmith, "Common Cold: Prevention and Treatment with Ascorbic Acid Not Effective," *Journal of the American Medical Association*, Vol. 216, No. 2 (April 12, 1971), p. 337.

human subjects.[15] It is doubtful if this amount will maintain optimal health. Studies of the actual utilization of ascorbic acid in the adult male indicate that 30 mg per day is sufficient to replenish the ascorbic acid metabolized daily. The Food and Nutrition Board recommends 45 mg per day of ascorbic acid as an adequate supply for health in normal adult men and women, preadolescents, and adolescents.

Precise requirements for infants and early childhood are not known but 35 mg per day appears to meet requirements for infants. For children up to 11 years of age 40 mg per day is recommended. Ascorbic acid dietary allowances are increased in pregnancy to 60 mg per day, and to 80 mg per day for lactating women. Although the allowance for ascorbic acid is not increased for the elderly, during periods of stress and drug therapy, the amount may need to be increased.

The recommended dietary allowances of the Food and Nutrition Board for all ages, both sexes, and for pregnancy and lactation are cited in Table 14–1.

Sources of Vitamin C

Vitamin C occurs in plant tissues, but there is a wide range in ascorbic acid content of most common foods. One of the best sources is citrus fruits and their juices. Table 14–2 indicates the vitamin C content of various fruit juices. Other foods that are relatively high in vitamin C content are tomatoes and cabbage. And many do not realize that such foods as potatoes, green leafy vegetables, and fresh fruits in season can contribute considerable amounts to the daily diet.

The vitamin C content of a fruit or vegetable, more than that of any other vitamin, can be influenced by many factors, particularly growing conditions. Light, such as sunlight, accelerates synthesis of this vitamin. Thus fruit sheltered from the sunlight by dense foliage will not have as much vitamin C, nor will fruit grown in a season of many rainy or

[15] Food and Nutrition Board, *Recommended Dietary Allowances*, 8th ed., National Academy of Sciences—National Research Council, Washington, D.C., 1974, pp. 63–64.

TABLE 14–2

Ascorbic Acid Content of Fruit Juices

FOOD (8-oz portion)	ASCORBIC ACID (mg)
Apple juice, fresh or canned	3
Apricot nectar	7
Cranberry juice cocktail	5
Grapefruit juice	
Fresh	92
Canned, unsweetened	84
Sweetened	78
Frozen, reconstituted	
Unsweetened	96
Sweetened	82
Grape juice	Trace
Lemon juice, fresh	113
Lemonade, frozen, reconstituted	17
Lime juice, fresh	80
Orange juice, fresh	122
Canned, unsweetened	100
Frozen, reconstituted	112
Dehydrated, reconstituted	108
Orange and grapefruit juice	
Frozen, reconstituted	102
Peach nectar	1
Pear nectar	1
Pineapple juice	22
Prune juice	4
Tomato juice, canned	38

SOURCE: *Nutritive Value of Foods*, Home and Garden Bulletin No. 72, U.S. Department of Agriculture, Washington, D.C., 1971.

cloudy days. The way fruits and vegetables are handled can greatly influence the vitamin C content. It is especially important that the homemaker be constantly alert in regard to vitamin C value of foods. First, she should select foods that are in their best state so that they have not already lost the vitamin; second, she should store them properly at home; and finally, her food preparation procedures should ensure the maximum return for her money. Table 14–3 shows the vitamin C content of various noncitrus fruits and vegetables.

It is not difficult to obtain vitamin C. But the practice of omitting breakfast and not including breakfast items in the menus throughout the day may account for the surveys re-

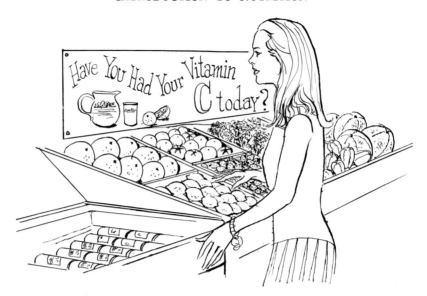

FIGURE 14–2. *Sources of ascorbic acid in the American diet.*

vealing that diets are low in this vitamin. Being familiar with the contributions that fruits (other than citrus fruits) and vegetables can make toward the vitamin C requirement is important. Note that dried fruits usually have less vitamin C than fresh fruits.

Nutritional Status

Findings of the *Ten-State Nutrition Survey*[16] indicated that black females from ages 17 to 59 years in the low-income-ratio states and black and white males over 60 years of age in the high-income-ratio states have a low prevalence of deficient values of vitamin C. Black and white males 17 to over 60 years of age in low-income-ratio states and Spanish-American males over 60 years of age have a medium prevalence of deficient values in vitamin C. All other age and ethnic groups of both sexes and income levels have only a minimal prevalence of deficiency in vitamin C. (See Table 2–2.)

The preliminary findings of the *First Health and Nutrition Examination Survey*[17] revealed that all age groups for both race and income levels had vitamin C intakes that approached 90 to 100 per cent of the standards or were above the standards. White children 1 to 5 years of age and white females 18 to 44 years of age tended to have a higher percentage of individuals who had vitamin C intakes less than the standards than did black individuals of similar age–sex–income groups. Corresponding percentages in the upper-income group were higher for blacks than for whites. In the age group 60 years and over, white adults in the lower-income group had a higher percentage of individuals with vitamin C intakes that did not meet the standard than did black adults of the same income group. On the other hand, black adults in the upper-income group had a higher percentage of individuals with less vitamin C values that did not meet the standard than did white adults. From the data of the two studies, it can be concluded

---

[16] *Highlights, Ten-State Nutrition Survey, 1968–1970,* DHEW Publication No. (HSM) 72–8134, Center for Disease Control, Health Service and Mental Health Administration, U.S. Department of Health, Education, and Welfare, Atlanta, Ga., 1972.

[17] National Center for Health Statistics, *Preliminary Findings, First Health and Nutrition Examination Survey, United States, 1971–1972, Dietary Intake and Biochemical Findings,* Health Resources Administration, Public Health Service, U.S. Department of Health, Education, and Welfare, Rockville, Md., 1974.

TABLE 14–3

Ascorbic Acid Content of Fruits and Vegetables

FOOD	PORTION	ASCORBIC ACID (mg)
Apple, raw	1 (2½-in. diam.)	3
Apricots, raw	3 (whole)	10
Dried	1 cup (40 halves)	19
Banana	1 (6 × 1½ in.)	10
Blackberries, raw	1 cup	30
Blueberries, raw	1 cup	20
Canteloupe	½ (5-in. diam.)	63
Cherries	1 cup	9
Dates, fresh and dried	1 cup	0
Figs, dried	1 large (2 × 1 in.)	0
Fruit cocktail, canned, heavy syrup	1 cup	5
Grapefruit, raw, medium	½ (4½-in. diam.)	50
Grapes, Concord	1 cup	7
Oranges, navel, California	1 (2½-in. diam.)	75
Papayas, raw	1 cup (½-in. cubes)	102
Peaches, raw	1 (2-in. diam.)	7
Dried, uncooked	1 cup	28
Pear, raw	1 (3 × 2½-in. diam.)	7
Pineapple, raw, diced	1 cup	33
Plums, raw	1 (2-in. diam.)	3
Prunes, dried, uncooked	4	1
Raisins, dried	1 cup	2
Raspberries, red, raw	1 cup	31
Rhubarb, cooked, sugar added	1 cup	17
Strawberries, raw	1 cup	87
Tangerines, raw	1 (2½-in. diam.)	26
Tomato	1 (2 × 2½ in.)	34
Watermelon, raw	1 wedge (4 × 8 in.)	26
Broccoli spears, cooked	1 cup	111
Collards, cooked	1 cup	84
Mustard greens, cooked	1 cup	63
Peppers, green	1 pod	79
Turnip greens, cooked	1 cup	87

SOURCE: *Nutritive Value of Foods*, Home and Garden Bulletin No. 72, U.S. Department of Agriculture, Washington, D.C., 1971.

that the lack of dietary intake of vitamin C is not as serious a problem as associated with other nutrients.

Consumption

The contribution of major food groups to the dietary intake of ascorbic acid for civilian consumption according to preliminary 1974 data[18] is as follows: meat (including pork fat cuts), poultry, and fish, 1.01 per cent; eggs, 0 per cent; dairy products, excluding butter, 4.0 per cent; fats and oils, including butter, 0 per cent; citrus fruits, 26.3 per cent; other fruits, 11.4 per cent; potatoes and sweet potatoes, 18.0 per cent; dark-green and deep-yellow vegetables, 8.3 per cent; other vegetables, including tomatoes, 27.6 per cent; dry beans and peas, nuts, soya flour, less than 0.05 per cent; flour and cereal products, 0 per cent; sugars and sweeteners, less than 0.05 per cent; and miscellaneous, 3.5 per cent.

[18] *National Food Situation*, Economic Research Service, U.S. Department of Agriculture, Washington, D.C., November 1974, p. 28.

SELECTED REFERENCES

Alfin-Slater, Roslyn, "Fats, Essential Fatty Acids, and Ascorbic Acid," *Journal of the American Dietetic Association,* Vol. 64, No. 2 (February 1974), pp. 168–170.

Davidson, Stanley, R. Passmore, and J. F. Brock, *Human Nutrition and Dietetics,* The Williams & Wilkins Company, Baltimore, 1972, Chapter 12.

Food and Nutrition Board, *Recommended Dietary Allowances,* 8th ed., National Academy of Sciences—National Research Council, Washington, D.C. 1974.

Highlights, Ten-State Nutrition Survey, 1968–1970, DHEW Publication No. (HSM) 72–8134, Center for Disease Control, Health Services and Mental Health Administration, U.S. Department of Health, Education, and Welfare, Atlanta, Ga., 1972.

Hodges, Robert E., and Eugene M. Baker, "Ascorbic Acid," in Robert S. Goodhart and Maurice E. Shils (eds.), *Modern Nutrition in Health and Disease,* Lea & Febiger, Philadelphia, 1973, Chapter 5, Section K, pp. 245–255.

Margen, Sheldon, "Vitamin C and Colds," *Journal of Nutrition Education,* Vol. 2, No. 4 (Spring 1971), pp. 131–133.

McLeroy, Vera Joyce, and Harold Eugene Schendel, "Influence of Oral Contraceptives on Ascorbic Acid Concentrations in Healthy, Sexually Mature Women," *American Journal of Clinical Nutrition,* Vol. 26, No. 2 (February 1973), pp. 191–196.

"New Roles for Ascorbic Acid," *Nutrition Reviews,* Vol. 32, No. 2 (February 1974), pp. 53–55.

Pauling, Linus C., *Vitamin C and the Cold,* W. H. Freeman and Company, San Francisco, 1970.

Pelletier, O., and M. Keith, "Bioavailability of Synthetic and Natural Ascorbic Acid." *Journal of the American Dietetic Association,* Vol. 64, No. 3 (March 1974), pp. 271–275.

Rhead, W. J., and G. N. Schrauzer, "Risks of Long-Term Ascorbic Acid Overdosage," *Nutrition Reviews,* Vol. 29, No. 11 (November 1971), pp. 262–263.

"Vitamin C and the Common Cold," *Nutrition Reviews,* Vol. 31, No. 10 (October 1973), pp. 303–305.

15

An Overview of Minerals

Nutrients previously discussed were organic in nature. There are, however, a number of minerals or inorganic elements that play a vital role in nutrition. Although the terms *inorganic elements* and *minerals* are used interchangeably, neither gives a true description of these particular nutrients. The term *mineral* is generally applied to a substance mined from the ground. Actually, the minerals utilized by the body are drawn from the ground by plants. Man then either gets the minerals in his food from the plants themselves or from animals that had previously eaten the plants.

The term *inorganic* is also something of a misnomer, for these nutrients are seldom found as strictly inorganic compounds. Most of the minerals are actually associated with organic compounds. (Common salt, which is made up of sodium and chlorine, is an exception.) However, since authorities in nutrition have used these terms for a long period of time, *inorganic elements* or *minerals* will be used interchangeably in the discussion. Occasionally the term *ash constituents* is used. When foods are burned in experiments, the organic material disappears and the ash that is left is composed of the inorganic elements.

Discovery of Mineral Nutrients

The invention of the electric battery in the latter part of the eighteenth century led Sir Humphry Davy to the discovery of a number of the minerals that are important to nutrition. (Previously Lavoisier had listed 33 elements but had indicated that there were probably many more.) Davy, concerned about the nature of elements, would pass an electric current through a substance to determine if it were an element or a compound. He used common material such as caustic alkali, of which caustic potash is an example, and alkaline earths. Through his experimentation he brought about the discovery of potassium, sodium, calcium, magnesium, barium, and strontium.

Earlier Scheele had discovered that phosphorus was present in the bones. He and other investigators were aware of the fact that the bones also contained calcium in large quantities. But it was not until the latter part of the nineteenth century that Sidney Ringer, a famous English physiologist, began to ponder the possible role of minerals in the functioning of the body.

His first experiment was conducted by

201

bathing the heart of a frog or a turtle in a salt solution. He discovered that the heart kept beating for some time in this solution. When very small amounts of certain mineral salts were added to the solution, Ringer found that the heart beating could be prolonged. When sugar was substituted for salt, the beating stopped. This discovery was used to advantage. He would stop the beating of the heart by placing it in a sugar solution and then place it in another solution to which certain salts had been added. When calcium chloride, for example, was added, the contractions took place sooner and continued longer. This led to the conclusion that both sodium, which was in the common salt solution, and calcium were important to the beating of the heart. He found that the concentration of these various salts was very critical, and that if the salt solution had the same concentration of salts as did the blood of the animal, the heart beating could be restored. Ringer's work was of such stature that experimenters today refer to *Ringer's solution,* which means any of the chlorides in solution that will keep tissues alive.

From the research of Osborne and Mendel[1] at Yale, as well as others, the conclusion was reached that mineral elements are of vital concern in nutrition.

Classification of Minerals

Mineral elements that are required in relatively large amounts in the body are commonly grouped as major minerals. These are calcium, phosphorus, potassium, sulfur, sodium, chlorine, and magnesium. Sodium, chlorine, and potassium are identified as the major electrolytes of body water. Mineral elements required or present in the body in amounts less than 0.005 per cent are known as *trace elements.* In this group are iron, zinc, selenium, manganese, copper, iodine, fluorine, chromium, molybdenum, and cobalt.

There are mineral elements for which human requirements have not been established

although there is some evidence that they may participate in certain physiological functions.

Mineral Composition of the Body

Although the role of minerals in human nutrition is significant, the amounts present in the body are small. About 4 per cent of body weight can be attributed to minerals—for example, 6 pounds of the weight of a 150-pound man—most of which are in the bones. Table 15–1 shows representative amounts of minerals in the adult human body.

Functions of Minerals

The use of tracer elements has made possible the discovery of new information about the role of minerals in the body. These elements are chemically marked so that it is possible to study their paths throughout the body. This type of research may shed light on the function of the mineral, the need for the mineral, and its metabolism. Many unanswered questions may be clarified by this process.

TABLE 15–1

Approximate Composition of Elements in Human Adult Body

ELEMENT	PER CENT
Calcium	1.5–2.2
Phosphorus	0.8–1.2
Potassium	0.35
Sulfur	0.25
Sodium	0.15
Chlorine	0.15
Magnesium	0.05
Iron	0.004
Manganese	0.0003
Copper	0.00015
Iodine	0.00004
Cobalt	Trace
Zinc	Trace
Selenium	Trace
Molybdenum	Trace
Fluorine	Trace
Others	Trace

SOURCE: Henry C. Sherman, *Chemistry of Food and Nutrition,* 8th ed., Macmillan, New York, 1952, p. 227.

[1] T. B. Osborne and I. B. Mendel, "The Inorganic Elements in Nutrition," *Journal of Biological Chemistry,* Vol. 34, No. 1 (April 1918), pp. 131–140.

Several criteria determine whether a mineral is considered essential. According to Underwood,[2] they are as follows: (1) if a deficiency state occurs on a diet that is considered adequate in all other respects except for the mineral under study, (2) if there is a significant growth response in repeated demonstrations after supplements of the mineral under question have been given, and (3) if the deficiency state correlates with a subnormal level of that particular mineral in the blood or certain tissues of the body.

In general, minerals have two main functions. The first one is as an actual constituent of the body in both the hard and soft tissues. For instance calcium, magnesium, and phosphorus are very important in the structure of bones and teeth. Other minerals may be found in tissues and fluids of the body.

Examples of minerals involved in the structure of the body are iodine in the thyroid gland and in its secretion, thyroxine; magnesium in the muscles and some in the blood; and copper, frequently found in conjunction with iron in the liver and in other tissues. Potassium is an integral part of muscles and various body organs. Chlorine occurs in the hydrochloric acid in the gastric juices and when combined with sodium to form sodium chloride is an important constituent of blood and other body fluids. Many of the hormones, enzymes, and other aspects of body composition include minerals in their makeup. Examples are copper and iron in the enzyme cytochrome oxidase involved in energy metabolism and zinc in the protein-splitting enzyme, carboxypeptidase, an integral part of the intestinal juice.

Every cell of the body makes a continuous demand for minerals. Iron and phosphorus are found in every living cell—phosphorus in the nucleus and iron in the chromatin of the nucleus. The cytoplasm, or the body, of the cell has phosphorus and other nutrients. Minerals in the cell influence the vital processes of oxidation, secretion, and growth.

Certain cells have unique functions. The iron-bearing protein, hemoglobin, for example,

is essential for bringing oxygen to the tissues and removing carbon dioxide. The supply of minerals in the cell may deter or facilitate the processes of cellular metabolism or metabolic homeostasis.

In their second important role, minerals both act as regulators and are necessary to certain body functions. For example, the minerals are important to the functioning of nerves. The transmission of a nerve impulse is facilitated by an exchange of sodium and potassium ions in the nerve cells. If the concentration of minerals such as calcium, magnesium, sodium, and potassium in the fluids bathing nerve cells is altered, the ability to transmit nerve impulses will be disrupted.

The maintenance of acid–base balance, or neutrality, is related to certain minerals. Some minerals have the capacity to generate an acid medium, such as chlorine, phosphorus, and sulfur. These minerals are predominant in protein foods like eggs and meats and in cereal products. Basic-reacting minerals are calcium, iron, magnesium, potassium, and sodium, which are found largely in fruits and vegetables. Although fruits like oranges and lemons have an acid taste, their organic acids are metabolized to an alkaline residue. Some foods, milk, for example, have an internal balance of elements that are acid and alkaline in nature. Pure carbohydrates and other foods without minerals lack any influence on the acid–base balance of the body.

Certain foods, cranberries, rhubarb, spinach, cocoa, and tea, for example, contain acids like benzoic, oxalic, and tannic acid, which cannot be metabolized by the body and so must be listed as acid forming. The acids are present in such concentration that the base-forming potential in these foods is overbalanced.

The functioning and even the survival of body cells depend on the maintenance of body neutrality. However, the body has a number of mechanisms to neutralize an excess of acid or base. One mechanism is dilution through the large amount of body water—70 per cent of the lean body mass. Another way is for the body to buffer excesses through the use of carbonates, phosphates, proteins, ammonia, and the like.

An imbalance in the ratio of the acid–base

[2] E. J. Underwood, *Proceedings of the Cornell Nutrition Conference*, 1957.

balance is not the concern of an individual who consumes an adequate diet. The individual who eats a lopsided dietary, overemphasizing high-protein foods or consuming only vegetarian foods, for example, may burden his neutrality processes.

Another important function of minerals is their contribution to osmotic pressure and the movement of body liquids. The concentration of minerals, such as sodium, potassium, and chlorine, on either side of a membrane governs the passage of fluids from one side to another. This process is demonstrated when digested materials in the intestinal tract are transmitted into the bloodstream without having any of the blood reverse into the intestine. Waste materials of the cells in the blood are transported by the blood to the kidneys for excretion. Nutrients are carried by the blood to various organs and other areas of the body to be utilized.

Minerals contribute to the water and electrolyte balance of the body. Certain mineral particles are positively charged—sodium, potassium, and magnesium ions, for example—whereas chlorine, phosphate, and sulfate ions are negatively charged. The extracellular and intercellular fluids in composition are regulated in such precise manner that an osmotic equilibrium is maintained in spite of variations in electrolyte distribution.

Certain phases of digestion require a specific acidity or alkalinity. This condition is facilitated by minerals that provide an acid or alkaline medium to favor the digestive process. In the small intestine, for example, certain alkaline salts are important to the digestion of fat.

The contractility of muscles depends on the presence of calcium, sodium, potassium, and chlorides in the fluid that bathes the muscle. This is especially true of that most important muscle, the heart. Calcium is essential to the rhythmic beating of this organ.

Minerals serve as catalysts in a number of important physiological reactions. Although they are not a part of the end product of the process, the reaction could not take place without them. Examples are the catalyzing action of enzymes in the metabolism of carbohydrates and fats, the clotting of blood by calcium, and the synthesis of hemoglobin. The

production of insulin depends on the presence of zinc. Calcium facilitates the absorption of vitamin B_{12}. Pancreatic lipase is activated by calcium and magnesium. Sodium and magnesium are important in the absorption of carbohydrate.

Mineral elements seldom operate in isolation. They are interrelated and balanced to perform well. Calcium and phosphorus, for example, are in a definite relationship in the composition of bones and teeth. Certain minerals, such as zinc, molybdenum, and manganese, are important as activators for certain metabolic reactions including enzymes. Additional relationships could be cited, and active experimentation is going on to prove that there are still others.

Requirements for Minerals

Seven mineral elements are required in macro amounts: calcium, chloride, magnesium, potassium, phosphorus, sodium, and sulfur, according to Sandstead.[3] Eight minerals are required in micro amounts: cobalt, copper, iodine, iron, boron, manganese, selenium, and zinc. Chromium, fluorine, nickel, and molybdenum appear to have a significant role in human metabolism. The importance of other minerals is still being investigated. Minor elements that appear in biologic systems but for which physiologic functions have not been assigned are aluminum, antimony, arsenic, barium, boron, bromine, cadmium, galium, lead, lithium, mercury, nickel, rubidium, silver, strontium, tin, titanium, and vanadium.[4] Difficulty in measuring their concentration in body fluids is another problem. The daily requirement of many of these minerals has not been established. The Food and Nutrition Board has established recommended dietary allow-

[3] Harold H. Sandstead, "Present Knowledge of the Minerals," in *Present Knowledge in Nutrition*, 3rd ed., Nutrition Foundation, New York, 1967, Chap. 28.
[4] Li Ting-Kai and Bert L. Vallee, "The Biochemical and Nutritional Role of Trace Elements," in Robert S. Goodhart and Maurice E. Shils (eds.), *Modern Nutrition in Health and Disease*, Lea & Febiger, Philadelphia, 1973, Chap. 8.

ances for calcium, phosphorus, iodine, iron, zinc, and magnesium.

Underload and Overload

Undernutrition may be considered as to scope, cause, and degree, according to Mc-Laren.[5] General undernutrition refers to total reduction of food intake and partial undernutrition occurs from a deficiency of one or several nutrients. The *primary* cause of undernutrition is a dietary lack; *secondary* cause refers to conditions of the body, such as disease, that interfere with utilization of the nutrient or nutrients. Degree is determined by clinical or biochemical means. Sometimes terms such as mild, moderate, or severe are used. Mineral deficiencies may be considered under several categories. Phosphorus, copper, cobalt, and chromium underloads seldom occur because there is an abundant supply of these nutrients in food. A lack of iron, iodine, selenium, or manganese in the diet do cause specific symptoms. Fluorine is related to the amount available in drinking water. Underload may be associated with certain conditions. With calcium, there may be a relationship to rickets; with magnesium, to loss in body fluids, such as gastrointestinal fluids; potassium deficiency is often associated with abnormal loss in the body such as from vomiting and diarrhea; and zinc underload may be facilitated by the incidence of alcoholic cirrhosis.

Overnutrition or mineral overload,[6] in addition to excessive amounts in the diet, may result from other sources of intake, such as alcoholic beverages, cooking utensils, water, drugs, and from pollution and contamination, such as mercury from industrial wastes in seafood.

Seldom does an individual suffer from a mineral overload from dietary sources. Certain physiological and pathological conditions may lead to hyperabsorption, a gross metabolic error in which there is a large deposition in the tissue; or accidental excessive intake, such as of iron or sodium may occur. Environmental influences may be a cause, such as excess fluorine leading to mottling of teeth.

Mertz[7] urges caution in the consideration of overload and underload in minerals. Only when mineral deficiencies are well defined can underloads be identified. A recognition of symptoms for overload of minerals is equally urgent. The *Recommended Dietary Allowances* indicates a "safe" intake. Dietary intakes of a mineral in appreciably lower quantities than recommended may lead to deficiency symptoms; excessive intake may adversely influence the availability of other minerals and result in imbalances.

Criteria for Food Sources

Mertz[8] contends that nutrients, including minerals, must be obtained from a wide variety of foods. Grossly imbalanced diets can result from food fads or ignorance about the constituents of an adequate diet. One problem in planning the daily diet is the lack of knowledge of the biologic availability of a mineral in specific foods. In some instances more extensive data are available for feeding animals than for feeding man.

Losses in preparation and cooking of food may decrease the mineral contribution to the diet. Soaking foods and cooking in large quantities of water, for example, when minerals are soluble, may reduce mineral content. The refinement of cereals may deprive an individual of a number of minerals. Schroeder[9] indicates that from 60.0 to 87.7 per cent of five bulk minerals, calcium, phosphorus, magnesium, potassium, and sodium, are removed in the milling process and from 40.0 to 88.5

[5] D. S. McLaren, "Undernutrition," in Miloslav Rechcigl, Jr. (ed.), *Food, Nutrition and Health,* Vol. 16, S. Karger, Basel, 1973, pp. 142–177.

[6] Charlotte M. Young, "Overnutrition," in Miloslav Rechcigl, Jr. (ed.) *Food, Nutrition and Health,* Vol. 16, S. Karger, Basel, 1973, pp. 180–198.

[7] Walter Mertz, "Recommended Dietary Allowances Up to Date—Trace Minerals," *Journal of American Dietetic Association,* Vol. 64, No. 2 (February 1974), pp. 163–167.

[8] Ibid., p. 166.

[9] Henry A. Schroeder, "Losses of Vitamins and Trace Minerals Resulting from Processing and Preservation of Foods," *American Journal of Clinical Nutrition,* Vol. 24, No. 5 (May 1971), pp. 562, 573.

per cent of seven essential trace minerals, chromium, manganese, iron, cobalt, copper, zinc, and molybdenum. Obviously, the use of whole-grain products is recommended. When a food is divided into component parts by extraction or refinement, the majority of trace elements goes with one part or the other. Marked losses of all trace minerals except copper occur when rice is polished. Corn oil, compared with corn, retained much chromium, little magnesium, and most of the original copper. Schroeder[10] concludes that raw foods are good sources of trace minerals, but that

persons subsisting on refined, processed, or canned foods may be receiving marginal intakes of these micronutrients, particularly chromium, manganese, and zinc.

In addition, Robinson[11] suggests that one must be aware of the nutrient density of minerals in foods that are selected and to note the amount of food that is actually consumed. Nutritional labeling showing the calcium and iron content of a product are useful to the consumer in buying and planning food for nutritious meals.

[10] Ibid.

[11] Corinne H. Robinson, *Fundamentals of Normal Nutrition*, Macmillan, New York, 1973, p. 104.

SELECTED REFERENCES

Davidson, Stanley, R. Passmore, and J. F. Brock, *Human Nutrition and Dietetics*, The Williams & Wilkins Company, Baltimore, 1972, Chapters 8, 9, and 10.

Goodhart, Robert S., and Maurice E. Shils (eds.), *Modern Nutrition in Health and Disease*, Lea & Febiger, Philadelphia, 1973, Chapters 6, 7, and 8.

Mertz, Walter, "Recommended Dietary Allowances Up to Date—Trace Minerals." *Journal of the American Dietetic Association*, Vol. 64, No 2 (February 1974), pp. 163–167.

News Digest, "Increase in Iron Enrichment," *Journal of the American Dietetic Association*, Vol. 63, No. 6 (December 1973), p. 669.

Rechcigl, Miloslav, Jr. (ed.), *Food, Nutrition and Health*, Vol. 16, S. Karger, Basel, 1973, pp. 142–202.

Robinson, Corinne H., *Fundamentals of Normal Nutrition*, Macmillan Publishing Co., Inc., New York, 1973, Chapters 8 and 9.

Schroeder, Henry A., "Losses of Vitamins and Trace Minerals Resulting from Processing and Preservation of Foods," *American Journal of Clinical Nutrition*, Vol. 24, No. 5 (May 1971), pp. 562–573.

16

Major Minerals

The minerals required in major, or macro, amounts are calcium, phosphorus, magnesium, potassium, sulfur, sodium, and chlorine. The development of sensitive and rapid methods of assaying minerals has increased the knowledge of their role in body functioning.

Calcium

The name *calcium* is derived from the Latin word *calx*, which means "chalk." Osborne and Mendel, near the close of World War I, were studying minerals by using young rats in their experimental laboratories. They discovered that young healthy rats seemed to be able to adapt to shortages of potassium, magnesium, chlorine, and sodium, but that they could not adapt to a shortage of phosphorus and calcium. There seemed to be a need for these minerals for normal growth. Sherman[1] substantiated these experiments and was noted for his studies on calcium, not only in experimental animals but also in children.

[1]H. C. Sherman and E. Hawley, "Calcium and Phosphorus Metabolism in Childhood," *Journal of Biological Chemistry*, Vol. 53, No. 3 (March 1922), pp. 375–399.

Importance of Calcium in Body Structure

There is more calcium in the body than any other mineral element. It is found largely in the bones and teeth. Without it, bones would be like rubber, and the ability to walk and to stand erect, and the protection given to vital organs such as the brain and liver, would be impossible. A simple experiment will demonstrate the importance of calcium. If a chicken drumstick bone is immersed in a bottle of vinegar or other acid and allowed to remain for a week or longer, all the calcium will have dissolved and the bone can be tied in a knot.

Although 99 per cent of calcium is found in the bones and teeth, the remaining 1 per cent plays a very significant role as a body regulator and as a constituent in body fluids and tissues.

Physical and Chemical Properties of Calcium

From the appearance of bones and teeth, it is obvious that calcium is a white substance. In its pure state it is powdery and chalk-like. It is stable to heat and light, but will dissolve in an acid medium.

Functions of Calcium

Calcium, in conjunction with phosphorus, is an important constituent in bone formation during growth and for maintenance. The mechanism involved in calcification is not fully understood. Normal bone function, of course, is not the sole responsibility of calcium and phosphorus metabolism. It is assumed that all the nutrients involved in growth affect bone formation, including vitamin A, magnesium, manganese, choline, and vitamin C, plus the important roles played by protein and vitamin D.

In the fetus, a matrix for bone formation is developed from the protein collagen. After birth, this matrix becomes more rigid as growth proceeds and the collagen is replaced by the deposition of calcium phosphate and calcium carbonate crystals. The ends of the bones have a porous structure known as *trabeculae*. The calcium in the trabeculae can be easily mobilized and sent to the part or parts of the body needing it. The calcium in the hard tissues, such as the bones and the teeth, is more metabolically stable, according to Hegsted.[2]

The calcium content of the blood is kept at a constant level. This mineral plays a very important role in the clotting of blood. It is also an important constituent of fluids that function in the rhythmic beating of the heart, in the response of nerve tissue to stimuli, in contraction of muscles, and in the control of the passage of fluids through cell walls. Calcium also plays an important role in the action of certain enzymes in metabolic processes and in the integrity of intercellular cement substances and various membranes.

Another important function of calcium is that it tends to be a kind of coordinator among inorganic elements. If excessive amounts of potassium, magnesium, or sodium are present in the body, calcium is capable of assuming a corrective role. If the amount of calcium is adequate in the diet, iron is utilized

to better advantage. This is another instance of "sparing action."

Calcium Deficiency

Although rickets in children is generally attributed to a lack of vitamin D, insufficient intakes of calcium and phosphorus, as well as an imbalance of these two minerals, may result in the disease. Osteomalacia, the adult rickets, may also be due to a calcium deficiency, but usually the situation is complicated by deficiency of phosphorus and vitamin D as well as other factors.

An increased incidence of osteoporosis (bone thinning) has attracted attention. It is more common among older people, among females, and among whites, according to Moldawer and others,[3] than among younger people, males, and nonwhites. Calcium, with other nutrients and various hormonal and environmental factors, is involved. A number of researchers, such as Rose[4] and Newton-John and Morgan,[5] agree that a relatively constant rate of bone loss occurs after the ages of 20 to 30 years. These same researchers also suggest that increasing the bone mass during the first 20 years of life is one way to reduce the possibility of osteoporosis in later life—an implication for emphasizing bone-growth nutrients in nutrition education.

Osteoporosis is characterized by other researchers as the most common systemic bone disease, with many unsolved problems in regard to its treatment.[6] Lutwak[7] suggests that

[2] D. M. Hegsted, "Present Knowledge of Calcium, Phosphorus, and Magnesium," in *Present Knowledge in Nutrition*, 3rd ed., Nutrition Foundation, New York, 1967, Chap. 33.

[3] M. Moldawer, S. J. Zimmerman, and L. C. Collins, "Incidence of Osteoporosis in Elderly Whites and Elderly Negroes," *Journal of the American Medical Association*, Vol. 194, No. 8 (November 1965), pp. 859–862.

[4] Alan G. Rose, "A Critique of Modern Methods of Diagnosis and Treatment of Osteoporosis," *Clinical Orthopology*, Vol. 55, Section 1 (January 1967), pp. 17–41.

[5] H. F. Newton-John and D. B. Morgan, "Osteoporosis: Disease or Senescence," *Lancet*, Vol. 7561, No. 1 (February 1968), pp. 232–233.

[6] "Nutritional Implications of Osteoporosis," *Dairy Council Digest*, Vol. 41, No. 5 (September–October 1970), pp. 26–28.

[7] Leo Lutwak, "Dietary Calcium and the Reversal of Bone Demineralization," *Nutrition News*, Vol. 37, No. 1 (February 1974), pp. 1, 4.

the sharp increase of phosphorus dietary intake has created a striking imbalance between calcium and phosphorus with a ratio of 1 to 4. This imbalance leads to decreased ability to absorb calcium as age increases. This, in turn, may lead to serious problems of skeletal health because bones have demineralized (as indicated by lower bone density), beginning with the jawbone, then the vertebrae, and finally other bones of the body.

Periodontal disease, which generally occurs before skeletal changes, affects any of the tissues surrounding a tooth but usually begins with a decrease in density in the alveolar bone. With continuous loss of calcium from this supporting bone, the teeth loosen, mastication may cause irritation, and gums become inflamed and infected with plaque. A dietary regime of adequate dietary calcium over the years should be a deterrent to this condition.

If the calcium content of fluids and blood becomes low, it may interfere with the response of nerves to stimuli. A marked decrease may actually result in tetany.

Absorption and Metabolism of Calcium

The calcium found in the diet is absorbed in the small intestine. A number of factors influence the amount absorbed. The body utilizes calcium, like other nutrients, very effectively when it is needed. In fact, the greater the need and the smaller the amount of calcium in the diet, the more efficiently is it absorbed. Absorption thus does not increase proportionately with liberal intakes or an increased level of calcium. Among the factors influencing absorption are the amount of vitamin D available and the degree of acidity of the digestive fluids. Since calcium is soluble in an acid medium, the hydrochloric acid of the gastric juice is very important in calcium absorption because it helps to dissolve the calcium so that it can be more easily absorbed from the small intestine directly into the bloodstream.

A low intestinal pH helps to keep the calcium in solution. If the medium in the small intestine is more alkaline than usual, absorption is impeded.

The particular food source of calcium also has an effect. The calcium in some foods is absorbed much more easily than the calcium in others. The lactose in milk, for example, facilitates its absorption. Adequate amounts of vitamin A and iron in the diet also foster calcium absorption, as do proteins and amino acids.

The presence of oxalic acid, which is found in certain foods, such as spinach and rhubarb, has an undesirable effect on calcium absorption and utilization. This acid combines with calcium to form a compound known as calcium oxalate, which passes through the intestine without being absorbed. The amount of oxalate formed will depend on the amount of oxalic acid in the food. (There is such a small amount of oxalic acid in chocolate that a concern over drinking cocoa is not justified; from a chemical standpoint these small amounts of oxalic acid combine with equally small amounts of calcium.) Phytic acid, found in the brown coats of certain cereal grains, also interferes in the same manner as oxalic acid. Large intakes of bran may also have an adverse effect. However, generous amounts of calcium in the diet will overcome these situations. Unwise use of laxatives is another factor that can interfere with absorption. And either an excess of fat in the diet or poor digestion of fats may also interfere because the calcium combines with the fat to form an insoluble soap that cannot be absorbed. A small amount of fat, on the other hand, appears to improve calcium assimilation. If for any reason the food mass is retained in the intestinal tract longer than usual, absorption is consequently delayed.

The age of an individual also has an influence on the utilization of calcium. Young children retain a higher percentage of calcium than do adults. The need for calcium due to very rapid growth is a possible explanation for this fact. Although a small amount of calcium is efficiently utilized when the need is severe, an individual who is undernourished, according to Stearns,[8] cannot absorb calcium as effectively as if he were well nourished.

[8] Genevieve Stearns, "Human Requirements of Calcium, Phosphorus and Magnesium," *Handbook of Nutrition*, Blakiston, Philadelphia, 1951, Chap. 4.

An adequate diet has been demonstrated to facilitate calcium utilization. After the calcium has been absorbed in the bloodstream, the blood takes it to whatever part of the body needs it. During growth, for example, calcium is drawn from the blood by either the bones or teeth. Vitamin D and ascorbic acid influence the incorporation of the calcium into the bones or teeth. The parathyroid gland, through its hormone, maintains the interchange of calcium between blood and bone so that a fairly constant level is maintained in the blood serum at all times. The hormone, calcitonin,[9] derived from "C" cells of the thyroid gland, has a positive control on the accumulation of calcium in the blood by inhibiting bone resorption. Once calcium is incorporated into teeth, it becomes static and is not withdrawn for other purposes. By contrast, the calcium stored in the bones is in a dynamic state. The ends of the long bones are particularly adapted for the storage of calcium. When needed, it can be transferred from the bones to other parts of the body.

The amount of calcium excreted in the urine varies somewhat among individuals. It may be influenced by the amount of water that is drunk during the day or by the level of intake of calcium. If the level is high, the kidneys may remove excess calcium. Any calcium found in the urine has been previously absorbed into the bloodstream. Research[10] indicates that the urinary excretion of calcium is related directly to protein intake; the higher the protein intake, the higher calcium urinary excretion will be.

Calcium is also excreted through the feces. Some of the calcium there has never been absorbed. Some of the absorbed calcium is returned to the feces by way of the digestive juices. The fecal calcium is also determined to a certain extent by the amount of calcium in the diet. If there is an excessive amount of calcium, more than is needed, it is generally excreted in the feces. Some calcium is also lost through perspiration.

Nutritive Needs for Calcium

The ratio of calcium need to body size is higher in infancy than at any other period of life. About 60 g are deposited during the first year. By the time a child reaches 4 or 5 years of age, the deposit rate will have dropped to as low as 20 g a year. By the time a child reaches 13 to 14 years of age, the deposit is greatly increased and it may amount to as much as 90 g a year, assuming that he weighs approximately 110 pounds. The greater the weight, the greater the deposit of calcium. These estimates of deposits are based on an adequate supply of calcium in the diet.

The recommended allowances for calcium for both sexes and all ages, plus pregnancy and lactation, are given in Table 16–1.

There are many factors that bear consideration in the determination of the recommended dietary allowance for a nutrient.[11] Approximately 320 mg of calcium are lost daily through excretion in the urine, feces, sweat, and by other means. Only 40 per cent of the dietary calcium is estimated to be absorbed. The FAO/WHO Committee on Calcium Requirements in 1962 recommended 400 to 500 mg per day as a "practical allowance" for an adult, based on the fact that countries whose inhabitants had intakes of this amount did not suffer from calcium deficiencies. The benefits of higher intakes of calcium have not been proved. Groups who appear to thrive on low calcium intakes live in tropical and semitropical countries where unrecognized sources of calcium may be available and there is abundant sunshine. The human body has the capacity with time to adapt to various calcium intakes. Calcium losses can be substantial when protein intakes are high over prolonged periods and this information bears attention.

By weighing all factors carefully, the al-

[9] Howard Rasmussen and Maurice M. Pechet, "Calcitonin," *Scientific American*, Vol. 223, No. 4 (October 1970), pp. 42–50.

[10] Sheldon Margen, J. Y. Chu, N. A. Kaufmann, and Doris H. Calloway, "Studies in Calcium Metabolism. 1. The Calciuretic Effect of Dietary Protein," *American Journal of Clinical Nutrition*, Vol. 27, No. 6 (June 1974), pp. 584–589.

[11] Food and Nutrition Board, *Recommended Dietary Allowances*, 8th ed., National Academy of Sciences—National Research Council, 1974, pp. 82–87

TABLE 16–1

Recommended Daily Dietary Allowances for Calcium, Revised 1974

Designed for the maintenance of good nutrition for practically all healthy people in the United States

	AGE (years)	WEIGHT (kg)	WEIGHT (lb)	HEIGHT (cm)	HEIGHT (in.)	CAL-CIUM (mg)
Infants	0.0–0.5	6	14	60	24	360
	0.5–1.0	9	20	71	28	540
Children	1–3	13	28	86	34	800
	4–6	20	44	110	44	800
	7–10	30	66	135	54	800
Males	11–14	44	97	158	63	1200
	15–18	61	134	172	69	1200
	19–22	67	147	172	69	800
	23–50	70	154	172	69	800
	51+	70	154	172	69	800
Females	11–14	44	97	155	62	1200
	15–18	54	119	162	65	1200
	19–22	58	128	162	65	800
	23–50	58	128	162	65	800
	51+	58	128	162	65	800
Pregnant						1200
Lactating						1200

SOURCE: Food and Nutrition Board, *Recommended Dietary Allowances*, 8th ed., National Academy of Sciences—National Research Council, Washington, D.C., 1974.

lowance of 800 mg per day for adult men and women seems a sensible interpretation for food consumption of all groups. Additional dietary calcium should be consumed during pregnancy and lactation to meet the needs of the mother, the growing fetus, and for producing human milk for the infant. Accordingly, the recommended dietary allowance for both pregnant and lactating women is 1200 mg per day. Some women with a high production of milk may require even higher allowances.

The recommended allowance for infants for the first 5 months of life is 360 mg per day; for the remaining months until 1 year of age, the recommendation is 540 mg per day. These allowances are for infants who are fed formulas. Breast-fed babies have calcium requirements fully met. For children from 1 to 10 years of age, the calcium allowances have been established at 800 mg per day. Healthy chil-

dren actually retain calcium above the minimum amount calculated for their age if their diet contains ample amounts of the mineral element. Based on unit of weight, growing children may need two to four times as much calcium as an adult. During the period of rapid growth typical of preadolescence and puberty (10 to 18 years of age), the intake is increased and the recommended dietary allowance for this age group is 1.2 g or 1200 mg per day, a level that will maximize calcium retention.

Since calcium is so often associated with growth, many adults feel that they do not need it. This is not true, because calcium is very important for the daily functioning of the body and for the replacement of calcium in the bones. It is also important that adults take the recommended daily dietary allowances of calcium each day, for individuals vary widely in their ability to use this mineral. Also, a number of factors influence the utilization and absorption of calcium. The recommended daily dietary allowance safeguards against such possibilities.

Sources of Calcium

Calcium is very unevenly distributed among foods. Milk and milk products are the richest source. If milk is not incorporated into the daily diet, it is almost impossible to provide an adequate amount of calcium. Two or three cups of milk are recommended for children under 9 years of age. Three or more cups (or 8-oz glasses) seem adequate for children from 9 to 12 years. During adolescence the need for milk may be increased to 4 or more cups. Adults are advised to have 2 or more cups in their diet daily. For pregnant women, 3 or more cups each day are recommended, and for nursing mothers it may be necessary to increase the amount of milk to 4 or more cups for adequate calcium.

Although not equal to milk in calcium content, green leafy vegetables contain a demonstrable amount of calcium. Mustard greens, kale, and broccoli are particularly rich. Unfortunately, these vegetables are not as frequently eaten in America as might be desirable.

The contribution of some common foods

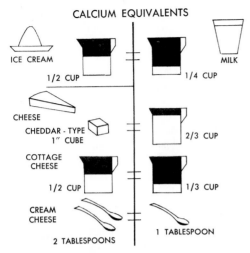

CALCIUM EQUIVALENTS

ICE CREAM
1/2 CUP

MILK
1/4 CUP

CHEESE
CHEDDAR - TYPE
1″ CUBE

2/3 CUP

COTTAGE
CHEESE
1/2 CUP

1/3 CUP

CREAM
CHEESE
2 TABLESPOONS

1 TABLESPOON

FIGURE 16–1. *Calcium equivalents of some dairy products in comparison with whole milk.* (Food 1959 Yearbook of Agriculture, USDA)

TABLE 16–2

Calcium Content of Some Common Foods

FOODS	SIZE OF SERVING	CALCIUM (mg)
Milk, whole	1 cup	288
Salmon, pink, canned	3 oz	167
Collards	½ cup	144
Turnip greens	½ cup	133
Cheese, American	1-in. cube	128
Pizza pie	⅛ of 14-in. pie	107
Broccoli	1 cup	132
Almonds, shelled	¼ cup	83
Oysters, medium	⅓ cup	75
Kale	½ cup	73
Orange	1 large	49
Figs, raw	3	40
Molasses, light	1 tbs	33
Roll, pan	1	28
Egg	1	27
Potato, French fries	10 pieces	9
Apple	1 medium	8

SOURCE: *Nutritive Value of Foods*, Home and Garden Bulletin No. 72, U.S. Department of Agriculture, Washington, D.C., 1971.

to the calcium allowance is shown in Table 16–2.

Many individuals are under the impression that they can get sufficient calcium in other food and do not have to drink milk. Even with calcium-rich foods, in order to get the calcium equivalent of 1 quart of milk, it would be necessary to eat these amounts of the following: 2 quarts of ice cream, 3½ pounds of cottage cheese, or 7 oz. of American cheese. In comparison with nondairy foods, 1 quart or four glasses of milk has the same amount of calcium as 6¾ pounds of cabbage, 27 pounds of potatoes, 28 oranges, 39 eggs, 7¼ pounds of carrots, or 4 pounds of escarole.

A low dietary intake of calcium is always associated with a low milk intake, since this is the best source of this mineral. The calcium in milk is available no matter what form the milk is in. In other words, the calcium of whole, skim, raw, pasteurized, homogenized, or chocolate-flavored milk, or in dry solids like cheese, is readily available to the body. Calcium in vegetables is not always as easily available.

Effect of Food Preparation on Calcium

Since calcium is quite stable, there is not the concern for its loss that there may be for other nutrients. If members of a family do not like to drink milk, it may be necessary to incorporate milk into other foods, such as creamed soups, sauces, or desserts. In recipes calling for boiled milk, the scum should not be removed because it is calcium caseinate. If removed, the calcium content of the food would be reduced. Often homemakers will remove bones from canned salmon or sardines. Actually these bones have been cooked so that they are very soft and can be eaten easily; they contribute considerable calcium to the daily diet.

If meat that contains bones is cooked in an acid medium, such as spare ribs prepared in the sweet-sour fashion, some of the calcium in the bones will dissolve in the sauce or gravy. This calcium will be lost, of course, unless the sauce is eaten. The use of lime in the preparation of corn for hominy or tortillas or in the making of soybean curd may add some calcium to the diet of those people who follow these particular practices.

Calcium Consumption

The contributions of major food groups to calcium consumption by civilians according to preliminary 1974 data are as follows: meat (including pork fat cuts), poultry, and fish, 3.5 per cent; eggs, 2.3 per cent; dairy products, excluding butter, 75.7 per cent; fats and oils, including butter, 0.4 per cent; citrus fruits, 0.9 per cent; other fruits, 1.2 per cent; potatoes and sweet potatoes, 0.9 per cent; dark-green and deep-yellow vegetables, 1.6 per cent; other vegetables, including tomatoes, 4.9 per cent; dry beans and peas, nuts, and soya flour, 2.8 per cent; flour and cereal products, 3.3 per cent; sugars and sweeteners, 1.5 per cent; and miscellaneous, 1.0 per cent.[12]

Phosphorus

Several men who were interested in alchemy had a hand in the discovery of phosphorus. A merchant in Hamburg by the name of Hennig Brand evaporated urine and distilled it. As heat was applied to the inorganic substance, Brand noticed a white, translucent, waxy substance with a very disagreeable smell. Furthermore, he was amazed that it gave off a bright light in his dark laboratory. For this reason it became known as *phosphorus*, which is the Latin for "morning star." Brand told a man from Dresden about his experiments, who, in turn, while traveling in England with his newly discovered substance found that Boyle had also prepared the element and filed a report on it.

Functions of Phosphorus

Phosphorus is generally found with calcium in the body, and it is important that a definite ratio be maintained between them. Both contribute to the supportive structures of the body. In addition, phosphorus does have a number of important functions of its own. It is important in certain metabolic processes, such as chemical reactions with proteins, fats, and carbohydrates, in order that the body may have energy. Phosphorus is present in cells and in the blood as soluble phosphate ion, as well as in lipids, proteins, carbohydrates, and energy transfer enzymes.[13] Many of the B vitamins are effective only when combined with the phosphate in the body. Phosphorus is an essential component in nucleic acids and the nucleoproteins responsible for cell division, reproduction, and the transmission of hereditary traits.[14] Phosphorus is also concerned with brain and nerve metabolism in normal blood chemistry. With calcium, phosphorus is necessary for normal response of nerves to stimulation and for the contraction of muscles. It also assists calcium in the maintenance of blood neutrality. Perhaps its most important function is in combination with calcium in giving rigidity to the bones and teeth of the body. Phosphorus is also an important constituent in enzymes and coenzymes, which are essential for tissue respiration. The importance of phosphorus in the body cannot be overestimated.

Nutritive Needs for Phosphorus

The Food and Nutrition Board has established recommended dietary allowances for phosphorus, as shown in Table 16-3.

Although the ratio of calcium to phosphorus is 2 to 1 in the bones, phosphorus is in a higher ratio in the soft tissues, so the dietary ratio is increased and the phosphorus requirement is equal to or exceeds the allowance for calcium for all age levels except for the young infant. In establishing the allowance for phosphorus for infant formulas, consideration must be given to the calcium-to-phosphorus ratio in cow's milk, 1.2 to 1, and in human milk, 2 to 1. The phosphorus content of cow's milk may contribute to the occurrence of hypocalcemic tetany during the first week of life. With this evidence, the calcium-to-phosphorus ratio in early infancy should be 1.5 to 1 or 240 mg per day, and for the 5- to 12-month period the recommended allowance is 400 mg per day. There is no evidence of a phos-

[12] *National Food Situation*, Economic Research Service, U.S. Department of Agriculture, Washington, D.C., November 1974, p. 28.

[13] *Recommended Dietary Allowances*, op. cit., p. 87.

[14] D. M. Hegsted, "Calcium and Phosphorus," in Robert S. Goodhart and Maurice E Shils (eds.), *Modern Nutrition in Health and Disease*, Lea & Febiger, Philadelphia, 1973, Chap. 6, Sec. A.

TABLE 16–3

Recommended Daily Dietary Allowances for Phosphorus, Revised 1974

Designed for the maintenance of good nutrition for practically all healthy people in the United States

	AGE (years)	WEIGHT (kg)	(lb)	HEIGHT (cm)	(in.)	PHOS-PHORUS (mg)
Infants	0.0–0.5	6	14	60	24	240
	0.5–1.0	9	20	71	28	400
Children	1–3	13	28	86	34	800
	4–6	20	44	110	44	800
	7–10	30	66	135	54	800
Males	11–14	44	97	158	63	1200
	15–18	61	134	172	69	1200
	19–22	67	147	172	69	800
	23–50	70	154	172	69	800
	51+	70	154	172	69	800
Females	11–14	44	97	155	62	1200
	15–18	54	119	162	65	1200
	19–22	58	128	162	65	800
	23–50	58	128	162	65	800
	51+	58	128	162	65	800
Pregnant						1200
Lactating						1200

SOURCE: Food and Nutrition Board, *Recommended Dietary Allowances*, 8th ed., National Academy of Sciences—National Research Council, Washington, D.C., 1974.

phorus deficiency in man to the extent that vital processes fail to function. Few studies have been done on animals to determine the biochemical effects of low phosphorus intake.

Sources of Phosphorus in Foods

In contrast to calcium, phosphorus is widely distributed in foods. Cereals and meats of all kinds are particularly rich sources. Whole-grain cereals provide more phosphorus than refined cereals. Legumes, nuts, meats, eggs, milk, and dairy products are all good sources, whereas vegetables and fruit on the whole are not. Protein-rich foods are especially high in phosphorus content. Table 16–4 lists the phosphorus content of some common foods.

Phosphorus Consumption

According to preliminary 1974 data, meat (including pork fat cuts), poultry, and fish contributed 26.2 per cent of the total phos-

TABLE 16–4

Phosphorus Content of Some Common Foods

FOOD	PHOSPHORUS (mg/100 g)
Cheese, cheddar	771
Almonds, roasted	504
Peanut butter	407
Salmon, pink	286
Liverwurst, smoked	245
Hamburger, cooked	230
Egg	207
Lima beans, cooked	121
Milk, whole, fluid	93
Bread, white, enriched	87
Rice, cooked	28
Banana	26

SOURCE: Bernice K. Watt and Annabel L. Merrill, *Composition of Foods, Raw, Processed, Prepared*, Agriculture Handbook No. 8, U.S. Department of Agriculture, Washington, D.C., 1971.

phorus from foods available for civilian consumption; eggs, 5.4 per cent; dairy products, excluding butter, 36.1 per cent; fats and oils, including butter, 0.2 per cent; citrus fruits, 0.7 per cent; other fruits, 1.1 per cent; potatoes and sweet potatoes, 3.9 per cent; dark-green and deep-yellow vegetables, 0.7 per cent; other vegetables, including tomatoes, 5.0 per cent; dry beans and peas, nuts, and soya flour, 6.2 per cent; flour and cereal products, 12.5 per cent; sugars and sweeteners, 0.3 per cent; and miscellaneous, 1.8 per cent.[15]

Magnesium

Although evidence of magnesium in the human body was demonstrated in the early 1930's, the importance of this major mineral has only recently been emphasized. Cumbersome and inadequate analytical determination was one cause of the lag.

Functions of Magnesium

One primary function of magnesium is to serve as an activator of many enzyme systems, including the system utilizing ATP (adenosine

[15] *National Food Situation*, op. cit., p. 28.

triphosphate), a compound that provides energy in the cells for muscle contraction, nerve impulses, and synthesis of vital cell constituents. Magnesium is also required for the activation of alkaline phosphatase, an enzyme important in calcium and phosphorus metabolism. Evidence is available that this mineral is essential for the functional and structural integrity of the heart muscle.[16]

Magnesium is the predominant cation in living cells. Maintenance of electrical potential in nerves and in muscle membranes are other functions.[17] Magnesium appears to share several control mechanisms with calcium, as is indicated by the influence of calcium on renal resorption of magnesium, which tends to vary inversely with that of calcium. Also, magnesium excretion in feces decreases as calcium is reduced. Magnesium is found in the bones, in body cells, and in extracellular fluid.

Magnesium Deficiencies

Magnesium deficiency may occur in the course of disease or stress. When intake is decreased, this mineral is lost from the body in larger amounts than usual. If a shift occurs in electrolyte balance, a magnesium deficiency may develop. Bone magnesium is not interchangeable, and is largely unavailable to replace magnesium deficits. Diseases or conditions that may precipitate a deficiency are renal therapy, protein-calorie malnutrition in infants, especially newborn, and children, postsurgical stress, diabetes, hyperthyroidism, acute alcoholism, burns, severe infections, gastrointestinal disorders, and diseases of the parathyroid. To pinpoint magnesium deficiencies is difficult because of association with disease or impaired body functioning, such as metabolic abnormalities, multiple dietary deficiencies, and the use of medications.[18] Symptoms of a magnesium deficiency are neuromuscular dysfunction as evidenced by pronounced personality changes, muscle spasms, convulsions (especially in infants), hyperexcitability, tremor, anorexia, nausea, apathy, and decreased tendon reflexes.

Magnesium Nutritive Needs

The Food and Nutrition Board of the National Research Council has established recommended dietary allowances of magnesium, as shown in Table 16–5.

Estimates for magnesium for adult men range from 200 to 700 mg per day. Based on these studies the recommended allowance for adult males is 350 mg per day and for adult females, 300 mg per day. The male adolescent requires an allowance of 400 mg per day for special growth and puberty needs. Allowances for pregnancy and lactation are 450 mg per

---

TABLE 16–5

Recommended Daily Dietary Allowances for Magnesium, Revised 1974

Designed for the maintenance of good nutrition for practically all healthy people in the United States

	AGE (years)	WEIGHT (kg)	WEIGHT (lb)	HEIGHT (cm)	HEIGHT (in.)	MAG-NESIUM (mg)
Children	0.0–0.5	6	14	60	24	60
	0.5–1.0	9	20	71	28	70
	1–3	13	28	86	34	150
	4–6	20	44	110	44	200
	7–10	30	66	135	54	250
Males	11–14	44	97	158	63	350
	15–18	61	134	172	69	400
	19–22	67	147	172	69	350
	23–50	70	154	172	69	350
	51+	70	154	172	69	350
Females	11–14	44	97	155	62	300
	15–18	54	119	162	65	300
	19–22	58	128	162	65	300
	23–50	58	128	162	65	300
	51+	58	128	162	65	300
Pregnant						450
Lactating						450

SOURCE: Food and Nutrition Board, *Recommended Dietary Allowances*, 8th ed., National Academy of Sciences—National Research Council, Washington, D.C., 1974.

---

[16] Mildren S. Seelig and H. Alexander Heggtveit, "Magnesium Interrelationships in Ischemic Heart Disease: A Review," *American Journal of Clinical Nutrition*, Vol. 27, No. 1 (January 1972), pp. 59–79.

[17] Maurice E. Shils, "Magnesium," in Robert S. Goodhart and Maurice E. Shils (eds.), *Modern Nutrition in Health and Disease*, Lea & Febiger, Philadelphia, 1973, Chap. 6. Sec. B.

[18] Shils, op. cit., pp. 288–292.

day. For the first 5 months of life, the infant requires 60 mg per day based on the content of magnesium in human milk, which in turn is adequate for the infant formula. Children from 1 to 10 years of age have an ascending allowance with age from 150 to 250 mg per day. The male from 11 to 14 years of age requires 350 mg per day. The preadolescent and the adolescent female have an allowance of 300 mg per day. Although allowances for children and adolescents are only estimates, consideration was given to increased needs for rapid bone growth during these periods.[19]

Sources of Magnesium

Good sources of magnesium in foods include whole-grain cereals, nuts, beans, and green leafy vegetables. Bran has a high content of this mineral, indicating that milling and processing reduce the content of magnesium. Dairy products, because of the amount consumed, make an important contribution. Powdered instant coffee, tea, and cocoa are rich sources in the dry state but of course are diluted when consumed, but still contribute an appreciable amount. Certain condiments such as curry powder and dried mustard are well endowed with this mineral, but amounts consumed by the population are limited. Bitter baking chocolate is a good source.

The magnesium content of many convenience, formulated, and processed foods is unknown, but because of the large amount of these types of foods that are consumed this information is very important and dietary intakes cannot be accurately determined until it is forthcoming. This situation, along with the decrease in cereal consumption and other changes in food habits, requires serious attention to the magnesium content of American diets. Table 16–6 lists some of the important sources of this major mineral.

Magnesium Consumption

According to preliminary 1974 data, meat (including pork fat cuts), poultry, and fish contributed 13.7 per cent of the total magnesium from foods available for civilian consumption; eggs, 1.3 per cent; dairy products, excluding butter, 21.6 per cent; fats and oils, including butter, 0.4 per cent; citrus fruits, 2.2 per cent; other fruits, 3.9 per cent; potatoes and sweet potatoes, 7. per cent; dark-green and deep-yellow vegetables, 2.1 per cent; other vegetables, including tomatoes, 10.4 per cent; dry beans and peas, nuts, soya flour, 11.7 per cent; flour and cereal products, 17.9 per cent; sugars and other sweeteners, 0.2 per cent; miscellaneous, 7.6 per cent.[20]

TABLE 16–6

Magnesium Content of Some Common Foods

FOOD (Edible Portion)	MAGNESIUM (mg/100 g)
Coffee, instant, dry powder	456
Wheat bran, added sugar and malt sugar	420
Cocoa, dry powder	420
Tea, instant, dry powder	395
Peanut butter	360
Mustard, dried	296
Chocolate, bitter or baking	292
Curry powder	284
Cashew nuts	267
Cowpeas, mature, dry	230
Spinach, raw	88
Whole wheat bread	78
Crackers, graham	51
Cheese, cheddar	45
Bananas, raw	33
Beans, snap, raw	32
Hamburger, cooked, broiled	21
Milk, cow, whole, fluid	13
Grapefruit juice, raw	12
Apricots, raw	12
Eggs, raw, whole	11

SOURCE: Bernice K. Watt and Annabel L. Merrill, *Composition of Foods, Raw, Processed, Prepared,* Agriculture Handbook No. 8, Consumer and Food Economics Research Division, Agricultural Research Service, U.S. Department of Agriculture, 1963, pp. 147–158.

Potassium

Ringer, in 1885, found that potassium with calcium and sodium in the form of chlorides

---

[19] *Recommended Dietary Allowances,* op. cit., pp. 88–89.

[20] *National Food Situation,* op. cit., p. 28.

could maintain the integrity of isolated animal tissues. The later work of Locke and Loeb established that the salt concentrations found in the blood were so designed for functional purposes.

Functions of Potassium

Potassium is primarily an intracellular cation. In large part, this cation is bound to protein and with sodium influences osmotic pressure and contributes to normal pH equilibrium.[21] It facilitates enzyme reactions related to protein and carbohydrate metabolism. The formation of glycogen, for example, requires potassium. The level of potassium in the body has been found to reflect body composition, so it has been used to determine lean body mass through the use of radioactive potassium.

Potassium is related to other minerals in metabolism. If a potassium deficiency exists, sodium retention may result. If potassium conservation in the renal tubule is to be facilitated, chloride must be present. Magnesium is closely related to this mineral in metabolism, for if there is a magnesium deficiency then potassium is depleted more readily.

Potassium Deficiency

A dietary lack is usually not the cause of a potassium deficiency. In 1941, Orent Keiles and McCollum produced the pathological state that results from a diet in which all nutrients except potassium are provided.[22] Body potassium may be depleted through fasting, starvation, infectious diarrhea, vomiting, or the administration of diuretics. Other complications, such as adrenal cortex malfunction, chronic lung disease that leads to alkalosis, severe protein-calorie malnutrition or diabetic acidosis, may result in potassium depletion, according to Sandstead.

Deficiencies may be manifested in such conditions as vomiting, diarrhea, muscle weakness, apathy, irritability, anorexia, and edema, according to Widdowson and Dickerson.[23]

Potassium Nutritive Needs

Plants and animals tissues are rich sources of potassium; thus a dietary lack is seldom found. The human body contains approximately 2.6 g of potassium per kilogram of fat-free body weight. The usual intake is 50 to 150 milliequivalents per day, according to the Food and Nutrition Board. Healthy adults need about 2.5 g per day of potassium.

Potassium is distributed among many foods. Some of the richest sources among meats are beef, veal, pork (fresh roasted), beef liver, light meat of chicken, and pink, canned salmon. Among fruits, banana, avocado, cantaloupe, watermelon, raisins, dried dates, figs, prunes, apricots, and peaches make the most valuable contributions. Among vegetables and legumes, cooked dry beans, defatted soy flour, peanut butter, potato, winter squash, and sweet potato are especially excellent sources. Milk makes a significant contribution to the potassium content of the diet. Cereal and cereal products make only a fair provision to the diet of potassium.[24]

Sulfur

Sulfur is found in the cytoplasm of every cell. Hair, skin, and nails are noted for sulfur content. Most of the sulfur in the body originates from the amino acids methionine and cystine. Other organic compounds containing sulfur are thiamin, insulin, biotin, taurine, a bile acid component, and heparin, an anticoagulant.

The main functions of sulfur include a role in the clotting of blood, in the development of bone, in muscle metabolism, and possibly as a growth factor. Certain sulfated polysaccharides serve as lubricants for the intestines. Sulfur is important in detoxication reactions by combining with the toxic substances to form a harmless compound.

[21] Harold H. Sandstead, "Present Knowledge of Minerals," in Present Knowledge of Nutrition, Nutrition Foundation, New York, 1967, Chap. 28.

[22] McCollum, op. cit., p. 339.

[23] Elsie Widdowson and J. W. T. Dickerson, "Chemical Composition of the Body," in C. L. Comar and Felix Bronner (eds.), Mineral Metabolism, Vol. 2, Part A, Academic Press, New York, 1964, Chap. 17.

[24] Elizabeth W. Murphy and Ann P. Mangubat, "Potassium in Common Foods," Family Economics Review, Consumer and Food Economics Institute, Agricultural Research Institute, U.S. Department of Agriculture (Highlights/Summer 1973), p. 22.

No human requirements have been established. If the protein requirement, including that for sulfur-bearing amino acids is met, the dietary need is met.

Sodium

The principal cation in extracellular fluid is sodium. Its functions are the maintenance of osmotic equilibrium and body-fluid volume, tissue formation, nerve transmission, and muscle contraction. Sodium is found on the surface of bone crystals, according to Pike and Brown.[25]

The body contains about 1.8 g of sodium per kilogram of fat-free body weight. The possibility of a sodium deficiency in human beings is quite remote. The mineral is widely distributed in foods, with plants containing less than animal sources. Many food processes, such as drying, flavoring, canning, and tenderizing, may add salt.

The Food and Nutrition Board recommends a sodium chloride intake of 6 to 8 g per day.

The body content of sodium is under homeostatic control so excretion is flexible, more with moderate loads and less if there are low levels of sodium. Disorders occur only when this mechanism becomes out of control, when the load is excessive, or when losses are beyond body control.

[25] Ruth L. Pike and Myrtle L. Brown, *Nutrition: An Integrated Approach*, Wiley, New York, 1967, pp. 92–93.

Sodium losses may occur during vomiting, renal disease, adrenal insufficiency, diarrhea, the use of diuretics, or profuse sweating. In cases of water intoxication, weakness, apathy, twitching, and the like may occur. If sodium loss is accompanied with water loss, the volume of blood will be decreased, muscle cramps will occur, and blood pressure may be low.

Sodium consumption may be restricted in the treatment of such conditions as edema or cardiac failure. The use of excessive salt in the diet may have implications for hypertensive diseases in man. No scientific evidence is available to confirm this effect of salt in humans. The large consumption of salty foods by Orientals and their possible effects are challenging tentative hypotheses.

Chloride

Chloride is an important anion generally considered in connection with sodium because these two ions function in the maintenance of pH of extracellular fluid, osmotic equilibrium, and electrolyte balance. In addition, chloride is essential for the formation of hydrochloric acid in the gastric juice and is an activator in a certain stage of carbohydrate metabolism. Chloride is associated with protein and other substances.

In healthy individuals, the chloride dietary intake is not a matter of concern. Chloride may be depleted in the same manner as sodium.

SELECTED REFERENCES

"Cost of Calcium from Different Milk Products," *Journal of the American Dietetic Association*, Vol. 62, No. 5 (May 1973), p. 541.

Dahl, Lewis K., "Salt and Hypertension," *American Journal of Clinical Nutrition*, Vol. 25, No. 2 (February 1972), pp. 231–244.

Davidson, Stanley, R. Passmore, and J. F. Brock, *Human Nutrition and Dietetics*, The Williams & Wilkins Company, Baltimore, 1972, Chapter 9.

Feeley, Ruth M., Patricia E. Criner, Elizabeth W. Murphy, and Edward Toepfer, "Major Mineral Elements in Dairy Products," *Journal of the American Dietetic Association*, Vol. 61, No. 5 (November 1972), pp. 505–510.

Food and Nutrition Board, *Recommended Dietary Allowances*, 8th ed., National Academy of Sciences—National Research Council, Washington, D.C., 1974.

Hankin, Jean H., Sheldon Margen, and Naomi Goldsmith, "Contribution of Hard Water to Calcium and Magnesium Intakes of Adults," *Journal of the American Dietetic Association*, Vol. 56, No. 3 (March 1970), pp. 212–224. (Excellent reference for calcium and magnesium content of foods.)

Hegsted, D. M., "Major Minerals, Calcium and Phosphorus," in Robert S. Goodhart and Maurice E. Shils (eds.), *Modern Nutrition in Health and Disease*, Lea & Febiger, Philadelphia, 1973, Chapter 6, Section A.

Hopkins, H. T., E. W. Murphy, and D. P. Smith, "Minerals and Proximate Composition of Organ Meats," *Journal of the American Dietetic Association*, Vol. 38, No. 4 (April 1961), pp. 344–349.

"Hypomagnesemia in Protein-Calorie Malnutrition," *Nutrition Reviews*, Vol. 29, No. 4 (April 1971), pp. 89–90.

Moon, Wan-Hee, Jean L. Mazer, and Helen E. Clark, "Phosphorus Balances of Adults Consuming Several Food Combinations," *Journal of the American Dietetic Association*, Vol. 64, No. 5 (April 1974), pp. 386–390.

Odland, Lura M., Rossie L. Mason, and Anne I. Alexeff, "Bone Density and Dietary Findings of 40 Tennessee Subjects. 1. Bone Density Considerations," *American Journal of Clinical Nutrition*, Vol. 25, No. 9 (September 1972), pp. 905–907.

Schroeder, Henry A., "Losses of Vitamins and Trace Minerals Resulting from Processing and Preservation of Foods," *American Journal of Clinical Nutrition*, Vol. 24, No. 5 (May 1971), pp. 562–573.

Shils, Maurice E., "Magnesium," in Robert S. Goodhart and Maurice E. Shils (eds.), *Modern Nutrition in Diet and Disease*, Lea & Febiger, Philadelphia, 1973, Chapter 6, Section B.

Singh, P. P., L. K. Kothari, D. C. Sharma, and S. N. Saxena, "Nutritional Value of Foods in Relation to Oxalic Acid Content," *American Journal of Clinical Nutrition*, Vol. 25, No. 11 (November 1972), pp. 1147–1152.

Tewell, Janice E., Helen E. Clark, and Jean M. Howe, "Phosphorus Balances of Adults Fed Rice, Milk, and Wheat Flour Mixtures," *Journal of the American Dietetic Association*, Vol. 63, No. 5 (November 1973), pp. 530–535.

Walker, Alexander R. P., "The Human Requirement of Calcium: Should Low Intakes Be Supplemented," *American Journal of Clinical Nutrition*, Vol. 25, No. 5 (May 1972), pp. 518–530.

17

Trace Elements

Interest in trace elements in human nutrition has been heightened for several reasons. Increasing consumption of highly refined or fabricated foods substantially reduces the intake of important microminerals unless these nutrients have been replaced. In addition, our rapidly deteriorating environment has exposed individuals to certain heavy minerals for which no essential human function has been discovered. The problem is to avoid imbalances and the extremes of excessive or deficient intakes.

Seventeen trace elements have been identified as important for biological functioning in animals. These micronutrients may eventually prove essential for man. Present knowledge indicates that the following trace minerals are critical for life: chromium, cobalt, copper, iodine, iron, manganese, molybdenum, selenium, and zinc. It is not intended that this list be considered exclusive but rather a reflection of the present state of information about human needs for trace elements.[1]

Iron

Historically, Boyle in 1684 published his observations on an analysis of blood; he noted that the ash was brick red but did not suspect that it was iron, according to McCollum.[2] Menghini in 1747 established proof of the presence of iron. Since that time, and particularly in the twentieth century, there has been considerable research on the role of this mineral, which is found in very small quantities in the body.

Functions of Iron

Like phosphorus, iron is found in every living cell. It is an important constituent of chromatin; in addition, it stimulates vital processes in the cell itself.

The highest percentage of iron is found in the hemoglobin of red blood cells. The chief function of hemoglobin is to carry oxygen from the lungs to the tissues, where it is released; there it absorbs carbon dioxide and returns it to the lungs. The cycle is continuous.

---

[1] Food and Nutrition Board, *Recommended Dietary Allowances*, 8th ed., National Academy of Sciences—National Research Council, Washington, D.C., 1974, pp. 91–92.

[2] Elmer V. McCollum, A *History of Nutrition*, Houghton Mifflin Company, Boston, 1957, pp. 344, 347, 349.

220

There are many interesting facts about red blood cells. From a study using radioactive isotopes it has been discovered that they can be formed in only a few hours, but last about 120 days. It is almost impossible to conceive of the number of red cells found in the human body. There are estimated to be 25 trillion in the adult body. When they deteriorate, the iron is very carefully saved and used again.

Iron is also found in muscle cells in the form of myoglobin, whose function is to store the oxygen necessary for muscle operation or contraction. And iron is present in, but is not actually a constituent of, the plasma—it is there only because it is being transported to places where it is needed. This iron in the plasma generally comes from three sources—it may be absorbed through the gastrointestinal tract, salvaged from worn-out cells, or released from the storage places in the body as needed.

Iron is a constituent of certain tissue enzymes that aid in energy metabolism. They facilitate the oxidation of carbohydrates, proteins, and fats.

Factors Influencing Absorption, Metabolism, and Utilization of Iron

Iron absorption occurs primarily in the upper part of the small intestine where the mucosa remains attuned to current needs for iron, according to Conrad.[3] The exact mechanisms for regulating iron transport across the intestinal mucosa are unknown. Research is active in this area.

A number of factors that influence iron absorption have been identified. The absorption of iron depends both on mucosal uptake of dietary iron by intestinal absorptive cells and the transfer of this iron into the body. This absorption further depends upon an ample supply of dietary iron being exposed to the absorptive cells of the small intestine for a sufficient interval of time for the action to take place. The iron must be in a physiochemical form that permits absorption to the extent that body requirements will be fulfilled.

Thus the quantity and quality of iron in the diet, the physiochemical form of dietary iron, intestinal secretions, intestinal motility, and the kind and amount of parasites present are all factors that influence absorption.

The physical and chemical form of dietary iron is critical. More iron, for example, is absorbed from meats than from vegetables of similar iron content. Hemoglobin iron is absorbed more efficiently than inorganic iron. Ferrous iron is better absorbed than ferric iron. Certain dietary constituents, such as amino acids and amides, sugars, and ascorbic acid, generally facilitate absorption. Food constituents that tend to decrease absorption are phosphates, phytates, oxalates, and carbonates. Sodium bicarbonate (baking soda) is an example of a compound that precipitates and polymerizes iron, preventing absorption. When self-administered by individuals for such conditions as hyperacidity or other conditions, it may lead to poor absorption of this important mineral.

Parasites that cause intestinal bleeding, such as hookworm, interfere with absorption through the intestinal mucosa. *Intestinal motility* may be affected by the intake of certain drugs that increase or decrease the duration of time in which iron is exposed to the intestinal mucosa. Drugs that prolong the time facilitate absorption, but drugs that decrease the time will deter the absorption. Prolonged chronic diarrhea interferes with absorption.

Increased red cell production enhances iron absorption into the body. In contrast, depleted stores of red blood cells, as found in starvation, blood transfusion, or the effect of radical changes in altitude, decrease iron absorption.

A delicate balance is maintained between iron absorption and iron excretion. The quantity of body iron remains at a fairly constant level, according to Conrad. Most of the iron in the body is present in the circulating hemoglobin and a small amount is distributed as a component in the bone marrow, hemoglobin, myoglobin, and respiratory enzymes. The remaining iron is stored as ferritin or hemosiderin in the tissues. Prolonged dietary deficiencies, loss by bleeding, or gastrointestinal pathology will disturb this equilibrium.

[3] Marcel E. Conrad, "A Primer on Iron Metabolism," in William Crosby (ed.), *Iron*, Medicom, Inc., New York, 1972, pp. 8–17.

Under normal circumstances, little iron is lost from the body. Some loss occurs from the feces, urine, bile, and sweat, and some may be lost from skin cells and by cutting of hair and nails.

Iron is held with tenacity by the body, and iron released from hemoglobin breakdown re-enters the body iron pool and is carefully reutilized in later hemoglobin synthesis.

Iron Deficiency

Iron deficiency anemia is probably the most widespread form of malnutrition in the United States.[4] A decrease in the amount of dietary iron leads to less available iron in the body and results in iron deficiency.

The diagnosis of iron deficiency should include laboratory investigations of the size and shape of red blood cells, measurement of serum concentration, estimation of iron storage in tissues, and the response of an individual to iron therapy, according to Conrad. When the diet is adequate in iron content, then an iron deficiency is generally caused by bleeding. When the diet has little meat, refined cereals, and few green vegetables, iron deficiency is usually prevalent. Factors such as growth, pregnancy, hookworm or other parasitic infestation, infection, and malnutrition contribute to and complicate a lack of dietary iron.

An iron deficiency is most commonly found among women during reproductive years. Blood losses from menstruation and greater nutritive demands during childbearing increase iron needs. Iron deficiency in the third trimester of pregnancy of a majority of women is strong evidence that most women enter pregnancy with inadequate iron stores, according to de Leeuw[5] and others. Iron deficiency is especially serious for adolescent girls, who often enter pregnancy with low stores of iron coupled with the additional demands of growth.

Not only is an iron deficiency precarious in pregnancy, but a shortage of iron in infancy is equally serious. Sturgeon[6] in a study discovered that half the infants showed chemical evidence of iron deficiency. Infants during the first year of life revealed an incidence of anemia from 8 to 64 per cent, according to a report of the Committee on Iron Deficiency[7] of the American Medical Association. Birth size is critical in determining the iron endowment of an infant, and subsequent needs are influenced by rate of growth and concomitant increase of red cells.

The one unequivocal systemic manifestation of iron deficiency is anemia, according to Wheby.[8] In this situation, either the number of red blood cells is reduced or they are incapable of carrying adequate oxygen, which in turn results in faulty body functioning. The red blood cells become pale in appearance, and consequently the person has a pallor of skin and tissues. This is generally accompanied by weakness, a tendency to easy fatigue, headache, palpitation, and other symptoms. This iron deficiency may be attributed either to a lack of iron in the diet or to poor absorption.

Some mothers become overzealous in feeding milk to their children. Granted, milk is a nutritious food; but when it pushes other nutritious foods from the diet, deficiencies may result. The overuse of milk can thus lead to anemia.

Wheby hypothesizes other systemic manifestations that appear unique in patients with iron deficiency anemia. Some of these patients have a history of pica, the consumption of nonfood items such as starch, ice, clay, and other materials. The correction of this defi-

---

[4] "Absorption of Dietary Iron in Man," *Nutrition Reviews*, Vol. 29, No. 5 (May 1971), pp. 113–115.

[5] N. K. M. de Leeuw, L. Lowenstein, and Y. A. Hsieh, "Iron Deficiency and Hydremia in Normal Pregnancy," *Medicine*, Vol. 45, No. 4 (July 1966), pp. 291–315.

[6] P. Sturgeon, "Studies of Iron Requirements in Infants and Children, IV. Recommended Daily Dietary Allowances," in R. O. Wallerstein and S. R. Mettier (eds.), *Iron in Clinical Medicine*, University of California Press, Berkeley, Calif., 1958, pp. 183–203.

[7] Clement A. Finch et al., "Iron Deficiency in the United States," *Journal of the American Medical Association*, Vol. 203, No. 1 (January 1968), pp. 119–124.

[8] Munsey S. Wheby, "Systemic Effects of Iron Deficiency," in William H. Crosby (ed.), *Iron*, Medicom, Inc., New York, 1974, pp. 39–45.

ciency usually relieves this abnormal craving. Pica practice in the southern United States may be a cultural pattern and not due to iron deficiency. The same is true of pica practice in infants and small children with whom the problem is more complex. A long-held clinical impression that iron deficiency may lead to cardiac effects has not been proved. Enlargement of the heart has been associated with severe chronic anemia, and iron administration has been helpful in some cases if no underlying heart disease was manifested. Brittle fingernails, excessive loss of head hair, or poor quality of head hair have been complaints of some iron-deficient women; in this deficiency, iron treatment will usually improve the condition. Additional controlled studies and other research are needed.

Certain drugs cause alimentary bleeding, and thus loss of iron. About 70 per cent of patients taking aspirin show evidence of blood loss. Examples are patients with rheumatoid arthritis and osteoarthritis who take aspirin and related compounds. Another category is anticoagulant drugs that occasionally cause bleeding.[9]

Anyone who contributes large amounts of blood as a blood donor should scrutinize his diet very carefully to be certain that extra large amounts of iron are included. A physician may prescribe iron salts in this particular instance.

A number of methods are used in the diagnosis of iron deficiency and anemia. Hemoglobin concentration and hemacrit were measures used to assess anemia, particularly iron deficiency anemia, in the *First Health and Nutrition Examination Survey*.[10] Both measures are general rather than specific indicators of anemia, and there are close relationships between the two measures. Serum iron and transferrin saturation were measures to assess nutritional iron status. Examination of the bone marrow for "stainable iron" is a reliable index of the body's storage iron, according to Crosby.[11]

Iron Nutritive Needs

Wide variations in body losses of iron, lack of pertinent information about the physiological availability of iron in specific foods and in a mixed diet, a dearth of knowledge about body mechanisms for absorbing iron from the intestinal mucosa, and insufficient data to determine the response of individuals to increased iron intake in instances of deficiency make it difficult to determine appropriate iron dietary allowances.[12] Three stages in life in which iron intake are frequently inadequate are infancy, reproductive life period of females (losses from menstruation), and during pregnancy.

The recommended allowance for iron for infants during the first 5 months of life is 10 mg and increases to 15 mg for the period up to 3 years of age. For children from 4 to 10 years of age, 10 mg is recommended. For preadolescent and adolescent males and females (11 to 18 years), the allowance is 18 mg. Males from 19 to 51+ years have an allowance of 10 mg. An allowance of 18 mg has been made for females from 18 to 51+ years and during lactation. Allowance for pregnancy is 18+ mg. The Food and Nutrition Board emphasizes that, in establishing iron allowances for child-bearing women, the goal to allow for a sufficient margin above average physiological requirement to cover variation among essentially all individuals in the general population cannot be met by the iron in a typical American diet. See Table 17–1 for complete information about recommended dietary allowances for iron.

Although the iron in the body is used again and again in a very efficient manner, some losses do occur. Experiments to determine the

---

[9] Sheila Callender, "Pursuing the Iron Lead: GI Bleeding," in William H. Crosby (ed.), *Iron*, Medicom, Inc., New York, 1972, pp. 42–45.

[10] National Center for Health Statistics, *Preliminary Findings, First Health and Nutrition Examination Survey, United States, 1971–1972*, Dietary Intake and Biochemical Findings, DHEW Publication No. (HRA) 74–1291–1, Health Resources Administration, Public Health Service, U.S. Department of Health, Education, and Welfare, Rockville, Md., 1974.

[11] William H. Crosby, "Pathogenesis of Iron Deficiency," in William H. Crosby (ed.), *Iron*, Medicom, Inc., New York, 1972, pp. 18–25.

[12] *Recommended Dietary Allowances*, op. cit., pp. 92–94.

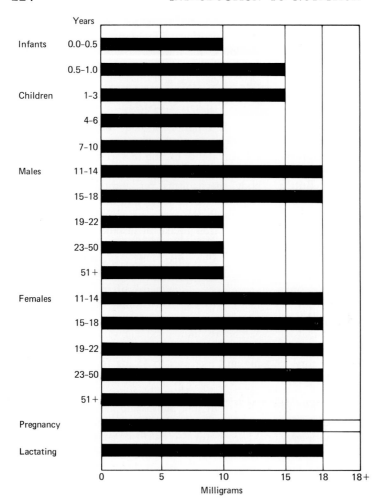

FIGURE 17–1. *Comparison of recommended daily dietary allowances of iron between various ages, both sexes, and for pregnancy and lactation. (Adapted from* Recommended Dietary Allowances, *8th edition,* Food and Nutrition Board, National Research Council—National Academy of Sciences, 1974)

iron requirement of individuals are tedious and require great skill.

Iron Nutritional Status

Two national nutrition surveys have provided information about iron nutritional status in United States. In the *Ten-State Nutrition Survey*[13] there was a high prevalence of deficient values of iron among blacks at all ages and for both sexes in the low-income-ratio states. Whites and Spanish-Americans of all

ages and both sexes in the low-income-ratio states had medium prevalence of deficient values in iron. Blacks and Spanish-Americans of all ages and both sexes in high-income-ratio states had medium prevalence of iron deficiencies. Whites of all ages and both sexes in the high-income-ratio states had a low prevalence of deficiencies in iron.

A high prevalence of low hemoglobin and hematocrit values was found throughout all segments of the population. These low levels of hemoglobin were associated with low levels of serum iron and serum transferrin saturation. Lower hemoglobin levels tended to be associated with low dietary iron intakes. An unexpected finding was a high prevalence of low hemoglobin levels among adolescent and

[13] *Ten-State Nutrition Survey, 1968–1970,* IV—Biochemical, DHEW Publication No. (HSM) 72-8132, V—Dietary, DHEW Publication No. (HSM) 72-8133, Center for Disease Control, Health Services and Mental Health Administration, Department of Health, Education, and Welfare, Atlanta, Ga., 1972.

TABLE 17-1

Recommendations for Daily Dietary Allowances for Iodine, Revised 1974

Designed for the maintenance of good nutrition for practically all healthy people in the United States

	AGE (years)	WEIGHT (kg)	(lb)	HEIGHT (cm)	(in.)	IRON (mg)
Infants	0.0–0.5	6	14	60	24	10
	0.5–1.0	9	20	71	28	15
Children	1–3	13	28	86	34	15
	4–6	20	44	110	44	10
	7–10	30	66	135	54	10
Males	11–14	44	97	158	63	18
	15–18	61	134	172	69	18
	19–22	67	147	172	69	10
	23–50	70	154	172	69	10
	51+	70	154	172	69	10
Females	11–14	44	97	155	62	18
	15–18	54	119	162	65	18
	19–22	58	128	162	65	18
	23–50	58	128	162	65	18
	51+	58	128	162	65	10
Pregnant						18+
Lactating						18

SOURCE: Food and Nutrition Board, *Recommended Dietary Allowances*, 8th ed., National Academy of Sciences—National Research Council, Washington, D.C., 1974.

adult males. This may indicate that standards for males should be revised or that anemia was a heretofore unappreciated problem among males. The low levels of hemoglobin in the total population appear to arise largely from a nutritional iron deficiency. One solution to this problem for many segments of the population may be to provide marketable foods with a higher iron-to-kcalorie ratio than presently available. (See Table 2-2.)

In the *First Health and Nutrition Examination Survey* (HANES),[14] preliminary findings indicate that the diets of the three age groups in both races (white and black) and both income groups (income below poverty level and income above poverty level) were below the standards for iron intake—children of ages

[14] National Center for Health Statistics, *Preliminary Findings, First Health and Nutrition Examination Survey*, op. cit.

1 to 5 years, adolescents of ages 12 to 17 years, and females of ages 18 to 44 years. In the lower-income group, blacks of ages 6 to 11, 45 to 59, and 60 years and over had mean iron intakes that did not meet the standards. A similar pattern was found among whites of similar ages and income level, except that those of 6 to 11 years of age met the standard. In the 6 to 11, 45 to 59, and 60 and over age groups in the income above poverty level, whites and blacks either approached or were above the standards. Males of ages 18 to 44 years for both race and income groups had mean iron intakes that exceeded standards. The cumulative percentage distribution data for children 1 to 5 years and females 18 to 44 years for both race and income groups showed that an average of 95 per cent of the individuals had iron intake values less than the standards. Corresponding values for persons 60 years of age and over averaged about 60 per cent of the individuals below standards.

Although all males of ages 18 to 44 years had mean iron intakes that met the standards, there were large proportions of black males at these ages with iron values that fell below the standards: blacks in the low-income group, 41 per cent; blacks in the high-income group, 25 per cent; whites of both income groups, about 15 per cent.

Mean iron intakes per 1000 kcalories were higher for black persons in most age groups than for white persons regardless of income. The highest mean intakes for iron per 1000 kcalories were found among black persons of both income groups in the age group of 45 years and over. The ratios of iron to kcalories for whites and blacks in the older age group, regardless of income, suggested that differences in iron between groups were related to selection of good food sources of iron rather than total kcaloric intake.

For biochemical findings, measurements were made of serum iron and transferrin saturation to evaluate nutritional iron status. These determinations gave some indication of the amount of iron in the blood. With only one exception, whites had higher mean transferrin saturation levels than blacks for all age groups regardless of income level. Mean serum iron levels were generally higher for whites than for blacks in all age groups for both income groups.

In children of ages 1 to 5 years, males of 18 to 44 years, and adults of ages 45 to 59 years, the mean serum iron levels for both whites and blacks were higher in the income level below poverty than in the income level above poverty. In general, blacks had a slightly higher percentage of low serum iron values than whites in the 1 to 5, 6 to 11, and 12 to 17 year age groups for both income levels. Blacks of ages 1 to 5 years in the income group above poverty level had 22.1 per cent low transferrin saturation values, which was the highest percentage for any group. Blacks had a higher percentage of low transferrin saturation values than whites in this age group for both income levels. In the 6- to 11-year age group, whites had a higher percentage of low transferrin saturation values than did blacks for both income levels. In the 12- to 17-year age group the percentage of low transferrin saturation values for blacks was higher than for whites. This situation was similar to observations in the 1- to 5-year age group.

Females, aged 18 to 44 years, had a higher percentage of low transferrin saturation values than did males for both races and income levels. The only group to have less than 3 per cent low values for percentage of transferrin saturation values was blacks 60 years of age and over. These biochemical findings provide evidence of iron deficiency for children and adolescents 1 to 17 years of age based on the relatively high percentage of low transferrin saturations. This information was not demonstrated in adult groups, particularly for black adults of 60 years and over.

Racial differences were apparent in these findings, but income was not an important factor except in the older income groups who usually had lower values in these iron measurements. The roles of folate or other deficiencies were not considered at the time these data were treated. The findings of these surveys indicate an iron deficiency problem in the United States.

Sources of Iron in Foods

One of the richest sources of iron is liver. Of those that reach the American table, pork liver contains the highest amount and chicken liver the lowest amount. All of them, however, are excellent sources. Other meat products, particularly organ meats, are excellent to good sources. The iron content in a serving of meat is decreased according to the amount of fat and bone. Egg yolk is a very good source, and for that reason is wisely incorporated into the infant's diet. Green leafy vegetables also make a very good contribution. The greener the leaf, the richer the source of iron. It is important to bear this in mind when selecting salad greens.

Certain dried fruits such as apricots and prunes furnish a good supply of iron. Fresh and canned fruits contain some, but they are not considered good sources. Whole-grain cereals are an inexpensive source, and enriched cereals and breads also contribute a significant amount to the day's requirement. Dried legumes, particularly beans, make a good contribution of iron to the diet and are also inexpensive.

Certain factors have had an influence on lowered iron intake in the diet. Iron cooking utensils have been replaced by stainless steel, aluminum, and nonstick varieties; hence iron contamination of foods from cooking utensils is almost nil. Cans for food have been enameled or detinned, thus reducing the possibility of securing iron from this source, according to White.[15] These factors, together with the fact that there are relatively few naturally rich sources of iron, necessitate a conscientious effort to include sufficient amounts in the daily diet.

Account must be taken of the losses of iron in processing and preparation of food, of the variability as well as availability of iron in foods for different individuals, and the possible interaction of foods upon each other. Additional research is required for further enlightenment. Table 17–2 indicates the iron content in an average serving of some common foods.

An examination of the table may bring certain surprises. The large amount of iron in

---

[15] Hilda White, "Iron, Nutrition—1972," cassette, The American Dietetic Association, Chicago, 1972.

TABLE 17–2

Iron Content of Some Common Foods

FOOD	SIZE OF SERVING	IRON CONTENT (mg)
Liver, pork, cooked	3 oz	26.1
Liver, lamb, cooked	3 oz	16.1
Liver, calf, cooked	3 oz	12.7
Liver, beef, cooked	3 oz	7.9
Clams, raw	4 oz	7.8
Liver, chicken	3 oz	7.6
Kidney, lamb	3 oz	6.6
Oysters, raw, medium	½ cup	6.6
Endive	⅛ lb	4.5
Spinach, cooked	½ cup	4.0
Liverwurst	2 oz	3.2
Hamburger, cooked	3 oz	2.7
Figs, dried	4	2.4
Chicken, with bone	1 leg, 4.2 oz	1.8
Apricots, dried, cooked	4 halves, 2 tbs juice	1.6
Collards	½ cup	1.1
Egg	1 medium	1.1
Prunes	4 large	1.1
Molasses	1 tbs	0.9
Potato	1 medium	0.8
Oatmeal, cooked	½ cup	0.7
Broccoli, cooked	½ cup	0.6
Bread, white, enriched	1 slice	0.6
Apple	1 medium	0.4
Carrots, cooked, diced	½ cup	0.3
Peanut butter	1 tbs	0.3
Milk	1 cup	0.2
Watercress, raw	5 sprigs	0.1

SOURCE: *Composition of Foods, Raw, Processed, Prepared,* Agriculture Handbook No. 8, U.S. Department of Agriculture, Washington, D.C., 1963.

oysters and clams is not generally realized. Molasses too, particularly dark molasses, is an excellent source, but a neglected one because it is not commonly eaten. A wider use of molasses might well be encouraged.

To ensure an adequate amount of iron in the diet each week, emphasis should be placed on such excellent sources as green leafy vegetables and liver. Although the iron found in milk is very small in quantity, the quality is excellent. And milk is frequently combined with foods that are high in iron content, such as whole-grain or enriched cereals or with meats, as in a cream sauce.

In October 1973, the Food and Drug Ad-

ministration ordered the nation's bakeries to increase the iron content of enriched white bread, enriched rolls, and enriched flour. The new level for enriched flour will be 40 mg per pound, compared to a present range of 13 to 16.5 mg; for enriched bread it will be 25 mg, compared to the present level of 8 to 12.5 mg. The Council of Foods and Nutrition of the American Medical Association backed the proposal. The purpose of the enrichment is to reduce the growing problem of iron deficiency anemia.

The proposal has had considerable opposition. William Crosby, for example, regretted that no research had been undertaken to prove that more iron in bread is sage or effective. Excessive iron intake could be harmful to the liver, the heart, and the pancreas, according to Crosby.[16]

Iron Consumption

The contribution of major food groups for nutrient supplies of iron available for civilian consumption from preliminary data for 1974 indicate that meat (including fat pork cuts), poultry, and fish were responsible for 29.1 per cent of the iron intake; eggs, 5.1 per cent; dairy products, excluding butter, 2.3 per cent; fats and oils, including butter, 0 per cent; citrus fruits, 0.8 per cent; other fruits, 3.3 per cent; potatoes and sweet potatoes, 4.4 per cent; dark-green and deep-yellow vegetables, 1.6 per cent; other vegetables, including tomatoes, 9.0 per cent; dry beans and peas, nuts, soya flour, 6.4 per cent; flour and cereal products, 28.9 per cent; sugars and other sweeteners, 7.4 per cent; and miscellaneous, 2.4 per cent.[17]

Copper

In 1924, Hart of the University of Wisconsin initiated a study of the nutritional factors influencing hemoglobin formation. Other workers were Elvehjem, Wadell, Herrin, and later Steenbock.[18] They were baffled by the fact that experimental animals (rabbits and rats) were not able to utilize iron in the synthesis of hemoglobin. But very small amounts of dried liver, dried kidney, dried muscle tissue, wheat, and corn added to the diet were found to be quite effective in helping the animals make hemoglobin.

In studying the ash samples from these foods, a pale blue color was frequently noted, and that gave rise to the idea that perhaps copper salts were involved. Consequently, a supplement of copper sulfate was added to the diet of a single anemic rat. There was a prompt response in hemoglobin formation. Additional tests with copper verified the need for copper in hemoglobin synthesis. Minerals such as zinc, nickel, arsenic, and manganese were tested either alone or in combination, but none of them could help to form hemoglobin.

Elvehjem established that copper is an essential nutrient for the human body. A deficiency is expressed as anemia, skeletal defects, defects in pigmentation, reproductive failure, cardiovascular lesions, and alteration of the structure and color of hair. A deficiency of copper is rare in man. Other evidences of deficiencies are diminished strength of elastin and collagen and degeneration of the nervous system. Copper deficiency has been noted in protein-kcalorie malnutrition, sprue, and nephrotic syndrome.[19] Premature infants fed exclusively on modified cow's milk formula for several months may have some of the above indications of a copper deficiency.[20]

The concentration of copper in the body is highest in the liver, kidney, heart, and brain. During growth, the highest concentration of copper is in the rapidly developing structures. Most of the copper in the body is associated with ceruloplasmin, the serum copper protein. Some copper is found in red blood cells. A small amount of the plasma copper is bound to amino acids and some to albumin. The potential of biochemical association of copper with other tissues and fluids is not well defined.[21] Dietary copper is absorbed from the upper intestinal tract. Acid facilitates absorption. Serum copper in healthy individuals is constant and is independent of age, sex, menstrual cycle, seasonal influences, and tissues

---

[16] "Iron in White Bread Doubled by F.D.A.," *The New York Times,* October 13, 1973, p. 14.

[17] "Contribution of Major Food Groups to Nutrient Supplies Available for Civilian Consumption, 1957–59 average and 1974," *National Food Situation,* Economic Research Service, U.S. Department of Agriculture, Washington, D.C., November 1974, p. 28.

[18] McCollum, op. cit., p. 339.

[19] *Recommended Dietary Allowances,* op. cit., p. 95.

[20] R. A. Al-Rashid and J. Spangler, "Neonatal Copper Deficiency," *New England Journal of Medicine,* Vol. 285, No. 15 (October 1971), pp. 841–843.

[21] Ting-Kai Li and Bert L. Vallee, "The Biochemical and Nutritional Role of Trace Elements," in Robert S. Goodhart and Maurice E. Shils (eds.), *Modern Nutrition in Health and Disease,* Lea & Febiger, Philadelphia, 1973, Chap. 8, Sec. B.

stores. Copper is stored in bone marrow, liver, and other organs. The range of copper in the body is from 75 to 150 mg in the adult. Women taking contraceptive medication have elevated serum copper concentrations. Nutritional implications are unknown.

Ordinary diets contain from 2 to 5 mg of copper per day, according to Leverton and Binkley.[22] An intake of 2 mg per day will maintain a copper balance in adults. Infants and children require 0.05 to 0.10 mg per kilogram per day; preadolescent girls, 1.3 mg per day.

There is little concern that adults may have a deficiency of copper since it is widely distributed in foods and generally there is an adequate supply. The richest sources of copper in foods, according to Pennington and Calloway,[23] are shellfish, especially oysters and canned crab; liver, particularly calf's liver; nuts and seeds, especially Brazil and hickory nuts and sesame and sunflower seeds; dry beans, notably navy, soy, kidney, and lima; bitter and sweet chocolate; all varieties of molasses; curry powder; cocoa powder; caffeine-free ground coffee; tea; and dried yeast.

Iodine

The element iodine has a very dramatic and colorful history. There is evidence that in early times certain people in iodine-poor sections of the world ate burnt sponges to counteract goiter. They did not realize that it was the iodine content of the sponges that overcame the deficiency causing the condition. The people in Savoy on the Italian-French border expected everyone to have goiter; the thyroid gland enlarged as the child grew. In the days of Gay-Lussac, in the early nineteenth century, some people were known to have painted their goiters with iodine. This gave some relief.

Iodine was first isolated by Courtais, a manufacturer of saltpeter, in 1811. He found it in the mother liquors that had been left after the extraction of saltpeter from seaweed. He noted that it had a violet color and smelled like chlorine. Condet, a Swiss physician, used iodine in the treatment of goiter as reported in 1820. Chatin, a French chemist, studied the occurrence of iodine in water and soil between 1850 and 1896. Baughman in 1895 discovered that iodine was a normal constituent of the thyroid gland.

One of the most important investigators in America was Marine.[24] In his early studies (1905–1910) he indicated the strong resistance to the acceptance of this early work about iodine and particularly to the idea that goiter resulted from a deficiency. He studied goiter found in fish living in iodine-poor waters. Other investigators had diagnosed this condition as cancer, but Marine was of the opinion that it was due to a lack of iodine. He reinforced his argument by using dogs in his study and demonstrating the same condition he had found in fish.

Marine and Kimball[25] tried to demonstrate the results of this deficiency in human beings. In large-scale studies in Akron, Ohio, they performed an interesting experiment. Over 2000 girls at the susceptible age of puberty were given iodine supplements in their drinking water twice weekly for a month during two periods of the year. The same number of girls of the same age served as controls and did not receive the iodine. In the experimental group, only five of the girls had goiter; but in the control group, about 500 developed goiter.

Functions of Iodine

Iodine is found in the thyroid gland, where it is utilized as an essential component of the thyroid hormone known as *thyroxine*. Thyroxine was isolated by Kendall[26] in 1915. Its

[22] Ruth M. Leverton and E. S. Binkley, "The Copper Metabolism and Requirement of Young Women," *Journal of Nutrition*, Vol. 27, No. 1 (January 1944), pp. 43–53.

[23] Jean T. Pennington and Doris Howes Calloway, "Copper Content of Foods," *Journal of the American Dietetic Association*, Vol. 63, No. 2 (August 1973), pp. 143–153.

[24] D. Marine, "The Physiology and Principal Interrelationships of the Thyroid," *Journal of the American Medical Association*, Vol. 104, No. 10 (November 1935), pp. 2250–2256.

[25] O. P. Kimball, "The Prevention of Goiter in Michigan and Ohio," *Journal of the American Medical Association*, Vol. 108, No. 3 (March 1937), pp. 860–864.

[26] McCollum, op. cit., p. 391.

chemical structure was determined by Harrington, who found that iodine combines with the amino acid tyrosine to form thyroxine, which regulates the basal metabolism rate.

Iodine in the diet is converted in the gastrointestinal tract to iodide and absorbed rapidly and completely and distributed through the extracellular fluid, according to Cavalieri.[27] Concentration of the iodide is found largely in the thyroid gland and to a lesser degree in the tissues of salivary glands, gastric mucosa, and mammary glands during lactation. In the thyroid gland, the iodide is utilized with the amino acid tyrosine in the synthesis of the thyroid hormones, thyroxine and triiodothyronine, which is the more active of the two although in lesser amount. The primary function of iodine as manifested in the thyroid hormones is to regulate basal metabolism.

A lack of iodine results in a condition known as simple goiter. The thyroxine level of the blood is lower than normal, and consequently the thyroid gland becomes overstimulated to compensate for this deficiency, which in turn causes enlargement of the gland. Boys and men are less susceptible to goiter than girls and women.

The thyroid hormone is essential in growth and development. The deficiency may be indicated by goiter, which becomes more severe as a child grows older. In extreme cases, children may fail to mature both physically and mentally.

Cretinism occurs if there has been a very serious deficiency in the thyroid secretion in childhood. This deficiency may be present at birth and during infancy. Growth is retarded and children develop very coarse features that give them an ape-like appearance. Not only are there physical evidences of retardation, but mentally these children are decidedly below normal.

Iodine is very important for normal reproduction and lactation. Many evidences of this need were found in livestock. Pigs with a lack of iodine produced young without hair.

---

[27] Ralph R. Cavalieri, *Trace Elements, Section A, Iodine*, in Robert S. Goodhart and Maurice E. Shils (eds.), *Modern Nutrition in Health and Disease*, Lea & Febiger, Philadelphia, 1973, Chap. 8.

Horses, cattle, and sheep developed enlarged thyroids during pregnancy. Similar evidences of abnormalities have been found in man. Sterility may result if individuals suffer from a prolonged deficiency of iodine.

Certain stresses, like the adolescent period for young girls, increase susceptibility to goiter. The stress of pregnancy may promote thyroid enlargement. Goiter also occurs more frequently during the menopause of women than during other years. Exposure to cold appears to have some bearing on enlarged thyroids. This condition may have some relationship to the greater energy requirement of a colder atmosphere. During such stress periods, it is especially important to have an adequate supply of iodine in the diet.

Endemic Goiter

The word *endemic* as applied to goiter denotes that the condition is peculiar to those areas of the world where the soil or water is low in iodine content. Figure 17–2 indicates such areas.

Before the cure was discovered, the regions in the United States where goiter was most prevalent were in the states surrounding the Great Lakes and the states in the Pacific Northwest. One interesting fact about the Pacific Northwest was that individuals, although living relatively close to the coast, still had goiter. This is explained by the fact that the high mountains prevented the iodine-rich air from moving to this area so that the soil would have the advantage of it.

In other parts of the world, the most seriously afflicted areas have been the Alps, Himalayas, and certain regions of New Zealand; in South America certain areas of Brazil, Chile, Peru, Ecuador, Colombia, and Uruguay are most seriously affected. Other afflicted areas include the northern part of Spain, inland areas in Sweden, parts of India and Tibet, a large area in interior China, Madagascar, and the African countries of Nigeria, Abyssinia, West Africa, Rhodesia, and Morocco. Endemic goiter continues to be a worldwide problem and one found in a few areas in the United States. The severity varies among population groups whose source of dietary iodine is limited.

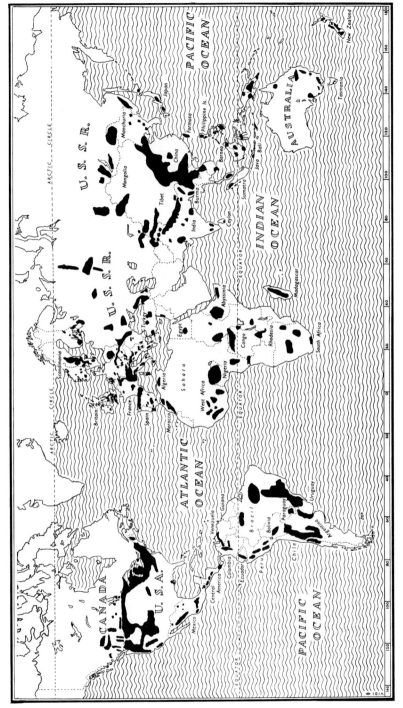

FIGURE 17-2. Goiter areas of the world. (Chilean Iodine Educational Bureau, London)

231

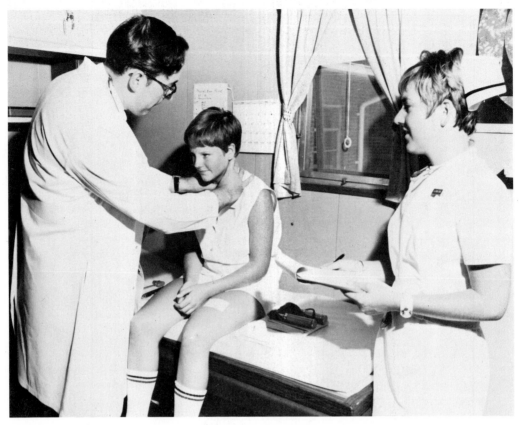

FIGURE 17–3.   *A physician examining a participant in a national nutrition survey for evidence of goiter.* (HANES)

Workers are exploring the possibility that other causes of goiter in addition to a lack of iodine in the diet be considered in endemic areas. Factors suggested are defects in the enzymes responsible for thyroid hormone biosynthesis, dietary goitrogens, and infectious agents. Dietary goitrogens are found in some foods. Such substances have been isolated from vegetables of the cabbage family, such as turnips, and rutabagas. Goiter due to goitrogens is unusually rare. The caution is offered that consumption of large amounts of goitrogens in an iodine-deficient environment might contribute to goiter, according to Cavalieri.

Iodine Nutritive Needs

The recommended dietary allowances of the National Research Council are based on research that includes balance studies. The daily requirement for adults is approximately 50 to 75 μg, or 1 μg per kilogram of body weight. Growing children, as well as pregnant and lactating mothers, need more. Table 17–3 shows the recommended dietary allowances for iodine.

Iodine Nutritional Status

The previous high incidence of iodine deficiency in endemic areas of the United States has decreased sharply with the introduction of iodized salt. The data from the *Ten-State Nutrition Survey*[28] showed no evidence of iodine deficiency. When goiter was prevalent, a relationship between this condition and iodine deficiency could not be demonstrated, suggesting that the goiter developed from

---

[28] *Ten-State Nutrition Survey*, op. cit., p. 12.

other causes. Goiter was less prevalent and smaller than during periods of iodine deficiency before the advent of iodized salt. Iodized salt was not regularly available or used in all the communities that were surveyed.

TABLE 17–3

Recommended Daily Dietary Allowances for Iodine, Revised 1974

Designed for the maintenance of good nutrition for practically all healthy people in the United States

	AGE (years)	WEIGHT (kg)	(lb)	HEIGHT (cm)	(in.)	IO-DINE (µg)
Infants	0.0–0.5	6	14	60	24	35
	0.5–1.0	9	20	71	28	45
Children	1–3	13	28	86	34	60
	4–6	20	44	110	44	80
	7–10	30	66	135	54	110
Males	11–14	44	97	158	63	130
	15–18	61	134	172	69	150
	19–22	67	147	172	69	140
	23–50	70	154	172	69	130
	51+	70	154	172	69	110
Females	11–14	44	97	155	62	115
	15–18	54	119	162	65	115
	19–22	58	128	162	65	100
	23–50	58	128	162	65	100
	51+	58	128	162	65	80
Pregnant						125
Lactating						150

SOURCE: Food and Nutrition Board, *Recommended Dietary Allowances*, 8th ed., National Academy of Sciences—National Research Council, Washington, D.C., 1974.

Recent studies have indicated high and increasing amounts of iodine in the American diet. In the *Ten-State Nutrition Survey*, preschool children and the 9- to 16-year-old children showed high levels of urinary iodine excretion. Dietary sources for these high iodine intakes have not been well identified. Iodized salt and seafoods do not appear to account for these higher levels of iodine excretion. One possibility are effects from food technology. Recent reports indicate that bread, milk, and certain food dyes may be among these sources of iodine. (See Table 2–2.)

Kidd and others[29] did a study on a sample of goitrous and nongoitrous children, ages 9 to 16 years, selected from a population screened for goiter in four states. A dietary frequency history from the children and food samples were analyzed for iodine. Data revealed no difference in intake of high iodine foods between goitrous and nongoitrous children.

Highest urinary iodine excretion occurred in children consuming iodated bread made by the continuous mixing process (iodate is a conditioner). The amount of milk consumed daily and the high iodine content of the milk samples affected the iodine excretion. The amount of seafoods consumed was low. Iodized salt was used in two thirds of the homes. Iodine excretion was higher for users than nonusers. The contribution of milk and bread to iodine intake has not been generally recognized nor well quantified. These and other unrecognized sources may contribute large amounts of iodine to the diet.

The public health implications of these relatively high iodine intakes have not been adequately defined. In the *Ten-State Nutrition Survey*, goiter prevalence was higher among participants excreting higher levels of urinary iodine than among those excreting median urinary levels. Children in the survey with mild thyroid enlargements were growing normally and there was no evidence of thyroid dysfunction. However, evidence is inadequate to make conclusions about adverse effects on health. Kidd and co-workers suggest that an iodine deficiency in the United States generally is unlikely, but the possibility of an iodine deficiency in some areas and among certain individuals cannot be discounted.

Sources of Iodine

The amount of iodine in food reflects the amount of iodine found in water or soil. Near the sea, the water and soil are generally much richer in iodine than they are inland. Seafoods are excellent and a consistent source of iodine. The content of eggs and dairy products de-

[29] Peggy S. Kidd, Frederick L. Trowbridge, James B. Goldsby, and Milton Z. Nichaman, "Sources of Dietary Iodine," *Journal of the American Dietetic Association*, Vol. 65, No. 4 (October 1974), pp. 420–422.

pends upon the composition of the animal feed. Vegetable products generally contribute little iodine. A sufficient intake of iodine in the diet can best be assured by the use of iodized salt.

Although the use of iodized salt is generally considered a safeguard against iodine deficiency, it is a protection only if it is actually used. People who use little or no salt either in food preparation or at the table might run the risk of an iodine deficiency.

The belief that sufficient iodine can be secured in drinking water is erroneous. The iodine content of drinking water varies considerably, depending on the source of the water, and cannot be a strictly reliable source. Even food grown in iodine-rich soil cannot be completely dependable. Iodine can be depleted from the soil and this lack is reflected in the produce.

Iodized salt cannot be used by persons on low-salt or salt-poor diets, which are often prescribed by physicians for hypertension or during pregnancy. Some other forms of iodine should be introduced into the diet for purposes of safety in these particular situations. On the other hand, iodine may be restricted by the physician in certain skin diseases, such as acne.

It is difficult to indicate the iodine content of common foods, since it varies with the area of the country where the foods originated. With the advent of fabricated and processed foods, the consumer does not have as much control over the use of iodized salt because salt sold to manufacturers, schools, and restaurants in bulk is usually not iodized. However, food technological processes may be adding iodine, as previously discussed.

Zinc

Zinc is an essential nutrient for plants and for man. One of its major functions is as a constituent of enzymes involved in protein and carbohydrate metabolism and RNA synthesis.[30] A large number of these zinc metalloenzymes have been isolated from the tissues

of many organs, pointing to the important role of this trace element. Zinc is vital for growth and development.

Zinc deficiency in infants is manifested by failure to grow (in severe deficiency, dwarfism may result), loss of appetite, testicular atrophy, and skin lesions. Low zinc hair levels may be characteristic. Loss of appetite and skin lesions may be found in adolescents and adults. Impairment of taste and smell acuity may be treated with zinc, indicating that these are symptoms of deficiency.[31] Patients in hospitals may have zinc-deficiency wounds and in the elderly a deficiency may result in leg ulcers.

Dietary allowances recommended for zinc are 15 mg per day for adults and adolescents and an additional 5 mg per day for pregnancy and 25 mg per day for lactation. An allowance of 10 mg per day is recommneded for young children and preadolescents. The basis for determining zinc requirements is not available. The allowance for the first 6 months of life is suggested as 3 mg per day, and 5 mg per day for the second 6 months. See Table 17–4.

The zinc nutritional status of the population of the United States has not been determined. Some experts believe that zinc deficiencies have been largely limited to inadequacies of this trace element complicating chronic illness or of zinc malabsorption.[32] Mertz,[33] however, contends that an optimal intake of zinc cannot be assumed. Periods when individuals are most vulnerable to zinc deficiency are during periods of rapid growth; in infancy, if fed formulas that do not include a zinc allowance; and during hospitalization, especially if patients indicate zinc-deficiency symptoms, such as wounds or anorexia. A report on zinc in human nutrition in a summary of a workshop of the Food and Nutrition Board indicates that many dietaries, although not grossly deficient in zinc, do not provide

---

[30] Ting-Kai Li and Bert L. Vallee, op. cit., pp. 382–389.

[31] Walter Mertz, "Recommended Dietary Allowances Up to Date—Trace Minerals," *Journal of the American Dietetic Association*, Vol. 64, No. 2 (February 1974), p. 165.

[32] "Growth and Zinc Deficiency," *Nutrition Reviews*, Vol. 31, No. 5 (May 1973), pp. 145–146.

[33] Mertz, op. cit., p. 165.

TABLE 17–4

Recommended Daily Dietary Allowances for Zinc, 1974

Designed for the maintenance of good nutrition for practically all healthy people in the United States

	AGE (years)	WEIGHT (kg)	WEIGHT (lb)	HEIGHT (cm)	HEIGHT (in.)	ZINC (mg)
Infants	0.0–0.5	6	14	60	24	3
	0.5–1.0	9	20	71	28	5
Children	1–3	13	28	86	34	10
	4–6	20	44	110	44	10
	7–10	30	66	135	54	10
Males	11–14	44	97	158	63	15
	15–18	61	134	172	69	15
	19–22	67	147	172	69	15
	23–50	70	154	172	69	15
	51+	70	154	172	69	15
Females	11–14	44	97	155	62	15
	15–18	54	119	162	65	15
	19–22	58	128	162	65	15
	23–50	58	128	162	65	15
	51+	58	128	162	65	15
Pregnant						20
Lactating						25

SOURCE: Food and Nutrition Board, *Recommended Dietary Allowances*, 8th ed., National Academy of Sciences—National Research Council, Washington, D.C., 1974.

for a margin of safety to meet the daily allowance or for periods of special stress.[34] One deterrent to meeting zinc allowances is the problem of individuals and families who may be using vegetable and cereal sources of protein because of low incomes or as an attempt to cope with inflation. The zinc in these sources is not as available as animal sources.

The best sources of zinc in foods are seafoods, especially oysters and canned tuna and sardines; meats, particularly beef round and lamb chops; whole-grain cereals and seeds; vegetables, notably legumes, and roots (white turnips are good), which are slightly higher than leafy vegetables; eggs, with the yolk be-

ing higher than the whole egg; soy lecithin, with a very high content; nuts, which are especially rich in this trace element, with pecans and Brazil nuts being exceptional; and such condiments as black pepper, ground mustard, and cinnamon, which have generous amounts.[35,36]

When foods rich in phytic acid, such as some cereals, are consumed, the availability of zinc is seriously decreased. Cereals that contain soya products also have a reduced zinc availability. Zinc content of grains and vegetables depends upon the zinc content of the soil in which they are grown.

Chromium

No dietary allowance has been established for chromium although there has been considerable evidence that this trace element is essential for man. Investigations of chromium-responsive disturbances of glucose intolerance indicate that marginal deficiency status may exist in the United States.[37]

Chromium is concentrated in many tissues in man. This trace element decreases in amount in the tissues with age. There is evidence that chromium is involved in carbohydrate and lipid metabolism, particularly in the utilization of glucose, and is associated with RNA.[38] Repeated pregnancies result in a significant decrease in hair chromium. Premature infants have low hair chromium content. The concentration of chromium in blood serum or plasma is not indicative of nutritive status.

Other chromium deficiencies noted are impairment of oral or intravenous glucose tolerance of the type that is associated with im-

---

[34] Food and Nutrition Board, "Zinc in Human Nutrition," in *Summary of Proceedings of a Workshop*, December 4–5, 1970, National Academy of Sciences—National Research Council, Washington, D.C., 1971.

[35] Harold H. Sandstead, "Zinc Nutrition in the United States," *American Journal of Clinical Nutrition*, Vol. 26, No. 11 (November 1973), pp. 1251–1260. (Table on zinc content of foods on p. 1257.)

[36] Dace Osis, Lois Kramer, Emilie Wiatrowski, and Herta Spencer, "Dietary Zinc Intake in Man," *American Journal of Clinical Nutrition*, Vol. 25, No. 6 (June 1972), pp. 582–588. (Table on zinc content of foods on p. 587.)

[37] Mertz, op. cit., p. 165.

[38] Li and Valee, op. cit., pp. 393–394.

provement with an increase of chromium intake, absence of a sharp rise in serum chromium following a challenge with insulin or glucose, and a low concentration of chromium in the urine. Chromium deficiency has been associated with protein-kcalorie malnutrition in some areas of the world.

Daily chromium intake in this country depends upon dietary preference. Meats, whole-grain cereals, and brewer's yeast are the best sources in foods. Fish, vegetables, and sugars are poor sources. On the whole, chromium is poorly absorbed. Estimates of absorption from some food sources are between 10 to 15 per cent of a stated amount.[39]

The manner in which chromium is combined influences its availability for absorption, tissue distribution, access to specific metabolic pools, and placental transport in pregnancy.[40] There are large qualitative and quantitative differences between simple chromium salts, on the one hand, and the organic chromium compounds found in food.

Cobalt

A need for this trace element was discovered when investigators found that it prevented a wasting disease among cattle and sheep in certain localities in Australia and New Zealand. These studies were further reinforced by similar ones for the same disease in Florida, Kenya, Scotland, and parts of England.

Although deficiencies of this mineral have been found in cattle and sheep, they have not been produced in rats, rabbits, or guinea pigs. However, there has been some evidence that cobalt will contribute to growth in rats and chicks. Colbalt deficiency is unknown in man.

The primary function of cobalt is as a constituent of vitamin B_{12}. It also contributes to

the formation of red blood cells. This mineral is readily absorbed in the intestinal tract, and excretion of most of the absorbed mineral is by way of urine. There is little retention in the body.

Cobalt is distributed widely among foods; hence it is readily available to man. However, there is no known human requirement for it. Apparently a sufficient amount for the vitamin B_{12} component is ingested with foods.

Fluorine

The requirement of fluorine as an essential trace element for optimal tooth health has been documented. Fluorine is especially important in dental health of infants and small children. The daily fluoride intake in many parts of the United States is not adequate to provide this protection. The addition of fluoride to water supplies has been standardized at 1 mg per liter, which is considered a safe, economical, and efficient method for reduction of the incidence of tooth decay. Evidence cites that dental caries have been decreased by 50 per cent among children.[41]

Fluorine is highly toxic when consumed in excessive amounts, but to achieve this condition requires 20 to 80 mg or more of the trace element. The daily intake of fluorine in the diet exclusive of drinking water ranges from 0.3 mg in low-fluoride areas to 3.1 mg in high-fluoride areas. Although no correlation could be established, Kramer and others[42] found the fluoride of the diet three times greater in fluoridated areas than nonfluoridated areas.

Manganese

The most important functions of manganese are as an essential constituent for bone structure, for reproduction, and for normal functioning of the nervous system. This trace element is also a part of the body enzyme

---

[39] Anna M. Baetjer, Chairman, Committee on Biological Effects of Atmospheric Pollutants, Division of Medical Sciences, National Research Council, "Chromium in Nutrition," in *Chromium*, National Academy of Sciences, Washington, D.C., 1974, Chap. 5.

[40] Report of a WHO Expert Committee, *Trace Elements in Human Nutrition*, World Health Organization Technical Report Series, No. 532, World Health Organization, Geneva, 1973, pp. 20–24.

[41] *Recommended Dietary Allowances*, op. cit., pp. 98–99.

[42] Lois Kramer, Dace Osis, Emilie Wiatrowski, and Herta Spencer, "Dietary Fluoride in the United States," *American Journal of Clinical Nutrition*, Vol. 27, No. 6 (June 1974), pp. 590–594.

system. The human requirement for manganese is unknown and deficiency symptoms in humans have not been established.

Nuts and whole grains are the richest sources of manganese. Vegetables and fruit rate next in content. Meat and poultry products contribute a little, and seafood and fish have the lowest amounts of this micromineral.

Molybdenum

Molybdenum has been found to be a part of the molecular structure of two enzymes that are involved in the metabolism of proteins and are important in oxidation. This trace element is considered as probably essential, but demonstrations still need to be made. No human requirement has been established.

The molybdenum content of foods varies greatly. Beef kidney, some cereals, and some legumes appear to be good sources.[43]

Selenium

The physical and chemical properties of selenium resemble sulfur, according to Li and Vallee.[44] This trace element is considered essential for humans, but little information is available about its biochemical reactions, functions, and dietary requirement. In animals, selenium appears to have functions related to vitamin E. Foods high in selenium content are seafood, kidney, meat, and, if the soil

composition is favorable, rice and grains. Vegetables and fruits are relatively poor sources.[45] Limited data indicate that processed or refined foods contain less selenium.

Other Trace Elements

The occurrence of *nickel* in human tissues and the fact that nickel deficiency has been produced in chickens and rats suggests some possibility of a human need for this trace element. In the controlled environment of a space vehicle there has been some evidence that a nickel deficiency may occur.

Information about the metabolic role or dietary need for *tin* is lacking. The tin content in dietary intake of man has decreased considerably. This is partially explained by lacquer coating replacing tin in cans, aluminum replacing tin in foil, and other changes in packaging in which tin has been replaced.

No evidence is available that *cadmium* is essential for man. Rather, the effects of an accumulation of this trace element as a food contaminant in undesirable amounts in the body is a matter of concern. Deficiencies of *silicon* have been produced in experimental animals, suggesting a possible human requirement, but implications for human nutrition are lacking. The paucity of evidence of a possible nutritional requirement for *vanadium* as well as a lack of knowledge of intakes prohibits a discussion of this trace element. Further research on man's requirements for essential nutrients is needed.[46]

---

[43] *Recommended Dietary Allowances*, op. cit., p. 102.

[44] Li and Vallee, op. cit., pp. 391–393.

[45] Report of a WHO Expert Committee, op. cit., pp. 24–29.

[46] Report of a WHO Expert Committee, op. cit., pp. 36–43.

SELECTED REFERENCES

GENERAL REFERENCES

Borenstein, B., "Micronutrient Consideration in Nutrient Labeling," *Food Technology*, Vol. 27, No. 6 (June 1973), pp. 32–34.

Davidson, Stanley, R. Passmore, and J. F. Brock, *Human Nutrition and Dietetics*, The Williams & Wilkins Company, Baltimore, 1972, Chapter 10.

Food and Nutrition Board, *Recommended Dietary Allowances*, 8th ed., National Academy of Sciences—National Research Council, Washington, D.C., 1974.

Gormican, Annette, "Inorganic Elements in Foods Used in Hospital Menus," *Journal of the American Dietetic Association*, Vol. 56, No. 5 (May 1970), pp. 397–403. (Excellent tables of trace element content in foods.)

Mertz, Walter, "Recommended Dietary Allowances Up to Date—Trace Minerals," *Journal of the American Dietetic Association*, Vol. 64, No. 2 (February 1974), pp. 163–167.

Nielsen, F. H., Newer Trace Elements in Human Nutrition," *Food Technology*, Vol. 28, No. 1 (January 1974), pp. 38–44.

"Nutritional Trace Element Research," *Nutrition Reviews*, Vol. 29, No. 4 (April 1971), pp. 90–93.

Report of a WHO Expert Committee, *Trace Elements in Human Nutrition*, World Health Organization Technical Report Series, No. 532. World Health Organization, Geneva, 1973.

Young, Charlotte M., "Mineral Overload," in Miloslav Rechcigl, Jr. (ed.), *Food, Nutrition and Health*, Vol. 16, S. Karger, Basel, 1973, pp. 194–202.

IRON

"Absorption of Dietary Iron In Man," *Nutrition Reviews*, Vol. 29, No. 5 (May 1971), pp. 113–115.

"Availability of Iron," *Nutrition Reviews*, Vol. 29, No. 10 (October 1971), pp. 234–237.

Bing, Franklin C., "Assaying the Availability of Iron," *Journal of the American Dietetic Association*, Vol. 60, No. 2 (February 1972), pp. 114–122.

Burroughs, Ann L., and Ruth L. Huenemann, "Iron Deficiency in Rural Infants and Children," *Journal of the American Dietetic Association*, Vol. 57, No. 2 (August 1970), pp. 122–128.

Crosby, William H., *Iron*, Medicom, Inc., New York, 1972.

Goldsmith, Grace A., "Iron Enrichment of Bread and Flour," *American Journal of Clinical Nutrition*, Vol. 26, No. 2 (February 1973), pp. 131–132.

Monson, Elaine R., "The Need for Iron Fortification," *Journal of Nutrition Education*, Vol. 2, No. 4 (Spring 1971), pp. 152–155.

Report of a Joint FAO/WHO Expert Group, *Requirements of Ascorbic Acid, Vitamin D, Vitamin B_{12}, Folate, and Iron*, World Health Organization Technical Report Series, No. 452, World Health Organization, Geneva, 1970.

Todhunter, E. Neige, "Iron, Blood, and Nutrition," *Journal of the American Dietetic Association*, Vol. 61, No. 2 (August 1972), pp. 121–126.

COPPER

Butler, Lillian C., and Janet M. Daniel, "Copper Metabolism in Young Women Fed Two Levels of Copper and Two Protein Sources," *American Journal of Clinical Nutrition*, Vol. 26, No. 7 (July 1973), pp. 744–749.

Gollan, John L., Peter S. Davis, and Donald J. Deller, "Binding of Copper by Human Alimentary Secretions," *American Journal of Clinical Nutrition*, Vol. 24, No. 9 (September 1971), pp. 1025–1027.

Hambidge, K. Michael, "Increase in Hair Copper Concentration with Increasing Distance from the Scalp," *American Journal of Clinical Nutrition*, Vol. 26, No. 11 (November 1973), pp. 1212–1215.

IODINE

Gillie, R. Bruce, "Endemic Goiter," *Scientific American*, Vol. 224, No. 6 (June 1971), pp. 93–101.

Kevany, John, and Joginder G. Chopra, "The Use of Iodized Oil in Goiter Prevention," *American Journal of Public Health,* Vol. 60, No. 5 (May 1970), pp. 919–925.

Koutras, D. A., P. D. Papapetrou, X. Yataganas, and B. Malamos, "Dietary Sources of Iodine in Areas with and Without Iodine-Deficiency Goiter," *American Journal of Clinical Nutrition*, Vol. 23, No. 7 (July 1970), pp. 870–873.

Kuhajek, Eugene, and Howard W. Fiedelman, "Nutritional Iodine in Processed Foods," *Food Technology*, Vol. 27, No. 1 (January 1973), pp. 52–53.

Thilly, C. H., F. Delange, and A. M. Ermans, "Further Investigations of Iodine Deficiency in the Etiology of Endemic Goiter," *American Journal of Clinical Nutrition*, Vol. 25, No. 1 (January 1972), pp. 30–40.

ZINC

"Growth and Zinc Deficiency," *Nutrition Reviews*, Vol. 31, No. 3 (May 1973), pp. 145–146.

McBean, Lois D., James T. Dove, James A. Halsted, and J. Cecil Smith, "Zinc Concentration in Human Tissues," *American Journal of Clinical Nutrition*, Vol. 25, No. 7 (July 1972), pp. 672–676.

———, Mohsen Mahloudji, John G. Reinhold, and James A. Halstead, "Correlation of Zinc Concentrations in Human Plasma and Hair," *American Journal of Clinical Nutrition*, Vol. 24, No. 5 (May 1971), pp. 506–509.

Murphy, Elizabeth W., Barbara Wells Willis, and Bernice K. Watt, "Provisional Tables on the Zinc Content of Foods," *Journal of the American Dietetic Association*, Vol. 66, No. 4 (April 1975), pp. 345–355.

O'Dell, Boyd L., "Effect of Dietary Components upon Zinc Availability," *American Journal of Clinical Nutrition*, Vol. 22, No. 10 (October 1969), pp. 1315–1322.

Osis, Dace, Lois Kramer, Emilie Wiatrowski, and Herta Spencer, "Dietary Intake in Man," *American Journal of Clinical Nutrition*, Vol. 25, No. 6 (June 1972), pp. 582–588.

Prasad, Ananda S., "A Century of Research on the Metabolic Role of Zinc," *American Journal of Clinical Nutrition*, Vol. 22, No. 9 (September 1969), pp. 1215–1221.

Sandstead, Harold H., "Zinc, a Metal to Grow On," *Nutrition Today*, Vol. 3, No. 1 (March 1968), pp. 12–17.

———, Verne C. Lanier, Glenn H. Shephard, and David D. Gillespie, "Zinc and Wound Healing," *American Journal of Clinical Nutrition*, Vol. 23, No. 5 (May 1970), pp. 514–519.

"Zinc in Hair as a Measure of Zinc Nutriture in Human Beings," *Nutrition Reviews*, Vol. 28, No. 8 (August 1970), pp. 209–211.

CHROMIUM

Hambidge, K. Michael, "Chromium Nutrition in Man," *American Journal of Clinical Nutrition*, Vol. 27, No. 5 (May 1974), pp. 505–514.

———, and J. David Baum, "Hair Chromium Concentrations of Human Newborn and Changes During Infancy," *American Journal of Clinical Nutrition*, Vol. 25, No. 4 (April 1972), pp. 376–379.

Li, Ting-Kai, and Bert L. Valee, "The Biochemical and Nutritional Role of Trace Elements," in Robert S. Goodhart and Maurice E. Shils (eds.), *Modern Nutrition in Health and Disease*, Lea & Febiger, Philadelphia, 1973, pp. 393–394.

18

Water and Nutrition

The story of man is colored by his quest for water. His earliest prayers were incantations for rain. Water is a prime requisite of life, second only to oxygen. Man has made adaptations for clothes and shelter and can live for a time without food but can survive only a few days without water. Clearly, water is an essential nutrient that is often ignored in planning for adequate nutrition.

Distribution in the Body

Water is found in every cell of the body. Many variables influence the amount of body water. At birth, the body water in relation to body weight of an infant is over 70 per cent. By adulthood, water content is around 65 per cent and decreases with age. Sex is a variable. Males during the growth period tend to decrease the water content of the body more slowly than females, who usually have greater fat storage. Lean adults and children account for a higher per cent of body water than obese adults and children who may have 10 per cent less water. The bodies of athletes have a higher percentage of water than non-athletes.[1] There is considerable variation in the concentration of water in the various tissues of the body. The water content of teeth is approximately 5 per cent; bone, 25 per cent; adipose tissue, 10 to 35 per cent; red blood cells, 60 per cent; striated muscle, 70 to 80 per cent; and blood plasma, 92 per cent.

The water of the body is divided into two major body compartments, the intracellular and the extracellular. The intracellular fluid, that within the cells, accounts for the major portion of the body weight. The extracellular compartment is subdivided into the intravascular, which comprises the water in the blood plasma, and the extravascular, which comprises the interstitial fluid found surrounding each cell.

Functions of Water

Water enters into almost every function of the body: it is essential to the digestive proc-

[1] H. T. Randall, "Water, Electrolytes, and Acid–Base Balance," in Robert S. Goodhart and Maurice E. Shils (eds.), *Modern Nutrition in Health and Disease*, Lea & Febiger, Philadelphia, 1973, Chap. 7.

240

ess; it is the vehicle that carries food to the tissues and carries away waste; it controls body temperature.

Each step of the process of converting the food eaten into tissue and energy is facilitated by water. First, the digestive secretions are largely water. This water acts as a solvent for nutrients; it softens, dilutes, or liquefies the food so that it can be digested more easily. It also helps to move the food along the alimentary canal. Then, the differences in fluid concentration on either side of the intestinal wall facilitate the absorption process. Finally, the blood and lymph carry these nutrients (either in suspension or solution) to the cells where they are needed.

In this metabolic process, water has an important chemical function. It forms one of the end products after fats, carbohydrates, and proteins are metabolized.[2] If this water is not used in body processes, it is excreted. The body is very efficient, however, in making use of it whenever necessary.

Equally important is the role of water in excretion. The blood and lymph that carry nutrients to the cells carry away waste materials from those cells. The largest amount of this waste is excreted as urine by the kidneys. However, appreciable amounts of water are excreted through other organs.

For example, the lungs exhale water along with carbon dioxide—as much as ⅓ quart (⅔ liter) of water each day in an adult. This moisture is visible when we breathe on a mirror or glass or, on a cold day, when we can "see our breath."

The skin disposes of waste and excess water through perspiration—under normal conditions, as much as 1 pint or about one-half liter a day. This increases, of course, and is more apparent in warm weather. During strenuous exercise, like baseball, football, or basketball, an athlete may lose as much as 8 to 15 pounds

or 3.6 to 6.8 kilograms of weight, most of it water.

Through perspiration, water not only rids the body of waste but acts as a thermostat. As a person perspires, the moisture evaporates and cools his body. Scientists tell us that the evaporation of 1 quart or 1.25 liters of sweat will disperse the heat from 580 kcalories. (High humidity causes discomfort because it impedes evaporation.)

Another important function of water is that it serves as a lubricant, cushion, and protector. The fluid surrounding the joints reduces friction and facilitates their motion. Internal organs, such as the small intestine, have fluids around them permitting them to glide easily without harm. Even tears serve as a lubricant. Water also keeps all air passages moist. Digestibility may be facilitated and fatigue relieved by water.

Sources of Water

Liquids like water, tea, coffee, carbonated beverages, or soups furnish the largest amount of water to the body. "Solid" foods vary greatly in their water content. Few people realize that, except for a few foods such as lard, practically all food contains some water. Figure 18–1 gives some indication of the variation in water content of some of our common foods. It is interesting to note that milk does not contain any more water than an orange. Cucumber, celery, and lettuce, which appear to be quite solid, actually contain a very high percentage. Some individuals may be surprised at the large amount of water in cooked spaghetti. Water from the metabolism of nutrients is another source of water for the body.

Effect of Water on Nutritive Value of Food

The amount of water in a food has a definite effect upon its kcaloric value as well as upon other nutrients. For instance, fruit juices have fewer kcalories than dried fruit, where some of the water has been removed. Besides being low in kcalories and supplying water needed by the body, a certain number

---

[2] The amount of water derived from each nutrient after it has been ingested and metabolized will vary. Scientists estimate that 1 g of protein yields 0.41 g of water; carbohydrate, 0.6 g; and fat, 1.07 g. Although these are only estimates, a person who knows how many grams of these nutrients he has had in his diet for a day can get an idea of the amount of water produced.

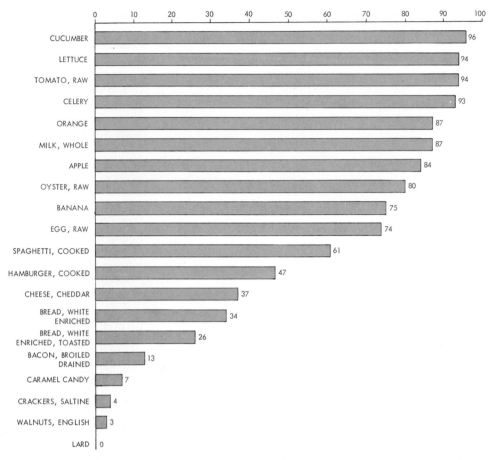

FIGURE 18–1. *Percentage of water content of some common foods.* (*Adapted from* Composition of Foods, Agriculture Handbook No. 8, USDA, 1963)

of foods of high water content is essential for palatability and for variety.

The point is that the amount of water does affect the total kcaloric value because of dilution. The same is true of protein. Although milk contains only 3.5 per cent protein, this figure can be somewhat misleading because milk contains 87 per cent water. Actually, then, milk is not a low-protein food but has an excellent protein contribution to make if consumed in sufficient volume. Cheese, for another example, has a higher concentration of protein and fat than lean meat because it has less moisture than meat. The addition of skim milk solids can increase the nutritive value of milk and other foods because of its very low moisture content.

Daily Water Requirement

For ordinary purposes, the body has a built-in control or guide for the amount of water needed daily—thirst—although sometimes people are prone to ignore this summons. However, infants cannot indicate their need for water, and ill persons, particularly those with fever, may have an abnormal desire for water. The physician must decide the amount of water in these cases.

Water requirements vary with age. The greatest fluid requirement is during infancy, about 110 ml per kilogram of body weight. The body water content is reduced rapidly between the first and fourth years, a fact that is reflected in water requirements. For adults,

1000 ml are recommended for every 1000 kcalories required.

Most authorities agree that six to eight glasses of water should be drunk daily by an adult. Fruit or vegetable juices, soups, coffee, tea, and other liquids can be counted for part of this water. Since it is so important to the body, it is essential that individuals make some plan for getting their daily quota. When the amount of available water in the body is curtailed, digestion and metabolism may be undesirably affected.

A question frequently arises about drinking water during meals. There are no harmful effects unless the water is used to wash the food down or drunk in excessive amounts so that saliva and other digestive juices are unduly diluted. Children sometimes drink water and then do not masticate food adequately. The temperature of the water may also be important. Large amounts of extremely cold water, particularly in warm weather, are not recommended.

The amount of water a person drinks during the day is determined by a number of factors and hence may vary considerably. The environment, particularly temperature and humidity, is an important factor. Less water is needed in a cold climate than in a hot climate. The amount of activity needs to be considered: a person who is extremely active would need much more water than a person who spends a good deal of time at a desk. More sleep and rest will also lessen the amount of water needed. Buskirk and Mendez[3] have studied the impact of physical activity and climate (chiefly temperature and altitude) on kcaloric and water requirements. It was concluded that water requirements were influenced by environmental conditions, such as vapor pressure and altitude, and by physical activity.

Workers and athletes may become fatigued because of insufficient water in the body. Periodic breaks for workers to drink some form of liquid may increase production. Some athletic coaches are encouraging the consumption of water during time outs or breaks in athletic events.

Johnson[4] has studied water economy on survival rations. He concluded that water and osmotic balance are mutually related. An osmotic deficit leads to a water deficit because the kidney's ability to retain water has been reduced. Under identical conditions of environment, physical work, water supply, and diet, there is a large interindividual variation but a consistent intraindividual pattern in water economy. Furthermore, individuals cannot be trained to get along with decreasing amounts of water. Even the best survival ration can only slow down functional deterioration. Consideration must be given to the length of the survival period. Survival for a day obviously has different water requirements than survival for a week or a month. The old, the young, the sick, the injured, and pregnant women are in particular need of water in the event of crises.

The physical environment and the work load have a marked effect on water requirements. Food intake, especially the ratio of protein to carbohydrate, to fat, and to the intake of salts, affects water requirement. Increased protein in the diet increases water needs because additional fluid is required to eliminate nitrogen by-products in the urine. Salt and water requirements are closely interrelated, according to Margen.[5]

Deviations in Water Metabolism

Any disturbance that leads to a reduction or accumulation of water in the cells may lead to serious consequences, because the cell functions best with a specific concentration of nutrients. Conditions such as diarrhea, nausea, or high fever may cause an abnormal loss of cell fluid and result in dehydration. Edema and similar deviations may result in increased water in the cells, thus interfering with functioning. Defective absorption in the intestine

[3] E. R. Buskirk and J. Mendez, "Nutrition, Environment and Work Performance," *Federation Proceedings*, Vol. 26, No. 6 (November–December 1967), pp. 1760–1767.

[4] Robert E. Johnson, "Water and Osmotic Economy on Survival Rations," *Journal of the American Dietetic Association*, Vol. 45, No. 2 (August 1964), pp. 124–129.

[5] Sheldon Margen, *Progress in Nutrition*, Avi Publishing, Westport, Conn., 1971, p. 127.

or other parts of the body may lead to a water disturbance. A deviation of 10 per cent, above or below, from the ideal water content of the body will result in difficulties.

If large amounts of water are lost through perspiration during work in high temperatures or under similar conditions, the loss of sodium may result in weakness and other debilitating symptoms. The use of salt tablets may be recommended by a physician.

The World's Water Supply

A WHO survey[6] indicated that only 11 per cent of the present urban population had good or fair water supplies, leaving 89 per cent

[6] "Water," *World Health*, July–August 1964, pp. 12–33.

with water supplies that were "unsatisfactory" or "grossly unsatisfactory." Furthermore, in most of the 75 countries surveyed, efforts to remedy the situation and also to prepare for the rising population fall far short of both objectives.

The need to make adequate provision for this important nutrient is greatest in South Central Asia, Southeast Asia, Africa south of the Sahara, and tropical South America. Individual countries in direst need are India, Indonesia, the Philippines, Nigeria, Brazil, Pakistan, the Republic of Korea, and Taiwan.

The earth has as much water now as it has ever had, but because of greater requirements for living, many other aspects must be considered. Efforts to tame the rivers, to prevent contamination of water, and to provide water needed to grow food for the increasing popula-

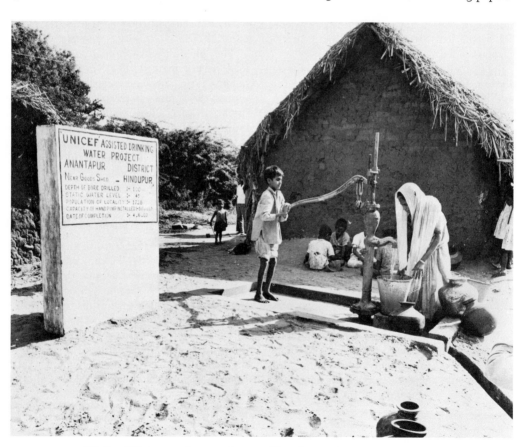

FIGURE 18–2. *Water supply must be considered with food supply for developing nations.* (UNICEF Photo/Buss)

tion are needed. Berg and others[7] contend that a mass improvement in the water supply of a developing nation needs to be emphasized with a food supply. A good diet may be of little avail if people are drinking contaminated water that results in diseases which undermine their health. Food may be contaminated if water is added as an ingredient during wash-

ing, if food is cooled by ice, or if cannery cooling water enters defects in the seams of cans.[8] To predict rainfall accurately, to turn the world's arid zones into productive areas, to reclaim land from the sea, to desalinate seawater for human consumption, and to develop new ways for treating, storing, and collecting water are other ways to ensure a clean, plentiful, and convenient water supply to the peoples of the world.

[7] Alan Berg, Nevin S. Scrimshaw, and David Call, *Nutrition, National Development, and Planning*, MIT Press, Cambridge, Mass., 1973, pp. 259–260.

[8] *Health Hazards of the Human Environment*, World Health Organization, 1972, Geneva, p. 73.

SELECTED REFERENCES

Albanese, Anthony A., *Newer Methods of Nutritional Biochemistry*, Academic Press, Inc., New York, 1972, p. 102.

Astrand, P. O. "Nutrition and Physical Performance," in Miloslav Rechcigl, Jr. (ed.), *Food, Nutrition and Health*, Vol. 16, S. Karger, Basel, 1973, pp. 75–77.

Berg, Alan, Neven S. Scrimshaw, and David Call, *Nutrition, National Development and Planning*, The MIT Press, Cambridge, Mass., 1973.

Davidson, Stanley, R. Passmore, and J. F. Brock, *Human Nutrition and Dietetics*, The Williams & Wilkins Company, Baltimore, 1972, Chapter 8.

Health Hazards of the Human Environment, World Health Organization, Geneva, 1972, Chapter 2.

Margen, Sheldon, *Progress in Human Nutrition*, Avi Publishing Company, Westport, Conn., 1971, pp. 119–120.

Randall, H. T., "Water, Electrolytes, and Acid–Base Balance," in Robert S. Goodhart and Maurice E. Shils (eds.), *Modern Nutrition and Disease*, Lea & Febiger, Philadelphia, 1973, pp. 324–361.

Robinson, Corinne H., *Fundamentals of Normal Nutrition*, Macmillan Publishing Co., Inc., New York, 1973, Chapter 9.

Robinson, James, "Water the Indispensable Nutrient," *Nutrition Today*, Vol. 5, No. 1 (Spring 1970), pp. 16–21, 28–29.

Nutrition and Dental Health

Throughout history man has been plagued by miseries concerning his teeth and gums. For example, in 1500 B.C. Egyptian pharaohs often had severe tooth and gum disease, as shown by X rays of the royal mummies. England's Queen Elizabeth I suffered from constant toothaches during her reign from 1558 to 1603. A possible cause was her fondness for honey. George Washington had a great deal of trouble with his false teeth, which were carved from wood and ivory.

Tooth decay is one of the most common diseases of mankind. This condition is so common that most individuals do not consider dental decay as a disease but rather as one of the inevitable hazards of living. Nutritional factors are often mentioned as causative or therapeutic agents for this condition.

Prevalence of Dental Caries

The picture of dental health in this country is alarming. According to government statistics, over 95 per cent of all Americans suffer from some form of dental disease. Approximately 25 million Americans are toothless, and there is a 50 per cent chance that persons reaching 60 will have lost all their teeth. Approximately one third of the population do not receive dental care. Low income and limited education correlate highly with little or no dental care. Many small children have one or more decayed teeth, and by school age approximately 90 per cent of our children are afflicted with dental caries. By the age of 15, many youth have dental caries in their permanent teeth and have lost on the average of at least two teeth. American mouths have an estimated 1 billion unfilled cavities, in spite of the population spending billions of dollars for dental care. The *Ten-State Nutrition Survey*[1] discovered poor dental health associated with low levels of dental care in many segments of the population.

Population Survey of Dental Health

Dental caries appear to be a disease of civilization. When native tribes are exposed to our refined foods, dental caries increase. When Eskimo groups lived near trading posts and the diet was changed to be comparable to that of the traders, the incidence of dental

[1] *Highlights, Ten-State Nutrition Survey, 1968–1970,* DHEW Publication No. (HSM) 72–8134, Center for Disease Control, Health Services and Mental Health Administration, U.S. Department of Health, Education, and Welfare, Atlanta, Ga., p. 10.

caries was extremely high: 83.3 per cent of the males and 90.5 per cent of the females.

A study of primitive tribes revealed a relationship of dental caries to diet. Orr and Gilks[2] found that an African tribe, the Masai, living mainly on milk, meat, and blood, had a very low caries rate. But another African tribe, the Kikuku, that lived largely on cereals, roots, and fruit had more dental decay.

Population studies were made of children in a number of European countries during World War II. There was a marked decrease in the incidence of caries among Norwegian children during the war period. This was attributed to the reduced consumption of sugar, refined flour, candy, and soft drinks. Fewer dental caries were also found among children in England; this was probably due to better general nutrition resulting from various distribution and fortification programs. In both England and Norway there was increased consumption of unrefined grain products, vegetables, and fish.

In 1952 the National Research Council of the National Academy of Sciences made a survey of all the literature[3] that had been published on the prevalence of tooth decay and possible causative factors. Over 2,000 studies were examined. The significant conclusion was that both heredity and environment have a strong effect on the incidence of decay.

This survey also indicated that an increase in the consumption of highly processed cereals and sugar leads to a concurrent increase in the rate of tooth decay. Guttorm Toverud of the Norwegian Dental Schools stated that dental caries decreased when sugar and sugar products were restricted. Studies showing a reduction in tooth decay after food habits were changed to a lower consumption of sugar and sugar products have also been reported in Great Britain, Hungary, Belgium, France, Germany, Italy, Switzerland, the Netherlands, and the United States.

In studies of primitive population, according to Shaw,[4] it is difficult to determine whether populations or specific individuals are caries-resistant genetically, because of good nutrition during tooth development, or if bacterial and other environmental factors were not present. For many decades the Indian population appeared to be caries-resistant genetically. Dunning and Shaw[5] raised the question of unconsidered variables, such as high fluoride levels in the enamel and dentine of Indian teeth, infrequency of eating, low availability of monosaccharides and disaccharides, deficient supply of kcalories, and an abundance of sunshine throughout the year. All these factors would contribute to a low incidence of dental caries.

In these population studies, one factor seems to have an important impact, the amount of the fluorine in the water supply. People living in areas where there were minute amounts of fluorine in the drinking water had significantly lower rates of dental caries. At least 16 countries reported similar, uniform results when fluoridated water supplies were used.

Five of the western agricultural stations in the United States have studied dental health of children as related to research of nutritional status. Dietary differences were ruled out, but the fluorine in the water supply was the most important factor in dental protection. In addition, it was noted that the hardness of the water had a favorable relationship.

Dental health surveys in the United States, according to Nizel,[6] indicate that the people in

---

[2] J. B. Orr and J. L. Gilks, "Studies of Nutrition: The Physique and Health of Two African Tribes," *Medical Research Council Special Report Series No. 155*, His Majesty's Stationery Office, London, 1931.

[3] Committee on Dental Health, A *Survey of the Literature of Dental Caries*, Publication 225, National Academy of Sciences—National Research Council, Washington, D.C., 1952.

[4] James H. Shaw, "Present Knowledge of Nutrition and Dental Caries," in *Present Knowledge in Nutrition*, 3rd ed., Nutrition Foundation, New York, 1967, Chap. 10.

[5] J. M. Dunning and James H. Shaw, "Variables Influencing Resistance to Dental Caries," in G. Blix (ed.), *Nutrition and Caries Prevention*, Swedish Nutrition Foundation, Stockholm, 1965.

[6] A. E. Nizel, "Nutrition and Oral Problems," in M. Rechcigl, Jr. (ed.), *Food, Nutrition and Health*, Vol. 16, S. Karger, Basel, 1973, pp. 228–230.

the New England and northwestern areas of the country have about twice the dental caries as the inhabitants of the south central states. The favorable conditions for dental health may be due to natural fluorides or the presence of other trace elements that exert cariogenic or cariostatic activity in the water supplies used by southern natives. Sunshine, humidity, and temperature may be influential environmental factors. Genetic factors and endocrine balance are other influences.

In some areas of Africa, Indochina, and Asia there is little evidence of dental caries. Ethiopia has the lowest mean of decayed, missing, or filled teeth of a number of populations that have been surveyed; the Aleuts in Alaska have the highest mean. Americans show the highest incidence of dental caries. Evidence for this chronic condition of dental health is usually characterized by a general state of malnutrition based on excesses, particularly sugar, and possible imbalances and deficiencies of essential nutrients.

Nutrition and Tooth Formation

The kind of diet a mother had before conception will be reflected in the teeth of her children. Certainly the quality of teeth is markedly influenced by the adequacy of the diet during pregnancy. Prenatal factors affect the deciduous teeth (baby teeth) far more than factors after birth.

At the early stage of the fourth fetal week, the tooth buds of the first teeth form. Calcification begins at about 20 weeks on the dentine and enamel of deciduous teeth. Obviously, tooth buds must be formed even before that time. Most of the tooth buds for the permanent teeth are formed before birth. The nutrients for these teeth must naturally be supplied through the mother's diet.

Children whose mothers had very poor diets are usually rated very low from a pediatric standpoint. They have a low resistance, which results in a greater number of illnesses during the first few months of their life. These

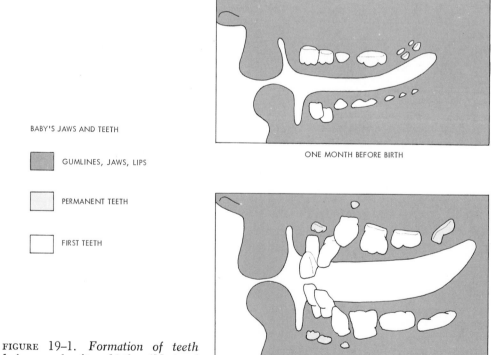

BABY'S JAWS AND TEETH

GUMLINES, JAWS, LIPS

PERMANENT TEETH

FIRST TEETH

ONE MONTH BEFORE BIRTH

NINE MONTHS AFTER BIRTH

FIGURE 19-1. *Formation of teeth before and after birth.* (*National Dairy Council*)

illnesses or even minor upsets will have an influence upon the quality of both baby and permanent tooth development.

That portion of the deciduous teeth which is formed after birth may show severe deformity. Two thirds of all pitting and irregular formation of enamel observed on permanent teeth occurs during this infancy period before the child is 10 months of age. Clinically, they are not observable until the child is 6 to 12 years old. It is difficult to realize that this early period has such an important influence on tooth health in later years.

Investigators are inclined to believe that these tooth disturbances are more frequent when the mother has had a poor prenatal diet. Caries susceptibility, therefore, seems to be influenced greatly by the nutrients received by children during the entire period of development, including the prenatal period.

The role of nutrition is important in determining if an individual will have good oc-clusion of his teeth—that is, whether the teeth will be arranged in the jaw so that they will function efficiently. Nutrition is important for the proper growth and development of bones and teeth. If tooth eruption is retarded owing to severe dietary deficiency, there may be some effect upon tooth arrangement in the jaw. If dental caries occur and one tooth is lost, partially destroyed, or chipped, the occlusion of the teeth will be unfavorably influenced.

There are a number of unanswered questions about the relation of nutritional status to dental development. More research has been done on bone development than dental development, according to Garn and Russell.[7] It is known that tooth eruption is slightly delayed in malnourished individuals. Tooth formation is advanced among individuals who are fatter or ahead developmentally. In nutrition surveys, however, it is important, according to these researchers, to pinpoint the phenomena at particular ages that reflect nutritional decay.

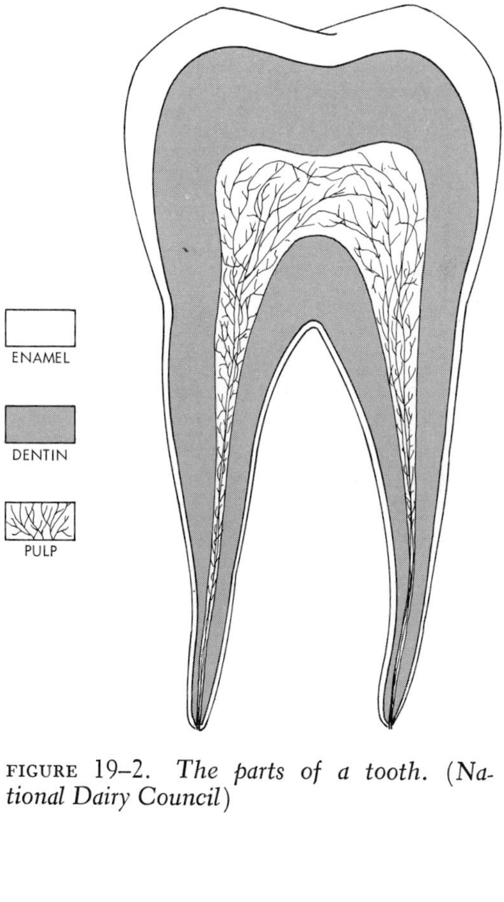

Supporting Structure of Teeth

In considering dental health, some attention needs to be given to the supporting structures of the teeth, sometimes called tooth settings. These structures are the jaw and the gums. Dentists and scientists refer to these structures as the periodontal tissues.

The periodontal tissues have metabolic processes similar to those of bone or soft tissue elsewhere in the body, according to Mayer.[8] These tissues react to aging, deficiencies, infection, disease, or body changes. In addition, allergies, irradiation, poisons, and psychosomatic disorders have an influence on these supporting structures of the teeth. Diseased periodontal tissues, in turn, may influence the health of other parts of the body. Discomfort in eating often interferes with the consumption of an adequate diet.

Authorities indicate that inadequate nutrition has long been considered a contributory

ENAMEL

DENTIN

PULP

FIGURE 19–2. *The parts of a tooth.* (*National Dairy Council*)

[7] Stanley M. Garn and Albert L. Russell, "The Effects of Nutritional Extremes on Dental Development," *American Journal of Clinical Nutrition,* Vol. 24, No. 3 (March 1971), pp. 285–286.

[8] Jean Mayer, *Human Nutrition,* Charles C Thomas, Springfield, Ill., 1972, pp. 511–512.

cause of difficulties in these structures because periodontal tissues are especially susceptible to an inadequate diet. Food can perform two important functions as far as tooth settings are concerned. First, food supplies the nutrients so essential for replacement. Second, the physical character of the food has a decided bearing on these tissues. Soft foods, sticky foods, or foods requiring little mastication may cause bacterial action. Foods that cling to the teeth, especially at the gum line, are to be avoided. Dentists sometimes refer to coarse fibrous foods, which require vigorous chewing, as detergents. The periodontium appears to be more severely disturbed by metabolic upsets than the tooth itself.

The health of the gums is particularly important. Surveys indicate that the major cause of loss of teeth after age 30 is gum disorders. The tissue gradually becomes detached from the tooth, and with this loss of support, teeth may become loose and extraction may be necessary.

Theories About Dental Caries

Dental caries are caused by the interaction of the metabolic products of oral microorganisms and the tooth substance, which results in tooth decay, according to Shaw.[9] These bacteria colonize in the pits and fissures of the occlusal surfaces in areas where teeth touch each other, and in some instances, on the smooth surfaces as well. Carbohydrates that ferment are essential for the metabolism of these bacteria. This process, in turn, creates acidic products that facilitate dental decay.

The bacterial origin of dental caries has been established beyond reasonable doubt, not only in animal experimental studies but also in man. These microorganisms can be transmitted from one animal with active lesions to another of the same species having no previous evidence of caries activity and can produce caries in the latter. This fact points to the necessity of giving dental attention to any cavity.

Dreizen[10] reports that the caries process begins on the surface of the tooth and progresses inward toward the pulp. Reference is made to the term *plaque*, a gelatinous accumulation of oral bacteria and salivary mucin that forms on the teeth. Areas of teeth that harbor microorganisms so they are undisturbed during mastication or cleaning are danger points. The type of oral flora related to dental caries has the capacity to convert ingested food into specific acids. When the concentration of these acid end products is sufficiently high, dental caries are activated.

The single most important dietary influence, according to Dreizen, is frequent, liberal intake of carbohydrate in a form that has the capability of penetrating the dental plaque and of undergoing microbial fermentation with acid formation. Direct measurements of acid production within the dental plaque following a carbohydrate meal indicate that harmful effects may begin within 4 minutes after food is taken into the mouth and may be maintained for 30 to 45 minutes. The production of caries is sporadic rather than continuous and is directly related to the quantity of carbohydrate intake. Human and animal experimentation has proved that tooth decay occurs only with diets containing carbohydrates.

The type and form of the carbohydrate are important, as well as the frequency of intake. Sucrose seems most conducive; starch is the least. Solid sugars are more cariogenic than those in liquid form. Carbohydrate foods that remain in the mouth for a very short period of time have a lower caries-producing capacity than foods, such as hard candies, that are retained in the mouth for considerable periods of time. Many acid foods and fruits with low sugar concentration are relatively noncariogenic. The rate of flow and the neutralizing power of saliva, particularly when coupled with mastication, tend to depress the development of caries.

This theory about carbohydrates has a special bearing on in-between meals and

[9] James H. Shaw, "Diet Regulations for Caries Prevention," *Nutrition News*, Vol. 36, No. 1 (February 1973), pp. 1, 4.

[10] Samuel Dreizen, "The Role of Diet in Dental Decay," *Nutrition News*, Vol. 29, No. 1 (February 1966), pp. 1–4.

TABLE 19–1

Sugar Content of Common Foods

FOOD	SERVING	AMOUNT OF SUGAR (tsp)
Angel or sponge cake	1 average piece	6
Chocolate cake, two-layer, iced	1 average piece	15
Apple pie	1 medium piece	12
Candy bar	5 oz.	20
Cherry pie	1 medium piece	14
Custard or coconut pie	1 medium piece	10
Pumpkin pie	1 medium piece	10
Ginger snap	1 medium	1
Molasses cookie	3 (½-in. diam.)	2
Brownie	1 average	3
Doughnut, plain	1 average	4
Cream puff, iced, custard filled	1 average	5
Custard, baked	½ cup	4
Gelatin	½ cup	4
Jam	1 tbs (level)	3
Jelly	1 tbs (level)	2 ½
Marmalade	1 tbs (level)	3
Chocolate fudge	1½-in. square	4
Chewing gum	1 peppermint stick	1–2
Hard candy	1 piece	1–3
Marshmallow	1 average	1–4
Maple syrup	1 tbs (level)	2½
Ice cream	1 cone or bar	5–6
Chocolate milk	1 cup (5 oz)	6
Sweet cider	6-oz glass	4½
Soft drinks	6-oz bottle	4
Fruit cocktail	½ cup	5

SOURCE: Dental Public Health Committee of the Academy of Dentistry, Toronto, Canada.

snacks. The use of candy, gum, soft drinks, doughnuts, and Danish pastry would be particularly injurious to teeth. Many people are completely unaware of the large sugar content of foods (see Table 19–1). From this information about the sugar content of some common foods one can understand how the American people consume much more sugar than is necessary.

Another aspect of the theory that carbohydrates may have a large bearing upon dental caries is the fact that sugar may replace more wholesome food. When a sweet dessert is eaten instead of fruit, or when a soft drink is consumed instead of milk, certain dietary essentials may be lacking. An inadequate diet may be reflected in tooth health.

Other factors influence the incidence of dental caries. Residents in highly developed countries appear to be more susceptible to caries than people in some of the primitive societies. The genetic factor has possibilities. The saliva is important.

The whole environment, Shaw believes, has a strong bearing on the incidence of caries. Parameters to consider are quantity and types of available foods, dietary patterns, economic status, actual hours of sunshine, humidity, type and amount of clothing worn, oral hygiene, composition of water supplies, and dental health facilities. Focus is on the food component, carbohydrate, with an emphasis on those types that are most cariogenic, sugar, for example. The consumption of sweets and the frequency of eating are vital factors to be considered.

The use of fluorine seems to have considerable value in reducing dental caries among children. This was discovered after a study of teeth that became mottled because of an excess of fluorine: the enamel of the tooth became pitted and appeared chalky white and stained, or corroded, in appearance. However, these teeth did not have caries. Experimentation revealed that a considerably smaller amount of fluorine in the water would prevent dental caries and avoid the mottled look. Since then, surveys in many parts of the world have showed that, where one part of fluorine is added to 1 million parts of water, teeth will be formed that are much more caries-resistant than teeth in areas where the fluorine content of the water is lower.

Later demonstrations in the United States and other countries with a consideration of racial, economic, and dietary factors revealed, according to Shaw,[11] that optimal ingestion of fluoride resulted in major reductions of dental caries in children which was reflected in later adult life. Studies of various types gave conclusive evidence that levels of fluoride conducive to the prevention of dental caries had no harmful effects on the human body. This evidence led to increased adoption of fortification of water supplies with fluoride as an inexpensive, safe, and effective control, and to reduction of dental caries. About 60 million people in the United States are using controlled fluoridated water supplies.

Less malocclusion as a result of fluoridation has been reported by Erikson and Graziano[12] in a 10-year study comparing the incidence of malocclusion in a community with fluoridated water and in a neighboring control community. Periodontal disease was also less prevalent in the fluoridated area than in the control community.

Fluorides are incorporated into the apatite crystals that form the calcified structure of the tooth, according to Nizel,[13] establishing a high resistance to the action of acids produced by cariogenic microorganisms. After the eruption of the crown of the tooth, it is impossible to incorporate the fluoride ion into the apatite structure. With less effect, the fluoride ion may be incorporated after eruption by applying fluoride solutions to the surface layer of the enamel of children or by brushing the teeth with a fluoride-containing dentifrice three or four times a day immediately after meals.

Nutrients for Dental Health

There seems to be considerable evidence that teeth are largely living tissue which must be nourished like other tissue. Special tooth-forming cells have to be fed nutrients to make healthy teeth. The jaws, gums, and other supporting structures need them also. Although all nutrients are needed for good tooth health, several do play a unique role. Among them are vitamins A, C, and D, calcium, fluoride, phosphorus, and protein.

Cellular development and the appearance of teeth is affected by the adequacy or inadequacy of vitamin A in the diet, according to Dreizen.[14] The enamel-forming cells in the developing tooth form defective enamel if there is a deficiency of vitamin A. In infants, the enamel and dentin may be poorly calcified. A vitamin A deficiency while the molars are developing during pregnancy has resulted in small molars in the infant.

Vitamin C is required for healthy dentin and periodontal tissues. Not only is there a degeneration of the cellular layer forming the dentin if vitamin C is deficient, but the same is true of enamel-forming cells, resulting in defective enamel of teeth. Gums become inflamed, spongy, and bleed easily.

The first and most prominent change be-

[11] James H. Shaw, "Present Knowledge of Fluoride," in *Present Knowledge in Nutrition*, 3rd ed., Nutrition Foundation, New York, 1967, Chap. 30.

[12] D. M. Erikson and F. W. Graziano, "Prevalence of Malocclusion in Seventh-Grade Children in Two North Carolina Cities," *Journal of American Dental Association*, Vol. 73, No. 2 (February 1966), pp. 124–128.

[13] Abraham E. Nizel, "The Contribution of the Science and Practice of Nutrition to the Prevention and Control of Dental Caries," *Food and Nutrition News*, Vol. 41, No. 4 (January 1970), pp. 1, 4.

[14] Samuel Dreizen, "The Importance of Nutrition in Tooth Development," *Nutrition News*, Vol. 35, No. 1 (February 1972) pp. 1, 4.

cause of a lack of vitamin D is the appearance of disturbed calcification of the dentin, followed by retardation of dentin formation. The ability to calcify the matrix structure of the predentin layer of the developing tooth is impaired. The formation of the enamel layer is also affected. The bony structures supporting the teeth are weakened by a lack of vitamin D, according to Shaw and Sweeney.[15] There appears to be a definite correlation between the mean annual hours of sunshine and the average incidence of dental caries among children. A possible explanation is that exposure to sunshine made available a greater amount of vitamin D. The role of vitamin E in human tooth formation has not been defined, but animal experimentation leads to speculation that this vitamin may contribute to dental health.

Calcium is an important constituent of teeth. During human tooth development, enamel has a priority for available calcium and dentin has preference over bone. Calcium is required for the bony structures supporting the teeth. A desirable calcium–phosphorus ratio during development of teeth is essential to proper calcification of enamel and dentin. Phosphates when added to animal diets appeared effective in the reduction of dental caries. The mechanism is not clear.[16] The role of magnesium has not been documented for human dental health, but a speculative role is indicated to prevent disturbances of mineralization, according to Dreizen,[17] plus malformation of the enamel. The need for trace elements other than fluoride has not been demonstrated.

A relationship between protein metabolism and oral health is contended by Cheraskin.[18]

Within the limits of brief observations, there appear to be significant parallelisms between oral health and protein metabolism. The relevant fact is that protein is an essential ingredient in the development of the osteoid matrix. In a study of the gingival state of dental students, the group receiving protein supplementation showed evidence of striking positive changes, according to Cheraskin.

Multiple Factors in Control of Dental Caries

Nizel[19] recommends a broad and all-encompassing approach to the patient with dental caries. To lean on any one theory is narrow and insular. Of the possible variables influencing the control of caries, Nizel is of the opinion that nutrition is the least applied and the most neglected in dental education.

Recommended Diet for Healthy Teeth

When people eat the recommended foods in the daily diet, there is considerable assurance that they are counteracting dental caries. If the daily diet, particularly during the growing period, contains 3 to 4 cups of milk, an egg, a glass of citrus fruit juice, and servings of other fruits and green-leafy and dark-yellow vegetables, plus butter, fortified margarine, and some chewy foods, the diet should be adequate. Candy, soft drinks, cakes, cookies and the like should be eaten in moderation. The same might be said about desserts. It is much wiser to have fruit for dessert than rich, sweet dishes.

The physical character of food, according to the American Dental Association, provides the exercise required by the teeth and jaw muscles. Mastication, by forcing unrefined, raw, and coarse foods over the teeth and gums, aids in cleansing them. Fibrous, granular foods like fresh fruits and vegetables are recommended. Foods such as white bread, jams, or mashed potatoes tend to cling to the surface of the teeth and to impact between the teeth. Cutting down on the consumption of sweetened beverages, candy, syrups, jams and jellies, or other confections during and between meals is advised.[20]

[15] James H. Shaw and Edward A. Sweeney, "Nutrition in Relation to Dental Medicine," in Robert S. Goodhart and Maurice E. Shils (eds.), *Modern Nutrition in Health and Disease*, Lea & Febiger, Philadelphia, 1973, pp. 745–746.

[16] Robert S. Harris, "Phosphates: A Promising Agent for Use in the Control of Dental Caries," *Nutrition News*, Vol. 34, No. 1 (February 1971), pp. 1, 4.

[17] Dreizen, op. cit., p. 1.

[18] E. Cheraskin, "Protein and Oral Health," *Food and Nutrition News*, Vol. 38, No. 5 (February 1967), pp. 1, 4.

[19] Nizel, op. cit., p. 1.

[20] Nizel, op. cit., p. 1.

The frequency of eating, particularly of adherent, plaque-forming carbohydrate snacks, is closely related to the incidence of caries in teen-agers. Further research is suggested to appraise the caries-producing ability of individual foods.[21]

Maintaining Dental Health

The dental profession agrees that good dental health habits will contribute a great deal to the reduction of dental caries and to giving a child a better chance for retaining his natural teeth. Baby teeth demand special attention so that permanent teeth will be well spaced and formed. It is equally true that a child who grows up in an environment of dental neglect may, with a degree of certainty, have difficulty with his teeth.[22] The work of Sweeney, Saffir, and de Leon,[23] demonstrates the relation of malnutrition to oral health. Among Guatemalan children with severe malnutrition, 73 per cent had dental problems. Related problems were low socioeconomic status, infectious diseases, and neglect of oral problems because they were not life-threatening. Good dental health requires

persistent individual effort, plus the professional assistance of a dentist.

The American Dental Association recommends the following measures:

1. A well-balanced diet for the growth of teeth and supporting structures.
2. Restriction of sweets, with an emphasis on reducing the present consumption. Avoid frequent snacking.
3. Brushing teeth immediately after eating, or rinsing the mouth with water if brushing is impossible.
4. Regular visits to the dentist every 6 months or as often as the dentist recommends.
5. Fluoridation of community water supply.

It must be remembered that keeping a mouth healthy is a lifetime job. People should not wait until they have a toothache before going to the dentist.

Relation of Dental Health to Total Health

The health of an individual reflects many complex factors. There is no question, however, that teeth which are functioning properly can contribute a great deal to the total health of the individual. They have an important function in preparing food for the first stage of the digestive process. There is a quite striking psychological effect on an individual whose teeth are in such condition that he cannot masticate his food well. Doctors have noted that illness may be reflected in the condition of the gums or even in the teeth. Healthy teeth are to be prized.

---

[21] "Frequency of Eating and Dental Caries Prevalence," *Nutrition Reviews*, Vol. 32, No. 5 (May 1974), pp. 139–141.

[22] "Malnutrition and Oral Health of Children," *Nutrition Reviews*, Vol. 32, No. 2 (February 1974), pp. 44–47.

[23] Edward A. Sweeney, Arthur J. Saffir, and Romeo de Leon, "Linear Hypoplasia of Deciduous Incisor Teeth in Malnourished Children," *American Journal of Clinical Nutrition*, Vol. 24, No. 1 (January 1971), pp. 29–31.

SELECTED REFERENCES

Davidson, Stanley, R. Passmore, and J. F. Brock, *Human Nutrition and Dietetics*, The Williams & Wilkins Company, Baltimore, 1972, Chapter 53.

"Dental Caries Prevalence and Trace Elements Other Than Fluoride," *Nutrition Reviews*, Vol. 32, No. 4 (April 1974), pp. 120–122.

Dreitzen, Samuel, "The Importance of Nutrition in Tooth Development," *Nutrition News*, Vol. 35, No. 1 (February 1972), pp. 1, 4.

Goodhart, Robert S., and Maurice E. Shils (eds.), *Modern Nutrition in Health and Disease*, Lea & Febiger, Philadelphia, 1973, Chapter 27.

Harris, Robert S., "Phosphates: A Promising Agent for Use in the Control of Dental Caries," *Nutrition News*, Vol. 34, No. 1 (February 1971), pp. 1, 4.

Hearings Before the Select Committee on Nutrition and Human Needs of the U.S. Senate, Ninety-third Congress, First Session, *Phosphate Research and Dental Decay*, Part 6, April 16, 1973, U.S. Government Printing Office, Washington, D.C., 1973.

"Malnutrition and Oral Health in Children," *Nutrition Reviews*, Vol. 32, No. 2 (February 1974), pp. 44–47.

Mayer, Jean, *Human Nutrition*, Charles C Thomas, Publisher, Springfield, Ill., 1972, Chapter 56.

Nizel, A. E., "Nutrition and Oral Problems," in Miloslav Rechcigl, Jr. (ed.), *Food, Nutrition and Health*, Vol. 16, S. Karger, Basel, 1973, pp. 226, 252.

——————, "Nursing Bottle Syndrome—Rampant Dental Caries in Young Children," *Nutrition News*, Vol. 38, No. 1 (February 1975), pp. 1, 4.

Report of a WHO Scientific Group, *The Etiology and Prevention of Dental Caries*, World Health Organization Technical Report Series, No. 494, World Health Organization, Geneva, 1972.

Shaw, James H., "Diet Regulations for Caries Prevention," *Nutrition News*, Vol. 36, No. 1 (February 1973), pp. 1, 4.

20

Geography, Culture, and Nutrition

Food gives meaning to life, according to Lee.[1] It serves as the root of meaningful behavior: as a center for social warmth as families prepare food together or share it with guests, as a point of relatedness, such as giving gifts of food, or as a means of creativity.

Mead[2] comments that when Americans travel to the homes of others, whether to the heart of Africa, a peasant community in Europe, a village in the Near East, or the like, they are asked to eat a set of foods that may be unfamiliar and in combinations that seem unreasonable. In these days of great human mobility, an understanding of the meaning of cultural values in relation to people's food habits can be rewarding. Each individual, according to Bernays,[3] is born into a culture or

group matrix that influences the formation of a tenacious pattern of foods consumed. In the effort toward better world understanding, an appreciation of international food cultures might be a good beginning.

Frame of Reference

It is erroneous to refer to a typical American, French, Indian, or East African diet. The diet of each nation, because of agricultural, economic, and social influences, varies from region to region and actually from family to family. Only generalizations on some of the common foods and indicated trends in eating patterns can be made. Each food pattern must be examined with caution and with the realization that it is not absolute, but relative.

There are many influences on the eating habits of a group or nation. Queen[4] points out that in a primitive, isolated society people subsist on whatever food is available to them. When the society advances in civilization and

[1] Dorothy Lee, "Why Do People Eat What They Eat?" *Proceedings Annual Food Forum*, sponsored by the United Fruit Company, New York, November 5, 1954.

[2] Margaret Mead, "Cultural Patterning of Nutritionally Relevant Behavior," *Journal of the American Dietetic Association*, Vol. 25, No. 8 (August 1949), pp. 677–680.

[3] Edward L. Bernays, "The Study of Man and His Food Habits," *Proceedings of the Sixth Annual Food Forum*, sponsored by the United Fruit Company, New York, November 8–9, 1956.

[4] George S. Queen, "Culture, Economics, and Food Habits," *Journal of the American Dietetic Association*, Vol. 33, No. 10 (October 1958), pp. 1044–1052.

256

transportation develops, diets may be modified and enriched by the introduction of a new cereal, a new farm animal, or a more modern method of agricultural production. Income, however, may continue to limit the food choices of families.

A geographic approach to food prejudices, according to Simoons,[5] can facilitate the understanding of cultural food patterns. The avoidance of fish, for example, appears sporadically from the western regions of the Sahara Desert to Tibet and Mongolia. The avoidance of fish in Africa is not associated with organized religions. Rather, it is due to indifference or to the belief that fish is an unclean food. In Tibet and Mongolia, the practice is related to the Buddhist reluctance to take life. Many of these areas have abundant fish supplies that could contribute to the nutritive quality of their dietaries.

Westerners have reacted strongly to the eating of dogs and insects because such practices would violate their sensibilities. Although scientists have urged consideration of the use of termites and grasshoppers with their high nutritive value, especially protein, the idea has low acceptance.

Emphasis on vegetarianism has strong historical roots as well as geographical implications and stems from a love of life and a reluctance to destroy it. Religious ties are noted with Hinduism, Buddhism, Jainism (an Indian variant), and some aspects of Christianity. Many of the questions regarding the geographical origin of vegetarianism remain unanswered. For example, do various types of vegetarians have common roots and how has the idea spread?

There is a strong aversion to milk and milk products in parts of India, Southeast and East Asia, and Africa. Some people view milk as unclean as well as a disgusting bodily secretion. However, milk bars for young people are becoming popular in Southeast Asia, and dried and canned milk is more acceptable today as an infant food. Regional differences still need to be explored.

[5] Frederick J. Simoons, "The Geographic Approach to Food Prejudices," *Food Technology*, Vol. 20, No. 3 (March 1966), pp. 42–44.

Regional Impact on American Food Patterns

Regional dietary patterns are becoming less sharply defined because of a heightened trend in family mobility and travel as well as other influences. Regional foods are now enjoyed in other parts of the nation. Such variations as exist stem from prevalence of native foods due to climate, soil, type of farming, and other dominating aspects; the impact of ethnic, religious, socioeconomic, and other aspects of background; local customs; urban or rural living, although the differences are narrowing; and similar influences. American Indians have unique food patterns that incorporate native foods. Some of these foods are found in contemporary diets. The nutrition student should become alert to nutritional strengths and shortcomings of food patterns.

In the South, there is an emphasis on such foods as hot breads, especially biscuits and cornbread; vegetable greens cooked with pork fat (often overcooked); pot liquor; fruit, especially oranges and watermelon; sweet potatoes; corn pone and hominy grits; nuts; fried chicken; ham; and fish and seafood. Groups within this region may have unique ways of preparing these foods. Food combinations may appear in culturally determined clusters, ac-

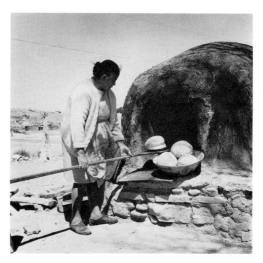

FIGURE 20–1. *A Jemez Indian baking traditional bread in a homemade oven.*

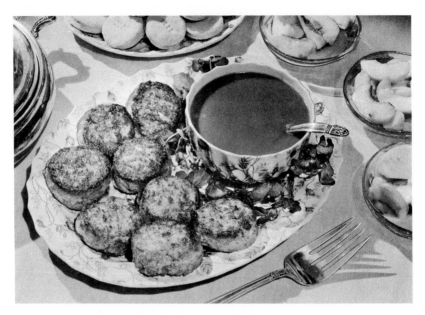

FIGURE 20–2. A plantation breakfast of beaten biscuits, sausage and pan
gravy, and fruit. (Armour and Company)

cording to Dickens[6] in a study done in the
Delta cotton belt. Biscuits, for example, were
more frequently eaten with boiled dried beans
and canned English peas, whereas cornbread
was consumed with turnip greens and boiled
field peas.

The influence of French and Creole cookery
is prevalent in Louisiana, particularly in New
Orleans and surrounding areas. Rice, too, is
eaten in this area. The people of the South
have clung to many of their specialties and
derive pleasure from serving these foods.

Spanish influence is dominant in the Southwest, and foods such as tamales, pinto beans,
tortillas, chili, and corn products may be a
part of the daily diet. In the Far West, the
abundance of fresh fruit and vegetables led to
the highlighting of salads in the daily diet. In
California, the influence of Oriental foods, including Hawaiian, is obvious. On the West
Coast, advantage is taken of the abundant supply of fish and other seafood.

Immigrants from Sweden, Germany, Poland, England, Switzerland, and other European countries have left an impact on the food
consumed by residents of the Midwest. Milk
and milk products, beef, pork, fruits and vegetables, especially in season, potatoes, wheat
products, eggs, and butter are among the
dominant dietary items. River and lake fish are
utilized. Many other foods have become available to this region through rapid transportation.

The food of people of the Eastern shoreline
has historical overtones, for this area was the
first to be settled. Fish, seafood chowders,
baked beans, brown bread, turkey, Indian pudding, and the like are typical menu items. The
foods of many ethnic groups, such as the
Irish, Italians, and Jews, also are part of the
daily eating patterns.

Other Cultural Food Patterns

National food patterns are developed largely
by what an individual's intimates in early life
enjoyed and considered wholesome to eat.
The emotional attachment to certain national
or group foods cannot be overestimated. It is

[6] Dorothy Dickens and B. Gillaspie, "Menu Patterns in the Delta Cotton Area," Journal of Home
Economics, Vol. 57, No. 6 (June 1965), pp. 431–
433.

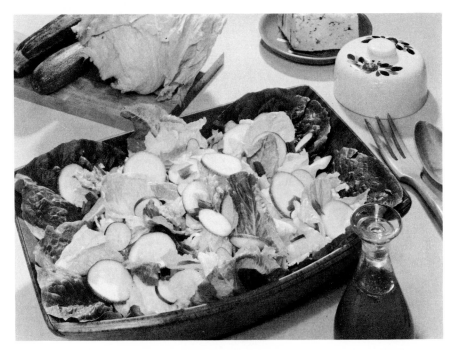

FIGURE 20–3. *Abundance of vegetables in the Far West leads to the frequent incorporation of a variety of salads in the diet.* (*Western Growers Association*)

sensible to incorporate these foods whenever possible in planning nutritious meals. It is easier for a person to make some modifications in his diet if there is the security of familiar foods.

The following descriptions must be considered as general points of departure and with a realization that many adaptations are typical.

Some African Food Habits

To discuss the food consumption of an entire continent is an unseemly assignment. There are 111 different ethnic groups identified for Africa south of the Sahara—the true Africa according to Grant.[7] Apart from the urban centers, people produce their own food. Most of the diets are characterized by an abundance of one or more foods high in carbo-

[7] Faye W. Grant, *Some Cultural Factors That Influence Food Habits in Parts of Africa*, A Talk presented at the Foods and Nutrition Agents of North Carolina Training Conference, Betsy Jeff Penn Training Center, Reidsville, N.C., April 20, 1966.

hydrate, such as cereals, including a variety of millets, sorghum, pennisetum, and Guinea and Indian corn (called *maize, mais*, and the like); rice and teff; and a variety of roots and tubers, such as white sweet potatoes, large white yams—unrelated to the American yam, tasting more like our white potato—cassava, and cocoyam (sometimes called *taro* in the Pacific islands). Plantain, a large variety of banana that is quite starchy and does not become sweet upon ripening, is used in many tropical areas. These foods constitute about 65 to 80 per cent of the energy value of the diets.

The amount and kind of meat consumed depends upon what is indigenous to the area in which individuals live. Developed areas consume the most. The following types have been identified with African foods: beef, lamb and mutton, pork, horse, camel, birds, palm squirrels, lizards, hedgehogs, fish, and burrowing squirrels. The meat that is used is incorporated into a sauce or a soupy stew, usually cooked in an iron pot, and accompanies

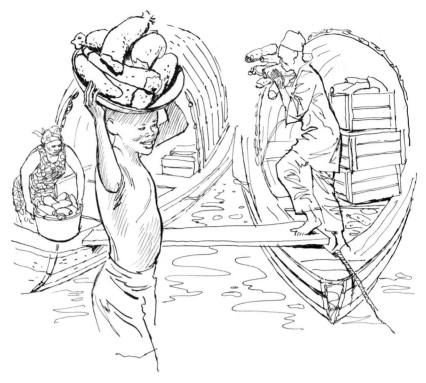

FIGURE 20–4. *Yams are an important item in the diet of many Africans.*

the stable carbohydrate food that is generally boiled or steamed, according to Grant.

Fruits included are bananas, oranges, avocadoes, grapefruit, papaya, pineapple, wild berries, guavas, mangoes, coconut, pawpaw, and melon. Children sometimes pick fruit on their way to school and eat it. The nutritive value of fruit appears to be largely unappreciated. Vegetables are tomatoes, peppers, onions, okra, eggplant, and some varieties of the squash family. Their availability depends on the amount of rainfall. Several varieties of beans and cowpeas are used in the stews and contribute to the nutritive value of the dietary. Peanuts (groundnuts) are widely used in some areas. Vegetable fats, such as oil from palm nuts, groundnuts, and coconuts, are used in cooking and to flavor foods.

Modern convenience foods have been developed such as instant *fufu* powder[8] made from cassava, which is used like potatoes in Ghana. This quick food saves the Ghanaian housewife the arduous and time-consuming task of preparing the cassava roots. The expense, no doubt, is greater.

Nichol[9] of the Nutrition Division of FAO made a survey of the protein and caloric concentration of diets in West Africa. The energy requirements of peoples in the Sahelian Zone, who consume sorghum and pennisetum, were considerably in excess of the requirements of the FAO Reference Man and Woman, in spite of their strenuous activity of herding cattle and walking miles for water. The protein requirements were met in excess of 200 per cent. In the Tropical Rain Forest Area (where manioc and dioscorea are consumed) a vast bulk of starchy roots are consumed, and yet the needs of protein and energy for those over 12 years of age were barely met. The

[8] Margaret Morris and Helen Strow, "Africa Tour," *Journal of Home Economics*, Vol. 66, No. 5 (May 1974), pp. 6–10.

[9] B. M. Nichol, "Protein and Caloric Concentration," *Nutrition Reviews*, Vol. 29, No. 4 (April 1971), pp. 83–88.

energy expenditure of these people may be less than the FAO Reference Man and Woman because the cultivation of root foods is done close to home and is easy.

In the younger age group in the sorghum–millet areas the situation differs from the excellent protein-kcalorie dietary intake of adults. Four-to-six-year-olds are often not given adequate food to meet their energy needs because parents are not aware of their high nutritional needs. Their protein intake is usually above requirements if the area has not suffered from drought or an epidemic disease. The preharvest time may be another critical period, sometimes identified as "hungry time." The "starchy root" consuming children of this age achieve only 70 to 80 per cent of their respective protein and kcalorie requirements. The low-quality dietary protein and the difficulty of consuming large amounts of this bulky and unattractive food account for the hindrances. Increasing the number of meals might improve the dietary intakes, but this plan is not compatible with lifestyles. Adequate vitamins and minerals are a separate problem to be solved in the form of fruits and vegetables, but the additional bulk increases the dilemma.

Greek Food Habits

A Greek meal is a family ritual, according to Valassi.[10] Bread is always on the table because each bite of food is accompanied with bread, even rice and spaghetti. Preparation of food is often time-consuming.

A variety of vegetables, raw or cooked, is consumed, including green beans, peas, cabbage, cauliflower, summer squash, cucumbers, okra, eggplant, tomatoes, spinach, and carrots. They are often cooked in meat broth and seasoned with onions, tomato paste, olive oil, and parsley. Sometimes meat is cooked with the vegetables. The main dish generally consists of vegetables, so these are eaten in generous amounts. Salads are an important part of the meal and are made from chopped,

shredded, or thinly sliced vegetables seasoned with oil and lemon or vinegar.

Fruits are consumed in large quantities, and include apricots, cherries, figs, melons, pears, plums, and quinces. They serve as the everyday dessert of the Greeks. The most popular meat is lamb, although considerable pork is consumed in northern Greece. Organ meats, as well as poultry and fresh fish, are well liked. Eggs are eaten more frequently at meals other than breakfast. Legumes are used extensively, especially among the lower-income groups. The most commonly used are beans, peas, lentils, and chick-peas. They are accompanied by olives and pickled relishes and often cooked with onions, tomatoes, celery, or carrots.

Greek bread is generally made from wheat, but it may be mixed with other cereals, such as barley, rye, and oats, according to Valassi. Large quantities of bread are consumed; thus the energy value of the diet comes largely from this source. Bread is usually eaten plain. Butter, jam, jelly or other spreads are seldom used.

Little fluid milk is consumed, but large amounts of yogurt are used. It may be eaten at the beginning of a meal with diced cucumber and olive oil, as a dessert, or as a topping on some vegetables or rice. Greeks are cheese eaters and incorporate it into their meals at all stages. Fresh feta cheese is incorporated into salads or added to the diet in other ways.

Italian Food Habits

Eating is an important part of the life of an Italian, according to Cantoni.[11] There are a number of different characteristics within this ethnic group, for each state or region holds traditions dearly. Northern Italians eat less pasta than southerners and may vary in other ways. From a homogeneous point of view, here are some generalizations about their food habits.

Milk is used in coffee but little is drunk or used in cooking. Goat's milk is preferred. An important ingredient in Italian meals, how-

[10] Kyriake V. Valassi, "Food Habits of the Greek-Americans," *American Journal of Clinical Nutrition*, Vol. 11, No. 9 (September 1962), pp. 240–248.

[11] Marjorie Cantoni, "Adapting Therapeutic Diets to the Eating Patterns of Italian-Americans," *American Journal of Clinical Nutrition*, Vol. 6, No. 5 (September–October 1958), pp. 548–555.

ever, is a wide variety of cheeses—parmesan, mozzarella, provolone, ricotta, and casicavallo. Bread is the leading food and is white, crusty, and varied in shape according to the part of Italy from which it originates. Pasta includes the macaroni, spaghetti, and egg noodles so characteristic of this group. Cornmeal is used in polenta, a thick mush served with meat and vegetables or in a casserole with sausage, tomato sauce, and cheese. Rice and cornmeal are characteristic dishes of northern Italians, whereas pasta is more popular in the south.

Meats are served frequently: roast or baked chicken, seasoned with oil and garlic; veal, as cutlets or scallopine; meat balls or loaf; Italian sausage; and chops, roasts, organ meats, and stews. Fish are popular. Vegetables include such favorites as broccoli, escarole, string beans, zucchini, other squash, asparagus, eggplant, artichokes, peppers, tomatoes, and many varieties of salad greens. Salads are eaten at least once a day and sometimes twice. Salad dressing consists of oil, vinegar, salt, pepper, and garlic. Fresh fruits in season are eaten as dessert.

Dietary calculations of typical northern and southern Italian diets indicate that nutritive requirements are adequately met on the whole, according to Cantoni.

Jewish Food Habits

The Orthodox Jewish dietary laws are based on Biblical and rabbinical regulations. The origin of these ideas has emerged from concepts about wholesomeness and appropriateness of foods for this faith. Foods used in accordance with these strict laws are designated *kosher*, known as *kashrut*, according to Siegel, Strassfeld, and Strassfeld.[12] This term has a threefold meaning: the food is fit or proper; the food can be eaten in accordance with Jewish dietary laws, that is, which foods are kosher and which are not; and it refers to the separation of milk from meat. Conservative and Reform Jews may be less ardent than the Orthodox Jew in the observance of these dietary laws.

Foods typical of the country of origin are often incorporated into their diet to the extent that adherence to dietary laws is possible. Most American Jews come from Russia, Poland, Czechoslovakia, or Germany.

One important distinguishing characteristic of a kosher diet is that food containing milk and food containing meat are not consumed at the same meal.[13] Furthermore, a separate set of dishes is used for milk or meat meals. Pareve foods, such as cereal without milk, fruit, vegetables, eggs from kosher birds, such as chicken, turkey, pigeons, tame ducks and geese, and tame doves,[14] and fish that are permitted, are considered neutral and may be eaten with either milk or meat meals.

Milk and milk products include milk, cottage and cream cheese, and sour cream. All are eaten in abundance. Sweet butter is preferred. Kosher meat comes from the forequarter and organs of beef, veal, or lamb. All meat and poultry must be slaughtered by the *schochet* (ritual slaughterer). Pork is forbidden. Poultry may be eaten but only fish with both fins and scales may be used. Shellfish is not allowed. Lox, a smoked salmon, is included as protein in dairy meals. Smoked whitefish and pickled herring are used in the same manner. Stuffed fish (gefilte fish) is a combination of whitefish, pike, and carp that is usually served chilled as an appetizer. Another very popular appetizer is chopped chicken liver. Chicken is a staple in most Jewish family dietaries. A classic Friday evening meal (Shabbat) is chicken soup followed by chicken prepared from a wide choice of recipes.

Vegetables are used generously in the kosher diet. Most of them are root vegetables and potatoes. Tomatoes and green peppers are often used in the preparation of meat dishes. Cucumber, lettuce, and tomatoes are combined in salads. Vegetable dishes include braised kale, beets mixed with prunes, sweet-and-sour red cabbage, fried eggplant, honeyed

---

[12] Richard Siegel, Michael Strassfeld, and Sharon Strassfeld, *The Jewish Catalog,* Jewish Publication Society of America, Philadelphia, 1973, pp. 18–36.

[13] M. Kaufman, "Adapting Therapeutic Diets to Jewish Food Customs," *American Journal of Clinical Nutrition,* Vol. 5, No. 6 (November–December 1957), pp. 676–678.

[14] Ibid., p. 20.

carrots, nahit (chick-peas) and rice, hot sauer-kraut, squash and rice, stuffed peppers, stuffed cabbage, and *tzimmes*, which is any combination of meat or vegetables or fruit, such as brisket, carrots, and sweet potatoes with brown sugar. If vegetables are cooked in milk in a *milchik* (refers to any food that contains or is derived from milk) pot (utensil used only for milk dishes), they are no longer pareve but must be considered as milk dishes. All fruit is considered pareve.

Breads include rye bread, pumpernickel, and white seed rolls. Bread products are cheese pancakes, potato *latkes* (pancakes), buckwheat pancakes, potato muffins, *challah* (braided egg bread) used on Shabbat and holidays (except Passover, which demands unleavened bread), fried matzo, bagel (boiled or baked dough shaped like a doughnut), and homemade noodles of several varieties, some of which are stuffed with meat, kasha, cheese, or potato. *Knishes* are raw dough, filled with pot cheese, ground chicken, or potato, then baked. Blintzes are a kind of crepe filled with vegetables, cheese, apple, or other fruit.

Buying Kosher Foods

When buying kosher foods, ask the clerk to identify the kosher symbol.[15] The buyer should check all products for the inclusion of milk or items of meat origin. Many breads and margarines, for example, contain milk. Read labels for inclusion of dried milk in other products, for example, some of the "natural" cereal products. The use of rennet in the making of cheese is objectionable to some rabbis because rennet is a secretion that comes from the stomach lining of pigs, calves, and other animals. Rennet from kosher animals that have been ritually slaughtered is acceptable. Gelatin products, according to some rabbis, are considered of animal origin. Jews are encouraged to consult with their rabbis about kosher and nonkosher foods.

Mexican Food Habits

Some characteristics of the Mexican diet are described here. Milk is often lacking ex-cept for a small amount of evaporated milk for infants. Meat, although well liked, is eaten infrequently. Beef, pork, cold cuts, goat, and chicken are emphasized. Fish is seldom eaten. Eggs may be consumed two or three times a week. Pinto beans are often and widely eaten.

Other Mexican dishes with protein content that may be listed in the meat group are described here.[16] Tacos are made from tortillas, which in turn are made from *masa* (dried corn, heated and soaked in lime water, washed and ground into a putty-like dough), or wheat flour, usually enriched, made into thin pancakes that are fried and stuffed with meat, poultry, or cheese, or eaten as is or with sauce and chilies. *Burritos* are made from 7-inch tortillas that are filled with green or red chilies and diced cooked meat and folded. *Enchiladas* are small tortillas, dipped in tomato sauce, fried quickly, and filled with shredded chicken, turkey, beef, or sausage, topped with cheese and served with the remaining sauce.

Tamales are ground meat spread on lime-treated corn, wrapped in corn husks, steamed, and served with the popular chili sauce. *Chili con carne* is ground beef, beans, chili peppers, seasoned with garlic—another protein dish. A *mole poblano* mix of chili powder, wheat flour, peanut butter, sugar, cocoa, salt, cotton-seed oil, cinnamon, and spices is used for making sauces and gravies that are frequently served with chicken and turkey. Sometimes bitter chocolate is used instead of the cocoa; raisins, nuts, and herbs may be added. An edible portion can contribute as much as 14 g of protein and 16 g of fat, some of which contains unsaturated fatty acids, according to Kight and others.

The breads and cereals used are corn in various forms, some wheat, rice, and macaroni. The corn is largely made into tortillas. Corn is also eaten fresh and dried on the cob. Vegetables and fruit include chili peppers, pumpkin, beets, peas, potatoes, squash, wild

---

[15] "Kosher Foods Described," *Journal of the American Dietetic Association*, Vol. 57, No. 3 (September 1970), p. 238.

[16] Mary Ann Kight, B. L. Reid, Janice I. Forcier, Carol M. Donishi, and Martena Cooper, "Nutritional Influences of Mexican-American Foods in Arizona," *Journal of the American Dietetic Association*, Vol. 55, No. 6 (December 1969), pp. 557–561.

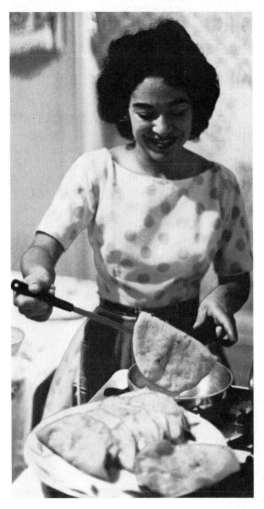

FIGURE 20–5. *A Mexican young woman preparing tortillas to be made into tacos.* (Forecast)

greens, sweet potatoes, string beans, pumpkin, turnips, tropical greens, bananas, apples, oranges, apricots, peaches, and *chayotes*. *Nopalites* are prepared from the leaf and stem of the prickly pear cactus, diced and served as a vegetable. Mexicans are fond of sugar and other sweets, as well as of highly seasoned foods.

NUTRITIONAL STATUS The health status, including nutritional status of Mexican-Americans is not well defined according to Bradfield

and Brun.[17] Few recent studies are available in the literature. Larson and others[18] found consumption of foods from the fruit, vegetable, and milk groups to be low among Mexican-American children of migrant families. Vitamin D and iron intakes were below recommended allowances. There was biochemical and clinical evidence of a vitamin A deficiency. Protein intake was high. The low income of many Mexicans limits their food consumption.

Near Eastern Food Habits

Families in the Near East have many common eating habits. Goat's, sheep's, or camel's milk and milk products are frequently used in the form of yogurt, fermented milk, sour cream, and cheese. Meat is primarily lamb and mutton that is barbecued or made into shish kebabs, stews, ground, and prepared in other ways. Kid and camel are eaten in some areas. Pork is seldom consumed for religious reasons and beef is generally too expensive because there is inadequate grazing grounds and feed. Grape leaves are stuffed with rice, bulgur, seasonings, and meat. Chicken, fish, and eggs are included. Nuts, such as chestnuts, peanuts, and hazelnuts, are a source of protein. Lentils are cooked with bulgur, rice, potatoes, homemade noodles, or vegetables such as tomatoes and green peppers, and seasoned with onions fried in olive oil. Cold, boiled beans may be served for breakfast seasoned with oil and vinegar. Chick-peas are ground, mixed with bulgur and spices, and deep fried, called *felafel*, and usually stuffed into bread. The popular vegetables are leeks, onions, tomatoes, squash, okra, peppers, broccoli, spinach, peas, green beans, dandelions, cucumbers, legumes, olives, peppers, eggplant, grape leaves, artichokes, and cabbage. Fruits, such as melons, dates, figs, grapes, cherries, oranges, raisins,

[17] Robert B. Bradfield and Thierry Brun, "Nutritional Status of California Mexican-Americans," *American Journal of Clinical Nutrition*, Vol. 23, No. 6 (June 1970), pp. 798–806.

[18] Lora Beth Larson, Janice M. Dodds, Donna M. Massoth, and H. Peter Chase, "Nutritional Status of Children of Mexican-American Migrant Families," *Journal of the American Dietetic Association*, Vol. 64, No. 1 (January 1974), pp. 29–35.

and apricots, are most commonly eaten. A wide variety of cereals are consumed—barley, rice, whole and cracked wheat, and breads shaped into thin, flat rounds. Bulgur or burghul, a favorite food, is made from wheat that has been boiled, dried, and cracked. Fats are used generously—sheep's butter, olive oil, and fat from other meats—in frying vegetables and other foods.

American Black Food Habits

The diet of the American black reflects the part of the world from which he comes. Most American blacks are in or come from the South or from the West Indies. Blacks in higher-income levels have diets similar to those of their white counterparts. Meats favored by many include chicken, salt pork, ham, bacon, and, occasionally, sausage. Fish such as mullets, spots, trout, croakers, perch, and butterfish are prized by some. Salt cod and salmon are made into patties, and salt herring is used among some families. According to Mayer,[19] catfish and other fish are caught in the rivers. Along the seashore, crabs, shrimp, clams, and crayfish are collected. Squirrels, rabbits, and other game are hunted during special seasons, but are not found in urban diets.

Milk and milk products include buttermilk, whole milk, evaporated milk, butter, and ice cream. There is little consumption of cheese. Breads and cereals consist largely of hot breads, hominy or grits, and white rice with sauce on top. Cornbread, biscuits, and muffins are widely used. Cookies, pastries, and cakes are also favorite foods.

Vegetables are plentiful in the black diet through the use of kale, mustard and turnip greens, collards, and cabbage cooked with salt pork, ham, or bacon. The pot liquor from these vegetables is consumed; thus some of the minerals and vitamins are salvaged. Other vegetables are onions, green pepper, cucumbers, and tomatoes. A wide variety of fruits is incorporated into the daily eating. Considerable fat is used in cooking. Molasses is used on breads and in other ways.

Soul food is a term often associated with foods eaten by blacks. The word soul is used in reference to other aspects of living such as "soul singing." It is used with food to connote dishes that give a sense of well-being, that are enjoyed, and that are associated with sentiments or feelings. Soul foods have vestiges of American Indian foods, such as hominy and mush, game, fish, oysters, and succotash. The poor white colonists by bringing hogs to the country contributed to the emphasis on pork. The blacks of Africa provided the foundation of soul food, according to Vogel,[20] with seasoned sauces and gravies, okra, watermelon, and beans. It was a diet that not only reflected the above impacts but an attempt to make the most of the discards of plantation owners. Some typical dishes are peas and rice, known as Hoppin' John, dried beans with tomatoes, and onion and fish in a savory stew. From the hog came foods such as chitterlings from the entrails; hog maws from the stomach lining; boiled pig's feet, tails, ears, and snout, sometimes made into scrapple; hog jowl; and neck bones. Desserts include sweet potato and pecan pies.

Mayer analyzes the nutritive status of Southern black dietaries and characterizes them as monotonous and low in "protective foods." Kcaloric requirements are usually met, but protein requirements for children are borderline. Calcium is low for 25 to 35 per cent of the population, and iron intake is inadequate for approximately half the population. Vitamin intakes of thiamin, riboflavin, and niacin are low in 12 to 15 per cent, vitamin A in about 50 per cent, and vitamin C is grossly inadequate, especially for the urban group for several months of the year. Information about Northern black nutritive intake is limited, and studies are badly needed.

Gladney,[21] in a study of black Americans in Los Angeles County, which actually repre-

[19] Jean Mayer, "The Nutritional Status of American Negroes," Nutrition Reviews, Vol. 23, No. 6 (June 1965), pp. 161–164.

[20] Marilyn Vogel, "Soul Food Is as American as Apple Pie," What's New in Home Economics, Vol. 38, No. 3 (March 1974), pp. 12–13.

[21] Virginia M. Gladney, Food Practices of Some Black Americans in Los Angeles County, Community Health Services, County of Los Angeles Department of Health Services, Los Angeles, Calif., 1972.

sented individuals from many parts of the United States, found changes in the traditional diets. There was an increased use in meatier cuts of meat, wild game was uncommon, cornbread and biscuits were still popular, the practice of frying foods had continued, and a substantial breakfast was important.

In regard to the basic four food groups, the use of more milk needs to be encouraged and less consumption of soft drinks. For meats and meat alternates, the use of less fried meat and eggs and smaller amounts of pork appears justified in light of overweight problems and diets high in saturated fatty acids. Some meat should be included in meals of greens and cornbread. More greens and citrus fruits should be included. Enriched and whole grains need to be emphasized.

Oriental Food Habits

Because of a shortage of fuel, many foods in the Orient are prepared in a short period of time. That is, they are cooked quickly. Cooking vegetables in this manner tends to preserve nutrients. Most foods are cut into small pieces. The use of lime water in the preparation of soybean curd contributes some calcium to the diet.

Food preferences include rice as the dominant food and principal cereal. Some wheat, barley, millet, and corn are included. Egg rolls are served in many parts of China. Noodles are popular in some areas and hot noodle shops provide snacks in Japan during the wintertime.

Little milk is consumed except for small amounts that are given to children and the ailing. A negligible amount of cheese is eaten, except a white cheese resembling farmer's cheese. Meats include fish and shellfish, especially shrimp, which are sometimes eaten raw; lamb; goat; pork; poultry, of which such parts of the carcass as spinal cord, blood, brains, and other organs are also used. Duck, pigeon, and chicken eggs are often preserved for use. Soybeans, other legumes, and almonds are also ingredients of the diet.

Vegetables are sliced thinly and cooked in oil for a short period of time. Favorites are cabbage, turnips, carrots, onions, bamboo shoots, celery, leeks, scallions, snow peas, greens such as shepherd's purse, spinach, and radish leaves, large radishes, water chestnuts, seaweed, dried mushrooms, potatoes—usually sweet—and bean sprouts and curd. Fruits include pears, tangerines, apples, mulberries, and persimmons. Little butter is used, but peanut, soy, and sesame oils are widely consumed, as well as lard.

The Oriental diet is often low in kcalories, calcium, riboflavin, iron, and thiamin if the rice is not enriched. The lack of milk in the diet of children is a serious deficiency.

Puerto Rican Food Habits

The staple foods of many Puerto Rican families as indicated by a study of Roberts and Stefani[22] are rice, beans, starchy vegetables (*viandas*), dry salted codfish, lard, sugar, and coffee.

Little milk is consumed. This lack is serious for growing children and explains the low-calcium dietary content. Other milk products are seldom used. The favorite meat is dried salted codfish, which is served with the *viandas* with oil and vinegar. Meat is liked, and when the income is increased, more is incorporated in the diet. Cooked legumes, such as chickpeas, navy beans, dried peas, pigeon peas, and red kidney beans (the favorite), are combined with *sofrito*, a mixture of tomatoes, green peppers, onion, garlic, salt pork, lard, and cooking herbs. All of this is eaten with rice seasoned with lard. Rice is prepared with chopped Vienna sausages, pork sausages, or codfish. Rice is also cooked with chicken and is eaten with stewed red beans, according to Torres.[23] Rice and beans are served frequently, sometimes twice a day.

The *viandas*, or starchy vegetables, include green bananas and green plantain, served like potatoes with fish or meat. A grayish-white variety of sweet potatoes, ripe plantain, and breadfruit (in some sections) are also eaten. Sometimes slices of raw onions and avocado

[22] Lydia J. Roberts and Rosa Luisa Stefani, *Patterns of Living in Puerto Rican Families*, University of Puerto Rico, San Juan, 1949.

[23] Rose Marina Torres, "Dietary Patterns of Puerto Rican People," *American Journal of Clinical Nutrition*, Vol. 7, No. 3 (May–June 1959), pp. 349–355.

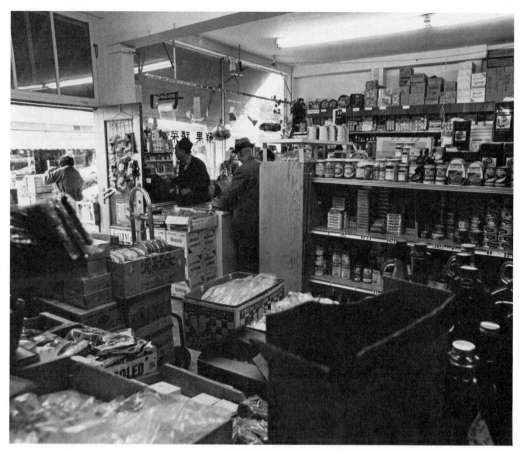

FIGURE 20–6. *Grocery stores that have predominantly Oriental foods are an enocuragement for the continuation of Oriental food patterns and for non-Orientals to incorporate some of these foods into their diets.*

in season are added to the boiled vegetable and codfish with vinegar and oil. Their vegetables, on the whole, are low in protein, calcium, and vitamin A except for plantain. When eaten in quantity, these vegetables do contribute fair to good amounts of iron and B vitamins, as well as kcalories.

Cereals other than rice are bread, noodles, spaghetti, oatmeal, and cornmeal (made into a mush). Cornmeal is occasionally substituted for rice. Oatmeal is usually cooked in milk. When milk is available, Puerto Ricans enjoy *café con leche*, made by adding a small amount of specially prepared coffee infusion to a cup of hot milk. Cocoa and chocolate, which are made with milk and generous amounts of sugar, are popular.

The more prosperous Puerto Ricans have stewed meats and steaks and use fewer *viandas*. Fruits are eaten between meals. Fruit pastes made from guavas, bitter oranges, pineapple, or mangoes are served with a native white cheese for dessert. The *acerola*, or Barbadoes cherry, is rich in vitamin C. Pineapple, oranges, grapefruit, and papaya are grown locally and contribute vitamin C when consumed.

Fernandez and others[24] did a nutritional study of the Puerto Rican population. Ac-

[24] Nelson A. Fernandez, Jose C. Burgos, Conrado F. Asenjo, and Irma Rosa, "Nutritional Status of the Puerto Rican Population: Master Sample Survey," *American Journal of Clinical Nutrition*, Vol. 24, No. 8 (August 1971), pp. 952–965.

cording to clinical data, there was a low prevalence of nutrition deficiencies. Dental caries were common in 62 per cent of the population. A vitamin A deficiency was found among 15 per cent of the sample. Only 9 per cent of the subjects showed signs of a vitamin C deficiency. A 15 per cent prevalence of riboflavin deficiency was noted. Only 7 per cent of the population indicated a thiamin deficiency. More deficiencies were found among the urban population than among rural inhabitants. There was a high prevalence of obesity, especially among urban women. A slight retardation of growth was noted among children. A low prevalence of anemias was observed, from 7 to 7.2 per cent. The severe forms of anemia were found among infants and preschool children. With the exception of the $5,000 to $5,999 income group, the highest percentage of deficient total proteins (range was from a mean 6.9 to 8.1 g of total proteins per 100ml) occurred among higher income levels rather than lower income groups. Intestinal parasites were found most frequently among children 2 to 14 years of age and in the lower income group.

Dietary findings showed that all age groups consumed at least 2 or more cups of milk daily, largely fresh milk, but this is inadequate for growing children. Breakfasts improved over a 1946 survey in that other foods had been added to the coffee, milk, and bread breakfast. Eggs were consumed at least three times a week. Codfish continued to be popular and was eaten 2 to 3 times a week. Poultry was a popular food and was included at least once a week at all income levels. Legumes had a high preference, but unfortunately pigeon and chick-peas with higher protein nutritive value were not used as often. Starchy vegetables, potatoes, green plantain, and green and ripe bananas made up the bulk of the diet and constitute a good source of kcalories, the vitamin B complex, and vitamin C. Fruit consumption was low. Oranges, pineapples,

and mangoes were eaten more often by the wealthier families. Rice was the favorite cereal and consumed daily at all income levels. Bread was used less frequently but crackers were eaten often. Lard is the preferred fat, but higher-income families preferred vegetable oil. Oil, butter, and margarine were consumed by all families. The favorite dessert was ice cream. Although this study was done in Puerto Rico, there are many implications for the diets of Puerto Ricans on the mainland, although the cost and availability of their favorite foods is a problem. The influence of the cities where they live will also affect diet.

Caution in Use of Cultural Dietaries

These cultural dietary reviews should be used with caution and discrimination. Every Italian, for example, does not eat spaghetti, nor do all Chinese eat rice. All foods could not be listed. Regional or other differences are not always included. Each summary was offered with the idea that some of these foods have been identified with these cultures at one time. Under no circumstances should an individual be stamped with a stereotype dietary.

A person will cling to these native dishes or grow away from them to the extent of his adaptability. In the case of mixed marriages or different backgrounds, an adult's eating pattern may reflect a number of food customs. All nationality dietaries usually have something good about them from a nutrition standpoint, and this fact should be respected.

The effect of inflation or recession, living in urban areas, and the availability of their cultural foods are making many changes in these food patterns. Rice and beans, for example, have had sharp price increases. The extent to which changes do take place under these and other influences makes a fertile area for future study.

SELECTED REFERENCES

Bailey, Marcelle A., "Nutrition Education and the Spanish-Speaking American," *Journal of Nutrition Education*, Vol. 2, No. 2 (Fall 1970), pp. 50–54.

Cussler, Margaret, and Mary L. De Give, *Twixt the Cup and the Lip*, Twayne Publishers, Inc., Boston, 1952.

Czajkowski, Janina M., *Chinese Foods and Traditions*, Connecticut Cooperative Extension Service, College of Agriculture and Natural Resources, University of Connecticut, Storrs, Conn., 1973.

Lowenberg, Miriam E., *Food and Man*, John Wiley & Sons, Inc., New York, 1974.

Natow, Annette B., Jo-Ann Heslin, and Barbara Raven, "Integrating the Jewish Dietary Laws into a Dietetics Program," *Journal of the American Dietetic Association*, Vol. 67, No. 1 (July 1975), pp. 13–16. (Note emblems that certify kosher products.)

Nickels, Harry G., *Middle Eastern Cooking*, Time–Life Books, New York, 1969.

Siegel, Richard, Michael Strassfeld, and Sharon Strassfeld, *The Jewish Catalog*, The Jewish Publication Society of America, Philadelphia, 1973.

Simoons, Frederick J. *Eat Not This Flesh*, University of Wisconsin Press, Madison, Wis., 1967.

Understanding Food Patterns in the U.S.A. American Dietetic Association, Chicago, 1969.

21

Nutrition
for Infants

Most mothers and fathers are anxious that their babies possess the priceless assets of health and happiness. Many of them, however, are unaware of the very important role that food plays in achieving these goals. Not only does it contribute to the child's nutrition, but it also relieves the annoying pain of hunger and creates an aura of security, comfort, and ease.

Parents must also realize that the baby has actually been nourished for 9 months prior to his birth and that the kind of nutrition he received then will have a great influence on his future well-being. It might be well to check important aspects of diet and pregnancy in Chapter 27.

Growth and Development of Infants

Growth rate is most rapid during infancy. The evaluation of body size during growth has been a contribution of anthropometry. Height is reflective of linear or skeletal growth. Increase in the amount of bone in contrast to cartilage indicates degree of maturation. Another dimension is weight, which includes body water, protein, and electrolytes, which are more or less constant, and fat, which varies.

Height and weight are generally compared to charts that depict the normal population. Recently efforts have been made to determine which scientific measurements, when integrated, of body size (such as anthropometric), body composition, and body cells will give the best prediction of normal growth.

Progress is being made to assess body composition in a simplified and standardized manner in living individuals, according to Fomon.[1] Some of the approaches for determining the body composition of the living infant are briefly cited here. The urinary excretion of hydroxyproline is considered a chemical index of growth. Hydroxyproline is mostly found in collagen, an integral part of skin, tendons, cartilage, blood vessels, connective tissue, organ capsules, and bone matrix. A rapid synthesis of collagen takes place during growth and is reflected in an increased rate of excretion of hydroxyproline. In contrast, excretion is decreased during periods of retarded growth.

A study of patterns of increase in cell number and size in organs or tissues of infants will provide insight about the nature as well as

[1] Samuel J. Fomon, *Infant Nutrition*, Saunders, Philadelphia, 1974, pp. 63–68.

270

failure of growth. Muscle cells of children with congenital heart disease were found by Cheek and Cooke[2] to be normal or somewhat larger in size but decreased in number. Winick[3] studied the tissues of children who died of malnutrition during the first year of life and found a marked reduction in the number of brain cells. It can be assumed that cell number and size are indicators of growth.

Evidence points to a difference in size and body composition in infants according to sex. Owen[4] and others cite differences in a larger mean weight and length in males than females and more rapid rate of growth in males than females in early life.

Whitten and others[5] tested the validity of the assumption that infants who do not receive adequate mothering in the form of emotional warmth, social contact, physical handling, and sensory stimulation tend not to thrive or grow normally. This situation is identified as the *"maternal deprivation syndrome."* In investigations that reached this conclusion, no attempt was made to determine the adequacy of the kcaloric intake. In addition, the cause of growth retardation was ill-defined. In the research undertaken by these investigators, the conclusion was reached that physical growth may be recovered by adequate kcalories but the research does not indicate that psychological and mental development have been improved if infants have been maternally deprived. It is recommended that long-term studies are needed to determine the effects of maternal deprivation of infants and nutriture on their growth.

[2] Donald B. Cheek and Robert E. Cooke, "Growth and Retardation," *Annuals of Review Medicine*, Vol. 15, Copy 3 (1964), pp. 357–382.

[3] Myron Winick, "Nutrition and Cell Growth," *Nutrition News*, Vol. 26, No. 7 (July 1968), pp. 1–4.

[4] G. M. Owen et al., "Body Composition of the Infant. Part II: Sex-Related Difference in Body Composition in Infancy," in F. Falkner (ed.), *Human Development*, Saunders, Philadelphia, 1966.

[5] Charles F. Whitten, Marvin G. Pettit, and Joseph Fischoff, "Evidence That Growth Failure from Maternal Deprivation Is Secondary to Eating," *Journal of the American Medical Association*, Vol. 29, No. 11 (September 15, 1969), pp. 1675–1682.

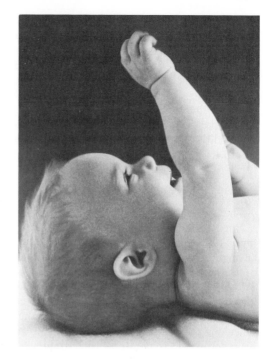

FIGURE 21–1. *In the complex of growth in an infant, nutrition is an important factor.* (*Courtesy Gerber Products Co.*)

How a Baby Eats

Eating is one activity in which a baby takes an important part. On the other hand, during bathing, clothing, or diapering, a very young baby is more or less helpless and has to have the tasks performed for him.

Three important mechanisms are vital to eating, and a baby is well-endowed with all three. They are rooting, sucking, and swallowing. Rooting is identified as that action in which a baby searches for the nipple. New parents are quite amazed at the adeptness with which a small baby can find the nipple. Once he has found it, the sucking process begins. He is aware that this is necessary in order to bring him milk. Infants will vary in the manner in which they perform the process of sucking. Some of them have a well-established rhythm in which they suck for a short period of time, then rest, and then start in again. Other babies may suck continuously until they are satisfied. Finally, there is the swallowing reflex. This is the last step in the eating process and is remarkably well coordinated with the breathing reflex. Swallowing takes place in such a way that the milk goes down the esophagus and not into the lungs, which would cause choking. This is accomplished largely through the fact that as the tongue pushes the milk to the back, it also prevents any additional milk from coming into the mouth.

Feeding Schedule

The kind of schedule for a baby has demanded considerable attention from time to time. *Self-regulation of feeding* appears to be highly recommended by most experts in contrast to a rigid set schedule of intervals of 3 to 4 hours. The latter method fails to take into account that the baby might not be hungry by the clock, and it also seems rather ridiculous to keep a baby crying for half an hour because it is not time to feed him. A disadvantage of the self-regulatory feeding is that a mother may be uncertain about such decisions as when a baby is hungry or when he has had enough. Although some kind of schedule seems appropriate, a mother is encouraged to be adaptable.

Eating and sleeping are closely related functions in babies. During the first weeks of life, sleep is light and often fitful. From 5 to 8 weeks of age, a baby begins a longer sleep period, so the night feeding may be eliminated. Later, when the long sleep period extends to 12 hours, feedings may be reduced to four a day.

The amount of food that is given in the self-regulatory schedule is equally important to the time interval between feedings. It is easy to determine when a baby is satisfied, but as he grows older and his stomach becomes larger, it will be possible for him to take greater amounts of food. Again the amounts of food will vary from baby to baby. Some babies are larger than others and have a larger frame, and consequently need more food. Some are more active; that is, they move their arms and legs frequently and are seldom still, and therefore require more food for energy purposes.

Infants vary, too, in the length of time it takes them to eat. This is true of bottle-fed as well as breast-fed babies. Some infants concentrate on the eating, whereas others take rest periods. In the case of a bottle-fed baby, it might be well to keep a chart of the times when a baby eats and the amount of formula he takes. In doing this for a period of time, it will be interesting to note if a pattern is developing. Sometimes the baby will not finish his bottle, but if he shows that he is satisfied, he usually has had sufficient food. If the baby is not getting enough to eat, he may awaken sooner than usual or he may give the hunger cry more frequently. This may specify a need for a change in his formula, which can easily be done upon the doctor's recommendation. It is amazing how an infant can communicate his wants and needs about how adequate his feeding is.

Food habits begin when food is first offered and an infant at the end of his first year may have accumulated many habits about the way he likes his food—temperature, texture, color, time of day, food preferences, willingness to experiment with new foods, preference for food preparation, and many others.

As there are many satisfactions to a baby during the feeding time, it cannot be overemphasized that it must be a pleasant time both for the baby and the mother.

Nutritive Needs of the Infant

The food given to an infant must be very nutritious. Nutritive requirements are higher in relation to size than at any other period in life. For that reason, it is imperative that the food be carefully selected to be small in quantity but high in nutritive value.

The recommendations for the nutritive needs of infants given by the Food and Nutrition Board of the National Research Council appear in Table 21–1.

Kcaloric needs of an infant are determined largely by basic kcaloric needs plus requirements for growth and muscular activity. A placid infant will obviously require fewer than an active one. A baby who cries often almost doubles his kcaloric needs. On the basis of body weight, an infant has approximately

TABLE 21–1

Recommended Daily Dietary Allowances for Infants, Revised 1974

Designed for the maintenance of good nutrition of practically all healthy people in the United States

	AGE	
	0.0–0.5	0.5–1.0
Weight, kg (lb)	6 (14)	9 (20)
Height, cm (in.)	60 (24)	71 (28)
Kcalories	kg × 117	kg × 108
Protein, g	kg × 2.2	kg × 2.0
Fat-soluble vitamins		
Vitamin A activity, RE[a]	420	400
Vitamin A, IU	1400	2000
Vitamin D, IU	400	400
Vitamin E activity, IU	4	5
Water-soluble vitamins		
Ascorbic acid, mg	35	35
Folacin, μg	50	50
Niacin, mg	5	8
Riboflavin, mg	0.4	0.6
Thiamin, mg	0.3	0.5
Vitamin B_6, mg	0.3	0.4
Vitamin B_{12} μg	0.3	0.3
Minerals		
Calcium, mg	360	540
Phosphorus, mg	240	400
Iodine, μg	35	45
Iron, mg	10	15
Magnesium, mg	60	70
Zinc, mg	3	5

SOURCE: Food and Nutrition Board, *Recommended Dietary Allowances*, 8th ed., National Academy of Sciences—National Research Council, Washington, D.C., 1974, p. 129.

[a] Retinol equivalents.

twice the body surface of an adult, so heat loss is greater. Fomon[6] warns that a mild excess of kcaloric intake is as undesirable as a slight deficiency. Weight gains are consistently greater in infants who receive concentrated formulas with higher kcaloric content.

Gross protein deficiency seldom occurs in technically advanced countries. To evaluate new infant formulas as they appear on the market, it is important, believes Fomon, to understand protein needs quantitatively and qualitatively. Exceptional requirements, as in phenylketonuria or defects in various aspects of protein metabolism, require adaptations.

Protein is essential for the very rapid development of the infant, particularly for maintenance, growth, and maturation of tissues. According to Holt and Snyderman,[7] the amount of protein required for the infant decreases to a greater extent in relation to body weight than do the kcaloric requirements as growth takes place. The reason is that infants are more active as they become larger. This function of activity, unlike growth and maintenance, does not require protein, but kcalories are needed. It is especially important that the essential amino acids be present in adequate amounts in the infant formula.

Fat in the diet makes a formula more palatable to the infant. However, Fomon expresses the opinion that, with the exception of the essential fatty acid, linoleic, which is necessary for growth and for the skin, fat is not absolutely necessary in the infant diet. Fat does carry certain fat-soluble vitamins and can increase the kcaloric value of the formula, thus reducing its volume.

On the whole, the vitamin content of most infant dietaries is adequate. Some concern has been expressed about undesirable effects of a slight overdosage of vitamin D. A mild deficiency of vitamin K in newborn infants is not uncommon. Rickets, due to a deficiency of vitamin D, occurs occasionally, and scurvy, due to a lack of ascorbic acid, is found in certain geographic areas. Iron deficiency anemia is commonly found, which indicates a possible folic acid deficiency also. The thiamin requirement parallels the increase of carbohydrate. In a similar manner, the need for vitamin B_6 increases with the increased requirement for protein, based on weight.

The major minerals are usually found in generous amounts in the infant's diet. Trace

---

[6] Fomon, op. cit., p. 20.

[7] Emmett Holt, Jr., and Selma E. Snyderman, "Nutrition in Infancy and Adolescence," in Robert S. Goodhart and Maurice E. Shils (eds.), *Modern Nutrition in Health and Disease*, Lea & Febiger, Philadelphia, 1973, Chap. 24.

elements are deficient more frequently. Iron deficiency is prevalent throughout the world and ranks next to fluoride as being most often deficient in the infant diet.

Breast Feeding

Milk is the most important food in an infant's diet. See Table 21–2 for a comparison of human milk and cow's milk.

There is an assumption that mother's' milk is always of high quality. Milk will vary from mother to mother. A poorly nourished mother, however, generally secretes much less milk and also secretes it for a shorter period of time. Malnutrition or other deviations in food intake will certainly have an influence on the mother's ability to supply milk of good quality.

Jelliffe and Jelliffe[8] admit that breast feeding has been a controversial topic but believe that new sociological and scientific developments demand a new look at the values of human milk. From a worldwide point of view the increase in the marasmus–diarrhea syndrome and the expensive and often unattainable cow's or other animal milk, not only in developing countries but in affluent countries in Europe and North America, is a problem that demands attention. In the search for new protein sources, nutrition planners may recognize that human milk, a food specifically designed for infants, has great potential, both economically and agriculturally, as a contribution to the protein gap. In addition, influential women's organizations have arisen to encourage breast feeding, possibly as a reaction to mechanized and dehumanized lifestyles. An example of such an organization is the La Leche League International (LLLI).

Human milk has many assets such as supplying linoleic acid, the essential fatty acid, and other unsaturated fatty acids; high levels of cystine, which can be handled more readily by the young infant than the methionine found in animal milks; and a great variety of nucleotides that are required indirectly for pro-

TABLE 21–2

Comparison of the Composition of Human Milk and Cow's Milk per 100 Grams

NUTRIENTS	HUMAN MILK	COW'S MILK
Water, g	85.2	87.4
Kcalories	77.0	65.0
Protein, g	1.1	3.5
Fat, g	4.0	3.5
Carbohydrate, g	9.5	4.9
Calcium, mg	33.0	118.0
Phosphorus, mg	14.0	93.0
Iron, mg	0.1	Trace
Sodium, mg	16.0	50.0
Potassium, mg	51.0	144.0
Vitamin A, IU	240.0	140.0
Thiamin, mg	0.01	0.03
Riboflavin, mg	0.04	0.17
Niacin, mg	0.2	0.1
Ascorbic acid	5.0	1.0

SOURCE: Bernice K. Watt and Annabel L. Merrill, *Composition of Foods*, Agriculture Handbook No. 8, Consumer and Food Economics Research Division, Agricultural Research Service, U.S. Department of Agriculture, Washington, D.C., 1963, p. 39.

tein synthesis, according to György.[9] Mata and Wyatt[10] state that breast-fed infants have greater resistance to gastrointestinal disorders and to a wide variety of other acute and chronic infections, such as respiratory and middle-ear infections and bouts with fever.

The presence of nucleotides in human milk facilitates protein synthesis. Higher levels of copper, ascorbic acid, and vitamin E are found in human milk than in cow's milk. The lactose level makes galactose easily available for growth and especially for brain development. Calcium in human milk is more efficiently absorbed and metabolized than the calcium in cow's milk. The curd tension of human milk

---

[8] Derrick B. Jelliffe and E. F. Patrice Jelliffe, "The Uniqueness of Human Milk," Introduction, *American Journal of Clinical Nutrition*, Vol. 24, No. 8 (August 1971), pp. 968–969.

[9] Paul György, "Biochemical Aspects," *American Journal of Clinical Nutrition*, Vol. 24, No. 8 (August 1971), pp. 970–975.

[10] Leonardo J. Mata and Richard G. Wyatt, "Host Resistance to Infection," *American Journal of Clinical Nutrition*, Vol. 24, No. 8 (August 1971), pp. 976–986.

facilitates digestion, metabolism, and efficient utilization of nutrients, which in turn encourages excellent growth in the infant. Anemia is less likely in the breast-fed infant than in those artificially fed because of the loss of ascorbic acid and folate in processed cow's milk preparations.

Certain immediate and long-term metabolic stresses and risks may be associated with cow's milk formulas. A low level of calcium may be found in the blood of the very young infant. A taste for sucrose may develop early (because some type of sugar is often added to a formula), which may lead to dental caries potential. If an infant is overfed on cow's milk (regulation of intake is easier with breast feeding), obesity may result. Allergies are more common in infants fed cow's milk. Human milk contains only one fifth as much strontium 90 as cow's milk but cow's milk has less DDT.

Newton[11] states that there is an increasing awareness of the emotional importance of close mother–child interrelationships. For the infant the initial experience of being fed is less traumatic generally with breast feeding than artificial feeding. Other advantages to breast feeding are that a baby's hunger can be relieved more quickly because a formula does not have to be prepared; greater oral satisfaction; more mother–child interaction; and more satisfying psychobiological and psychosocial communications and consequences. There are many economic considerations, according to McKigney.[12] The cost of artificial feeding is high with the purchase of either ready-prepared formulas or mixes that have to be prepared at home. Baby foods are expensive. Home-produced formulas and strained or chopped foods prepared from home-produced food can reduce costs considerably, particularly for the mother who must work and cannot breast feed her baby or only in a limited manner. The nursing mother must increase the nutrients in her diet and, in times of inflation,

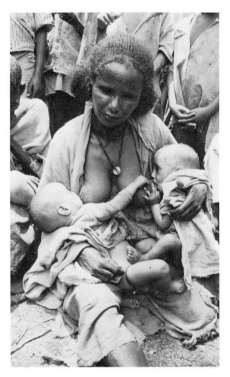

FIGURE 21–2. A refugee mother breast feeding two babies to keep them alive. (UNICEF/ Bill Campbell)

nutritious foods must be selected in terms of cost.

One recommendation of the White House Conference on Food, Nutrition and Health was as follows: "In implementing nutrition education activities, special efforts should be directed towards: 1. The pregnant women and the new mothers to encourage breast feeding, especially for the first 6 months of life."[13] Mayer[14] contends that a sweeping change in attitude is necessary for the implementation of this recommendation. The mother herself is the most vital factor in this decision. Although breast feeding has declined in the United States, Mayer believes that the trend

[11] Niles Newton, "Psychologic Differences Between Breast Feeding and Bottle Feeding," American Journal of Clinical Nutrition, Vol. 24, No. 8 (August 1971), pp. 993–1004.

[12] John McKigney, "Economic Aspects," American Journal of Clinical Nutrition, Vol. 24, No. 8 (August 1971), pp. 1005–1012.

[13] Jean Mayer (chairman), White House Conference on Food, Nutrition and Health, Final Report, U.S. Government Printing Office, Washington, D.C., 1970, p. 48.

[14] Jean Mayer, "Breast Feeding Might Be the Next New Status Symbol," The New York Daily News, August 23, 1973, p. 19.

may be reversing. Breast feeding has become more popular among mothers in the suburbs than anywhere else, especially among higher socioeconomic and better educated groups. The rate has been especially high among women married to students in the professional groups and in graduate college—about seven out of every ten. Some college women are making the decision to breast feed before they have their children. More (about half) private patients in hospitals tend to breast feed their babies. About one third of clinic patients breast feed their babies, although this is not an increase in number but rather a stationary statistic. With these women as pacesetters, breast feeding may become more popular.

Jelliffe and Jelliffe[15] conclude that it is not only human milk that must be considered but breast feeding itself, which is not only a physiological process that nourishes the infant but a powerful psychosocial communication between a mother and her child.

Formulas

Milk-based formulas supply most of the nutritional needs of an infant during the early weeks and months of his life. These formulas continue to be the major source of kcalories and essential nutrients even after other foods are introduced into the diet. A wide variety of infant formulas—some in powder form to be reconstituted by the addition of water and others in liquid form, and some in disposable nursing bottles—are available in the United States and Europe, according to Brown.[16] Although these products are carefully tested and offer great convenience, the consumer pays for this service.

Cow's milk differs from human milk in the greater concentration of protein and minerals and lower concentration of lactose. See Table 21-2. The high casein content of cow's milk is the source of a relatively large mass of

    [15] Derrick B. Jelliffe and E. F. Patrice Jelliffe, "An Overview," *American Journal of Clinical Nutrition*, Vol. 24, No. 8 (August 1971), pp. 1013–1024.

    [16] Roy E. Brown, "Breast Feeding in Modern Times," *American Journal of Clinical Nutrition*, Vol. 26, No. 5 (May 1973), pp. 556–562.

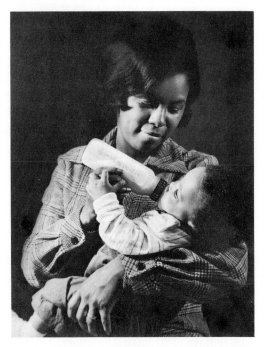

FIGURE 21-3. *Feeding an infant a milk-based formula. (Evenflo Products, Division of Pyramid International, Inc.—A Questor Company)*

somewhat indigestible curds. Dilution, addition of an acid, or heating (usually to 145 to 161°F) will reduce the curd tension and produce a softer, flocculent curd that facilitates enzymatic action in the digestive tract. The fat of cow's milk contains several saturated fatty acids that are less well tolerated than human milk fat, not only by infants of low birth weight but by full-term infants during the first weeks of life.

One major difference between the feeding of human milk and cow's milk, according to Fomon, is that the former is consumed directly from the breast so that nutrients are transferred without loss. Cow's milk, in contrast, through collection, processing, transportation, delivery, and storage, may facilitate losses in vitamins particularly.

The forms of cow's milk used in formulas are whole or skim, pasteurized, homogenized, evaporated, condensed (seldom used because of high carbohydrate content), freeze-dried, or dried. Of these milks, evaporated milk is used for 80 per cent of the bottle-fed babies in the United States. Advantages are sterility, less cost, and avoidance of curd indigestion. Goat's milk is widely used in some parts of the world and is considered nutritionally adequate. The fat of goat's milk is more easily digested than that of cow's milk. This milk has a lower content of folic acid, which must be taken into consideration.

A baby's formula is best planned by the physician to meet the specific needs of a particular infant, including ingredients and amount. Variations may include amount of activity, size, age, sex, amount of other liquids included, and if other foods or supplements are to be added.

A number of formulas prepared with cow's milk, added carbohydrate (it may be lactose, corn sugar, cane sugar, maltose–dextrin, or mixtures), minerals, vitamins, and sometimes fat, are prepared commercially. Few are fortified with iron and vitamin C. For infants of low birth weight, formulas have been developed of nonfat cow's milk, vegetable oils, such as corn oil, and carbohydrate, which is usually lactose or corn sugar. Most of these formulas provide adequate nutrients. One type of formula marketed as a powder combines nonfat cow's milk and whey proteins in a ratio to casein, so that the protein more closely resembles human milk.

For infants with allergies, special milk-free formulas are utilized. These formulas contain protein, fat, and carbohydrate from soybeans. Corn and coconut oils are also used. Sucrose or corn sugar is included. Certain of these formulas appear to be as adequate nutritionally as a milk-based formula.

Additions to the Infant's Diet

Additions to an infant's diet will depend on the doctor's recommendation based upon the nutritional needs of the child and his ability physiologically and otherwise to handle them. The strong trend to earlier introduction of additional foods has been under scrutiny. The appeal in the marketing of special infant foods may be a contributing factor to a mother's belief of a sound feeding regimen. In the case of a bottle-fed baby some vitamin C should be added, for heating the milk may partially destroy this vitamin. Unless the nursing mother has an ample amount of vitamin C, it is also well to protect the breast-fed baby with some supplement. Citrus fruit juices are generally given to supply this need—orange, grapefruit, or tomato juice. It must be borne in mind that orange juice contains approximately 15 mg of vitamin C to the ounce, whereas tomato juice contains a little less than 5 mg per ounce. The juice is generally diluted with warm water and fed from a bottle with a nipple.

In some marginal regions where it is difficult to get citrus fruits, Stearns[17] recommends pot liquor. Concentrated liquid in the pot in which greens are cooked is cheap and a good source of vitamin C. Acerola juice, an excellent source of vitamin C, is used in Puerto Rico. A syrup made from rose hips is used in some countries and is also an excellent source. The crystals or tablet of ascorbic acid can be used but must be dissolved in water. Sometimes this is given to babies found to be allergic to natural forms.

The fruit juices that may be given may be fresh, frozen, or canned. They should be very carefully strained under all circumstances. The water added to fruit juice should have been previously boiled and cooled to lukewarm or cool.

Taking fruit juice is a new food experience for a baby and might be considered one of the first steps in growing up. From now on he will be learning new tastes and new consistencies, and in time will need to learn how to chew and to use his tongue. All these experiences should be pleasant and free from worry to prevent food problems.

The acceptance of new foods will depend a great deal on how the mother offers them to the infant. If she is relaxed and offers the food in a reassuring manner, the baby will generally respond in a like fashion. The mother is urged to go slowly and patiently in introducing anything new to the baby, and to make it seem as though it is a part of the regular routine. Under no circumstance should she force the

---

[17] Genevieve Stearns, "Infants' and Toddlers' Food," *Food, The Yearbook of Agriculture, 1959,* U.S. Department of Agriculture, Washington, D.C., 1959, pp. 283–295.

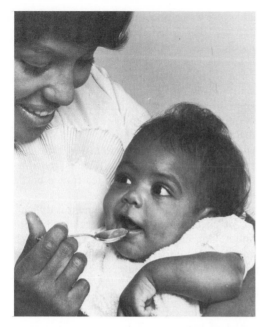

FIGURE 21–4. *Additions to an infant's diet are based on nutritional ·needs. (Courtesy Gerber Products Co.)*

child or introduce fear. If a mother will bear in mind that each step should be a pleasurable one to both the mother and the baby, there should be few difficulties. If the infant seems to resist the first time, it might be well to stop at that point and to introduce the food again later.

Another nutritional need is some form of vitamin D. In the case of the bottle-fed baby, some of the milks used are already fortified with vitamin D, so the baby is certain of securing a certain amount. To ensure that the infant receives an adequate amount, the physician generally prescribes some form of vitamin D. The amount given at the beginning is generally very small and mothers are urged to be particularly cautious in following doctors' directions, since an overdose of vitamin D can be very serious. All babies need 400 units daily; this will prevent rickets and encourage growth. It is a good plan to give vitamin D at the same time each day so that it will not be forgotten. In the summertime the sunlight can make vitamin D in the baby's skin. However, this is an uncertain matter and cannot

be counted on, so it is well to use a vitamin D preparation. This vitamin is essential for the utilization of calcium and phosphorus for strong bones.

It is important to know whether the preparation of vitamin D can be given with milk or by medicine dropper or spoon. Some preparations do not dissolve in milk or water and may be left on the side of the bottle. Consequently, the infant will not receive the benefit of them.

The doctor advises the mother about the first food fed by spoon. As all the baby's food up to this time has been liquid in nature, this is a very important step for him. Some babies accept the food from a spoon much more readily than others; again this is a matter of individual difference. The food should be the consistency of cream soup to run off the end of the spoon easily. Spoon feeding should not be forced too early or feeding problems will result. The first food may be cereal, egg yolk, or strained mild fruit, to be offered as early as 4 to 6 weeks. The cereal should be highly refined but enriched. Ready-prepared cereals are quite inexpensive and save a mother's time. Labels should be checked for enrichment, especially iron, because some combinations of cereals with fruit, egg yolk, or bacon have not been enriched.

A physician will generally recommend at which time of the day or at which feeding this new food should be introduced. The 10 A.M. feeding is the one commonly chosen, but the choice will vary from baby to baby. Some mothers have found the 6 P.M. feeding the best. Still other questions need to be answered. Should the cereal or new food be given before or after the milk? Or should the baby be given some milk first, then the new food, and the remainder of the milk? Each mother will have to decide which is the best way to do it and may need to do some experimenting with her baby to find out when he appears to like it best.

By the time an infant is 6 months of age, or earlier, he may have whole-grain cereal, which is very nutritious. Also, it is possible to begin to vary the kinds of cereal so that he will become accustomed to difficult types. Precooked dry cereals are commercially prepared for infants. Formula may be added to the cereal to facilitate feeding. For older infants, milk may be used. Some of the cooked cereal that the family has may be offered to him. This is one way of introducing him to cereals that he may eat even after he is an adult. Sometimes a doctor will recommend that the cereal be interchanged with potato. The potato must be cooked thoroughly by baking, boiling, or pressure cooking. It should be carefully peeled and then mashed very finely with a fork. A small amount of milk that has been heated, or some of the formula, may be added to the potato.

Most babies like fruit. In fact, this is one reason why fruit rather than cereal may be preferred as a first "solid" food. It may be fresh, stewed, or dried, unless prepared baby foods are used. All fruits must be very carefully sieved. Well-strained apple sauce or mashed banana, which have a very mild taste, are usually introduced as the first fruits. Banana is one of the few fruits a baby can eat raw. It should be very ripe and mashed very finely. The skin of the banana should be quite dark, which indicates that it is ripe; if it is not ripe, it is difficult for the baby to digest. If fruit is stewed at home, it is wise to refrain from adding sugar. Fruits are naturally sweet, and it does not seem necessary to develop the sweet taste of the baby.

The baby may be fed the fruit with a teaspoon at the beginnng or the end of the feeding period. Again the 10 A.M. or the 6 P.M. feeding seems a desirable time. Very small amounts of the fruit, not more than a teaspoon, should be offered at the beginning, and gradually increased as the baby learns to like the food.

If the baby is eating only a small amount of fruit, it might be well to strain some which the family is eating. In using the small jars of prepared fruit for babies, it must be remembered that it can be kept safely in the refrigerator only for 2 or 3 days after it is opened. Some infants like having the same fruit for several days in succession; others prefer change. It is important that the baby be introduced to many different kinds of fruit. Most babies, however, will disclose very decided preferences for certain fruits. This should

not discourage the mother, however, from introducing the infant to other types. Fruits contribute kcalories, as well as vitamins C and A. Fruits, with the exception of prunes and plums, are considered poor sources of iron.

Vegetables are generally recommended by the doctor some time between 4 and 6 months. This food should be introduced at a feeding when the baby is not taking either cereal or fruit. Vegetables may be purchased in the cans or jars specially prepared for babies, or the vegetables that are used for the family may be modified for infant use. It is well to begin with those that are mild in flavor. This category would include green beans, carrots, spinach, asparagus, summer and winter squash, peas, beets, tomatoes, and chard. When the baby is older, cauliflower, cabbage, turnips, parsnips, broccoli, and lima beans are usually added, but they are not recommended among the first vegetables to be introduced.

Vegetables are often introduced in the same manner as other foods, that is, by giving the baby a taste. A small amount is allowed for the first few days and then gradually increased to two or three tablespoons. Sometimes it is possible to buy mixed vegetables. This does give the baby variety, but is not recommended as a steady diet because it is important for babies to learn to identify different vegetables and to associate certain flavors with them.

A baby may express strong likes and dislikes in vegetables as he has with other foods. Fortunately, green and yellow vegetables can be used interchangeably for vitamin A value, and since there is a wide variety of these foods, it should not be difficult to make a selection.

Leftover vegetables, either home cooked or canned, spoil easily and should not be kept more than a few days. They might be used in the family meals in some manner. Before the end of the first year it is well to change over to coarsely mashed or chopped vegetables. Babies are generally ready for the coarser foods at 9 months of age. This is the transition from the sieved vegetables to the whole food. If the baby is kept on strained vegetables too long, it becomes quite difficult for him to accept vegetables in the coarser form. He should be permitted to use his judgment in regard to the amount of food that he can eat.

Whole-grain cereals and green vegetables supply iron. In addition, it is important to add egg yolk, not only for its iron but also for additional protein. Egg yolk is generally introduced anywhere from 3 to 5 months of age. Usually the egg white is not given until the baby is older. It is quite watery and does not give as much nutritive value as the egg yolk, and sometimes it does not agree with infants.

Egg yolk must be thoroughly cooked. It may be served in several ways—mashed with a fork, added to the cereal or to the vegetables, or even added to the milk. A small amount may be offered on a teaspoon without any other food. As soon as the baby becomes accustomed to its flavor, the amount of egg yolk is generally increased until he is receiving the whole yolk. Mothers may find prepared egg yolk baby food more convenient. From the age of 9 months to a year, the doctor may suggest giving the baby the whole egg. In that case, it may be soft cooked or poached and can be given to him at breakfast or at supper. Egg can be used interchangeably with meat or fish.

Meat may be added in a finely ground or strained form, as the baby can utilize it well. It is generally introduced during the second half of the baby's first year, although he doesn't actually need the protein if he is given a whole egg and milk. However, there is a great difference of opinion about the time when meat should be introduced. Finely ground liver is sometimes given as early as 3 months of age. Others recommend that an infant wait until 9 months, and still others suggest 6 months of age as a good time. At any rate, it is good to acquaint him with different flavors of meat fairly early.

It seems wise to buy the small cans of meat prepared especially for babies. It is difficult to prepare meat for a baby in the home, and it is generally much cheaper to buy the canned variety.

Meat should be introduced to a baby for the first time in the same manner as other foods, by offering him a small amount on a teaspoon. The flavor and texture of meat are so different from the other foods he has had that there may be some reaction to it. A mother should not be discouraged but should give him his other foods and try again the next day. Once a child has become accustomed to meat, he is usually very fond of it. Beef is often used to introduce meat for the first time, and after that lamb, veal, liver, lean pork, ham, and chicken may be tried. Babies cannot tolerate very much fat. If the meat is prepared at home, fat should be removed. If pork is cooked at home, it must be cooked very thoroughly. Some strained meats provide 1 to 4 mg of iron per 100 g. Soups, meat combinations with vegetables, and "dinners" provide less iron. Meat contributes protein and niacin, too.

Fish is not added to an infant's diet until he is about 12 months of age. At the beginning only fresh, white fish is used, such as haddock, halibut, cod, and flounder; this is because these fish are very low in fat. Dark-meat fish, such as mackerel, contain considerable oil. The fish may be baked, steamed, or boiled. All bones should be carefully removed, especially the tiny or second bones; the fish can be flaked with the fork to help find them. It may then be served as meat is.

Infants do not have special desserts prepared for them. Toward the end of the first year, however, for variety the baby may occasionally have gelatin—particularly if it has been prepared with milk or egg, rice pudding, and custard or other milk dessert. If possible, sugar should be omitted.

Many questions have been raised about commercial baby foods. For example, the protein content of these foods varies considerable, according to White.[18] Four-and-three-quarter-ounce dinners, such as "High Meat Dinners" (consisting of ham with vegetables and macaroni, or macaroni, tomato, beef, and bacon), contain 9.5 g of protein. Protein content of other foods are pure strained meats, 19 g; junior meats, 25 g; soups and one-dish meals, 3 g; and cottage cheese mixtures, 9.5 g. The

---

[18] Philip L. White, "Let's Talk About Food," *Today's Health*, Vol. 49, No. 1 (January 1971), p. 11.

likes and dislikes of the infant and the price are other considerations in the purchase.

It is important to read all baby food labels carefully. Some jars contain as much as 50 per cent water, especially meats. If water is the first ingredient listed, there is more water than any other ingredient. A random check of baby food labels listed such ingredients as vanilla, cinnamon, brown sugar, dehydrated onion, shortening, broth, cream, sugar, celery extractive, modified tapioca starch, and other modified starches. There is a question about the digestibility of the starches, and the other ingredients contribute little to the nutritive intake and their inclusion is questionable.

There is controversy about the amount of salt that baby foods should contain. Dahl[19] is firmly convinced that excessive salt is unnecessary and may contribute to hypertension, as has been demonstrated in rat experiments. In his laboratory, Dahl has analyzed baby foods with meat that contained five to six times as much salt as fresh table meats, and vegetables that contained six to sixty times as much as fresh vegetables. Some authorities point to the dilemma that unsalted foods may prompt a mother to salt the food at home.

Filer[20] provides another viewpoint about the salt content of infant foods in a review of the report of the Subcommittee on Safety and Suitability of MSG and Other Substances in Baby Foods of the Food Protection Committee of the Food and Nutrition Board of the National Academy of Sciences. In summary, the subcommittee did not find any evidence that, insofar as healthy infants are concerned, addition of sodium chloride, at current levels, is either harmful or beneficial to the infant. In the viewpoint of the subcommittee no valid scientific evidence was available in support of the contention that the addition of salt contributed to the development of hypertension nor was there valid evidence that the practice is not harmful or that

salt levels now consumed by American infants overburden excretory functions. Present salt intakes of infants, however, do provide substantially more sodium than is required by the infant. Therefore, limiting the total intake of salt seems reasonable. There is no good basis for recommending salt at any level in processed baby foods on the assumption that salted foods appear to be more satisfying to the taste of the mothers of infants.

The addition of sugar to commercial baby foods or to foods prepared at home is questionable because the sugar dilutes the nutritive density of the food and encourages a sweet taste for foods in later life. The trend in marketing fancier baby foods, such as pie or cobbler, that have the ingredients of a pastry is a dubious nutritive contribution to a young child's diet.

To reduce costs many mothers use family foods such as fruits and vegetables and put them in the blender until they reach the proper consistency. Some foods need to be strained in addition. Family cereals are usually much less expensive than baby-food types. Cream of wheat and cream farina, for example, are fortified with iron and can be used. Labels for oatmeal and grits must be checked for fortification.

Nutritional Status of Infants

The most comprehensive investigation of the nutritional status of infants was done in the *Ten-State Nutrition Survey*.[21] The findings indicated that mean dietary intakes for infants 6 to 11 months of age were sufficient to meet the standards for all nutrients except iron. However, the cumulative percentage distribution revealed a wide range of intake, with many infants consuming much lower intakes of kcalories, iron, vitamin A, and vitamin C than standards. White infants from 6 to 11 months of age in the high-income-ratio states

---

[19] Lewis K. Dahl, "Notes," *Nutrition Reviews*, Vol. 26, No. 4 (April 1968), pp. 124–125.

[20] Lloyd J. Filer, Jr. (Committee Chairman), "Salt in Infant Foods," *Nutrition Reviews*, Vol. 29, No. 2 (February 1971), pp. 27–28.

[21] *Ten-State Nutrition Survey, 1968–70, V—Dietary*, DHEW Publication No. (HSM) 72-8133, Center for Disease Control, Health Services and Mental Health Administration, U.S. Department of Health, Education, and Welfare, Atlanta, Ga., 1972.

had the most satisfactory diets; black and Spanish-American infants had lower dietary intakes for most nutrients.

Specifically, for kcalories, 6- to 11-month-old black infants tended to have the lowest mean kcaloric intake in low-income-ratio states and Spanish-Americans in high-income-ratio states. Mean protein intakes were exceptionally high for 6- to 11-month-old infants; but this may reflect errors in recall. However, in the low-income-ratio states, 8 to 10 per cent of the infants had mean protein intakes below standard compared to 5 to 8 per cent in high-income-ratio states. Differences in protein intake were primarily dependent on total food intake. Calcium and riboflavin were also well above dietary standards. Again, milk consumption may have been overestimated. Six per cent of the infants had a mean calcium intake below standard.

Iron was the only nutrient with mean intakes generally below the dietary standard. Almost half of the white 6- to 11-month-old infants in both income levels had an intake below standard. Almost three fourths of the black and Spanish-American infants had iron intakes below standard. The high mean intake of iron among white infants may reflect the use of iron-fortified foods.

Approximately 15 per cent of the 6- to 11-month-old infants had vitamin A intakes below standard. No consistent differences existed among ethnic groups. Dietary intakes of thiamin were above standard. Mean intake for this age of infant was higher than for older-age-group children. Riboflavin intakes were much higher than dietary standards but decreased with age. Only 5 per cent of the infants had mean intakes below standards in the low-income-ratio states and only about 2 per cent in high-income-ratio states. Between 50 to 60 per cent of the infants had vitamin C intakes of less than 30 mg per day. The prevalence of below-standard vitamin C intakes in the high-income-ratio states was slightly lower than in the low-income-ratio states. An examination of the distribution data revealed that for most nutrients a large number of infants had intakes below dietary standards. (See Table 2–2.)

Infant mortality rates are another indication of poor nutritional status although other factors are also responsible. Lowe[22] addresses himself to the continuing high level of infant mortality, about 20 per 1,000 live births, placing the United States fourteenth among advanced nations. In spite of the low position, progress has been made because the infant mortality rate in 1950 was 30 per 1,000 live births. Although the infant mortality rate has continued a slow fall, the prematurity rate, births under 2500 g has continued to rise and is now over 8.2 per cent. An analysis of the infant mortality data reveals that three fourths of the deaths occur in the first month, doubtless owing to premature birth. The nutritional status of the mother is an important factor in these statistics.

Ho and Brown[23] studied the food intake of infants attending well-baby clinics in Honolulu. Except for iron, nutrient intakes met at least two thirds of the recommended allowances for most infants. Intakes of protein were well above recommended levels. The iron intakes for slightly more than half the infants were below 50 per cent of the recommended allowances for this age. Sodium intakes were above recommendations for growth, and some of the infants consumed amounts of sodium that were near or exceeded maximum levels suggested. The level of intake is serious because of possible relation to hypertension.

Burroughs and Huenemann[24] investigated the frequency and severity of iron deficiency anemia among infants in Southern California. In general, infants whose weights were in the lowest percentiles had low dietary intakes of kcalories and other nutrients and showed less favorable blood findings. There was an extremely large variation in iron intake at various

[22] Charles U. Lowe, "Research in Infant Nutrition: The Untapped Well," American Journal of Clinical Nutrition, Vol. 25, No. 2 (February 1972), p. 250.

[23] Claire Hughes Ho and Myrtle L. Brown, "Food Intake of Infants Attending Well-Baby Clinics in Honolulu," Journal of the American Dietetic Association, Vol. 57, No. 1 (July 1970), pp. 17–21.

[24] Ann L. Burroughs and Ruth L. Huenemann, "Iron Deficiency in Rural Infants and Children," Journal of the American Dietetic Association, Vol. 57, No. 2 (August 1970), pp. 122–128.

ages. Infants from 6 to 11 months of age had a mean iron intake of 8.6 mg per day with a standard deviation of 4 mg and a coefficient of variation of 47 per cent. In terms of the 1968 recommended allowances, the mean intake of iron represented 57.3 per cent. In regard to other nutrients, ascorbic acid, vitamin A, thiamin, riboflavin, calcium, phosphorus, kcalories, and protein mean intakes were above recommendations. No significant correlations between the nutrient intakes and blood variables appeared consistently at each age grouping.

The researchers point to many unanswered questions in relation to this type of study. For example, the hemoglobin concentrations and blood measurements that are compatible with health and growth have not been determined. The minimum iron intake to prevent iron deficiency anemia and the maximum intake that will produce undesirable effects have been barely outlined. Information about the utilizable iron available from various foods or body losses under various conditions is limited.

Studies of vitamin A and iron content of infant diets in Israel revealed that no diet contained more than 60 per cent of the iron recommended and over 40 per cent of the diets provided only 60 per cent of recommended vitamin A.[25] Davis[26] in a study of vitamin E adequacy in infants' diets found a wide range of vitamin E intake daily, from 0.94 to 16.95 IU. Infants had low stores of vitamin E in their bodies and deficiencies could develop if the diet did not contain foods that supply adequate vitamin E. Many formulas contain less than recommended allowances of this vitamin. A high percentage of formulas do contain 5 or more IU of vitamin E but do not meet the proper ratio of this vitamin to polyunsaturated fatty acids. Jelliffe[27] contends

that so much stress has been placed on the need for adequate protein in the infant's diet that the adequacy of kcalories has been overlooked—so important in use of protein to the best advantage.

The need for additional research on the nutritional status of infants is urgent. From a survey of the studies cited here, iron appears to be the nutrient that is lacking most frequently in the infant's diet. Evidence of low vitamin A, ascorbic acid, and vitamin E intakes are other areas of concern. When kcalories are insufficient, protein and perhaps other nutrients are inadequate also. The quality of the diet in the first year of life is reflected in the quality of living in later years.

Nutrition and Brain Development and Behavior

Evidence to date indicates that malnutrition[28] per se and as an integral part of environmental influences may indirectly or directly produce adverse effects on brain development and behavior. Malnutrition never appears alone; it occurs in conjunction with poverty, disease, genetic disadvantages, familial disorganization, apathy, a lack of stimulating experiences, a mother with a low IQ and/or little education, ignorance, despair, and other variables.[29,30] Investigators have not determined if malnutrition as such contributes more or less than deprived social and environmental conditions. The periods in life when malnutrition is most serious are during pre-

[25] A. Goldberg and A. Reshef, "Vitamin A and Iron in Infants Diets in Israel," *Journal of the American Dietetic Association*, Vol. 60, No. 2 (February 1972), pp. 127–30.

[26] Karen C. Davis, "Vitamin E: Adequacy of Infant Diets," *American Journal of Clinical Nutrition*, Vol. 25, No. 9 (September 1972), pp. 933–938.

[27] D. B. Jelliffe, "Nutrition in Early Childhood," in Miloslav Rechcigl, Jr. (ed.), *Food, Nutrition and Health*, Vol. 16, S. Karger, Basel, 1973, p. 5.

[28] David B. Coursin (chairman), Richard H. Barnes, Herbert G. Birch, Robert Klein, Myron Winick, Paul R. Pearson, and Merrill S. Read, "Present Knowledge of the Relationship of Nutrition to Brain Development and Behavior," excerpts from the position paper on "The Relationship of Nutrition to Brain Development and Behavior" of the Subcommitttee on Nutrition, Brain Development and Behavior of the Food Nutrition Board of the National Academy of Sciences, *Nutrition Reviews*, Vol. 31, No. 8 (August 1973), pp. 242–246.

[29] Herbert G. Birch, "Malnutrition, Learning and Intelligence," *American Journal of Public Health*, Vol. 62, No. 6 (June 1972), pp. 773–775.

[30] Margaret R. Stewart, "Nutrition and Learning—Implications for Schools," *Nutrition Program News*, March–April 1971, pp. 1–4.

natal and early postnatal life (see Chapter 27).

When children have been severely malnourished in early life, tests at school age show that these children do less well than well-nourished controls who have not had a previous history of malnutrition. Some studies are in conflict with these results, raising the possibility of the impact of social–familial factors as abetting or retarding school performance. Chronic undernutrition into the school years leads to a suboptimal level of intellectual functioning, responsiveness, attentiveness, and vitality, according to Birch.[31] A state of adequate nutrition is essential for appropriate and sensitive responsiveness to the environment. Continued study is in order to identify and document more clearly the effects of interaction between nutrition and other environmental factors in the cognitive development of children. An overall effort to improve all facets of life, including nutrition, can contribute to intellectual growth and achievement of disadvantaged children.

Feeding the Premature and Low-Birth-Weight Infant

The premature baby, usually one who weighs from 2 to 5 pounds, demands special attention in feeding. The control of vital functions, such as sucking, coughing, and breathing, is incomplete. Nutrients he had formerly received from his mother's blood in a form ready for immediate use must now be ingested, digested, and absorbed, and with a rather defective apparatus this is a problem. Because of the difficulty in sucking and swallowing, the baby often regurgitates and may aspirate his food with serious results. There are few, if any, nutritional reserves, and almost inevitably the infant suffers from some form of anemia.

Most of these infants have to be hospitalized and fed through a tube. What to feed these infants is debatable. In a research study[32] three groups of low-birth-weight infants were each

fed one of the following milk preparations: mother's expressed breast milk, a proprietary low protein adapted cow's milk, or a half-cream and partly skimmed evaporated cow's milk. Each milk fed had an energy value of 65 kcalories per 100 ml. The protein content in the feeds were, respectively, 1.2, 1.5, and 4.1 g per 100 ml. The mean weight gain of each group of babies was at least 230 g per week during the third week of the trial. There were no symptoms of low blood calcium and at the end of 24 hours of life the blood glucose concentration was normal. There was no evidence of milk aspiration in any baby.

Ghadimi and others[33] made several observations about the nutritional management of low-birth-weight infants. Undernutrition is perhaps the most serious problem. Research is needed to determine the long-term effects of undernutrition at this age. The loss of weight after birth should not be accepted as it is for full-term infants, because nutritive reserves are very limited or nil. Conventional feeding methods cannot be employed.

Snyderman and Holt[34] indicate a number of nutritional problems of the premature infant: kcaloric requirements are higher, vitamins and fats are absorbed poorly, and there is a greater need for vitamin C, especially when high protein feedings are given. Brody[35] reports of studies done in New York and Finland indicate that the premature baby cannot handle cow's milk or a prepared infant formula because he cannot synthesize cystine, the amino acid that is lacking in cows' milk. Human milk has a good supply of cystine and one suggestion is to tube feed this kind of milk to these infants.

Babies born too soon and too small are more susceptible to death in the weeks after birth than full-term infants. Much prematurity and low birth weight are linked with

---

[31] Birch, op. cit., p. 781.

[32] "Feeding the Baby of Low Birth Weight," *Nutrition Reviews*, Vol. 31, No. 1 (January 1973), pp. 14–15.

[33] H. Ghadimi, K. Arulanantham, and M. Rathi, "Evaluation of Nutritional Management of the Low Birth Weight Newborn," *American Journal of Clinical Nutrition*, Vol. 26, No. 5 (May 1973), pp. 473–476.

[34] Snyderman and Holt, op. cit., pp. 673–675.

[35] Jane E. Brody, "Standard Diet for Premature Babies Is Questioned," *The New York Times*, July 8, 1970, p. 20.

teen-age pregnancy because the mother's body is not fully mature, she is at an age when nutritional demands of her own are urgent, and she may be malnourished. Low-income-level mothers often have premature and low-birth-weight babies. Premature babies of drug-addicted mothers have additional risk of complications from withdrawal symptoms such as vomiting, convulsive tremors, restlessness, and breathing problems.

Undernutrition in Infants

Malnutrition in the infant has a complex etiology; various important factors are assumed to be involved and potential interrelationships among these factors have been analyzed in many ways, according to Hegsted.[36] Authorities usually include quality and quantity of food, undesirable psychological and physical environment, parents or persons responsible for children who are ignorant of appropriate infant care, and inadequate health services.

The capacity for compensation of nutritional deficiencies is questionable, if a lack of nutrients occurs at a critical period of growth. Although further research is required, evidence is mounting that physical, mental, and biochemical handicaps are found in young children from undernutrition. Stunted growth, apathy, defective learning, reduced intelligence, and altered biochemical and immunologic responses are possible evidences. Obviously, the severity of nutritional deprivation, the time of life it occurs (critical periods are prenatal and early infancy), associated complications of infection, and the degree of chronicity are important considerations.

Social deprivation may be as devastating in effect as nutritional inadequacies. Children from minority groups, low socioeconomic classes, migrant families, institutions, and from depressed rural areas or metropolitan slums are indicated as high risks in development. Manifestations are impaired intellectual capacities, smaller physical size, higher mortality rates, and poor psychosocial adjustments.

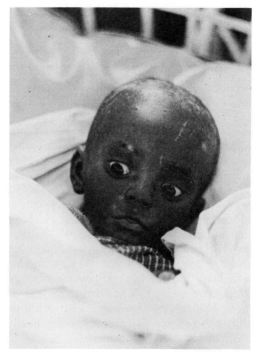

FIGURE 21–5.   *Refugee baby in Biafran emergency hospital suffering from severe nutritional deprivation.* (UNICEF)

Concomitant changes in the social environment, as well as other influences, must accompany nutritional improvement to be effective.

A particular concern about mental development has emerged. The brain and nervous system are dependent on nutrients for structure and function. Winick[37] has approached this problem by studying the increase in cell number and cell size in organs. Restricted nutrition results in a decreased cell number. Cell division ceased earlier in the brain than in other organs. Mönckeberg[38] contends that severe malnutrition during the first months of life provokes damage to the central nervous system. Malnutrition also leads to a diminishing of the brain size. A follow-up study of children

[36] D. M. Hegsted, "Deprivation Syndrome or Protein-Calorie Malnutrition," *Nutrition Reviews*, Vol. 30, No. 3 (March 1972), pp. 51–54.

[37] Winick, op. cit., p. 1.

[38] Fernando Mönckeberg, Susana Tisler, Sonia Toro, Vivian Gattas, and Lucy Vega, "Malnutrition and Mental Development," *American Journal of Clinical Nutrition*, Vol. 25, No. 8 (August 1972), pp. 766–772.

up to 7 years indicated a marked retardation of physical and psychomotor development.

Overnutrition in Infants

A surplus of kcalories leads to obesity in infants, which generally remains in childhood and often into adulthood. A survey[39] of infants in the first year of life showed a high incidence of overweight and obesity. One contributing factor suggested was early weaning and early introduction of solid food (some infants were offered food during the first week of life, 40 per cent by 4 weeks of age, and 93 per cent by 13 weeks of age) to the infant's diet, which resulted in a mean energy intake of 140 kcalories per kilogram of body weight—significantly above recommended allowances. Protein, carbohydrate, and fat intakes were also higher than recommended. The low incidence of breast feeding may have had a relationship to obesity. A high correlation was found between obese babies and obese parents.

Fomon[40] is concerned about the practice in some parts of the United States of feeding skim milk to infants beginning at 4 to 6 months of age as a means of treating real or imagined obesity or to prevent atherosclerosis. Although skim milk may be reasonably consumed in later childhood, it is unsatisfactory for infants in Fomon's estimation. Reasons offered are that, when skim milk is the major source of kcalories, kcaloric and fat intake are at undesirably low levels and protein and lactose are in contrast at too high levels. When kcaloric intake is less than 90 kcalories per kilogram of body weight per day between 4 and 8 months of age, there may be a curtailment of growth or activity or both. The low fat may interfere with the myelination of the nervous system.

An excessive amount of nutrients other than

kcalories may have undesirable effects on growth and development. A balance among the nutrients in amounts that yield an optimal diet is a good goal.

Infant Nutrition Around the World

Although the United States and other developed countries have the advantage of high-quality milk and other foods that help infants to grow and develop, this is not true in other parts of the world. In the developing countries, on the whole, infants are breast fed. The results are fairly satisfactory at the beginning, but if breast feeding is prolonged and the mother is poorly nourished, both the child and mother suffer. In a few instances extra foods may be given to mothers during pregnancy and lactation, but this is the exception rather than the rule. In addition, there are many restrictive taboos that present a nutritional disadvantage. In some countries, for example, there is a superstition about the eating of eggs.

Many types of animal milks have been used in these developing countries, but they are highly expensive and the supply is poor. Unfortunately, when fresh milk is bought, it is usually watered and adulterated and may even be further diluted by the mother to make it go further. Sweetened condensed milk is used in some areas because of its keeping qualities, but here again it is employed more as a flavoring than as a food.

In many countries semisolids are introduced at a very early age. In Malaya and other nearby countries, for example, rice may be given in the first days or weeks of life. Generally, however, they are added to the diet between the sixth and twelfth month, although variations occur, depending on the situation. In many cultures, the starchy food in the adult diet is prepared in such a manner that only the very soft portions of it are fed to the infant, but in some instances this is highly unsuitable. A paste is often made of rice, corn, or banana. In general, there is little transition between the infant diet and the adult diet. In many parts of the world, the infant diet is predominantly carbohydrate, with the addition of few other foods when available.

---

[39] "Overfeeding in the First Year of Life," *Nutrition Reviews*, Vol. 31, No. 4 (April 1973), pp. 116–118.

[40] Samuel J. Fomon, "Skim Milk in Feeding," *Commentaries on Infant and Child Nutrition*, Maternal and Child Health Service, Public Health Service, U.S. Department of Health, Education, and Welfare, Washington, D.C., January 1973, pp. 1–5.

Of great concern is the small amount of protein given to infants. Infectious diarrhea has many serious consequences at this age level. In some instances, all protein foods are withdrawn, which paves the way for kwashiorkor, the protein-deficiency disease. In rural Guatemala, for example, available figures reveal that at least 5 per cent of all children under 5 years of age at any given time are suffering from diarrhea, and evidence also discloses that for children at 1 year of age this condition occurs on an average of five times per year. When infants suffer from malnutri-tion, the result is the beginning of a vicious cycle. Malnutrition produces children and adults with depleted energy, shortened life spans, and lack of enterprise, all of which impede the physical, mental, and economic growth of the people of a nation. The nutrition efforts of specialized agencies of the United Nations, such as WHO, FAO, UNICEF, and UNESCO, have been of enormous assistance in solving this problem. The goal of sturdy healthy children in all countries of the world is indeed an admirable one.

SELECTED REFERENCES

Berg, Alan, *The Nutrition Factor*, The Brookings Institute, Washington, D.C., 1973, Chapters 2 and 7.

Cowell, Catherine, Ethel Maslansky, Margaret Grossi, Ruth Dash, Susan Kayman, and Morton Archer, "Survey of Infant Feeding Practices," *American Journal of Public Health*, Vol. 63, No. 2 (February 1973), pp. 138–141.

Cravioto, Joaquin, "Infant Malnutrition and Later Learning," in Sheldon Margen (ed.), *Progress in Human Nutrition*, The Avi Publishing Company, Westport, Conn., 1971, Chapter 8.

———, and Elsa R. DeLicardie, "Nutrition and Behavior and Learning," in Miloslav Rechcigl, Jr. (ed.), *Food, Nutrition, and Health*, Vol. 16, S. Karger, Basel, 1973, pp. 81–96.

Fomon, Samuel F., and Thomas A. Anderson, *Practices of Low-Income Families in Feeding Infants and Small Children with Particular Attention to Cultural Groups*, Maternal and Child Health Service, Public Health Service, U.S. Department of Health, Education, and Welfare, Washington, D.C., 1972.

———, Margaret G. Phillips, Mary C. Egan, and Nancy Haliburton, *Nutrition and Feeding of Infants and Children Under Three in Group Day Care*, Maternal and Child Health Service, Public Health Service, U.S. Department of Health, Education, and Welfare, Washington, D.C., 1971.

———, *Infant Nutrition*, W. B. Saunders Co., Philadelphia, 1974.

Food and Nutrition Board, *Recommended Dietary Allowances*, 8th ed., National Academy of Sciences—National Research Council, Washington, D.C., 1974.

Hegsted, D. M., "Deprivation Syndrome or Protein-Calorie Malnutrition," *Nutrition Reviews*, Vol. 30, No. 3 (March 1972), pp. 51–54.

Jelliffe, D. B., "Nutrition in Early Childhood," in Miloslav Rechcigl, Jr. *Food, Nutrition and Health*, Vol. 16, S. Karger, Basel, 1973, pp. 1–21.

Jelliffe, Derrick B., and E. F. Patrice Jelliffe (guest eds.), Symposium, "The Uniqueness of Human Milk," *American Journal of Clinical Nutrition*, Vol. 24, No. 8 (August 1971), pp. 968–1024.

Kallen, David J., "Nutrition and Society," *Journal of the American Medical Association*, Vol. 215, No. 1 (January 4, 1971), pp. 94–100.

King, Maurice, Felicity King, David Morley, Leslie Burgess, and Ann Burgess, *Nutrition for Developing Countries*, Oxford University Press, New York, 1972.

"Malnutrition, Learning, and Behavior," *Dairy Council Digest*, Vol. 44, No. 6 (November–December 1973), pp. 31–34.

Snyderman, Selma E., and L. Emmett Holt, Jr., "Nutrition in Infancy and Adolescence," in Robert S. Goodhart and Maurice E. Shils (eds.), *Modern Nutrition in Health and Disease*, Lea & Febiger, Philadelphia, 1973, Chapter 24.

"A Special Number Marking the Eightieth Year of Cicely D. Williams," *Nutrition Reviews*, Vol. 31, No. 11 (November 1973), entire issue.

22

Nutrition for Children

The status of nutrition of children today will be reflected in the next and succeeding generations. Within recent years the significance of nutrition in childhood has become more widely appreciated. Malnutrition may result in a tragic waste of human resources, so a high priority should be assigned to facilitating adequate nutrition of the young.

Growth

The complex process of growth depends heavily on nutrition, genes, environment, and time, according to Cheek.[1] Growth as defined by this researcher is a physiologic accretion of new tissue that is reflected in an increase in size—length, weight, and volume. Vital to the growth process is the growth hormone (GH) produced by the pituitary gland. Chok Hao Li has synthesized the growth hormone—the largest molecule ever produced in a laboratory.[2] The growth hormone functions by increasing the rates of synthesis of proteins and other cellular elements although the process itself is unclear.

Certain anthropometric measures are used to determine evidences of growth. Height reflects linear or skeletal growth. Two aspects are observed by X ray; growth of cartilage (chondroplasia) for length, and growth of bone structure and epiphyseal development (osteogenesis) for degree of bone maturation. Weight includes body water, protein, and electrolyte components that are constant, whereas body fat may vary. Height and weight of a child are commonly compared with the normal population of the same age to determine similarities or deviations as indications of growth status.

Other indices of growth are body density (which may be determined by an underwater weighing technique[3]), skinfold thickness, and wrist and hand X ray. Malina[4] researched pos-

[1] Donald B. Cheek, *Human Growth*, Lea & Febiger, Philadelphia, 1968, p. 3.

[2] Sandra Blakeslee, "Human Growth Hormone Produced in Laboratory," *The New York Times*, January 7, 1971, p. 1, 23.

[3] Charlotte M. Young, Sonia Sipin, and Daphne A. Roe, "Body Composition of Pre-adolescent Girls and Adolescent Girls," *Journal of the American Dietetic Association*, Vol. 53, No. 1 (July 1968), pp. 25–31.

[4] Robert M. Malina, "Skin Fold–Body Weight Correlations in Negro and White Children of Elementary School Age," *American Journal of Clinical Nutrition*, Vol. 25, No. 9 (September 1972), pp. 861–863.

sible correlation between skinfold weight of black and white children and found these measurements to be highly correlated. Magnitude of skinfold weight correlations was reasonably similar for three skinfold sites studied longitudinally over a 1-year period.

In the *Ten-State Nutrition Survey*[5] there was a heavy representation of children; more than 50 per cent of the population was 16 years of age or less. Height, weight, and other body measurements were used in identifying populations where nutritional inadequacies were reflected in retarded growth and development. Results indicated an excess of underweight and undersized children in comparison to commonly used U.S. standards.

Retarded growth and development were generally more prevalent in low-income-ratio states than in high-income-ratio states. Within each state surveyed, growth among children was less adequate in low-income groups. Despite low-income levels, black children were taller than white children and more advanced in skeletal and dental development, indicating a need for appropriate standards for black children. Racially based as well as nutritional factors have implications for growth.

In the nationwide *First Health and Nutrition Examination Survey*[6] certain measurements were taken: height and weight, elbow breadth, upper arm girth, triceps and subcapular skinfolds, bitrochanteric breadth, and sitting height. Children from 1 to 7 years of age were also measured for head and chest circumferences. Results were compared with U.S. standards. All these measurements gave some indication of growth status.

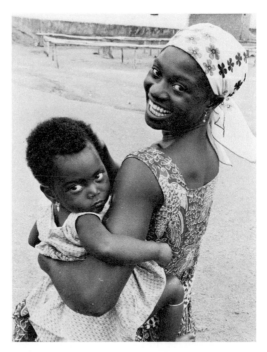

FIGURE 22–1. *Loving parental care may be a factor in healthy growth.* (UNICEF/Peter Larsen)

Factors other than nutrition have a bearing on growth. Emotional deprivation and trauma[7] have led some observers to the conclusion that these conditions generate a metabolic or hormonal dysfunction that is reflected in aspects of growth failure. Martin,[8] for example, found evidence of poor growth not due to organic causes as possibly associated with emotional deprivation, neglect, rejection of child by parents or peers, or poverty. Strong food dislikes, anorexia, and failure to thrive were important symptoms. Family–child interaction, suboptimal parental care, or emotional status may be at fault. Mata[9] and others

[5] *Highlights, Ten-State Nutrition Survey, 1968–1970*, DHEW Publication No. (HSM) 72–8134, Center for Disease Control, Health Services and Mental Health Administration, U.S. Department of Health, Education, and Welfare, Atlanta, Ga., 1972, p. 11.

[6] Vital and Health Statistics, Programs and Collection Procedures, *Plan and Operation of the Health and Nutrition Examination Survey, United States—1971–1973*, DHEW Publication No. (HSM) 73–1310 National Center for Health Statistics, Health Service and Mental Health Administration, Public Health Service, U.S. Department of Health, Education, and Welfare, Rockville, Md., 1973.

[7] "Emotional Deprivation and Growth Failure," *Nutrition Reviews*, Vol. 28, No. 2 (February 1970), pp. 36–38.

[8] Harold P. Martin, "Nutrition: Its Relationship to Children's Physical, Mental, and Emotional Development," *American Journal of Clinical Nutrition*, Vol. 26, No. 7 (July 1973), pp. 766–775.

[9] Leonardo J. Mata, Juan Jose Urrutia, Constantino Albertazzi, Olegario Pellecer, and Eduardo Arellano, "Influence of Recurrent Infections on

found that recurrent infections were reflected in deficient growth among low-income Guatemalan children. Important and lasting weight losses occurred consequent to infectious disease. Control of the disease as well as measures facilitating optimal nutrition are pertinent to desirable growth of children.

Martin contends that feeding and eating are the arena for acting out conflict between parent and child, and this information must be considered in addition to the dietary history. Nutritional status may reflect all aspects of life: physiological, psychological, and social.

Nutritional Status

Findings in the *Ten-State Nutrition Survey*[10] indicated a significant proportion of the child population surveyed was malnourished or was at high risk of developing nutritional problems. Income was found to be the major determinant of nutritional status, with factors such as social, cultural, and geographic differences also having an effect on the level of nutriture of a population group. Malnutrition was found most frequently among blacks, less commonly among Spanish-Americans, and least among whites. These findings reflect, in part, the lower income level of individuals living in the low-income-ratio states. (See Table 2–2.)

Preliminary findings of the *First Health and Nutrition Examination Survey* (HANES) in the United States[11] included information on kcalories, protein, vitamin A, vitamin C, and iron intakes for this age level. Intakes of less than 1000 kcalories were found in about 14 per cent of the white children 1 to 5 years of age and 23 per cent of the black children of the same age and in both income groups (be-

low and above poverty level). However, the overall mean intake of kcalories for children 1 to 11 years of age met 100 per cent of the standard for both blacks and whites in both income levels. Children of this age level for both race and income groups had calcium, vitamin A, and vitamin C intakes that met 90 to 100 per cent of the standard or were above the standard.

On the basis of mean intakes, iron was the nutrient most often found to be below the standard in population groups. Children 1 to 5 years of age had means that were 31 to 41 per cent below the standard in both income levels for blacks and whites. Black children from 6 to 11 years of age in the lower-income group consumed amounts of iron that were 19 per cent below the standard. Mean protein intakes per 1000 kcalories showed little or no variation by race or income, indicating that protein intake was closely related to total kcaloric intake. No protein problem appeared to exist in the 1 to 5 age group. In the 6 to 11 age group in the income level above poverty, white children had a greater percentage of low serum protein values (about 5 per cent) than did black children, who had about 1 per cent. No such change occurred in albumin values for this age level for which the percentage of low values was still zero.

Patterson[12] studied the food habits and physical development of fourth, fifth, and sixth graders of the Phoenix, Arizona, area; the children were of differing socioeconomic representation. Findings indicated that lower socioeconomic level children had more frequently occurring and more severe nutrient deficiencies than the higher socioeconomic group. Sixty-three per cent of the higher socioeconomic group and 71 per cent of the lower socioeconomic group had diets that failed to meet two thirds of the 1968 recommended dietary allowances for one or more nutrients. Nutrients most often below these recommended allowances in order of decreasing frequency were iron, vitamin A, calcium, thiamin, and ascorbic acid. Girls in the higher socioeco-

Nutrition and Growth of Children in Guatemala," *American Journal of Clinical Nutrition*, Vol. 25, No. 11 (November 1972), pp. 1267–1275.

[10] *Highlights, Ten-State Nutrition Survey*, op. cit.

[11] National Center for Health Statistics, *Preliminary Findings, First Health and Nutrition Examination Survey, United States, 1971–1972*, DHEW Publication No. (HRA) 74–1291–1 Health Resources Administration, Public Health Service, Department of Health, Education, and Welfare, Rockville, Md., 1974, pp. 1–25.

[12] Linda Patterson, "Dietary Intake and Physical Development of Phoenix Area Children," *Journal of the American Dietetic Association*, Vol. 59, No. 2 (August 1971), pp. 106–110.

nomic groups were larger in all measurements than the lower group. Boys in the higher socioeconomic group were taller and larger in hip widths than the lower socioeconomic group. Weights, leg girths, and skinfold measurements were fairly similar for both groups.

Ruffin and others[13] studied the nutritional status of preschool children of Marin County, California, welfare recipients. Findings revealed that growth retardation was evident in both white and black groups, particularly among the girls. There did not appear to be any distinct racial differences in the growth of equally impoverished children. It was impossible to isolate nutritional variables from other environmental factors. Although the dietary records showed low intakes of iron, the incidence of anemia was low. Serum protein values were within the normal limits. Dietary calcium, folacin, vitamin A, ascorbic acid, and vitamin B_{12} were low. The most outstanding biochemical defects were the low folacin levels in 36 per cent in the predominantly white groups and in 60 per cent of the chiefly black groups. Low hematocrit values were found in 18 per cent of the white group and 55 per cent of the black group. Another conclusion is that welfare allowances are grossly inadequate to purchase the quality of foods that provide adequate nutrition.

Larson and others[14] studied the nutritional status of Mexican-American migrant families. This 3-year study evaluated dietary, biochemical, clinical, and socioeconomic factors. The results were that mean vitamin A intake was generally adequate in comparison with recommended allowances when vitamin supplements taken by the children were included in the calculations. Vitamin D was considerably less than the allowances. Iron intake was slightly low, but protein intake was about twice the

recommended allowances. Intake of other nutrients generally exceeded the allowances. Biochemical and clinical evidence of vitamin A deficiency was found consistently in one third to one half of the children. Clinical evidence of vitamin D deficiency was present. Iron deficiency anemia was less common in 1972 than in 1970 or 1971. Low height and weight attainment in many of the children suggested the presence of nutritional problems.

A study of the nutritional status of black preschool children in Mississippi[15] has been made. Results were evaluated in terms of the mother's education. The average dietary intakes of kcalories and ascorbic acid, two of the more limited nutrients, were significantly greater if the mother's education was above the eighth grade. The percentage of children with "low" dietary intake of calcium paralleled the education of the mother, being significantly higher if the mother had more than an eighth grade education. Although protein intake was not a problem, again children of mothers with an education above the eighth grade had a significantly higher intake.

Dietary studies of preschool children in the North Central region revealed that approximately two thirds of 3,444 children were receiving the recommended allowances of kcalories and nearly all, the allowances for protein; calcium and phosphorus intakes compared favorably. Allowances fail to acknowledge the decrease of appetite and growth in the second year of life. Iron intakes were low as judged by 1968 recommendations.[16,17] In this as well

[13] Minnie Ruffin, Doris Howes Calloway, and Sheldon Margen, "Nutritional Status of Preschool Children of Marin County Welfare Recipients," *American Journal of Clinical Nutrition*, Vol. 25, No. 1 (January 1972), pp. 74–84.

[14] Lora Beth Larson, Janice M. Dodds, Donna M. Massoth, and H. Peter Chase, "Nutritional Status of Children of Mexican-American Migrant Families," *Journal of the American Dietetic Association*, Vol. 64, No. 1 (January 1974), pp. 29–35.

[15] Mary F. Futrell, Lois T. Kilgore, and Frances Windham, "Nutritional Status of Negro Preschool Children in Mississippi," *Journal of the American Dietetic Association*, Vol. 59, No. 3 (September 1971), pp. 224–227.

[16] Beth A. Fryer, Glenna H. Lamkin, Virginia M. Vivian, Ercel S. Eppright, and Hazel M. Fox, "Diets of Preschool Children in the North Central Region—Calories, Protein, Fat, and Carbohydrate," *Journal of the American Dietetic Association*, Vol. 59, No. 3 (September 1971), pp. 228–232.

[17] Hazel M. Fox, Beth A. Fryer, Glenna Lamkin, Virginia M. Vivain, and Ercel S. Eppright, "Diets of Preschool Children in the North Central Region—Calcium, Phosphorus, and Iron," *Journal of the American Dietetic Association*, Vol. 59, No. 3 (September 1971), pp. 233–237.

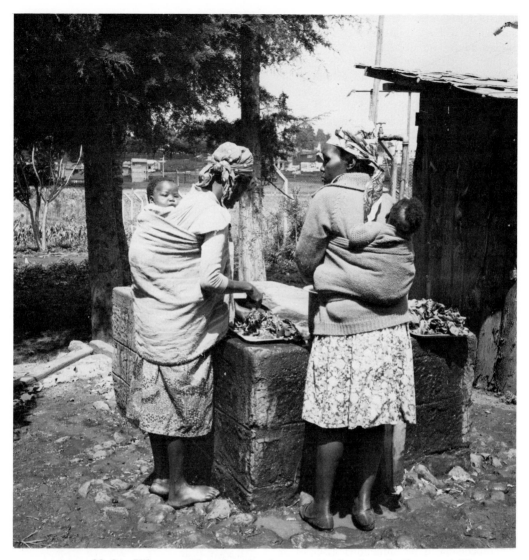

FIGURE 22–2. *Kikuyu mothers learning to prepare spinach and other vegetables for their malnourished children* (UNICEF/Alastair Matheson)

as other research cited here, iron is the nutrient that most frequently is short in dietary intake.

Lactose Intolerance

Low lactose intolerance among nonwhite populations in Asia, Africa, and among American blacks has been widely reported in contrast to a low prevalence among Caucasians. Most of the studies have been done on adults;

little information is available about the incidence among children. An examination as to whether lactose intolerance necessarily implies a milk intolerance was made by Reddy and Pershad.[18] These researchers studied the incidence of lactose intolerance and the levels of

---

[18] Vinodini Reddy and Jitender Pershad, "Lactose Deficiency in Indians," *American Journal of Clinical Nutrition*, Vol. 25, No. 1 (January 1972), pp. 114–119.

intestinal lactase in a group of Indian adults and children. Lactose intolerance was high in Indian adults, but lactase levels were higher in children. However, lactase levels decreased with age. Some children who exhibited low lactase activity did not manifest intolerance to lactose. The authors conclude that several factors, such as total lactase available, dose of lactose, and the amount of milk consumed at a time, are important in determining symptomatic response. One conclusion of the study was that some lactose-intolerant subjects can consume as much as 1 quart of milk daily if they drink small amounts throughout the day. Lactose intolerance is an important area of study in relation to nutritive status, because milk is recommended for all age levels for an adequate diet.

Risk Factors

Certain components of a child's diet, such as excess kcalories, fat, or sugar, may become risk factors leading to serious diseases in later life. Risk factor intervention programs, according to Friedman and Yanochik,[19] may reduce the potential of these conditions. Atherosclerosis, for example, is the basic cause for the number one national health problem, cardiovascular disease. This disease process may begin in the pediatric age as well as other associated risk factors, such as hypertension, obesity, and high levels of serum cholesterol. Screening children for overeating and inclusion of foods high in saturated fats and sugars appears desirable. Testing for the presence of hyperlipedemias is recommended. Lack of exercise and environmental factors, such as low income, unfavorable living conditions, and family–child relations, bear consideration. Parents and other adults responsible for children's health are often not aware that factors in a child's nutrition and life may have an impact on the quality of life in later years as well as the length of life.

[19] Glenn M. Friedman and Anita Yanochik, "Atherosclerosis and the Pediatrician," presented at the Symposium on Childhood Obesity in New York City, November 15 and 16, 1973, sponsored by the Institute of Human Nutrition, College of Physicians and Surgeons, Columbia University.

The Toddler Age

By the time the baby is 1 year of age, he graduates into the toddler class. At this age, his weight is about three times his birth weight, and his height is about one and a half times his birth length. He may have six to eight teeth. He can stand, at least with some support, and some 1-year-olds are able to walk. He makes some attempts at talking.

The toddler age, the period between 1 and 3 years, is noted for certain physical and mental changes. The rate of growth slows during the end of the first year and quite obviously after the first birthday. This may be alarming to parents, but it is normal. Another interesting facet is that the pattern of growth changes. For example, the legs and arms grow more than the trunk. Beginning at 18 months of age, or thereabout, there is usually a sudden surge in very rapid muscle growth. The skeleton itself may grow more slowly, but mineral is being deposited at quite a rapid rate so that the bones are stronger. This is necessary to support the greater weight of the child. As

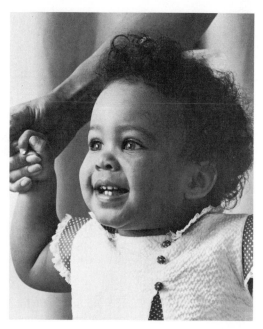

FIGURE 22–3. *A toddler with characteristics of excellent nutrition.* (*Courtesy Gerber Baby Foods*)

the muscles become larger, the child begins to look less and less like a baby. At the same time that these physical changes are taking place, there are corresponding changes in personality development. If a child is healthy and well nourished, the possibility of his being active, strong, happy, and friendly is good.

Nutritive Needs for the Toddler

Although the growth rate diminishes to its lowest childhood level at the toddler period, it is still extremely important to be aware of nutritive needs. Ample protein for the rapid growth of muscle is a primary consideration, but protein is also important for the growth of other body tissues. The National Research Council recommends that children 1 to 3 years of age have 23 g of protein daily.

The inclusion of 800 mg of calcium and 800 mg of phosphorus is important since these minerals are needed for increased mineralization of the bones, and it is essential that the bone strength keep pace with the growth of muscles. Iron also is a very important nutrient. The daily recommendation for iron for a child 1 to 3 years of age is 15 mg. This high requirement is to compensate for variations in availability of iron in foods and in absorption.

A child at this age level needs fewer kcalories for general body growth, comparatively speaking, than does the small baby. For instance, some children will not eat as many kcalories during their second year of life as they did during the second half of infancy. It is true that they need more kcalories for activity, but fewer for general growth.

The amount of activity varies greatly among children of this age. Very active children may consume as much as 2000 kcalories daily; very quiet children may consume around 1000 kcalories. The recommended allowance[20] for children 1 to 3 years of age is 1300 kcalories.

Recommended allowances for other nutrients for children from 1 to 3 years of age are 2000 IU of vitamin A, 400 IU of vitamin D, and 7 IU of vitamin E. Recommended allow-

[20] Food and Nutrition Board, *Recommended Dietary Allowances*, 8th ed., National Academy of Sciences—National Research Council, Washington, D.C., 1974.

ances for water-soluble vitamins for this age are 40 mg of ascorbic acid, 100 μg of folacin, 9 mg of niacin, 0.8 mg of riboflavin, 0.7 mg of thiamin, 0.6 mg of vitamin B_6, and 1 μg of vitamin B_{12}. Allowances for other minerals include 60 μg of iodine, 150 mg of magnesium, and 10 mg of zinc. All these nutrients are extremely important, and mothers who are inclined to become careless about food for a child at this age should be warned about the serious consequences of malnutrition. See Table 22–1 for recommended daily dietary allowances for children.

Food Requirements of the Toddler

Milk continues to be one of the most important foods in the toddler's diet. To provide adequate calcium, 2 to 3 cups of milk as a beverage and in foods such as cream soups, creamed dishes, milk desserts, and other types of milk dishes may be included. Milk also provides needed protein, phosphorus, large amounts of vitamin A and riboflavin, and some of the other B vitamins. Milk may be in any form acceptable to the child—fresh fluid whole, skim, dry (whole or nonfat), evaporated, or buttermilk. Cheese may be used in place of milk. (See Chapter 16 for equivalents.)

Other foods that will contribute to the protein requirement are 3 to 4 eggs a week and 1 to 2 tablespoons of meat a day. Occasionally mashed, cooked dried beans or peas or peanut butter may be substituted. Eggs may be scrambled, soft cooked, poached, steamed, or baked, but the important point is that they be cooked at low heat so that no crust forms on top. Children are very sensitive to the texture and consistency of eggs, and they are much more discriminating than adults in detecting off-flavors or differences in flavor. The eggs should be strictly fresh and kept well covered in the refrigerator so that there is little opportunity for them to absorb odors.

The meat may be beef, pork, lamb, liver, chicken, and boned fish. It can be made into patties or meat loaf and can be served in a tomato or white sauce. Special emphasis should be placed on frequent inclusion of liver to meet high demands for iron. The number of teeth the child has determines

TABLE 22–1

Recommended Daily Dietary Allowances for Children, Revised 1974

Designed for the maintenance of good nutrition of practically all healthy people in the United States

	AGE (years)		
	1–3	4–6	7–10
Weight, kg (lb)	13 (28)	20 (44)	30 (66)
Height, cm (in)	86 (34)	110 (44)	135 (44)
Kcalories	1300	1800	2400
Protein, g	23	30	36
Fat-soluble vitamins			
Vitamin A, IU	2000	2500	3300
Vitamin D, IU	400	400	400
Vitamin E, IU	7	9	10
Water-soluble vitamins			
Ascorbic acid, mg	40	40	40
Folacin, μg	100	200	300
Niacin, mg	9	12	16
Riboflavin, mg	0.8	1.1	1.2
Thiamin, mg	0.7	0.9	1.5
Vitamin B_6, mg	0.6	0.9	1.2
Vitamin B_{12}, μg	1.0	1.5	2.0
Minerals			
Calcium, mg	800	800	800
Phosphorus, mg	800	800	800
Iodine, μg	60	80	110
Iron, mg	15	10	10
Magnesium, mg	150	200	250
Zinc, mg	10	10	10

SOURCE: Food and Nutrition Board, National Research Council, *Recommended Dietary Allowances*, 8th ed., National Academy of Sciences, Washington, D.C., 1975, p. 129.

whether the meat is to be well ground, chopped, or cut into small pieces.

Some form of citrus fruit, such as oranges, grapefruit, or raw or canned tomatoes, needs to be given every day to meet the vitamin C requirement of the diet. And it is well to serve one other, noncitrus fruit. One serving of potatoes is important, and if boiled with the skin or baked, will contribute thiamin, niacin, and vitamin C in appreciable amounts. Two or more vegetables, especially green and yellow ones, are important for vitamins and minerals. There should be at least three servings of cereal or bread a day to contribute kcalories, iron, and B vitamins. A small amount

of table fat such as butter or margarine is important, too—generally a teaspoon is adequate. In regard to other foods like meat, fruit, and vegetables, 2 to 3 tablespoons is generally considered a serving for this age.

The diet pattern may vary in different parts of the country. In the South, for example, the use of beans and many kinds of greens provides an excellent source of iron. If cornmeal is used in bread, it is important that it be enriched.

Thus the foods for the 1- to 3-year-olds are very similar to those for the 1-year-old, but the variety is much greater and naturally the quantities are larger. Fresh ripe fruit may be added—the pulp of peaches, apricots, plums, pears, strawberries, blueberries, watermelon and canteloupe without seeds, and orange sections. Crisp raw vegetables like celery, leaves of lettuce, and strips of carrots can be introduced gradually. Bacon may be enjoyed also. All these foods should be bite sized or finger foods. Children like to feel as well as to see food, and enjoy it much more as a result.

It is extremely important at this age to avoid foods like corn, peanuts, nuts, raisins, large seeds of any kind, particularly watermelon seeds, cherry pits, gristle around chicken bones, and bits of tough fruit skin such as that on peaches and plums. The reason for this great care is that children can very easily inhale these foods into the windpipe, and this naturally could cause very serious trouble.

Other foods to be avoided are sugar, jams, jellies, marmalades, cake frostings, candy, and all types of soft drinks. They provide only kcalories and, since they are very sweet, tend to depress the appetite.

Children should be given an opportunity to learn new foods in order to recognize textures and flavors. Sometimes the mother of a child between 1 and 3 has a tendency to open cans of strained or chopped vegetables and mix them with other foods and make one big serving for the tot. This practice could be the beginning of violent dislikes for foods. Since changes from one texture to another take place during this age period, it is very important to make changes with the favorite fruit or vegetable first, if possible, and to select that time of day when the child seems to be hungriest. Children during this age can be rapidly moved to three meals a day with some snacks in between. See Table 22–2 for suggestions.

TABLE 22–2

Foods Included in Daily Diet for Children 1 to 3

FOOD[a]	AMOUNT[b] NEEDED DAILY	AVERAGE SIZE OF SERVING
Milk	2–3 cups	½–¾ cup
Eggs	1 medium egg, 3 to 4 times weekly	1 medium egg
Meat, poultry or fish	1 or more servings daily	2–3 tbs. Occasionally substitute cottage cheese, peanut butter, or cooked dried beans or peas.
Cereal[c]	1 serving a day	2 tbs cooked, or ⅓ cup ready to eat[c]
Bread	At each meal at which cereal is not served.	½ slice
Fruits and vegetables	4 or more servings (small). 1 serving every day of oranges or grapefruit, 1–2 servings every day of green or yellow vegetables. Cook vegetables and peel fruit. Include a wide variety of other fruits and vegetables.	1–2 tbs. If orange juice, 4 oz.
Butter or margarine	Some every day	Spread on bread or use in cooking

SOURCE: *Foods for the Preschool Child*, Office of Child Development, Children's Bureau, U.S. Department of Health, Education, and Welfare, Washington, D.C., 1970.
[a] Check foods for vitamin D content. The doctor may prescribe additional amounts.
[b] All measurements are level measuring cups and spoons being used.
[c] Cereals should be iron fortified and not sugar coated.

Feeding the Toddler

Not only are the foods for this age level important, but also the manner in which the child is fed. Often a child makes some attempt to feed himself before he is 1 year old. This is indicated when he reaches for the spoon, puts his fingers in the food, and attempts to carry it to his mouth. Managing a spoon when the muscles do not coordinate very well can become quite a task. Mothers should be very patient and give the child every possible encouragement. Sometimes children will even have difficulty in identifying which end of the spoon to use for eating. Some mothers, while feeding the child, have found it helpful to let him have a spoon too. This permits him to stir the food, to dip into it, and occasionally to attempt to feed himself. It is important that the spoon be of a size and shape that he can handle easily. Certainly a child cannot learn unless he has a chance to experiment; learning to handle utensils is not a spontaneous thing.

Other utensils need to be selected very carefully. A child during this age period will still encounter some difficulty in drinking from a cup. For that reason it might be well to use a small, unbreakable plastic cup. From 18 months of age to 3 years, children certainly

enjoy pouring their own fruit juice or milk from a small pitcher. Any responsibility that can be given to a child that makes him feel as though he is growing up or is participating is extremely helpful.

Children during this age period should not be expected to eat from a flat plate. Instead, the plate should have sides so that the child can run the spoon along the side and collect the food in that way for eating.

Eating habits are usually much better established if the child is fed apart from the family. The family table may offer too many distractions, and it is extremely important that a child of this age eat the food he requires. However, it may be wise to have the child eat an occasional meal with the family. At any rate, eating arrangements will vary with the family situation.

The child should not be fed in a part of the house where the mother is going to be concerned about damage to a new rug or to fresh wallpaper or the like. Not only will he get food all over himself and his high chair, or wherever he is sitting, but it may be distributed to other parts of the room. For that reason it is well to place the child's chair on a large piece of plastic material or the like, to protect the floor. Any anxiety that the mother shows about furnishings or even the

Suggested Menu for Child Aged 1 to 3

Breakfast	1 medium-sized orange in sections Cooked cereal 1 cup milk—part on cereal, remainder to drink
Midmorning snack	½ cup milk or small piece of fresh fruit or a cracker
Lunch	1 oz canned chopped liver Baked potato Mashed carrots, whole cooked carrots, or raw carrot strips Milk pudding ½ cup milk Bread
Midafternoon snack	½ Zwieback (enriched)
Supper	Scrambled egg Toast with butter or fortified margarine ½ cup milk to drink Banana *Size of servings is adjusted to age of child*

appearance of the child will be transmitted quickly. It may turn the process of feeding himself into a frustrating experience rather than a pleasant and exciting adventure.

A casual attitude is urged when a child accepts or rejects food. Comments by family members that are derogatory about a food or in contrast oversell a food may color a child's reaction toward specific foods. A child should not be forced to eat even a bite of food that he dislikes. Substitutes of foods similar in nutritive value may be offered.

Lowenberg[21] suggests that timing is important for successfully feeding the child. If possible avoid feeding children by the clock but rather have hunger determine mealtime. Knowing the individual child will help—when he is hungriest, amount of outdoor exercise, amount of sleep he has had, was play active or sedentary in nature, and how he feels—loved or rejected. The needs of the child as far as possible should determine the times for feeding.

A child gets many of his teeth during the toddler period. As teething is a painful experience, this may cause some fretfulness. Food should not be forced upon him. Some mothers have found that frequent small feedings are more acceptable; others have discovered that having something to chew on is a help. It may be necessary to change the consistency of foods, to serve them as soups or in other soft or liquid form.

Table 22–2 suggests the amounts of food that children from 1 to 3 should have each day, and a typical menu for this age level is suggested. The older child will naturally have larger servings than the younger one.

In-Between Feedings for the Toddler

The toddler usually has midmorning and midafternoon snacks. The snack will depend somewhat upon the kind of food served at other meals. But, in any case, essential foods should be included each day. Foods commonly served at this time are pieces of fresh fruit,

peeled and with seeds removed, Zwieback, tomato or fruit juice, milk, Melba toast, or graham crackers. These snacks should not in any way detract from regular meals.

Avoiding Food Problems for the Toddler

Persons responsible for feeding small children can do much to avoid serious food problems. Mealtime should be a pleasant time. Even small children will respond to a pretty table or gay dishes. Garnishes on food, such as a bit of chopped parsley or a sprinkle of hard-cooked agg, are inviting. Fruit may be hidden in the bottom of a pudding dish to serve as a surprise.

It is extremely important that the foods not be too hot or too cold. Certainly scorched foods or lumps in foods are very noticeable to children.

Toddlers gradually become more and more independent, and parents should encourage this trait. On the other hand, because they are learning so many new things, they can easily become discouraged. A calm and sympathetic attitude seems to be a good safeguard in most situations. Children will imitate their parents

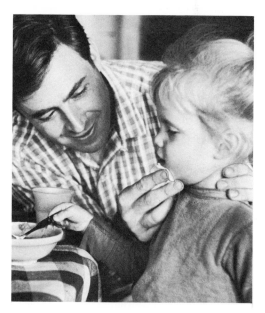

FIGURE 22–4. A father assists his child in developing good food habits. (Forecast)

[21] Miriam E. Lowenberg, "For the Young Child —Success Promotes Success in Eating," Food and Nutrition News, Vol. 40, No. 6 (March 1969), pp. 1, 4.

even at this age; hence desirable food habits on the part of their elders are important. New food should be introduced in small amounts and, if possible, in connection with the food that is well liked. Also, it is well to serve it at a time when the child is hungriest. Seeing other members of the family eat the food with relish can be a genuine incentive.

Parents must realize that children of this age may be dawdlers. Their attention is very easily distracted so it is advisable for them to eat in a quiet place, away from any other activities that may draw their attention. The mother must also be sensitive at realizing the point at which the child is weary and needs help in eating. If he begins to throw food on the floor and to play with it, he is usually indicating that he is not hungry. The food should then be removed promptly without scolding. A mother must learn to reduce all signs of anxiety about the child's eating. At times his appetite may seem very small. Some children are hungry once a day and eat little at other meals. And some days they eat much less than others. A healthy child will generally eat well if he has adequate exercise. Very rarely do children undereat consistently.

Parents or others responsible for feeding children of this age should bear in mind that their attitudes and efforts in handling eating situations are just as important as in other aspects of child rearing. Good eating habits can be achieved easily if the child is carefully handled and is given sympathy, interest, and praise for his accomplishment.

Adapting Family Meals for the Toddler

The family with children of toddler age need not be faced with the problem of different meals for different age levels. Food that is good for children is also good for adults. And some adult foods can be adapted for children. For example, if a cream pie is prepared for the older members of the family, the filling can be served to the children as their dessert. And sauces added to adult foods may be omitted from the children's food. Children can learn rather quickly that certain foods are only for grownups and accept the difference in a happy manner. Size of servings vary, of

course. It is difficult for adults to realize that servings for this age level are very small. It is much better to give toddlers small servings and have them ask for seconds than to overwhelm them with large servings. Excessive sugar and salt should be avoided.

Food for the Preschool Child

A child in the preschool period from 4 to 6 years continues to build food preferences and prejudices that may have a great influence upon his eating habits. By this time his senses have developed to the extent of influencing his behavior. In other words, if there are foods whose color, taste, texture, odor, or the like do or do not appeal to him, he will respond accordingly. His nutritional needs continue to be very important and it is imperative that they be met.

Nutritive Needs of Preschool Children

The nutrients recommended by the Food and Nutrition Board for children from 4 to 6 years of age are listed in Table 22–1.

Foods for the Daily Diet of the Preschool Child

Certain foods should be included in the diet each day. Among these food groups it is important to provide as wide a variety as possible to be absolutely sure that the child has an adequate diet.

The following foods are recommended for the preschool child:

MILK   Two to three cups, some of which may be used in cooking.

EGG   One egg three to four times per week, which may be prepared in many ways or combined with milk as a custard or other desert.

MEAT   An average serving of beef, lamb, poultry, fish, pork, or liver. Occasionally fish may be offered as a substitute for one serving of meat. An average serving of meat for this age is generally considered one level tablespoon per year of age, but this is not an inflexible rule and perhaps the entire amount should not be placed on the child's plate at once. He can ask for a second serving.

POTATOES One average serving.

VEGETABLES One or two servings including a green or yellow vegetable. Vegetables may include carrot, squash, lettuce, green peas, rutabaga, green peppers, celery, tomatoes, beets and beet greens, green and wax beans, broccoli, cauliflower, cabbage, spinach. Vegetable juices may be served to children and are usually enjoyed.

FRUITS At least two servings, if possible. One of these servings should be a citrus fruit such as orange or grapefruit or tomato juice (three times as much).

CEREALS One average serving of enriched or whole-grain cereal (iron-fortified recommended).

BREAD Three thin slices of whole-grain or enriched bread.

BUTTER Two level teaspoons of butter or margarine.

SOURCE OF VITAMIN D According to physician's directions.

These foods will provide the nutrients each day for the child. If he is extremely active and appears to need extra kcalories, it might be well to increase the bread, cereal, or fruits and vegetables.

Suggestions for Food Handling by the Preschool Child

Children of this age have developed many skills and are able to handle food much better than the toddler. Furthermore, they like to have some choice and to experiment with food. They are not adult by any means, espe-

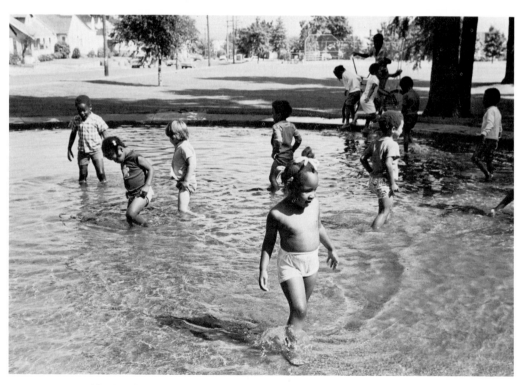

FIGURE 22–5. *Active children may need extra kcalories.* (USDA)

cially in the handling of food, and so for that reason it is well to have as many finger foods as possible. Bread or toast or sandwiches should be cut in strips. Lettuce and cabbage are much more easily eaten in leaf form than if they are shredded. Raw vegetables like carrots, green pepper, and celery can be in strips. Meat or liver, and even vegetables, cut into small pieces are much easier to manage.

Children enjoy change of texture in their food. They like crisp vegetables or chewy foods like lamb chop bones or potato skins. Cereals and puddings should be of a jelly-like rather than paste-like consistency.

At this age, children frequently go on "food jags," which should be treated in a nonchalant manner. They may go all out for liver or baked potatoes for a number of days and then scorn them completely and take up some other food or combination of foods. Bland foods with mild and delicate flavors are much to be preferred to strong-flavored foods.

Color appeals to them strongly, so that food with bright colors seems to make a child's plate much more attractive to him. Color can also be stressed in the utensils, such as cups, plates, and even the table mats.

Every attempt should be made to introduce the child to new foods periodically so that his repertoire will grow. However, it is advisable not to try more than one new food at a meal. It is too much to expect the child to face three or four new foods at the same meal with enthusiasm.

The temperature of food seems to be very important. Children generally prefer their food to be lukewarm, even milk. However, some 4- and 5-year-olds like their milk cold. This is a matter of personal preference.

The utensils used by young children should be convenient for them to handle. Children at this age level as well as toddlers prefer flat soup bowls or plates with curved edges so that they do not have to chase food around on a flat plate. Their fingers are too chubby and awkward to lift foods on a spoon or fork from a flat plate. Glasses should be low, squat, and light in weight. The size should be 4 oz, rather than 8 oz, which seems to be a little too large for a child to handle. Children are likely to spill easily at this age because their large muscles are developed much better than their smaller muscles. Providing individual pitchers so that they may pour their own milk is a great stimulant for drinking milk. Forks should have broad short handles and short blunt tines, and spoons should have shallow bowls.

Children, according to Lowenberg,[22] seem to resist eating fish. She was ingenious in developing a souffle incorporating the fish right in the white sauce and custard mixture, which children liked very much. She also recommends that creamed foods should not be put on pieces of toast, but rather that bite-sized pieces of toast be placed in the sauce—a much easier style for a youngster to handle.

Children like surprises in food. Sometimes they respond to interesting names for foods and in some cases they may like to name the foods themselves. In serving, it is important that all the tough parts be removed and that the food be cut into bite-sized pieces.

Needs will vary from child to child, but generally children need some kind of between-meal snack. This might be a small serving of orange juice, skimmed milk, or a cracker. It is extremely important that children be well rested before starting to eat. Many a child dawdles or seems to be uninterested in his food because he is tired and sleepy. If he is extremely weary at night, it might be better for him to miss the meal entirely and to go to bed. Sometimes it is good practice to have a short rest before mealtime. A child at this age thrives on schedules and responds well to regularity.

Some Don'ts for Preschool Children

Although many parents are under the impression that they do not force their child to eat, they may, in fact, be guilty of a number of faults. Some of the most common are as follows:

ENTERTAINMENT Frequently parents will indulge in all kinds of capers to interest their

---

[22] Miriam Lowenberg, "Food Preferences of Young Children," *Journal of the American Dietetic Association*, Vol. 24, No. 5 (May 1948), pp. 430–434.

child, such as dancing, singing, use of puppets, reading or telling a story, or permitting the child to eat and watch television. Such practices are wrong, for they distract the child from his food and cause him to focus his attention on anything but the food.

SCOLDING Constantly reminding a child that he is naughty because he is not eating leads only to tension and frustration.

COMPETITION Many a parent will hold up a brother or sister as an example to get a child to eat. They may resort to: "See, Susie is eating all hers. Why can't you eat yours?"

BRIBERY Many a parent will bribe a child into cleaning his plate. He may be given a choice toy or a promise of some kind of activity.

HURRYING Parents must be extremely patient and the mother who starts almost immediately to say, "Come on, come on, don't keep me here all day," or something similar is not providing the best eating environment for her child.

PLEADING Often mothers will use an imploring tone and practically beg their children to eat. This practice helps children to realize that eating can be an attention-getting device, and they will concentrate on that rather than on eating.

THREATS Occasionally mothers threaten their children with punishment or some other form of unpleasant reprisal if they do not eat.

These and many other procedures are to be condemned as leading to unwholesome food habits. Parents must learn to be casual in handling children while eating.

Adapting Family Meals for Preschool Children

Family meals can be easily adapted to this age level. The budget can also be kept down even though there are children of various ages

in the family. Sometimes parents are under the impression that only expensive food should be given to children. Fruits and vegetables in season, meat that gives the most lean meat for the money, canned vegetables that are often cheaper than fresh or frozen, tomatoes either home- or commercially canned, and such meats as ox tongue or beef heart are all good examples of wholesome food easily obtained at low cost. Sometimes fish can be purchased inexpensively and made into fish loaf.

The important point for parents to realize is that they can learn a great deal about their children by studying them. Children express their likes and dislikes very freely, and these should be observed and taken into consideration. There is a wide variety of ways to adapt meals to likes and dislikes. If certain vegetables are disliked, perhaps others that are

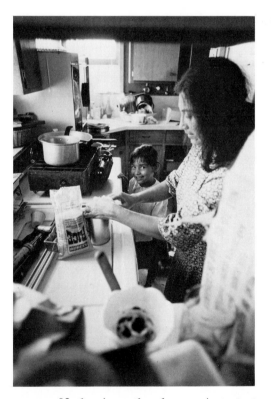

FIGURE 22–6. A mother has an important responsibility to plan a nutritious diet for her children. (USDA)

equally nutritious can be substituted, and in time the child may learn to like the food he disliked so heartily at one time. Parents must also realize that eating is a very important step in the child's development, and the kind of person that he will be for the remainder of his life may be strongly influenced by the good habits established at this period.

The impact of the frequency of eating on the dietary intake of children has had little attention. Eppright and others[23] made a study of preschool children in 12 North Central states. The findings were that eating schedules of preschool children were highly individual. No typical times were found for morning, noon, and evening meals. Snacks were eaten as frequently as meals. The majority of the children (71.2 per cent) ate four to seven times a day. Forty per cent of the meals were eaten with other members of the family.

The largest percentage of the children ate four to five times a day, including meals and snacks, and this frequency was established by the fourth, fifth, and sixth years. If eating occurred less than four times, the food energy intake was negatively affected; it was positively affected if eating took place six or more times a day. Eating less than four times a day had an unfavorable effect on calcium, protein, and ascorbic acid but not on protein or iron content of the diet.

The question is frequently asked if a child can be well nourished on a vegetarian diet. Adequate nutritive intake can be provided on a lacto-ovo-vegetarian diet if sufficient milk, eggs, and cheese are included to make provision for the needs for good-quality protein, vitamin B_{12}, vitamin A, calcium, iron, and other minerals; deficiencies may occur on a strict vegetarian diet without these foods. Green-leafy vegetables must be incorporated for folic acid and vitamin C. One problem of the vegetarian diet is the large amount of bulk, which may aggravate the functioning of the gastrointestinal tract. (See Chapter 29

for additional information on vegetarian diets.)

Sanjur and Scoma[24] in a study of food habits of low-income children in northern New York had findings of interest. More children than mothers had a diversified diet. Foods unfamiliar to the mother were also unfamiliar to the child. The contention that black families retain faith in a high number of erroneous beliefs about food and nutrition was negated. The mother's regional origin was the strongest predictor of family functioning.

Food habits of this age group may be influenced by mass media, especially television commercials on children's programs. A young viewer may see as many as 25,000 commercials a year. This stimulation of children's desires and subsequent buying has been discussed by Ward.[25] For example, 95 per cent of the mothers of children in the 5 to 7 age group and 88 per cent of mothers of the 8 to 10 group felt that children frequently request products and brands mentioned on television advertising.

Arena,[26] a physician, is concerned about the impression given that vitamin pills and medication are "just candy" and that their safe use is not highlighted. Overdoses can be serious. Some commercials imply that vitamin pills compensate for inadequate diets—an untruth. Television commercials could be informative nutritionwise and make a genuine contribution to the health of American children.

Pica Practices

Some young children in this age level indulge in pica practices. Ingestion of such non-food items as dirt, match ends, charcoal, cigarette ashes, bean clods, and pieces of clay

[23] Ercel S. Eppright, Hazel M. Fox, Beth A. Fryer, Glenna H. Lamkin, and Virginia M. Vivian, "The North Central Regional Study of Preschool Children, 3. Frequency of Eating," *Journal of Home Economics*, Vol. 62, No. 6 (June 1970), pp. 407–410.

[24] Diva Sanjur and Anna D. Scoma, "Food Habits of Low-Income Children in Northern New York," *Journal of Nutrition Education*, Vol. 2, No. 3 (Winter 1971), pp. 85–95.

[25] Scott Ward, "Children and Promotion: New Consumer Battleground," Preliminary Research Report, Working Paper, Marketing Science Institute, Cambridge, Mass., 1972, pp. 7–12.

[26] Jay Arena, "Vitamin Pills and Children," *The New York Times*, June 30, 1972, p. 35.

TABLE 22–3

Foods Needed Every Day for Ages 7 to 10

FOOD	AMOUNT	REMARKS
Milk	2–3 cups to 9 years of age; 3 or more cups at 10 years	May be served as a beverage and some incorporated into other foods.
Egg	1	At least 3 or 4 a week.
Meat, liver, fish, or poultry	3 oz	Liver should be served at least once a week
Citrus fruit or tomato	1 serving	Fruit or as juice. Three times as much tomato is needed as citrus fruit.
Fruit, other	2 servings	Fresh, frozen or cooked.
Potato, cooked	1 small	
Vegetable, green leafy or yellow	1 serving ⎫	In salad or cooked.
Vegetable, other	2 servings ⎭	
Bread or cereal, whole grain or enriched	3 servings	
Butter or margarine	1 tbs	Spread on bread.

pots were reported by Bruhn and Panghorn[27] in a study of incidence of pica among migrant families of Mexican and "Anglo" ancestry. In a number of incidences the mothers of these children also exhibited pica. In their review of the literature on this practice the authors indicate that pica has its basis in tradition, pleasure, and general living conditions.

The School Child

School days are among the most eventful periods in life. During the years from 7 to 10, boys and girls grow, mature, become socially independent, and expand their contacts and interests. The kind of food a child has during this period can do much to increase the quality of his living in general, as well as his life expectancy.

Nutritive Needs of Children 7 to 10

The nutritive needs for 7 to 10 age group are indicated in Table 22–1, as recommended

[27] Christine M. Bruhn and Rose Marie Panghorn, "Reported Incidence of Pica Among Migrant Families," *Journal of the American Dietetic Association*, Vol. 58, No. 5 (May 1971), pp. 417–420.

by the Food and Nutrition Board. The nutrients required for children of this age can readily be translated into everyday foods. Table 22–3 shows foods that these children should have every day.

Suggestions for specific foods under these various categories are offered here. In selecting leafy green and yellow vegetables, it is well to have them a deep yellow or a bright green. For citrus fruit, select canned, fresh, or frozen fruit, depending on local conditions and prices. In regard to milk, pasteurized or evaporated milk may be used in the diet of a child; dried or evaporated milk used in cooking reduces the food budget. All types of meat, fish, or poultry can be introduced into the diet, and special emphasis should be given to organ meats. Liver should be served once a week if possible. In the selection of bread and cereals, whole-grain or enriched products should be chosen. Margarine or butter may be included in the diet in many ways.

Suggestions for Meal Patterns

These foods lend themselves easily to a menu pattern for the day, as indicated in the suggested menu. In addition to the foods in-

Suggested Menu for Child Aged 7 to 10

Breakfast	Fruit or fruit juice (citrus fruit preferred) Cereal dry or cooked Egg (3 to 4 a week) Bread Milk
Lunch (carried to school)	1 to 2 sandwiches on whole-grain bread with a protein filling such as meat, cheese, fish, or peanut butter Raw vegetable sticks Fruit Milk Cookie
Dinner	Meat, fish, or poultry (sometimes cheese) Potato Green or yellow vegetable Salad Dessert (preferably with some fruit) Bread
Snacks	Fruit, milk, crackers, or raw vegetables make appropriate snacks for after school or in the evening.

dicated, others may be added for adequate kcalories, depending upon the lifestyle of the child.

By using this menu pattern, one can have endless variations in the days' meals. For breakfast, eggs may be prepared in many ways —soft cooked, poached, scrambled, or in an omelet. They should be served at least three times a week. Tomato juice may be substituted for the citrus fruit for breakfast, but three times the amount must be served to get the same vitamin C value. Potatoes can be prepared in many ways and in some cases might be combined with meat or cheese. The green or yellow vegetable may be the cooked vegetable for dinner, or served in the salad for dinner, or as vegetable sticks for lunch. Other items like desserts, salad dressings, soups, or sauces may be added to the diet for flavor and to increase kcalories.

The day's nutrients should be well distributed among the important meals. In other words, there should not be a light breakfast and a heavy lunch or dinner. If a child eats his lunch at home or in the school cafeteria, the menu plan should be adjusted accordingly. It is important that this meal carry its share of important nutrients. Each meal should contribute to the day's nutrients.

Children's Meals Are Family Meals

A child's meals are seldom different from the family meals. A mother or whoever is responsible for planning the meals, however, will wish to give special attention to the growing child so that he has adequate nutrients. This will require frequent checking on the food eaten outside of the home so family meals can compensate for any apparent nutritive shortcomings. Also, the family can do a great deal to help a child in learning how to select foods so that he will eat a nutritious meal whether he is at home or elsewhere. The kind of meals he has at home will determine to a large extent his food preferences as well as his feelings about food. Tasty and attractive food will facilitate good food habits.

School Life Affects Meal Plans

When a child starts to school, some adjustments are necessary if he eats his noon meal away from home—at school or near the school.

Most youngsters of school age do not lack an appetite. Sometimes this age is considered

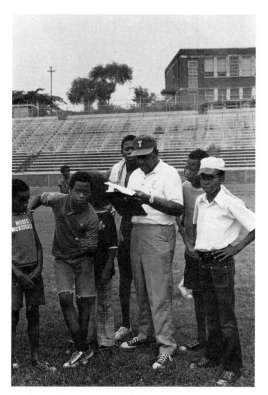

FIGURE 22–7. *A nutritious diet is helpful in promoting physical fitness for school athletics.* (USDA)

the healthiest time of life, for the mortality rate is lowest. However, a complex schedule, which sometimes accompanies a school program, may cause eating problems.

Hurrying through breakfast or skipping it, rushing through lunch, or permitting outside activities to interfere with the evening meal should be avoided at all times. The problem of undereating during this period can be serious. In every community the home must cooperate with the school to ensure an adequate nutrition and health program.

Food Habits of Children

Research and surveys show a noticeable trend toward poorer eating habits as the child grows older. Since the habits formed during this particular age may remain with a youngster throughout his entire life, every effort should be made to establish good eating habits.

Sheer ignorance of nutritional needs may be a major cause of poor food habits. Many parents are unaware not only of their children's needs in foods but also of other health requirements, like regularity of meals and adequate sleep and exercise.

When families are large and income is low, there seems to be a greater tendency toward poor food habits. Surveys show that there are fewer protective foods used in low-income families and the incidence of malnutrition among the children is greater.

On the other hand, it has been demonstrated that mere knowledge of nutrition does not ensure a good diet. Many other factors are involved. In many homes the children have not been helped to establish a taste for nutritious food, nor have food prejudices been discouraged. Parents seldom realize the importance of setting a good example. If father[28] does not like salad or does not drink milk, it will be difficult for his young son to follow a better eating plan. The dislikes of one individual are often imitated by other members of the family. Children especially tend to imitate the mother, who has a tremendous influence on family eating habits. Seldom will she prepare foods she dislikes, and consequently children may not be exposed to these foods unless they have them in their school lunch or on other occasions.

General family practices influence food habits in other ways. The cultural background is of prime importance. Attempting to make adaptations for foods they like a great deal is especially prevalent among families who have migrated to this country from other parts of the world. In other families, fad diets are popular, and as a result children become innocent victims.

Another serious food habit is simply having too little food. This may come about through scanty breakfasts or skipping certain meals.

[28] Marian S. Bryan and Miriam E. Lowenberg, "The Father's Influence on Young Children's Food Preferences," *Journal of the American Dietetic Association*, Vol. 34, No. 1 (January 1958), pp. 30–35.

Parents are not aware that active children do need adequate amounts of food.

A study of the food habits of Minnesota schoolchildren by Littman[29] and others revealed that the children endorsed milk, potatoes, bread, meat, butter, and eggs as everyday foods. Through the use of the Lewin Anchorage Point of Food Habits technique, children indicated that they were most likely to be scolded for eating sweet and confectionery foods and praised for the consumption of vegetables, dairy products, and the like. The mother was the most powerful influence in the sanctioning of food habits. Green and yellow vegetables and liver were little favored by these children.

Psychological Aspects of Children's Eating

Emotions are often associated with eating. The child's feelings toward his parents, particularly his mother, who is responsible for giving him food, may affect his food habits, especially if the relationship is not wholesome. The environment or locale in which a child lives may have an effect on his food choices. In many homes children develop a very strong feeling toward certain traditional foods, holiday foods, or foods for fast days. Often they also refuse to eat certain foods because they are not eaten by their playmates. The approval of one's peers is a very strong motivation.

In the minds of many children, the symbolic significance of food is more important than the food itself. Many children gain approval by giving food to others, for example, giving candy, sharing something in their lunch box, or bringing something from home that can be given to friends. Swapping foods from their lunch boxes or from their school cafeteria trays may deprive children of important nutrients and should be discouraged.

Feeding Handicapped Children

There are millions of handicapped children in the United States and family members and individuals responsible for them must be cognizant of their nutritional needs, according to Wallace.[30] A handicapped child has the same needs as other children, but, in addition, nutrition may be a factor in survival and development into useful and productive members of society.

Self-feeding is often one of the activities of daily living in the rehabilitation process. When a child can feed himself, it is an important step to independence not only in feeding but in other areas of life. A child's family plays an important role in this process, such as in planning nutritious food for the child and in helping him to learn to handle his food by himself.

Few studies have been done on the nutritional status of handicapped children. Bryan and Anderson[31] in a study of crippled children in North Carolina found that 45.7 per cent of the children had low nutrient intakes. For 72.2 per cent of the children, the cause was the poor diet of the family. Kripke and Sanders[32] noted that 13.4 per cent of the children had height measurements and 9.5 per cent had weight measurements below the third percentile. Some were anemic; 4.1 per cent had hemoglobin concentrations below 10.0 g per 100 ml.

Deaf children may be hampered because they are not exposed to cultural cues for learning about foods and nutrition as much as other children. The potential for interaction with

[29] Theodore J. Littman, James P. Cooney, and Ruth Stief, "The Views of Minnesota School Children on Food," *Journal of the American Dietetic Association*, Vol. 45, No. 11 (November 1964), pp. 433–440.

[30] Helen M. Wallace, "Nutrition and Handicapped Children," *Journal of the American Dietetic Association*, Vol. 61, No. 2 (August 1972), pp. 127–133.

[31] A. H. Bryan and E. L. Anderson, "Dietary and Nutritional Problems of Crippled Children in Five Counties in North Carolina," *American Journal of Public Health*, Vol. 55, No. 10 (October 1965), pp. 1545–1554.

[32] S. S. Kripke and E. Sanders, "Prevalence of Iron-Deficient Anemia Among Young Children Seen in Ambulatory Clinics," *American Journal of Clinical Nutrition*, Vol. 23, No. 6 (June 1970), pp. 716–724.

individuals in their world is lessened. Consequently, many deaf children are lacking in food and nutrition knowledge, according to Garton and Bass.[33] In a food and nutrition knowledge survey with deaf and hearing students, the hearing students answered 67 per cent of the questions correctly as compared to 47 per cent for the deaf children. Because deaf children do not hear the names of food spoken, they may fail to identify the name with the food; some foods, such as gelatin salad, were unknown to 18.4 per cent of the deaf children, and veal cutlets were not identified by 20.4 per cent of the group. Food preferences on the whole were similar to hearing students, with salads and vegetables receiving the lowest preference ratings. A special effort to teach the deaf with pictures of food and by placing food labels near foods served in the cafeteria to strengthen identification is under discussion.

Many suggestions[34] have been offered for the feeding of handicapped children. Some must be helped to learn to chew, to suck, to swallow, to control their tongues, or to guide hand movements while eating. Special equipment such as a bent spoon with a special handle, a spoon with an extended handle, a plate guard, using clay underneath as an anchor for a plate, and other devices are helpful.

Feeding the retarded child can present special problems. The mechanics of eating, such as learning to chew, masticating food adequately, and swallowing a little food at a time may prove to be a hurdle. These children may be obese, have poor digestion and constipation, as a result of the difficulty in learning to eat properly. Some retarded children appear to be greedy, gulping down large quantities of food at a time; others may refuse to eat. Parents must be especially vigilant in selecting an adequate diet for these children. Also, they must be patient and give considerable attention to assisting the child in the process of eating as well as in general motivation.

It must be borne in mind that many factors can cause eating problems. No eating problem is simple. Generally speaking, many aspects are involved. It behooves a teacher, parent, or anyone working with the child to determine and then eliminate possible causes or make necessary adjustments.

Developing Interest in Eating

Children have much more interest in their daily meals when they have a hand in preparing or planning them. When they have responsibilities for setting the table, preparing vegetables, fixing salads, or cooking simple desserts, they feel as though they have had a part in it and are much more interested in eating. These responsibilities should not have the onus of a chore, but rather should be regarded as a part of family cooperation. It should be considered fun to do these jobs.

Youngsters can attempt to prepare food at an early age. The first recipes might be ones that do not require any actual cooking, like simple milk shakes, salads, or some desserts. Frequently mothers are reluctant to have children in the kitchen because they may be untidy. However, the compensations for permitting a child to try his hand at recipes he likes can go a long way in broadening his food interests. Children might be encouraged to bring recipes from school, to have their own little cookbooks, or to be creative about cooking.

In many homes the mother will let the children help plan family menus, which adds to their enjoyment. They should have no more responsibility than they can handle. This may mean planning the dessert or some other part of the meal. They should also be encouraged to suggest things that they like to eat. In any case, it is well for parents to show appreciation for their children's help.

When it is possible, a garden of his own usually has a desirable effect on a child's eating

[33] Nina B. Garton and Mary A. Bass, "Food Preferences and Nutrition Knowledge of Deaf Children," *Journal of Nutrition Education*, Vol. 6, No. 2 (April–June 1974), pp. 60–62.

[34] *Feeding the Child with a Handicap*, Children's Bureau Publication No. 450, U.S. Department of Health, Education, and Welfare, Washington, D.C., 1967.

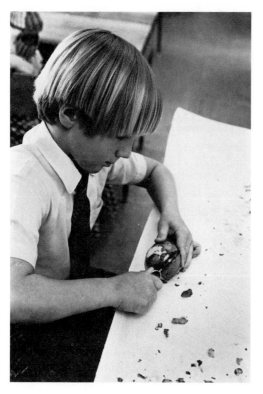

FIGURE 22–8.   *Learning to prepare foods may develop a new interest in eating.* (USDA)

habits. If children can grow foods that may be somewhat unfamiliar to them, they may develop a liking for them. Sometimes in school there are tasting periods when children bring unusual vegetables or other items that they have grown in their gardens to share with their friends. It is particularly encouraging for the child to see his family enjoy foods he has grown.

Another activity that can add considerable interest to eating is to help with the marketing. Surveys indicate that many children of this age have considerable responsibility for buying food. They can be encouraged to think of desirable foods for family meals and even to do comparative shopping. Developing an awareness of the types of foods different markets offer will do a great deal to develop a cosmopolitan taste for foods.

The preparation of food for camping, outdoor meals, or for guests may encourage an interest in nutritious foods. Learning about the foods of families of other countries can prove to be another incentive. Identifying wild plants[35] that are edible can become an exciting hobby and increase knowledge of nutritive values of these foods.

Undernutrition in Children

The U.S. Senate Committee on Nutrition and Human Needs estimates that approximately 4 million children in the United States are undernourished. Stunted growth, severe anemia, mental retardation, and mild to severe symptoms of nutritional deficiencies have been noted. In a broad sense, the underdevelopment of human resources, poverty, and malnutrition are involved in a vicious cycle that demand massive social programs to unlink them.

A lack of one or more nutrients in the diet of children may arise in a number of ways. The food consumed, for example, may not have been selected on the basis of nutrient density. In the preliminary findings of the *First Health and Nutrition Examination Survey*[36] it was revealed that the differences among groups in vitamin C intake were more related to nutrient density than to total food consumed.

Insufficient total food intake may lead to undernutrition because children do not consume adequate servings while eating or skip one or more meals. Kcalories are likely to be low and other nutrients lacking. If continued, weight loss, stunted growth, poor dental health, and symptoms of deficiency diseases may ensue.

An omission of one or more of the four food groups means that certain nutrients will probably be in short supply. Neglect of the cereal group, for instance, may reduce amounts of iron and important B vitamins. Unwise selection of snacks and frequent eating in fast-food restaurants may lead to a lack

[35] Euell Gibbons, *Stalking the Healthful Herbs,* David McKay, New York, 1966.

[36] *First Health and Nutrition Examination Survey,* op. cit., p. 10.

of fresh fruits, vegetables, and milk in a child's diet, especially if soft drinks are consumed.

If the environment is not conducive to pleasant eating, such as noise, confusion, hurry, crowdedness, quarreling, nagging, and a haphazard setting, the effect may be deleterious on the kind and amount of food that is consumed by children. The attitude of family members toward nutrition may be reflected in undernutrition if there is indifference or ignorance about the relation of nutrition to good health. The environment should provide for learning to prevent undernutrition now and later. Learning about food and nutritive contributions and to enjoy the taste, smell, color, and texture of food will increase an interest in food and hopefully lead to desirable food habits. The frequent lack of sociability, as when a child has to eat alone, may discourage eating. Eating is more than food, and a feeling of acceptance, recognition, and affection by the child is important.

Overnutrition in Children

Obesity in childhood is not a uniform condition, according to Bruch,[37] but may range from mild degrees of overweight during periods of decreased activity or overeating to severe weight excesses with poor functioning in all areas of life. Obesity may develop gradually from infancy, or there may be a sharp increase in weight in a short period of time. Families react differently to obese children; upper-class families usually are concerned about even slight overweight, but other-class families may be indifferent or accepting; some low-class families feel it is an indication of being good providers.

Obese children tend to be of large size with few exceptions. This fact was discussed as early as 1821 by Jaeger,[38] who noted that only tall children with a strong bone structure had a predisposition to becoming fat. Other disposing factors may be genetic in nature, and

there is evidence that the number and size of adipose cells are crucial.[39] Excessive nutrition early in life may result in an unusually high count of fat cells, which in turn may lead to obesity in later life or extend obesity throughout life. Bruch adds interaction with environmental factors as related to these predispositions, such as disturbed interpersonal relations —an overprotective or rejecting mother, quarreling parents, or other forms of discord.

Eppright and others[40] did an impressive study of the eating behavior of 3,444 preschool children and the related concerns of their mothers. Some of the results are of interest because of possible implications for overweight. For example, concern that their children ate too little applied to 19.9 per cent of the mothers, but only 4.9 per cent were concerned about their children eating too much. Some mothers used food for nonnutritional purposes, such as 23 per cent of them using food as rewards for good behavior. Reward foods in order of frequency were baked goods and desserts, 75 per cent; sweets, such as suckers and other candies, 39 per cent; and fruits, 32 per cent. In the same order, children were deprived of these foods for punishment. Bruch[41] contends that a mother's misperception of her child's needs and her own behavior are among the complex factors that lead to excessive feeding of a child. There continues to be some confusion and disagreement about the importance of emotional factors in childhood obesity, that is, if they contribute to the condition or if they are secondary to the social rejection that obese children encounter. Bruch believes that both facets intertwine. Furthermore, this researcher states that the only fat children who "outgrow" their obesity do so on their own initiative. The life of a child has

---

[37] Hilde Bruch, *Eating Disorders*, Basic Books, New York, 1973, Chap. 8.

[38] G. F. Jaeger, *Vergleighung einiger durch Fettigkeit oder kolassale Bildung aus gegeichneter Kinder und einiger Zwerge*, Metzler, Stuttgart, 1821.

[39] J. Hirsch and J. L. Knittle, "Cellularity of Obese and Nonobese Human Adipose Tissue," *Federation Proceedings*, Vol. 29, No. 4 (July–August 1970), pp. 1516–1521.

[40] Ercel S. Eppright, Hazel M. Fox, Beth A. Fryer, Glenna H. Lamkin, and Virginia H. Vivian, "Eating Behavior of Preschool Children," *Journal of Nutrition Education*, Prototytpe Issue (Fall 1968), pp. 16–19.

[41] Bruch, op. cit., p. 140.

many facets for consideration in a study of obesity. (See Chapter 10 for additional information.)

Overnutrition of any one nutrient can lead to serious health consequences. Overemphasis upsets the balance of nutrients that are required for an adequate diet.

World Nutrition of Children

More than two thirds of the world's children in developing countries are estimated to be malnourished or undernourished.[42] In industrialized nations there are large pockets of malnourished or undernourished children, particularly in poor families and among minority groups.

Food patterns and food availability vary from one part of the world to another. Nutritional status will depend on the degree to which nutrients are or are not available for an adequate diet. Protein-kcalorie malnutrition diseases exist according to physical and clinical evidence, such as kwashiorkor and marasmus, but milder forms of deficiencies can have long-term consequences for children. WHO considers malnutrition to be the greatest health problem of the world. Malnutrition leads to stunted growth rate, lower resistance to infectious diseases, poor general physique, and possibly poor mental development. Anemias are common in some parts of the world. Malnutrition and infections have a mutually aggravating effect. The deficiency of vitamins A and C contribute to this condition. Malnutrition reduces the resistance to infections. The lack of other nutrients varies in different parts of the world.

The possible damaging effect of malnutrition on brain development is another concern. Monckeberg[43] states that malnutrition coupled with sociocultural factors that interfere with adequate stimulation for intellectual growth result in a condition that interferes with individual development as well as society's growth. Among other social factors is low per capita income, which seriously limits food consumption. The trend of moving from rural to urban areas all over the world brings nutritional problems, especially for growing children because they may not have access to familiar foods. This change in food habits may lead to very deficient diets. The social and cultural organization of a country or community has an impact on food habits.

The 1-to-three-year period for children in developing countries is a transition from babyhood to childhood and is considered a most dangerous time because of a cessation of breast feeding and the beginning of a diet composed largely of carbohydrates and low protein content. This diet, coupled with exposure to infections and possible emotional upsets, often results in slow weight and growth gains. After

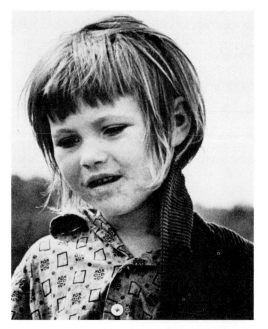

FIGURE 22–9. *There are hungry children in many parts of the world, including the United States. (Courtesy of National Institute of Child Health, U.S. Department of Labor)*

---

[42] Department of Economic and Social Affairs, *Report on Children*, United Nations, New York, 1971, pp. 20–27.

[43] Fernando Monckeberg, "Malnutrition and Mental Capacity," *Bulletin of the Pan American Sanitary Bureau*, Vol. 7, No. 1 (January 1973), pp. 87–93.

the third year the young child develops some resistance to infection and can handle a wider range of the family diet to greater advantage.

The problem of child nutrition in the world is related to food production and distribution. The kcaloric supplies in developed countries are 20 per cent above needs but are 6 per cent short in developing countries. To solve these and other problems of nutrition demands a comprehensive interdisciplinary action.

SELECTED REFERENCES

Birch, Herbert G., and Joan Dye Gussow, *Disadvantaged Children, Health, Nutrition, and School Failure,* Harcourt Brace Jovanovich, Inc., New York, 1970.

Coursin, David B., Richard H. Barnes, Herbert G. Birch, Robert Klein, Myron Winick, Paul B. Pearson, and Merrill S. Read, *The Relationship of Nutrition to Brain Development and Behavior,* Food and Nutrition Board, National Academy of Sciences, Washington, D.C., 1973.

Cravioto, J., and Elsa R. Delicardie, "Nutrition and Behavior and Learning," in Miloslav Rechcigl, Jr. (ed.), *Food, Nutrition and Health,* Vol. 16, S. Karger, Basel, 1973, pp. 80–96.

Department of Economic and Social Affairs, *Report on Children,* United Nations, New York, 1971, pp. 20–27.

Food for the Family with Young Children, Home and Garden Bulletin No. 5, Consumer and Food Economics Institute, Agricultural Research Service, U.S. Department of Agriculture, Washington, D.C., 1973.

Gussow, Joan, "Counternutritional Messages of TV Ads Aimed at Children," *Journal of Nutrition Education,* Vol. 4, No. 2 (Spring 1972), pp. 48–52.

Jelliffe, D. B., "Nutrition in Early Childhood," in Miloslav Rechcigl, Jr. (ed.), *Food, Nutrition and Health,* Vol. 16, S. Karger, Basel, 1973, pp. 1–21.

Martin, H. P., "Nutrition: Its Relationship to Children's Physical, Mental, and Emotional Development," *American Journal of Clinical Nutrition,* Vol. 26, No. 7 (July 1973), pp. 766–775.

McLaren, D. S., "Undernutrition," in Miloslav Rechcigl, Jr. (ed.), *Food, Nutrition and Health,* Vol. 16, S. Karger, Basel, 1973, pp. 142–177.

Moore, William M., Marjorie M. Silverberg, and Merrill S. Read, *Nutrition, Growth and Development of North American Indian Children,* DHEW Publication No. (NIH) 72–26, U.S. Government Printing Office, Washington, D.C., 1972.

Sims, Laura Smail, and Portia M. Morris, "Nutritional Status of Preschoolers. An Ecological Perspective," *Journal of the American Dietetic Association,* Vol. 64, No. 5 (May 1974), pp. 492–499.

Wyden, Barbara W., "The Fat Child Is Father of the Man," *The New York Times Magazine,* September 13, 1970, pp. 89–92, 97–99.

Your Child from 6–12, Children's Bureau Publication Number 324–1966, U.S. Government Printing Office, Washington, D.C., 1970.

23

Public and Private Feeding and Nutrition Programs

A public and private concern to safeguard the health and well-being of the people of the nation has led to the development of numerous feeding and nutrition programs directed to raise the level of nutrition among children and low-income households generally.[1]

Background

The elimination of hunger is one of the nation's most serious problems. This condition leads to malnutrition, which in turn impairs the quality of living of an individual not only as a child but in his future as an adult. The challenge is to develop means so that every person who is not receiving an adequate diet is provided with food to accomplish this end. Federal, state, county, and city governments, cooperatively or individually, have attempted to plan programs that would cope with this situation. These efforts will be discussed in this chapter. Private charitable

groups, mostly urban, according to Choate,[2] have served about 1 million meals to the poor, free or partially free. But many of the poor are not reached.

Complexity of the Problem

Hunger cannot be eliminated by increased production of food. The actual consumption of nutritious foods is influenced by incomes of families and individuals, the foods that are available to them, their food habits, and many other factors, according to Hegsted.[3] High-risk groups must be identified, such as pregnant women, infants and children, adolescents, and the elderly. Many members of low-income families need help. Groups must be recognized at the local level.

Many recent programs have not been evalu-

[1] Stephen J. Hiemstra, "Evaluation of USDA Food Programs," *Journal of the American Dietetic Association*, Vol. 60, No. 3 (March 1972), pp. 193–196.

[2] Robert Choate, "Special Programs for the Very Poor," in Jean Mayer (ed.), *U.S. Nutrition Policies in the Seventies*, W. H. Freeman, San Francisco, 1973, Chap. 18.

[3] D. Mark Hegsted, "A National Surveillance System," in Jean Mayer (ed.), *U.S. Nutrition Policies in the Seventies*, W. H. Freeman, San Francisco, 1973, Chap. 8.

ated and were discontinued because sufficient benefits could not be cited. Dietary surveys are helpful in the comparison of groups and provide useful statistics. If this information is fortified by measurements of the biochemical status of individuals, the evidence becomes stronger. These tests are expensive and not all nutrients can be surveyed. Some of the WIC (Women, Infants, Children) projects are being evaluated to aid in the justification of their existence.

It is difficult to protect the dignity of the individuals who are served. A man who gives food stamps at the checkout counter in a supermarket, the elementary school student who receives a free lunch, or a woman who receives a free meal from a charitable organization may do so reluctantly. Although some members of a family receive food, other members of the family who are also hungry are not so fortunate. Fomon and Egan[4] contend that the nutritional needs of other members of the family cannot be ignored. Policies must be developed that contribute to the solidarity and integrity of the family unit. Other basic needs such as shelter, clothing, education, emotional security, and income must be considered. Related to these ideas is the necessary planning for an adequate diet combining the food consumed at home with the nutritive contribution of meals eaten outside of the home, as is typical of many of these programs.

There are many political overtones to these projects. Financing must come from government and private sources. Attempts to balance the national budget, or a president, governor, or other important administrator who is disinterested or does not encourage expenditures may cause programs to suffer. Representatives and senators dedicated to the cause of the hungry may not be reelected and unfavorable repercussions may result. All this contributes to an instability of programs. Sometimes cooperation between federal, state, and local agencies is inadequate, or the state or local government cannot meet the demands for the required facilities, administration, or funds. In

some instances the pride of the poor who refuse services is a deterrent. Although many of the programs that have been launched are excellent, it has been impossible to secure adequate funds for expansion so that more can be served.

Another problem is that many of the needy do not receive the information necessary to participate. Others have difficulty because of a lack of transportation or a physical handicap that prevents them from going to the station where aid is available. Some are not only poor but have had little education and cannot understand the logistics of the program. Unfortunately, with many of these programs little nutrition education accompanies the feeding aspect. Attempts have been made with certain programs, such as food stamps, but the success of a program is limited if individuals and families do not have an opportunity to learn ways to improve their present diets. Inflation or recession is another reason for the need of education so that the food dollar may be spent as wisely as possible.

Feeding and nutrition programs will be discussed under three categories: (1) child nutrition; (2) women, infants, and children; and (3) family assistance. These programs are largely the joint venture of federal and state governments, local communities, schools, children, and parents. Some philanthropical organizations have programs, but the bulk of the programs are government oriented.

Child Nutrition Programs

All Child Nutrition Programs are administered by the Food and Nutrition Service of the U.S. Department of Agriculture (USDA) and operate at the federal, state, and local levels.[5] Included are the National School Lunch Program, School Breakfast Program, Special Milk Program, and Special Food Service Program for Children. Children in public and nonprofit schools, child-care centers, settlement houses, summer day camps, and recreation centers are eligible. Children in every

[4] Samuel J. Fomon and Mary C. Egan, "Infants, Children, and Adolescents," in Jean Mayer (ed.), *U.S. Nutrition Policies in the Seventies*, W. H. Freeman, San Francisco, 1973, Chap. 1.

[5] Joanne Pearson, "Child Nutrition Programs of the Food and Nutrition Service, U.S. Department of Agriculture," *Nutrition Program News*, May–June 1973, pp. 1–4.

state, the District of Columbia, the Trust Territory of the Pacific Islands, Guam, Puerto Rico, American Samoa, and the Virgin Islands benefit from the Child Nutrition Programs. Criteria for participation include operation of the nonprofit food service for all children regardless of race, color, or national origin; provision for free or reduced-price meals to children unable to pay the full price, without identification or discrimination of the children; and service of meals that meet the nutritional requirements established by the secretary of agriculture.

National School Lunch Program

Since 1946 the National School Lunch Program has enabled schools throughout the nation to serve wholesome, low-cost lunches to children each school day. All public and nonprofit schools of high school grade and under, including preschool programs that are operated as part of the school system, are eligible. Most programs are administered through the state Department of Education. Private schools in 21 states and child-care institutions in 16 states are directly administered by the Food and Nutrition Service, U.S. Department of Agriculture.

Federal assistance is in the form of cash reimbursements with a guarantee of a stated average rate per lunch that meets the minimum nutritional requirements; special cash assistance funds for free and reduced-price lunches for needy children; agricultural commodities; and nonfood assistance, such as equipment. Flexibility is permitted in special situations, such as areas where schools are particularly needy. Approximately 80 per cent of the food used in the school lunch program is purchased in local markets. Foods acquired by the USDA under three basic authorities—price support, surplus removal, and food purchases based on school needs—are generally available to all eligible nonprofit school lunch programs.

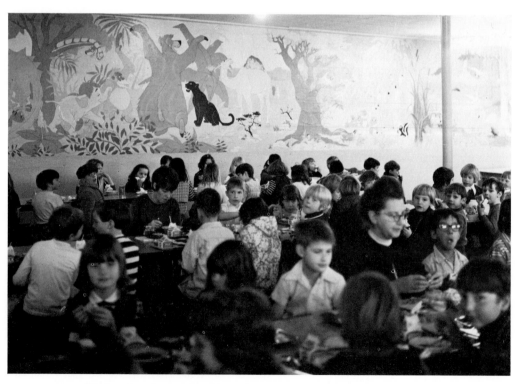

FIGURE 23–1. *An elementary school lunch program.* (USDA)

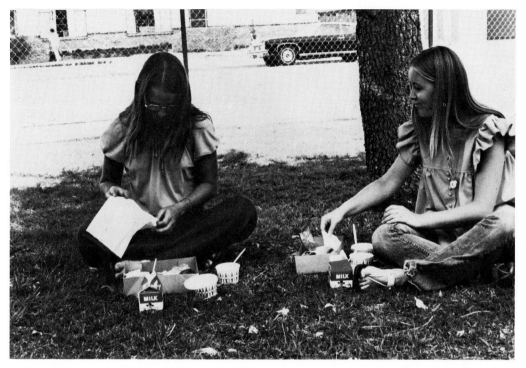

FIGURE 23–2. *Box lunches are another type of school lunch program.* (USDA)

The traditional food service is the cafeteria type. Satellite feeding from base or central kitchens is used when there are a number of schools in the system that do not have facilities for the preparation of food. Types of meals may range from cold food in box lunches; some food hot, for example, the main dish, with the remainder of food cold; or complete hot lunches in bulk containers or on individual insulated trays. Some receiving schools have small service kitchens; others have movable serving carts. Sometimes the food is delivered frozen, ready for heating. In other schools children may be bussed to schools that have a cafeteria. Canned-food entrees, called "lunch in a cupcan"[6] by students in a parochial school in Philadelphia, are used. A typical lunch might be chicken stew in a can, bread and butter, an apple, and a half-pint of milk. Foods are heated in a small oven. Or individual-sized serving cans of spaghetti and

meat balls, stew, or beans and franks are heated and served as the main dish and eaten directly from the can. In other schools, institution-sized cans of food are heated. Food-management companies and caterers are used by some schools to provide food for students. Some authorities question the food habits that are established with these procedures.

Nutritional Standards

Nutritional standards are met by serving a Type A lunch to each student. The goal is to provide approximately one third of the daily dietary allowances recommended by the Food and Nutrition Board of the National Research Council, National Academy of Sciences, for 10- to 12-year-old boys and girls. With the exception of milk, it is suggested that the quantities of other foods be adjusted appropriately for older or younger students. The following minimum amounts of foods are to be included.

WHOLE MILK   One half-pint of fluid whole milk served as a beverage. When whole milk

[6] "Reaching the Hard-to-Reach Schools," *Food and Nutrition*, Vol. 1, No. 2 (August 1971), pp. 5–7.

cannot be obtained, one half-pint of reconstituted evaporated or dry whole milk shall be served as a beverage. Alternates such as skim or cultured buttermilk, flavored or unflavored and low-fat milk may be offered. The milk must meet the minimum butterfat and sanitation requirements of state and local laws.

PROTEIN-RICH FOODS Two ounces (edible portion as served) of lean meat, poultry, or fish; or 2 oz of cheese; or one egg; or ½ cup of cooked dry beans or peas; or 4 tablespoons of peanut butter; or an equivalent quantity of any combination of these foods. It is nutritionally desirable to serve some cheese, meat, or peanut butter when dried beans or peas are served. To be counted in meeting this requirement, these foods must be served as a main dish or in a main dish with one other menu item.

VEGETABLES AND FRUIT A ¾-cup serving consisting of two or more vegetables or fruits or both. Full-strength vegetable or fruit juice may be counted to meet not more than ¼-cup of this requirement.

BREAD One slice of whole-grain or enriched bread; or a serving of cornbread, biscuits, rolls, muffins, or other bread product made of whole-grain or enriched meal or flour.

BUTTER OR MARGARINE One teaspoon of butter or margarine.

Options to Type A lunch menu planning have been considered. For schools that have computer support, menu planning may be easier through the designed nutrient standard for a school lunch. Computer Assisted Menu Planning (CAMP) involves recipes with variations that are costed out and measured in terms of nutritive values. Palatability requirements may be included. It is hoped that this plan will provide greater assurance of meeting nutritional requirements.[7]

Harper[8] developed a manual technique through an abacus-like device that tallied the nutrient contributions of a planned menu. The nutritive contributions of over 800 acceptable school lunch recipes were calculated in bead units that represented one tenth of the nutrient requirement for a lunch. Other adaptations are certain to follow in planning menus for school lunch programs.

Food scientists at Rutgers University advocate a food technological approach to school lunch planning. Lachance and his colleagues[9] contend that changing food habits is extremely difficult, so the obvious step is to change the food to contain desirable nutrients but to taste like the food that students prefer, such as spinach tasting like a potato chip. Nutrient requirements can be met with some nutrification of foods and nutrient-standard menu planning that requires simple food combination guidelines to meet a selected nutrient goal. By nutrifying at least one item in the menu the process is simplified.

Lachance and co-workers[10] believe that, prior even to the nutrients in a school lunch, such qualities as color, flavor, and texture which make food attractive to the student must be given top attention, because the food must be eaten if the nutrients are to be effective. This plan gives a great emphasis to acceptance.

Lachance and co-workers[11] give further warning that the school lunch menu should not reflect the faulty rationale that nutrient deficiencies in the Type A lunch will be compensated for in other meals eaten at home

[7] National School Lunch Program, 25 Years of Progress, Food and Nutrition Service, U.S. Department of Agriculture, Washington, D.C., 1971, p. 6.

[8] Judson M. Harper, "School Lunches on a Nutrient Standard," in a paper presented at the 56th Annual Meeting of the American Dietetic Association, Denver, Colo., October 24, 1973.

[9] "Rutgers Promotes Nutrient Standards," CNI Weekly Report, Vol. 2, No. 32 (November 9, 1972), pp. 6–7.

[10] Paul Lachance, Ruth Brown Moskowitz, and Henry H. Winawer, "Balanced Nutrition Through Food Processor Practice of Nutrification," Food Technology, Vol. 26, No. 6 (June 1972), pp. 30–40.

[11] Dorothy Miskimin, James Bowers, and Paul A. Lachance, "Nutrification of Frozen Prepared School Lunches Is Needed," Food Technology, Vol. 28, No. 2 (February 1974), pp. 52–56.

by the child. For many children the school
lunch meal is the only adequate meal consumed. For that reason a nutritive imbalance
in the school lunch cannot be tolerated.

Eligibility for Free or Reduced-Price Lunches

Children are identified for eligibility for
free lunches on the USDA family-size-family-
minimum-income criteria that are uniform in
the 48 contiguous states. Alaska and Hawaii
are considered separately. More students are
eligible therefore in states with lower incomes
such as Alabama and Mississippi and fewer
students are eligible in states with higher incomes such as New York and California. Emmons and others[12] raise a question about having these guidelines serve as the sole criteria.
Poor diets do appear more frequently among
low-income families but some children may
be poorly fed because of poor food habits, a
lack of home supervision, or other reasons although they come from a middle-class or
affluent home. These researchers sought to
determine if children eligible for free lunches
were also the most in need of the nutritional
benefits of the program. The results indicated
that one third of the students studied in school
lunch programs and identified as nutritionally
needy were not eligible for free school lunches.
Of the ineligible children, 25.2 per cent in
district A and 29.8 per cent in district B were
judged to have nutritionally adequate diets, so
their families, in spite of limited incomes, do
manage to have nutritious diets. However,
23.3 per cent of the ineligible children in
district A and 28.4 per cent in district B were
classified as nutritionally needy. Unless their
families paid for their lunches, these students
could not capitalize on a nutritious source of
food of which they were in need. In conclusion, only one third of the eligible children
were both economically and nutritionally
needy. Nutritional status appears to be an
important criteria for determining the need
for school lunches for certain children.

Nutritive Evaluation of the School Lunch Program

Studies of schoolchildren made in all regions
of the United States reveal that the frequency
of low intakes of nutrients was reduced among
children who participated in the school lunch
program. However, further efforts to improve
the diet of a relatively large number of children whose diets were found low in calcium,
vitamin A, and ascorbic acid are needed.

Murphy and co-workers[13] have made a series
of research studies on the nutritive contribution of the Type A school lunch. The total fat,
fatty acids, and total sterols were determined
by laboratory analysis on lunches served to
sixth graders in 300 schools. The lunches contained an average of 31.8 g of fat that contributed 39 per cent of the kcalories. On the
average, lunches contained 14.6 g of saturated
fatty acids; 10.2 g of monosaturated fatty
acids, of which 9.5 g was oleic acid; and 3.8 g
of polyunsaturated acids, of which 2.9 g was
linoleic acid (essential). In light of the recommendations of the Food and Nutrition Board
that Americans reduce the total fat intake and
substitute some polyunsaturated fats for some
saturated fat in the diet, this guideline might
well be applied to menu planning for school
lunches. From a practical sense this might be
accomplished by using fewer baked desserts
that are rich in shortening and by replacing
them with fruit-based desserts, puddings, and
gelatin desserts. Part of the solid fat used in
preparation might be replaced by vegetable
oils.

Another study was done by Murphy and co-
workers[14] on the calcium, phosphorus, magnesium, iron, sodium, and potassium in type
A lunches. Results indicated that none of the
lunches were seriously low in calcium content.

[12] Lillian Emmons, Marian Hayes, and David L.
Call, "A Study of School Feeding Programs, 1.
Economic Eligibility and Nutrition Need," *Journal
of the American Dietetic Association*, Vol. 61,
No. 3 (September 1972), pp. 262–268.

[13] Elizabeth W. Murphy, Louise Page, and
Percilla C. Koons, "Lipid Components of Type A
School Lunches," *Journal of the American Dietetic
Association*, Vol. 56, No. 6 (June 1970), pp. 504–
509.

[14] Elizabeth W. Murphy, Louise Page, and Bernice K. Watt, "Major Mineral Elements in Type A
School Lunches," *Journal of the American Dietetic
Association*, Vol. 57, No. 3 (September 1970), pp.
239–245.

Only 4 per cent failed to meet the nutritional goal of 400 mg of phosphorus per lunch. On the average, lunches failed to meet the magnesium requirement. Emphasis might be placed on vegetables and fruits that are excellent sources of this mineral, thus also enhancing the vitamin A and B_6 contributions to the lunch, nutrients that are often lacking. Iron appears to be the most serious problem, with less than 10 per cent of the lunches reaching the nutritional goal. Levels of sodium appeared to be compatible with California hospital standards. Potassium content appeared to be adequate. Proportions of all minerals were significantly related to kcaloric and protein values of the lunches.

Trace minerals were also analyzed by these USDA researchers.[15] Recommended dietary allowances had not been established for these trace elements at the time of the study although many are considered essential. Included in the study were chromium, copper, manganese, zinc (recommended allowance established for 1974 allowances), aluminum, barium, cadmium, boron, and strontium. Conclusions reached were that amounts of chromium and copper were low or marginal, manganese seemed adequate, zinc was probably adequate, aluminum values varied widely, and cadmium was near the lower levels of sensitivity. Little information is available on strontium so comparisons could not be made. Barium and boron were at the lower levels of sensitivity, and boron was much less than Underwood's lower estimate.

Emmons, Hayes, and Call[16] did a research study on the effects of school breakfasts and/or lunches on the nutritive intake, biochemical measurements, and the physical growth of elementary children during an academic year. Results indicated that adequate amounts of protein, calcium, vitamin A, riboflavin, and niacin were provided in the school lunches.

Kcaloric levels of lunches were slightly lower than the one third of the recommended daily dietary allowances used as a criterion. Ascorbic acid, iron, and thiamin were adequate in one district studied but not in the other. Some children brought bag lunches. Milk was either purchased at school or brought from home. A comparison of the nutritive values of the bag lunch with the school lunches indicated that school lunches were significantly higher in all the nutrients except kcalories and niacin equivalents. Differences were especially pronounced in protein, calcium, vitamin A, riboflavin, and ascorbic acid. With the exception of ascorbic acid, over- and underweight needy children did not have significantly different dietary intakes at home than at school.

Points for Discussion

One of the most serious problems facing the school lunch program is the steady climb in wholesale food prices. The protein foods have become especially costly. The energy crisis has increased the cost of operating various types of equipment used in the preparation of lunches. There is little hope that these prices will decrease in the future. If school lunch prices are increased, the number of paying students decreases proportionally and fewer students receive the benefits of the program.[17] The possibility of phasing out food donations by the USDA is being considered. Many schools are receiving the same amount or less funds than formerly. Increases in funding are tied to higher restaurant prices because of an escalator clause related to federal funding. A leveling off of federal financial support will halt the expansion of free and reduced-price lunches for the needy.[18]

Other problems are the double scheduling of school facilities so that all students may participate in the school lunch program. Time constraints thus interfere with adequate scheduling. Children who can afford to pay more

[15] Elizabeth Murphy, Louise Page, and Bernice K. Watt, "Trace Minerals in Type A School Lunches," *Journal of the American Dietetic Association*, Vol. 58, No. 2 (February 1971), pp. 115–122.

[16] Lillian Emmons, Marion Hayes, and David L. Call, "A Study of School Feeding Programs," *Journal of the American Dietetic Association*, Vol. 61, No. 3 (September 1972), pp. 268–275.

[17] "School Feeding Faces a Crisis," *CNI Weekly Report*, Vol. 4, No. 14 (April 4, 1974), p. 4.

[18] "Signs Point to Widespread Decline in School Lunch Program," *CNI Weekly Report*, Vol. 4, No. 12 (March 1974), pp. 1–2.

often go elsewhere to buy their lunch. The need for well-trained staffs, adequate personnel, and more research in the technology of delivery might be helpful. The Rutgers University food scientists[19] believe that greater political acceptance should be sought, including concrete data on the educational value of child feeding programs on performance.

Law and others[20] questioned students about their attitudes toward the school lunch. Students liked eating lunch at school for the following reasons (in descending order): talking to friends, convenient, economical, atmosphere, and other reasons. Reasons given for disliking to eat at school were waiting in line, not leaving school, insufficient time, not eating with friends, poor food, too crowded, small servings, dislike of foods, and the like.

Bettelheim[21] believes that nourishing food is of little avail unless it is eaten in an appropriate psychological environment. There should be an opportunity to share meals with friends and teachers. Food is a source of security and may help to fortify students to cope with their learning experiences.

Greater involvement of students and parents may have a positive effect. Students may elect representatives of their group to serve on an advisory committee for the school lunch program. The two-way communication process is helpful. Students contribute reactions of the student body about the foods that they like, complaints about the lunches, and innovative suggestions for improvement. The school lunch staff, in turn, can inform the students about the workings of the program, its limitations, its possibilities, and other aspects of operation. Students may help plan seating arrangements, or improve the appearance of the lunchroom through posters, murals, and other art devices. Integrating the school lunch program with the

total school program has educational potential, such as in nutrition (by having a table for students watching their weight, athletes, or vegetarians); in mathematics by determining how the school lunch dollar is spent and making surveys of students who eat in the school lunch; or in social studies by making an analysis of food habits as related to social factors.

If the menu can reflect ethnic food preferences, students may be more pleased with the fare offered to them. In some schools, for example, breads typical of a culture are served with the school lunch. In New York's famous lower East Side, whose population reflects many ethnic groups, foods were planned to represent these many backgrounds, according to Brand,[22] such as Chinese, Spanish, or "soul food." Montoya[23] describes the development of Mexican-American and Navajo Indian recipes for use in the school lunch programs in California, Utah, New Mexico, Arizona, and other states. Brand[24] describes how the school lunch program in a Jewish parochial school in the New York metropolitan area was able to provide kosher food for its students.

School Breakfast Program

Widespread hunger among school children in the morning impairs their ability to learn. Congress recognized this problem in 1966 and inaugurated the School Breakfast Program modeled after the National School Lunch Program. Some USDA studies indicate benefits of eating breakfast.[25] In Massachusetts, 3,500 high school students' breakfast habits were studied. Eleven per cent of the boys and 19 per cent of the girls had a poor breakfast. When breakfast was skipped, students took

---

[19] "Lunch Report Published," CNI Weekly Report, Vol. 2, No. 32 (November 9, 1972), p. 6.

[20] Helen M. Law, Harvye F. Lewis, Virginia C. Grant, and Dorothy S. Bachemin, "Sophomore High School Students' Attitudes Toward School Lunch," Journal of the American Dietetic Association, Vol. 60, No. 1 (January 1972), pp. 38–41.

[21] Bruno Bettelheim, "Why School Lunch Fails," School Foodservice Journal, Vol. 26, No. 3 (March 1972), pp. 36–39.

[22] Elaine Brand, "Type A—The Ethnic Way," Food and Nutrition, Vol. 3, No. 5 (October 1973), pp. 14–15.

[23] Benedicto Montoya, "Catching the Ethnic Flavor," Food and Nutrition, Vol. 3, No. 3 (June 1973), pp. 12–15.

[24] Elaine Brand, "Keeping Kosher with Chicken," Food and Nutrition, Vol. 3, No. 4 (August 1973), pp. 8–9.

[25] "FOR: Better Breakfasts, AGAINST: Skipping Breakfasts," Food and Home Notes, September 14, 1970, pp. 1–3.

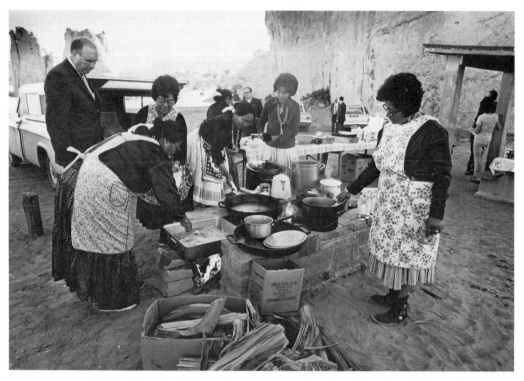

FIGURE 23–3. *Navajo Indian volunteers preparing breakfast for chlidren that emphasizes ethnic foods.* (USDA)

longer to make decisions, were less steady, and their work output was less. The school lunch supervisor reported to the U.S. Department of Agriculture that teachers observed many positive changes in children after the breakfast program was inaugurated such as less tardiness, less truancy, better attitudes toward school, more alert and awake students, and actual learning improvement among younger children. In Northampton County, North Carolina, teachers reported a marked improvement in student grades as well as an increase in attendance. Birch and Gussow[26] contend that a society genuinely concerned about the education of socially disadvantaged children must recognize that expanding learning facilities is only one aspect. The health of a child is an aspect of primary importance and breakfasts

at school are one means of contributing to his nutritive status.

Breakfasts served must meet standards set by the secretary of agriculture.[27] Each meal must include fruit or juice, bread or cereal, with meat or an alternate served as often as possible.

One area of controversy is the use of alternate or engineered foods in schools where facilities for preparation of breakfasts is lacking. Large baking companies sold fortified cream-filled cakes and other foods developed by food technologists that had nutritive values comparable to 4 oz of orange juice, 2 slices of bacon, 1 egg, 1 pat of butter, and 1 slice of bread. When served with a half-pint of whole milk, requirements are alleged to meet the USDA criteria for the school breakfast program.

Several criticisms are leveled at this practice.

[26] Herbert G. Birch and Joan Dye Gussow, *Disadvantaged Children, Health, Nutrition, and School Failure*, Harcourt Brace Jovanovich, New York, 1970, p. 9.

[27] Pearson, op. cit., p. 3.

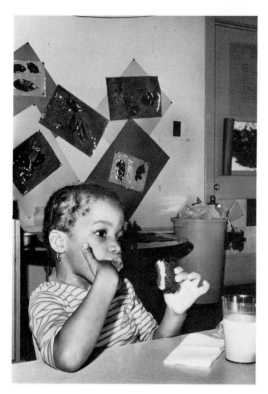

FIGURE 23-4. *Somewhat controversial engineered food in which a cake-like product is served with a glass of milk and meets USDA School Breakfast Program criteria.* (USDA)

Because many of these foods resemble cake, nutritionists question the effect on food habits. Dentists are concerned about the sugar content and possible relation to tooth decay. Ullrich[28] raises the question about the wisdom of fortifying foods or preparing fabricated foods because trace elements and other little known nutrients may be overlooked.

Participation in the school breakfast program is rapidly increasing but many needy children do not have access to the program. Gussow[29] recommends that if only one meal can be provided to hungry children, then breakfast is the most desirable meal so that children do not have to sit through a morning of classes on an empty stomach.

Special Milk Program

The purpose of this program is to encourage the consumption of milk by children and to create desirable milk-drinking habits so that their nutrition will benefit. Milk may be served throughout the day in schools and institutions eligible for the program, including mealtime, snacktime, recess, and before and after school. Approved types of milk are low fat, skim, or cultured buttermilk, unflavored or flavored, in addition to whole milk.[30] Funds for this program are provided to state agencies and eligible individual institutions in the form of reimbursement payments. Especially needy children may have free milk and schools may be reimbursed. The milk program is especially important to schools that do not have a regular food service because milk consumption by children is increased.

Special Food Service Program for Children

The purpose of this program is to assist child-care institutions in providing nutritious meals such as breakfast, lunch, dinner, and between-meal supplements. Institutions that are eligible include public and nonprofit private institutions, such as day-care centers, settlement houses, recreation centers, summer day camps, and other programs that provide nonresidential child care in low-income areas and areas with many working mothers.[31] Requirements are similar to those of the National School Lunch Program. Guidelines for various meals are the same as for school lunch and school breakfast. For between meals, milk, fruit or vegetable juice, and bread or cereal are approved. Participation in these programs

[28] Helen D. Ullrich, "The Right Way: In Whose Judgment," *Journal of Nutrition Education,* Vol. 5, No. 3 (July–September 1973), p. 184.

[29] Joan Dye Gussow, "Counter Advertising—The Handwriting on the Wall," address given at Advertising Age Creative Workshop, August 15, 1972.

[30] "USDA Revises Regulations on Use of Milk in Child Nutrition Programs," Food and Nutrition Service, Northeast Regional Office NEWS, U.S. Department of Agriculture, Washington, D.C., August 9, 1973.

[31] Pearson, op. cit., pp. 3–4.

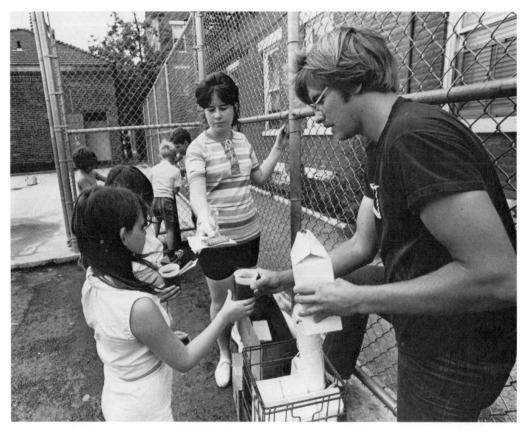

FIGURE 23–5. *Between meal food served to children in a Summer Food Service Program.* (USDA)

has increased each year. In addition to reimbursement, federal assistance includes donated commodities and financial help to buy or rent necessary food service equipment. Funds are disbursed by the state educational agency on a nondiscriminatory basis.

A few examples of how the program is implemented are cited here. In Portland, Oregon, in a neighborhood park small children come from a wading pool and older children who have been playing baseball come to have lunch. In a library in a low-income neighborhood, children come to have lunch and stay for a story hour afterwards. There were 80 program sites in Portland during the summer of 1972 that served 4,000 children lunch on weekdays. Eighty per cent of the cost was reimbursed by the USDA and the remainder

came from local contributions, such as of labor, facilities, and trucks.[32] In Cincinnati, Ohio, lunches and supplemental meals were served to approximately 9,000 children each weekday. All foods included in the lunch menu contributed nutritionally to the child's diet.[33] Migrant children have benefited from this program. In the Zellwood, Florida, Migrant Child Care Center support was received from the USDA and from the Department of Health, Education, and Welfare to serve breakfast,

---

[32] Benedicto Montoya, "Special Food for Summer," *Food and Nutrition*, Vol. 3, No. 2 (April 1973), pp. 2–3.

[33] Joan Luck and Milton Papke, "In Cincinnati," *Food and Nutrition*, Vol. 3, No. 2 (April 1973), pp. 4–8.

lunch, and midafternoon snack.[34] In a church basement in Minneapolis children from the surrounding low-income housing project came to a child-care center that with the help of the Minnesota Department of Education served breakfast, lunch, and two snacks. This experience enhanced the education of the children as well as contributing to their nutritive intake. Many of the children were hungry and malnourished.[35]

The USDA is examining ways to improve the summer program particularly so that food may be provided for a larger number of children. Administrative requirements are being made more flexible and in keeping with the particular situation. Improvement of menus is also encouraged.[36] Although participation in this program has increased, a great number of children, estimated at at least 2 million, are in particular need of this program, especially on a year-round basis.[37]

Programs for Adults, Families, and the Elderly

The USDA has two programs that assist needy adults and families, the Commodity Distribution Program and Food Stamps. The Administration on Aging has funding for elderly nutrition programs and supportive services. Feeding programs for women, infants, and children (WIC) are a USDA funded project.

Commodity Distribution and Direct Food Assistance

Originally, commodity distribution was designed to use surplus agricultural commodities that were purchased under a price support program and used to alleviate hunger among the poor. When surplus foods were no longer available, the government purchased foods for distribution known as donated foods. Foods are purchased through competitive bidding by food suppliers and processors and must meet federal specifications for quality equal to foods available in retail stores.[38] Foods available vary from time to time but may include canned meat and poultry, peanut butter, dry beans, instant mashed potatoes, instant dry milk, canned fruits and vegetables, table and cooking oils, enriched flour, enriched cornmeal, rice and other cereals, and prunes and other dried fruit. State and local agencies are offered sufficient food to supply each person in the family donation program with over 30 pounds of food per month.

This program is used to provide direct aid to needy families. To be eligible a family or individual must meet federal specifications, such as having access to cooking facilities and having such a low income that they cannot buy needed food. Recipients include those on public welfare, on Social Security, on very small pensions, the unemployed, or those who work part-time or for very low wages. Evidence of residence, monthly income received, and expenditures must be demonstrated.

The distribution of donated foods is extended to school lunch programs on Type A lunches, orphanages, homes for the aged, summer camps, child-care centers, and other charitable agencies. These donated foods have been used for relief of victims of natural disasters, such as floods, tornadoes, and hurricanes.

Some examples of the use of donated foods for direct assistance are cited here. Migrant workers who come·to work in the Walla Walla Valley to help in the harvesting of crops and in other parts of the country have benefited from having their children fed with donated foods in day-care centers.[39] On Drummond

[34] Ralph E. Vincent, "A Chance for Zellwood Children," *Food and Nutrition*, Vol. 2, No. 2 (April 1972), pp. 2–4.

[35] "Educare for Preschoolers," *Food and Nutrition*, Vol. 2, No. 2 (April 1972), pp. 4–5.

[36] "USDA Study Recommends Major Changes in Summer Lunch Effort," *CNI Weekly Report*, March 21, 1974, pp. 4–5.

[37] Select Committee on Nutrition and Human Needs, U.S. Senate, *Dollars for Food* (March 1973), U.S. Government Printing Office, Washington, D. C., 1973.

[38] "Food Assistance Provides Direct Relief," *Food and Nutrition*, Vol. 1, No. 1 (June 1971), p. 8.

[39] Benedicto Montoya, "A Happy Stopping Place," *Food and Nutrition*, Vol. 2, No. 6 (December 1972), pp. 4–5.

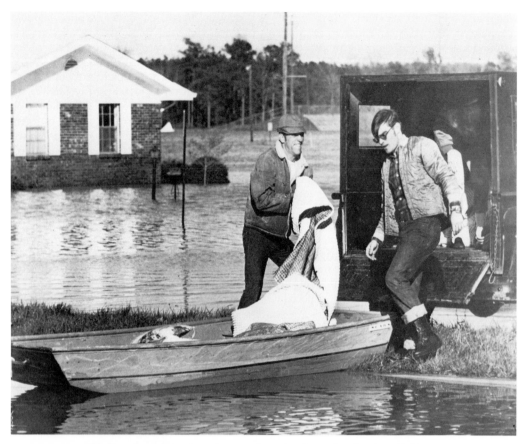

FIGURE 23–6. *A program for crises, such as floods, makes food available.*

Island in Chippewa County, Michigan, the school bus is used to bring donated foods to the needy in this isolated country in the winter. In a similar manner, 300 needy families in north-central Wisconsin receive donated foods in the wintertime.[40] In a housing project in Jersey City, New Jersey, USDA donated foods contribute to a program for providing an after-school snack for 4,000 children in nine public housing projects.[41] In the wake of Hurricane Agnes over 2½ million pounds of donated foods were distributed to those left hungry in the northeastern states.[42]

Nutritive Evaluation of Commodity Distribution Program

If the 20 foods listed for distribution are incorporated into the family diet, a diet that comes close to meeting full nutritional needs is provided. All the family's supply of protein, calcium, thiamin, and riboflavin are included and substantial amounts of iron and vitamins A, C, and D. Guthrie and others[43] studied the

[40] Charles T. Weirauch, "Food Returns to the Farmland," and "Fighting Hunger in the Wilderness," *Food and Nutrition*, Vol. 2, No. 6 (December 1972), pp. 6–9.

[41] "Time to Eat in Jersey City," *Food and Nutrition*, Vol. 2, No. 5 (October 1972), pp. 4–5.

[42] Elaine Brand, "The Northeast Recovers from Agnes' Wrath," *Food and Nutrition*, Vol. 2, No. 5 (October 1972), pp. 6–9.

[43] Helen A. Guthrie, J. Patrick Madden, Marion D. Yoder, and Helen Perrault Koontz, "Effects

effects of the Commodity Distribution Program on the nutritive intake of families. The conclusions were that the program was ineffective in improving the overall nutritive intake. However, participating families had fewer diets providing less than two thirds of the recommended dietary allowances of four or more nutrients and had more diets meeting the criterion for energy and vitamins that did similar families who did not participate in the Commodity Distribution Program. The relatively low subsidy (all available foods were not included) was another important factor to consider.

Problems in Commodity Distribution

High prices for foods have prevented USDA officials from purchasing some important items, such as fruit juices, vegetables, cheese, meat, and poultry on which needy families have depended. Because of supply and demand problems it is difficult to predict which foods and what quantities will be available. Serious questions have arisen if this particular program can continue. Some families and individuals could be shifted to the Food Stamp Program, but isolated areas and some Indian reservations would encounter difficult problems. Continuation of governmental approval is another concern. In some instances the USDA has authorized cash in lieu of commodities.

Food Stamp Program

The Food Stamp Act was passed in 1964 and provided a means for low-income households to buy more food of greater variety to improve their diets. Participants must meet federal criteria for household, income, resources, tax dependents, and work registration to buy food stamps. This information determines the ratio of money paid to the value of the food stamps, which may be used like money in participating food stores. The

amount of money that a family pays for food stamps is called the purchase requirement. The amount increases as the household income decreases.[44] In 1973 a family of four that earned $387 per month paid $92 for $116 of stamps while a family of four with an income of $100 a month paid $25 for $116 of stamps. Recipients of food stamps are families and persons on welfare or with small savings who get by on low salaries, pensions, or social security. In June 1972, 3,555,000 households were participating in the Food Stamp Program and received more than $330,-000,000 in coupons per month for approximately 12.5 million persons.[45] Food stamps may be purchased at banks, post offices, credit unions, community groups, and other facilities. During floods and other natural crises, the USDA has issued food stamps free to the survivors. Food stamps may be used to purchase garden seeds and plants to produce food for personal consumption. Recession, inflation, unemployment, and other adverse economic situations have increased the number of users of food stamps.

Nutrition Program for the Elderly

This program emerged as one of the recommendations of the 1971 White House Conference on the Aging. In March 1972 a nutrition bill was signed by President Nixon with recommendations for funding. Some of the important aspects of this program are discussed here.[46] States plan and establish their own criteria and give contracts to eligible projects. In the establishment of project areas and meal sites, the recommendation is that an attempt should be made to reach the 25

of USDA Commodity Distribution on Nutritive Intake," *Journal of the American Dietetic Association*, Vol. 61, No. 3 (September 1972), pp. 287–292.

[44] *Food Stamp Facts*, Food and Nutrition Service, U.S. Department of Agriculture, Washington, D.C., February 1972.

[45] Loretta Rowe and John Calvin, "A Profile," *Food and Nutrition*, Vol. 3, No. 6 (December 1973), pp. 10–11.

[46] "Rules and Regulations, Title 45—Public Welfare, Chapter IX—Administration on Aging, Social and Rehabilitation Service, Department of Health, Education, and Welfare, Part 909—Nutrition Program for the Elderly," *Federal Register*, Vol. 37, No. 162 (August 19, 1972).

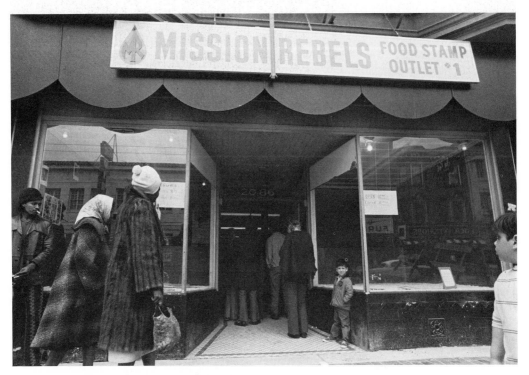

FIGURE 23–7. *A youth neighborhood organization sponsored the selling of food stamps to the poor.* (USDA)

per cent of the elderly with incomes below the poverty level. This criterion applies only to site selection and not to participant selection. Eligible individuals are those aged 60 or over who cannot afford to eat adequately, lack the skills or knowledge to select and prepare nourishing meals, have limited mobility that may impair ability to shop and cook for themselves, or have feelings of rejection and loneliness that obliterate the incentive to prepare and eat a meal alone.

Each state plan must provide that meals will be served in a congregate setting and at least one hot meal will be served 5 or more days a week. Each meal must meet at least one third of the recommended daily dietary allowances. Whenever feasible and appropriate, special menus should be available to meet particular dietary needs arising from health requirements, religious requirements, or ethnic backgrounds of participants. Supportive services such as transportation of individuals to and from meal sites, information and referral services, health and welfare counseling, nutrition education, shopping assistance, and recreational activities incidental to the project may be included. Each individual has the privilege of paying for the meal what he considers within his ability and may request a free meal if unable to pay. No individual should be denied participation in the nutrition program because of inability to pay. Settings for these projects are in public and private schools, recreation and community centers, public housing, social rooms of churches, homes for the aged, and senior centers. Reports from projects indicate that the elderly enjoy eating together.

Supplementary Food for Women, Infants, and Children (WIC)

Pregnant women, infants, and preschool children are among the high-risk populations

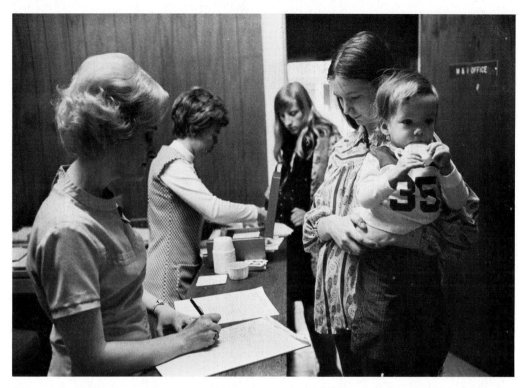

FIGURE 23–8.   *A pregnant mother and small son filling out an application for the WIC program.* (USDA)

from a nutritional standpoint, so the USDA program WIC makes a valuable contribution to the diet of individuals in these groups. Poor maternal nutrition and low birth weight appear to be factors in later manifestations of intellectual and educational deficits, according to a long-term study by Rubin[47] at the University of Minnesota. The continuation of WIC as one answer to this problem is urged.

In April 1974 there were 255 projects in 45 states, Puerto Rico, and the Virgin Islands. These projects have served 375,000 women, infants, and children up to 4 years of age. The following are eligibility criteria: participants must live in a project area, be qualified to receive medical treatment at reduced cost from a local health agency serving the project

area, and be certified by medical personnel to be in need of supplemental food.

Infants in the program may receive iron-fortified formula or milk, iron-fortified infant cereal, and fruit juice. Pregnant or nursing women and children over 1 year of age may receive milk, cheese, iron-fortified cereal, fruit juice, and eggs. One recommendation is that provision should be made that entire families be assured of an adequate diet so that these supplemental foods are used by the designated three groups and not shared with hungry fathers and older children of the family.[48] In April 1974 there were 20 projects that were participating fully in the medical evaluation component of the program. Other projects are evaluating to the extent of availability of funds. The results of these evaluations could

[47] "Low Birth Weight Linked to Disabilities," testimony at Senate Nutrition Committee hearings during week of April 1, 1974; reported in *CNI Weekly Report*, Vol. 4, No. 15 (April 11, 1974), p. 2.

[48] "USDA Announces New WIC Grantees," *CNI Weekly Report*, Vol. 4, No. 11 (March 14, 1974), p. 6.

make a valuable contribution to the health needs of this group and indicate the impact of improved nutrition.

Emergency Food and Medical Programs

Emergency programs are funded by the Office of Economic Opportunity in areas that indicate serious need. One grant for example has been given to Neighbors in Need, a network of 68 food banks serving the state of Washington. This organization was created by church groups in response to an acute hunger crisis by massive layoffs in Seattle's aerospace program. Although the problems of this situation have abated somewhat, Neighbors in Need has expanded its food banks to other areas of the state and feeds 60,000 to 70,000 individuals each month. Participants are families who are not reached by existing federal feeding programs. Puerto Ricans, Indians, and migrant families have benefited from emergency food and medical programs.

Challenges

Although the programs described reach many families and individuals in need, there continue to be millions of the hungry that do not have access to these programs. Solving this problem should have high priority. Furthermore, the continuation of some of the programs described here is in jeopardy. There is a need for enlightened citizens and communities to be sensitive to the needs around them and to be aware of the legislative steps necessary to stamp out hunger and related problems. Education must be a more vital force so that families and individuals can understand the nutritive aspects of the food served to them and can assume greater responsibility for their own nutritional status.

SELECTED REFERENCES

Bunting, Fredericka, and Robert Reese, "USDA Food and Nutrition Programs—A Progress Report," *National Food Situation*, Economic Research Service, U.S. Department of Agriculture (February 1975), pp. 34–42.

"Child Nutrition Programs," *Dairy Council Digest*, Vol. 45, No. 1 (January–February 1974), pp. 1–5.

Child Nutrition Programs, Food and Nutrition Service, U.S. Department of Agriculture, Washington, D.C., 1971.

Food Research and Action, *Out to Lunch*, A study of USDA's Day-Care and Summer Feeding Programs, Gazette Press, Inc., Yonkers, N.Y., 1974.

Head, Mary K., Roma J. Weeks, and Eleanor Gibbs, "Major Nutrients in the Type A Lunch," *Journal of the American Dietetic Association*, Vol. 63, No. 6 (December 1973), pp. 620–625.

Hiemstra, Stephen J., "Evaluation of USDA Food Programs," *Journal of the American Dietetic Association*, Vol. 60, No. 2 (March 1972), pp. 193–196.

Irvings, Mark, and Suzanne Vaupel, *If We Had Ham, We Could Have Ham and Eggs . . . If We had Eggs: A Study of the National School Breakfast Program*, The Food Research and Action Center, New York, 1972.

Maternal and Child Health Service Report, *Promoting the Health of Mothers and Children*, Public Health Service, Health Services and Mental Health Administration, U.S. Department of Health, Education, and Welfare, Washington, D.C., 1972.

National School Lunch Program, 25 Years of Progress, Food and Nutrition Service, U.S. Department of Agriculture, Washington, D.C., 1971.

Nichaman, Milton Z., and Gretchen E. Collins, "Nutrition Programs in State Health Agencies," *Nutrition Reviews*, Vol. 32, No. 3 (March 1974), pp. 65–67.

"Not by Enriched Bread Alone," Community Nutrition Institute, Washington, D.C., 1972.

Payne, Norman E., Avalon L. Dungan, and David L. Call, *The Economics of Alternative School Feeding Systems*, Department of Agricultural Economics, Cornell University Agricultural Experiment Station, New York State College of Agriculture and Life Sciences, Cornell University, Ithaca, N. Y., 1973.

Pearson, Joanne, "Child Nutrition Programs in the Food and Nutrition Service, U.S. Department of Agriculture," *Nutrition Program News* (May–June 1973), pp. 1–4.

Proceedings, Second Annual Joseph Despres Conference for Senior Citizens, *Meals for the Elderly Now!, Housing for the Elderly Now?* The Hudson Guild, New York, 1972.

Special Summer Food Service Program, Food and Nutrition Service, U.S. Department of Agriculture, Washington, D.C., 1973.

Todhunter, E. Neige, *Nutrition*, Background Issues, The Technical Committee on Nutrition, White House Conference on Aging, Washington, D.C., March 1971, U.S. Government Printing Office, Washington, D.C., 1971.

———, "School Feeding from a Nutritionist's Point of View," *American Journal of Public Health*, Vol. 60, No. 12 (December 1970), pp. 2302–2306.

"12 Million on Food Stamps—and a Lot More to Come," *U.S. News and World Report*, Vol. 75, No. 36 (September 10, 1973), pp. 55–56.

Vaupel, Suzanne, *Every School Has a Legal Right to the Revised School Breakfast Program*, Food Research and Action Center, New York, 1973.

Wolgamot, Irene H., Mary M. Hill, et al., *Nutrition Programs for the Elderly*, A Guide for Menu Planning, Buying, and the Care of Food for Community Programs, Consumer and Food Economics, Agricultural Research Service, U.S. Department of Agriculture, Washington, D.C., 1972.

Yeutter, Clayton, "How Can We Strengthen the School Food Service," *Food and Nutrition*, Vol. 3, No. 5 (October 1973), pp. 2–4.

24

Nutrition for Adolescence and Youth

The individual's stage of development is an important factor in determining nutrition requirements. In addition, other influences—economic status, education, ethnic background, knowledge of nutrition and concern about health on the part of parents of these young persons—are involved.

The age span of 11 to 22 years covers a wide range of developmental experiences, from those of late pre-teens to early adolescence to adolescence to postadolescence.

Social and Environmental Influences

Adolescents and youth represent a higher proportion of the total population in the 1970's than in the 1960's.[1] Their education is more extensive and consequently school enrollments for this age are higher in both high school and college. American youth are a mobile group, especially in the upper age levels. Many of the lower age group do some part-time work. Teen-agers 16 to 17 years of age are less likely to be in the labor market

than older youth. Seventy-five per cent of the men and about 60 per cent of the women in the upper age group were working in 1972. About one third of this group from 14 years and up was married. About 58 per cent of young men 14 to 19 years of age received incomes in 1971; but only 7 per cent were working year-round and full time, and only 38 per cent had incomes of $100 or more per week. Among persons 20 to 24 years of age, 94 per cent of the men and 76 per cent of the women had incomes in 1971.

Mead[2] lists the two outstanding aspects of adolescence and youth as becoming capable of reproduction and of full physical participation in work. Every individual, family, and society has come to grips with these aspects of development. The norm for maturity varies from group to group, and conflicts and anxieties arise if a young person does not meet the norm. Expectations of family and community are that certain responsibilities and activities of maturity can be assumed. Mead recommends readiness rather than chronological age

[1] U.S. Bureau of the Census, *Current Population Reports*, Series P-23, No. 44, "Characteristics of American Youth: 1972," U.S. Government Printing Office, Washington, D.C., 1973.

[2] Margaret Mead, "Adolescence in a Changing World," *UNICEF News*, Issue 79, 1974/1, pp. 3–11.

as a criterion. Gillette[3] believes that adolescents and youth have greater potential for mature and responsible action than parents, older sisters and brothers, teachers, and other adults realize. These culturally bound concepts and taboos should be removed or at least examined. Fresh and flexible approaches are needed to determine the role of the adolescent in society.

Growth and Physical Characteristics

Growth is a regular and highly regulated process according to Tanner.[4] Progress is not disorderly and unpredictable as many believe. The 11-year-old is on the threshold of puberty and is experiencing altered endocrine activities. The ages 12 to 16 are characterized by considerable alteration in growth rate. Body size increases rapidly, body composition and shape change, and there is a rapid development of the reproductive organs heralding the event of sexual maturity. Changes are complex and tremendous. Three determinants, genes, hormones, and the environment, and their interactions affect the process of growth and development, according to Valadian.[5]

Most changes are sex specific but a few are common to both sexes. Boys, for example, have a great increase in muscle size and strength accompanied with other physiological changes that produce an ability to do heavier physical work and to run faster and longer than girls. Bones of boys are longer, shoulders are broader, and stature is taller than girls on the whole. Girls have wider hips and more fat and mature 2 years earlier than boys. Both sexes mature earlier than formerly.

Different parts of the body grow at different rates and produce changes in body proportions. Growth may continue after adolescence.[6] According to some studies,[7] boys continued to grow for nearly 8 years after the peak of age height velocity and girls for 6 years. Deceleration of growth occurs earlier in girls than in boys. There is considerable variation in the tempo with which adolescents pass through the various stages of puberty. These differences are often the source of anxiety in the young. During the later years of the age group discussed in this chapter, the final stages of acquiring adulthood are experienced with a deceleration of growth and additional growth of muscle.

Nutritionwise, longitudinal studies of child health and development[8] have indicated the close relationship between growth in height and protein intake during the entire childhood and in specific periods, such as adolescence. In adolescence there was also an increase in kcaloric intake during rapid growth. The early-maturing individuals increase their kcaloric or protein intake sooner than late maturers. Girls curtail their kcaloric intake as soon as they reach their growth peak, with early-maturing girls curtailing intakes more and earlier. The wisdom of this action is questionable because other nutrient intakes such as protein are reduced as well. Adolescence is a key period for acquiring adult dietary patterns. Postadolescent dietary intakes are more highly predictive of adult intakes than dietary patterns of childhood. Improved nutrition, freedom from infectious diseases, and improved living conditions have contributed to faster maturing and larger children.

[3] Arthur Gillette, "The Young Adolescent: An Untapped Resource," UNICEF News, Issue 79, 1974/1, pp. 24–27.

[4] J. M. Tanner, "Sequence, Tempo, and Individual Variation in the Growth and Development of Boys and Girls Aged Twelve to Sixteen," Daedalus, Vol. 100, No. 4 (Fall 1970), pp. 907–930.

[5] Isabelle Valadian, "The Adolescent—His Growth and Development," in Youth—Nutrition —Community, Proceedings of National Nutrition Education Conference, Miscellaneous Publication No. 1254, U.S. Department of Agriculture, U.S. Government Printing Office, Washington, D.C., 1973, pp. 21–32.

[6] "Growth After Adolescence," Nutrition Reviews, Vol. 31, No. 10 (October 1973), pp. 314–315.

[7] A. F. Roache and G. H. Davilia, "Post Adolescence Growth," Pediatrics, Vol. 50, No. 6 (June 1972), p. 874.

[8] Isable Valadin, R. B. Reed, H. C. Stuart, et al., "Interrelationships Between Protein Intake, Illness and Growth as Manifested by Children Followed from Birth to 18 Years," paper presented at the Eleventh International Congress of Pediatrics in Tokyo, 1965.

Nutritive Needs

Nutritive requirements for boys and girls reach the maximum during the period of pre-adolescence and adolescence. Only during pregnancy and lactation do girls surpass their teen-age requirements. After 10 years of age, allowances for boys and girls are stated separately owing to their specific needs. Table 24–1 shows these nutritive needs.

In planning dietary allowances for the age groups of 11 to 14, 15 to 18, and 19 to 22 years, the Food and Nutrition Board[9] took into consideration growth periods, rate of maturity, size, body composition, activity, and related factors in a general manner. Individuals must bear these factors in mind in planning their own dietary intake and make necessary adjustments.

Nutritive requirements reflect the fact that girls complete their growth much earlier than boys. The kcaloric requirement for both boys and girls needs to be adjusted to their activity. If they tend to lose weight on this kcaloric intake, it is necessary for them to increase kcalories. If there is a tendency to overweight —and this is more often true with girls than with boys—then foods that are high in kcaloric value should be curtailed accordingly. Sleep, as well as activity, has an effect on the amount of kcalories needed. Many teen-agers get insufficient sleep. Consequently, their period of activity is prolonged so that even more energy is required.

One of the most critical nutrients for this age is calcium. It is estimated that the daily intake of calcium during this period must be enough to permit the storage of more than 1 pound of calcium. This may seem like a very small amount, but storage is difficult to accomplish because the daily diet will seldom furnish more than 1/400 pound, of which only 1/500 pound can be stored under the most favorable conditions.

Calcium is needed to provide material for the growth of the skeleton and the teeth and for other physiological functions. Owing to the

[9] Food and Nutrition Board, *Recommended Dietary Allowances*, 8th ed., National Academy of Sciences—National Research Council, Washington, D.C., 1974.

very uneven distribution of calcium in foods, an adolescent must use milk and milk products as the prime source. Some investigators have discovered that emotional stress and strain, which are quite characteristic of the adolescent period, may interfere with the retention of body calcium.

Iron for body tissue and blood is also essential. Since this age marks the onset of the menstrual cycle for girls, it is particularly important that they have an adequate supply.

The need for iodine is increased in adolescence, particularly for girls. If iodine intake is reduced to the point of inadequacy, thyroid difficulties will certainly occur. The use of iodized salt and iodine-rich foods will provide an adequate intake.

It is advisable for parents and others to bear in mind that although a young person may be of the same size as an adult, his nutritive requirements are much greater. Growth takes place in spurts, and it is particularly important that sufficient nutrients be provided during these rapid periods of growth.

Nutritional Status of Adolescents

There are few studies of this age group that combine clinical, biochemical, anthropometric, and dietary assessment in the analysis of nutritional status. Only one study, that of the *First Health and Nutrition Examination Survey* (HANES) of the National Center for Health Statistics, has nationwide representativeness. Preliminary reports of the first survey indicate that mean kcaloric intake was low for both white and black males and females in both income groups (income below and income above poverty level) for the ages discussed here. The mean protein intake was adequate for all ages, sexes, and incomes. The mean calcium intake was adequate for all ages, sexes, incomes, and races except for black females in the lower and upper income levels at ages 18 to 44 years. Mean iron intake was low for the 12- to 17-year-olds (approximately 70 per cent of the standard), low for white and black females in both income groups in the 18- to 44-year levels (about 55 to 60 per cent of the standard for the lower income and slightly higher for the income

TABLE 24-1

Recommended Daily Dietary Allowances for Males and Females Aged 11 to 22, Revised 1974

Designed for the maintenance of good nutrition of practically all healthy people in the United States

	11–14		15–18		19–22	
	MALES	FEMALES	MALES	FEMALES	MALES	FEMALES
Weight, kg (lb)	44 (97)	44 (97)	61 (134)	54 (119)	67 (147)	58 (128)
Height, cm (in.)	158 (63)	155 (62)	172 (69)	162 (65)	172 (69)	162 (65)
Kcalories	2800	2400	3000	2100	3000	2100
Protein, g	44	44	54	48	54	46
Fat-soluble vitamins						
Vitamin A activity, IU	5000	4000	5000	4000	5000	4000
Vitamin D, IU	400	400	400	400	400	400
Vitamin E activity, IU	12	12	15	12	15	12
Water-soluble vitamins						
Ascorbic acid, mg	45	45	45	45	45	45
Folacin, μg	400	400	400	400	400	400
Niacin, mg	18	16	20	14	20	14
Riboflavin, mg	1.5	1.3	1.8	1.4	1.8	1.4
Thiamin, mg	1.4	1.2	1.5	1.1	1.5	1.1
Vitamin B_6, mg	1.6	1.6	2.0	2.0	2.0	2.0
Vitamin B_{12}, μg	3.0	3.0	3.0	3.0	3.0	3.0
Minerals						
Calcium, mg	1200	1200	1200	1200	800	800
Phosphorus, mg	1200	1200	1200	1200	800	800
Iodine, μg	130	115	150	115	140	100
Iron, mg	18	18	18	18	10	18
Magnesium, mg	350	300	400	300	350	300
Zinc, mg	15	15	15	15	15	15

SOURCE: Food and Nutrition Board, *Recommended Dietary Allowances*, 8th ed., National Academy of Sciences—National Research Council, Washington, D.C., 1974.

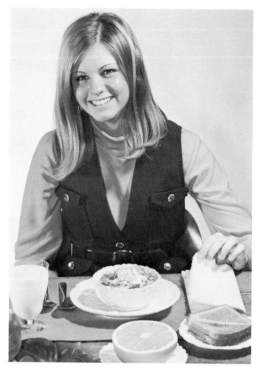

FIGURE 24-1. *Nutritious food is especially important during this age span. (Cereal Institute, Inc.)*

above poverty level), and above standard for black and white males in both income groups, with white males having a higher percentage above the standard.

The mean vitamin A intake was decidedly above standard in all income levels, age levels, and for males and females, except for black youth in the 12- to 17-year group at approximately the 95 per cent level of the HANES standards. Mean vitamin C intake was quite adequate for all age levels at both income levels and for males and females of both races. HANES standards were the same as those used in the *Ten-State Nutrition Survey.*[10]

[10] National Center for Health Statistics, *Preliminary Findings, First Health and Nutrition Examination Survey, United States, 1971–1972,* Dietary Intake and Biochemical Findings, DHEW Publication No. (HRA) 74–1219–1, Health Resources Administration, Public Health Service, U.S. Department of Health, Education, and Welfare, Rockville, Md., January 1974.

Findings of the *Ten-State Nutrition Survey*[11] for the 10- to 16-year-olds indicated that significant numbers had *kcalories* below standards set for their age, sex, and weight. Mean kcaloric intakes per kilogram of body weight decreased with age. Individuals in low-income-ratio states had lower mean intakes of kcalories than persons in high-income-ratio states.

Protein intakes for all subgroups exceeded dietary standards. Mean *calcium* intakes were higher for males than for females. Differences were greatest among 15- to 16-year-olds. Mean calcium intake tended to increase with age in males and decrease for females. White adolescents at all ages and at both income levels tended to have the highest mean intake. The cumulative percentage distribution data indicated that 20 to 54 per cent of adolescents had intakes less than the established standard of 650 mg.

Mean intakes of iron were lower than any other nutrient, particularly for females. Mean iron intakes for black and white adolescent females in low-income-ratio states were about half the amount established by the dietary standard. Spanish-American females in the low-income group had a somewhat higher iron intake. The cumulative percentage distribution data revealed that more than 80 per cent of the females of all age groups had iron intakes less than 18 mg. Mean iron intakes above the standard (10 mg) were found only for males 10 to 11 years of age.

Mean *vitamin* A intake exceeded dietary standards in most subgroups. Black adolescents generally had higher vitamin A intakes than did either white or Spanish-American participants. Mean intakes among blacks were almost twice as high as Spanish-American adolescents. Mean intakes tended to be higher for males than for females.

All adolescent participants approached or exceeded dietary standards for *thiamin.* With few exceptions, Spanish-Americans had the

[11] *Ten-State Nutrition Survey, 1968–1970,* DHEW Publication No. (HSM) 72–8134, Center for Disease Control, Health Services and Mental Health Administration, Department of Health, Education, and Welfare, Atlanta, Ga., 1972, pp. V–81 to V–85.

highest mean intakes and blacks had the lowest. Higher mean intakes were found in the high-income-ratio states. Within a given ethnic group, thiamin intakes increased slightly for males and decreased slightly for females.

Mean *riboflavin* intakes for all subgroups were above dietary standards. Little consistent relationship between ethnic group and mean riboflavin intakes was discovered except for white 12- to 14-year-olds, who had the highest mean intakes, and blacks, who had the lowest. Although mean values were high, the cumulative percentage distribution data revealed that large numbers of adolescents had low intakes. In all age groups the prevalence of low values was higher for females than for males. Adolescents in low-income-ratio states tended to have lower mean intakes of riboflavin.

All subgroups had higher mean *vitamin C* intakes than the dietary standard of 30 mg daily, often in the order of two to three times as much. In the low-income-ratio states, mean vitamin C intakes generally were higher for the Spanish-Americans than for either the white or black adolescents. In the high-income-ratio states there was less variation in mean values among ethnic groups. A trend to increased vitamin C intakes with increase in age was noted; however, intakes per kilogram of body weight decreased with age for all adolescents.

In summary, adolescents in low-income-ratio states generally had lower nutrient intakes than did adolescents in high-income-ratio states. Black adolescents tended to have the lowest nutrient intakes and whites had the highest. This was true of all nutrients except vitamin A, for which Spanish-Americans in low-income-ratio states had the lowest values. The prevalence of adolescent females with nutrient intakes below dietary standards tended to increase with age. Detailed information about the nutritional status of youth from 17 to 22 years of age was not available in this survey.

The *Ten-State Nutrition Survey* also produced information about growth and development for the 10 to 16 age group. In all income levels, ethnic groups, and for both sexes there was a low prevalence of deficiency status. (See Table 2–2.)

In the 1965 Household Food Consumption Survey of the U.S. Department of Agriculture,[12] an assessment of the food intake of approximately 1,400 youth, 12 to 19 years inclusive, was included. Average intakes of boys met or slightly exceeded recommended dietary allowances. Girls' mean intake of iron was 11 mg when 18 mg was the requirement. Vitamin A and thiamin were also slightly below the recommended amounts. Mean kcaloric intake (3049) for boys was highest for the 18- to 19-year-old group but only slightly higher than the 15- to 17-year-olds (2989). The 12- to 14-year-old girls consumed the most kcalories (2146).

From a review of the research it is apparent that adolescents and postadolescents have nutritional problems, according to Huenemann.[13] Dental caries, obesity, and anemia in girls and, though less, in boys are the major problems. Less than desirable amounts of dietary vitamins A and C are consumed according to analysis of food intake. This less than optimal nutritional status must be the concern of this age group and their families.

Young families with a teen-age mother are of special interest because nutritional inadequacies may occur. Van de Mark and Underwood[14] studied 100 families with a teen-age mother, a father living at home, and a baby for their dietary habits and food consumption patterns. Both husbands and wives fell below recommended dietary allowances for kcalories, protein (except for husbands 14 to 22 years of age), vitamin A, vitamin C (except for husbands 14 to 18 years of age), niacin (ex-

---

[12] Consumer and Food Economics Research Division, *Food Intake and Nutritive Values of Diets of Men, Women, and Children in the United States, Spring 1965.* Agricultural Research Service, U.S. Department of Agriculture, Washington, D.C., 1969.

[13] Ruth L. Huenemann, "A Review of Teenage Nutrition in the United States," *Proceedings of National Nutrition Education Conference,* Miscellaneous Publication No. 1254, U.S. Department of Agriculture, Washington, D.C., 1973, pp. 37–41.

[14] Mildred S. Van de Mark and Virginia Ruth Sherman Underwood, "Dietary Habits and Food Consumption Patterns of Teenage Families," *Journal of Home Economics,* Vol. 63, No. 7 (October 1971), pp. 540–544.

cept for husbands 22 to 28 years of age; those 18 to 22 years of age had 99 per cent), riboflavin (except for husbands 14 to 18 years of age), thiamin (except for husbands 18 to 22 years of age; wives 18 to 19 years of age had 99 per cent), calcium—seriously low, and iron (except for husbands 18 to 28 years of age).

Other results showed that dietary intakes were low for husbands and wives in the consumption of milk, meat, fruits and vegetables, or total kcalories. Race, annual income, age of homemaker, or educational levels of the husband and wife had little effect on the dietary intake of these young families. The results of this study give cause for serious consideration of possible solutions to this problem.

Food Habits

Huenemann[15] made a number of observations in the study of 1,000 high school students in Berkeley, California. Teen-agers tend to eat more than three times a day. Dinner was the meal eaten most consistently. Some subjects showed great variability from day to day. Lunch was omitted more than breakfast, particularly during summer vacations, probably owing to late breakfasts.

Differences among socioeconomic groups were less striking than those among ethnic groups. Boys ate more of all food groups than girls, and obese boys and girls ate smaller amounts of dairy products, vegetables and fruits, and were more frequent breakfast skippers.

Caucasians were the greatest consumers of dairy products; fats, oils, and nuts; and vegetables and fruits. Blacks ate the most desserts and sweets. Orientals led in the cereal group and were low in starchy vegetables because they ate rice in place of potatoes. In the meat and legume group, Oriental boys and black girls were the largest consumers.

The upper third of the socioeconomic group of these adolescents used more dairy products than the lower two thirds. All groups consumed generous amounts of the meat–legume foods. Oriental boys and girls ate the most fish, and blacks ate the most pork. Raw fruits and vegetables were consumed in greater quantities by girls than by boys. Boys preferred cooked fruits and juices. The smallest quantities of raw fruits and vegetables were consumed by black boys and girls. Black girls led in the consumption of cooked starchy vegetables.

Teen-agers are snackers. Frequent eating, according to research findings, is not detrimental to health, and little relationship is found to overall nutritive quality of the diet provided at least three meals per day are taken. When less than three meals are taken, there is usually a nutritive deficiency. When teen-agers eat most of their food after school and before going to bed, their diet is usually inadequate. The important point is that approval of snacking carries a responsibility for checking on total nutritive needs and does not condone overeating.

Food habits are strongly influenced by family. The mother appears to be an authority figure as revealed in studies of the food habits of girls. Findings indicated a striking correspondence with food patterns of mothers and their daughters.[16] Parents, particularly mothers, need to understand that the requirements of individual children do vary. Being unduly concerned can lead to feeding problems and undesirable food habits. Adolescents must understand the genesis of their own food habits, for at the end of the spectrum of this adolescent age level, they may be assuming parental responsibilities for the food of their children.

Good food habits at this age definitely relate to general life adjustment. The more mature the adjustment, the better the food habits.

Nutrition cannot be examined in isolation; the total person must be considered. Youngsters at this age are maturing rapidly in all areas and are trying to find a place for themselves in the world. As they emerge from

[15] Ruth L. Huenemann et al., "Food and Eating Practices of Teenagers," *Journal of the American Dietetic Association,* Vol. 53, No. 1 (July 1968), pp. 17–24.

[16] "Factors Influencing Adolescent Food Habits," *Dairy Council Digest,* Vol. 36, No. 1 (January–February 1965), pp. 1–2.

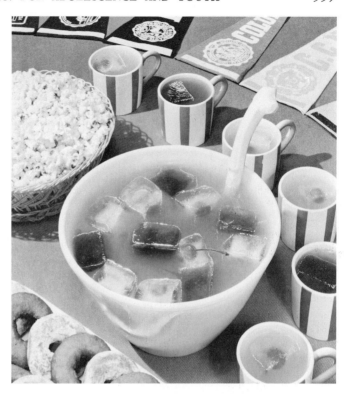

FIGURE 24–2. *Snacks of low nutrient density are often eaten by the young. (American Can Company)*

childhood to adulthood, they need careful and sympathetic handling. It must be realized that teen-agers try to identify with adults, for they want to be grown up.

Suggestions for Desirable Meal Patterns

The essential foods that should be included in the diet every day for teen-agers are suggested here:

MILK GROUP   Four or more cups every day and 2 or more cups if 20 years or post-adolescent. This might include whole milk, skim milk, buttermilk, dried milk, or cheese made from whole milk.

MEAT GROUP   Two or more servings every day. A choice may be made from meats of all kinds, poultry, or fish. Peas, beans, or nuts might be used if fortified with protein from animal sources. Pork occasionally in some form is recommended for its thiamin content. Organ meats such as liver and kidney are especially rich in nutrients. An egg should be included at least three or four times a week.

VEGETABLE–FRUIT GROUP   Four or more servings every day. These should include a dark-green or deep-yellow vegetable every day, a citrus fruit or generous serving of tomatoes, and other fruits and vegetables.

BREAD–CEREALS GROUP   Four or more servings a day. This may include breads of all types, quick breads, cooked or dry cereals, waffles and pancakes, hominy, macaroni, spaghetti, tortillas, noodles, and the like. Emphasis should be on whole-grain or enriched products made from wheat, corn, oats, rye, rice, or other cereals.

In addition, foods like butter, margarine, peanut butter, baked beans, ice cream, and puddings made with milk may be included in sufficient amounts to maintain weight.

The format for putting this guide into action is highly personal because it must fit

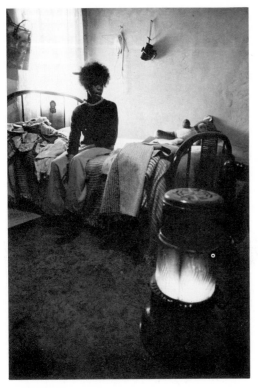

FIGURE 24-3. *A young migrant worker often has problems to secure an adequate diet.* (*USDA*)

into the lifestyle of the individual. It need not be traditional.

Like people of all ages, the adolescent should be interested in as wide a variety of foods as possible. The diversity will aid considerably in providing an adequate diet. Food should be wholesome, simply prepared, and appetizing. Most adolescents have a good appetite. Highly seasoned food and condiments such as catsup, relishes, and pickles should be used sparingly in the diet. It is not uncommon for an adolescent to put catsup or some other kind of sauce on almost everything that he eats. Such a habit should be discouraged.

It cannot be overemphasized that the need for food is great during most of this period. Adolescents should be encouraged to eat so that growth takes place in a normal manner and weight is maintained. To ensure adequate kcalories during strong spurts of growth, it may be necessary to plan a number of in-

between feedings that are high in nutritive value, including kcalories.

Eating Between Meals

Many youths do not give much consideration to the kind of food eaten between meals. A chocolate bar may have as much as 680 kcalories, yet contribute little else to the nutritive needs of the day. Doughnuts, whipped cream, and double malteds are high in kcalories. For adolescents who do not need to be concerned about weight, these foods may be eaten almost without restriction if other foods carrying the dietary essentials are included. But care should be taken that the foods eaten between meals do not hamper the appetite for the next meal, not only for adolescents but pre- and postadolescents as well.

Stasch[17] and others made a study of the food practices of college students and included snacking. Questions were asked about the snacks eaten most often at college and snacks eaten most often at home. Soft drinks were the most commonly chosen snack in both places. In college, greater use was made of coffee, candy, and hamburgers, and less use of milk, iced tea, fruit, cake, and cheese, which were more widely used at home.

Snacks at any age level in this group will be influenced not only by personal and peer preference but also by inflation, impact of vegetarianism, and interest in foods of one's heritage such as soul food, chili, spaghetti and macaroni, blintzes, and others.

Nutrition and Athletics

Many adolescents, and pre- and postadolescents, and youth have a strong interest in sports such as football, basketball, track, swimming, or tennis. The question is often asked, "What is the best food to eat?" The answer is, "A diet adequate in all required nutrients." One change will be more kcalories

[17] Ann R. Stasch, Mae Marth Johnson, and Glennell J. Spangler, "Food Practices and Preferences of Some College Students," *Journal of the American Dietetic Association*, Vol. 57, No. 6 (December 1970), pp. 523–527.

and, consequently, additional thiamin for this extra physical activity.

No particular foods have special merit for a diet for athletes. Some coaches are under the impression that a high meat diet is essential and even recommend steak for breakfast. No additional protein is required except where there is an unusual development of muscle (as discussed in Chapter 7). Most athletes need only sufficient high-quality protein foods, such as eggs, meat, fish, and poultry, to meet the daily needs.

Although athletes prefer high-protein diets, Consolazio[18] contends that ingestion of large amounts of protein requires additional water for metabolism, or dehydration and its debilitating effects may result.

The maintenance of water balance is essential to maximum physical performance, according to Mickelsen.[19] Many coaches restrict the amount of water consumed by athletes because there is a belief that "water logging" will occur. Sometimes coaches permit their players to rinse out their mouths with water but not to swallow any. There is considerable research to indicate that water consumed during an athletic event can be beneficial. Olympic cross-country skiers were reported to drink as much as 1 liter of water with glucose during a 3-hour meet. College football players receiving a 0.2 per cent sodium chloride solution that was drunk freely throughout a game that was played in a warm climate impressed spectators, television announcers, and the opposition with their performance. Fatigue accompanies dehydration, which is detrimental to action.

Another example is cited of exercise in extreme cold weather. When Sir Edmund Hillary conquered Mount Everest, an adequate water supply was planned for the final ascent by having adequate fuel to melt snow for drinking; this contributed to the success of the venture. The Swiss expedition a year earlier may have suffered from dehydration and accompanying fatigue because the amount of water available was only 1 pint per day for the last 3 days.

There is a great variation in the expenditure of energy among the various types of athletic performance. The capacity for prolonged muscle expenditure may be greater if there are ample glycogen stores prior to the exercise period. This conclusion was reached after experiments in which athletes were maintained on extremely high fat diets, on high carbohydrate diets, and on mixed diets. The endurance of athletes was greatest on the high carbohydrate diets, according to Van Itallie and others.[20]

A number of unfounded beliefs have been associated with milk in the diet of athletes. A condition of dry mouth, often referred to as "cotton mouth," was believed by some to be caused by the inclusion of milk in the pregame meal. Studies show that the dry mouth is related to saliva flow, the amount of perspiration, and the reduction of water content in the body and not to the milk in the diet, according to Fait.[21]

The pregame meal should consist of highly digestible foods and should be consumed not less than 3 hours before the athletic activity. Athletes frequently are under strain and stress prior to a game or contest and digestion may be prolonged. Replacing a solid pregame meal with a kcalorie-rich meal of liquids has been tried and found to be sound from the practical and physiological points of view. Individual food preferences should be respected, for an athlete knows from experience the foods he tolerates best.

There are other myths about the specific effect of certain foods being especially beneficial, according to Darden.[22] Many athletes

[18] C. F. Consolazio, "Nutrition and Athletic Performance," in Sheldon Margen (ed.), Progress in Nutrition, Avi Publishing, Westport, Conn., 1971, Chap. 12.

[19] Olaf Mickelsen, "Nutrition and Athletics," Food and Nutrition News, Vol. 41, No. 7 (April 1970), pp. 1, 4.

[20] T. B. Van Itallie, L. Sinisterra, and F. J. Stare in W. R. Johnson (ed.), Science and Medicine of Exercise and Sports, Harper, New York, 1960.

[21] H. F. Fait, What Research Shows About the Effects of Milk in the Athlete's Diet, School of Physical Education, University of Connecticut, Storrs (undated).

[22] Ellington Darden, "Olympic Athletes View Vitamins and Victory," Journal of Home Economics, Vol. 65, No. 2 (February 1973), pp. 8–11.

depend upon quick energy foods such as dextrose, honey, sugar, or other sweets. This practice may be detrimental because water is drawn to the gastrointestinal tract from other parts of the body, and if losses of water are great because of sweat, as in endurance-type sports, dehydration may occur. An adequate diet and adequate water intake appear to be the critical nutritional factors in maximal athletic performance.

Davidson and others[23] offer a number of valuable suggestions for the diet of the athlete. None of the ordinary foods are of special value or harmful in athletic training. Special preparations of vitamins and minerals have not improved performance. If an athlete prefers a vegetarian diet, adequate protein sources, such as eggs and dairy products, must be emphasized. There are large losses of fluid during strenuous exercise, and it is urgent that these losses be made good promptly so that muscle efficiency is not impaired.

Obesity and Underweight

There is considerable evidence that obese children do not grow out of this condition but tend to become obese adults. Although obese children tend to be above average height upon entrance into adolescence, their ultimate height may be below standard. Obese children appear to grow somewhat faster. Body fatness gradually increases in a girl, increasing in early adolescence and accelerating during the sixteenth and seventeenth years. The adolescent boy, in contrast, becomes leaner. By the midtwenties, the young man begins to add body fat slowly, whereas the young woman adds it more rapidly.

The obese adolescent is in a particularly vulnerable position from a developmental point of view. Obesity produces additional stress on the normal developmental processes. Adolescent obesity is among the more severe and resistant forms. There is some speculation that there may be more than one body compositional type among obese teen-agers. The

proportion of boys who are overweight or obese is much less than the corresponding proportion of girls.

One of the big problems among adolescent girls is an undue concern for a trim figure. The teen-age girl is much more zealous in her desire to have a slim figure than many of her elders. As a result, she may tend to starve, eat too little, or at least fail to get many of the essential foods at mealtime.

These girls try to reduce in a number of ways. One of the most common is to skip breakfast. Another way is to skip other meals or to eat very lightly, particularly at lunchtime.

A girl of this age easily becomes the victim of faddish diets. Because of the extravagant claims made for them, teen-agers often succumb to these diets more readily than older people. The omission of certain foods, such as potatoes, milk, and other nutritious fare, is also a dangerous practice. Many teen-age girls invent their own dietary regimen, which usually leaves much to be desired from the standpoint of nutrition.

Girls need help in distinguishing between slenderness and emaciation. Our culture is somewhat to blame, for we place such a high value on subnormal weight. Many girls are not aware of the fact that being well nourished can enhance one's appearance. And they fail to realize that heredity played an important role in the kind of figure they now have. Little can be done about certain unique characteristics like body build, height, and type of legs. Also, every girl has her own timetable for growth and development.

A study[24] of overweight adolescent girls revealed that underactivity is as critical to overweight as eating too much. Frequently, when girls are heavy, they do not participate in sports or even dancing as readily as their slimmer sisters. Many girls of this age compound the problem by eating for psychological compensation because they are not as attrac-

[23] Stanley Davidson, R. Passmore, and J. F. Brock, Human Nutrition and Dietetics, Williams & Wilkins, Baltimore, 1972, Chap. 58.

[24] Ruth L. Huenemann, Leona R. Shapiro, Mary C. Hampton, and Barbara W. Mitchell, "Teen-agers Activities and Attitudes Toward Activity," Journal of the American Dietetic Association, Vol. 51, No. 5 (November 1967), pp. 433–440.

tive and not admired as much by the opposite sex as slimmer girls.

Nutrition and Complexion

One of the first symptoms of malnutrition is often found in the skin. The plague of many adolescents is a poor complexion—pimples and acne. When they are afflicted with this condition, it is well to check on their diet. Of course, poor nutrition may not be the cause of a bad complexion—exercise, fresh air, and recreation must also be considered.

Eating Away from Home

Many adolescents leave home before they have completed their growth—to get jobs, be married, or attend college. It is extremely important that they be well grounded in desirable food habits and have some knowledge of nutritional requirements so that they can select food wisely. Skeletal and muscular development of their bodies may continue in post-adolescence or until they are at least 25 years of age.

Here are suggestions on adequate nutrition that the adolescent away from home might bear in mind.

1. Be certain that the day's diet includes all the dietary essentials.
2. Try to have meals fairly well balanced in the amount of food as well as in dietary essentials.
3. Eat regularly.
4. Do not omit any meals.
5. Watch weight—this means watch for both overweight and underweight—and adjust calories accordingly.
6. Remember when selecting food that cost does not indicate nutritive value. In other words, inexpensive food can be nutritious.
7. Make mealtime a pleasant occasion.

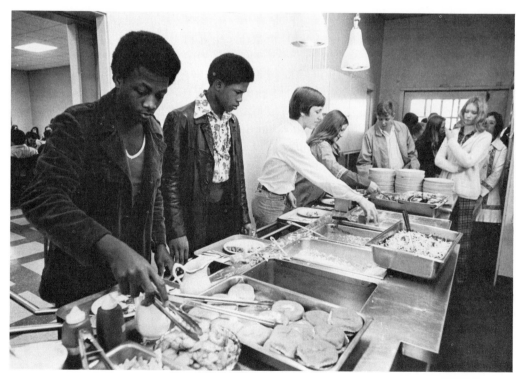

FIGURE 24–4. *Meals eaten away from home must contribute to the total nutritive intake.* (USDA)

Influence of the Adolescent Diet on Later Life

Individuals of this age group eat nutritious food everyday to facilitate good health, but they must realize that optimal nutrition today will have an influence on their health tomorrow. This is particularly true of the adolescent girl. The possibility of tuberculosis at this age level is a serious concern. And the strains and stresses of pregnancy can be met much more readily if a girl has maintained adequate nutrition throughout adolescence.

For the young man, good nutrition during the period of adolescence and postadolescence will tend to give him strength and stamina, which he needs in a competitive world. Also, he must serve as a good example to his children.

There is abundant evidence from research, too, that optimal nutrition will do a great deal to reduce disease and disability in later years. In fact, good nutrition can do much to prolong creative and productive years in an individual's life. Although Americans are taller and eat better than people did 50 years ago, the poor food habits of the younger generation could swing this pendulum backward.

SELECTED REFERENCES

"Adolescence: The Neglected Years," *UNICEF News*, Issue 79 (1974/1).

Consolazio, D. F., "Nutrition and Athletic Performance," in Sheldon Margen (ed.), *Progress in Human Nutrition*, Avi Publishing Company, Inc., Westport, Conn., 1971, Chapter 12.

Current Population Reports, Special Studies, Characteristics of American Youth; 1972, Bureau of the Census, Social and Economic Statistics Administration, U.S. Department of Commerce, Washington, D.C., 1973.

Graubard, Stephen R., "Twelve to Sixteen: Early Adolescence," *Daedalus*, Vol. 100, No. 4 (Spring, 1971).

A Handbook for Coaches, *Nutrition for Athletes*, American Association for Health, Physical Education, and Recreation, Washington, D.C., 1971.

"Nutrition and Athletic Performance," *Dairy Council Digest*, Vol. 46, No. 2 (March–April 1975), pp. 7–11.

Proceedings, *National Nutrition Education Conference*, Theme: Youth—Nutrition—Community, Miscellaneous Publication No. 1254, U.S. Department of Agriculture, Washington, D.C., 1973.

Snyderman, Selma E., and L. Emmett Holt, Jr., "Nutrition in Infancy and Adolescence," in Robert S. Goodhart and Maurice E. Shils (eds.), *Modern Nutrition in Health and Disease*, Lea & Febiger, 1973, Philadelphia, Chapter 24.

25

Nutrition for Adults

In the years from age 23 to 50, people experience some of the most significant events of their lives. This is the time a home and family are established, and children are reared to assume their own role in life. These are the work years—the greatest income-producing period. The kind of living done during these years will have a bearing on nutrition.

Adults

During the early stages of this age span, most young people leave home and learn to be independent. They may have finished school and most are working. At the lower end of this age scale, the young adult may be discovering that the process of assuming adulthood is strenuous.

Many men and women are married during this age period and may become parents. The wife and mother faces a serious and heavy responsibility. Not only must she select nutritious foods for herself, but she is also responsible for her husband's nutritional welfare. She should be well equipped to buy and to prepare nutritious meals.

Even more important is the ability of this wife to feed her children well. Evidence is cited repeatedly of the important role the mother plays in establishing good food habits. This is a vital step in health and adjustment to life itself. The trend to early marriages raises the question of the effect of stress and strain on the nutritional status of young folk. They must assume responsibilities that require maturity and considerable adjustment.

Adults are in important productive years during which they are making their commitment to society. They must bring up their children and establish their socioeconomic status. The tensions of this period may be severe, especially for people who are ambitious or have heavy family responsibilities. Many of the women will work. Some of the men will hold two jobs to increase income. The family may have to move a great deal, and, on the whole, the financial burdens of buying a home, educating children, and keeping up with status demands may be trying. Certainly the adult must be equipped with good health to face these stresses.

Nutritive Needs of Adults

The Food and Nutrition Board of the National Research Council recommends the daily dietary allowances given in Table 25–1. The

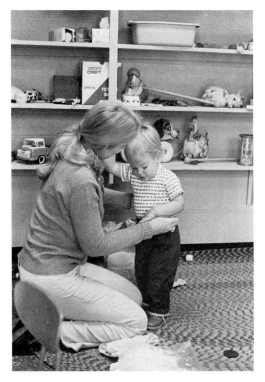

FIGURE 25-1. *Young mothers lead active lives and are responsible for an adequate diet for their family.* (*Children Today*)

kcaloric requirement for women is lower because they are smaller and consequently the need is less. The protein requirement is also less for women because it is related to size. On the other hand, the iron requirement is greater for women because of menstrual losses and other stresses. The differences in thiamin required for men and women can be attributed to the differences in kcaloric requirements.

The same guidelines for good nutrition, like the basic seven or daily food guide, apply at this age level as at earlier periods of life. It is well to remember that a good diet will foster a vigorous maturity and can do much to delay the characteristics of old age. Men and women should scrutinize their daily food carefully to see that their dislikes do not eliminate important nutrients. Inadequate amounts of certain nutrients in the diet in earlier years, if continued at this age, may have serious repercussions.

People at this age do not have to include nutrients for growth and the strenuous activities of youth. But their diet must provide means for maintaining body tissue so that its integrity is not threatened. This means adequate protein, minerals, and vitamins, with a sufficient amount of kcalories to maintain a desirable body weight. Good nutrition as well as other health habits should be stressed.

Influences on the Adult's Diet

The food required by adults may vary with their activities. Some people lead extremely active lives; others are somewhat sedentary.

First, the type of occupation must be considered—whether the person works in an office, in industry, or is studying. This factor will affect not only what he needs to eat but also the times at which he may eat.

Then, too, the type of recreation he chooses will affect his food needs. If he is very active in sports, or even dancing, he may need additional food both to maintain his weight and to supply enough nutrients. On the other hand, this supplement will not be required if his recreation is limited to the movies or spectator sports.

For many people the mode of living may lead to rather bad food habits. Eating too little, skipping meals, and eating at irregular hours are some of the shortcomings that may appear. And the quality of the meals may be affected. Indulging in highly seasoned fare or using large amounts of food accessories like catsup, pickles, and relish may distort the desire for wholesome food. Often they develop an exaggerated appetite for sweets, which needs to be checked. If they eat large quantities of candy, desserts, cake, or pies, their consumption of nutritious foods like milk, fruits, and vegetables may be critically reduced.

Men and women of middle age have matured and should be enjoying one of the most interesting periods of their lives. Most married couples at the upper level of this age scale are living alone again, for their children have married or left home. People in this group are on the way to or have reached the peak of their earning capacity and adapt their living standards accordingly. Job security is generally assured. It would seem to be a time

TABLE 25–1

Recommended Daily Dietary Allowances for Men and Women Aged 23 to 50, Revised 1974

Designed for the maintenance of good nutrition of practically all healthy people in the United States (allowances are intended for people normally active in a temperate climate)

	MALES	FEMALES
Weight, kg (lb)	70 (154)	58 (128)
Height, cm (in.)	172 (69)	162 (65)
Kcalories	2700	2000
Protein, g	56	46
Fat-soluble vitamins		
Vitamin A activity, IU	5000	4000
Vitamin D, IU	—	—
Vitamin E activity, IU	15	12
Wate-soluble vitamins		
Ascorbic acid, mg	45	45
Folacin, μg	400	400
Niacin, mg	18	13
Riboflavin, mg	1.6	1.2
Thiamin, mg	1.4	1.0
Vitamin B_6, mg	2.0	2.0
Vitamin B_{12}, μg	3.0	3.0
Minerals		
Calcium, mg	800	800
Phosphorus, mg	800	800
Iodine, μg	130	100
Iron, mg	10	18
Magnesium, mg	350	300
Zinc, mg	15	15

SOURCE: Food and Nutrition Board, *Recommended Dietary Allowances*, 8th ed., National Academy of Sciences—National Research Council, Washington, D.C., 1974.

when life could be freer of tensions and strain. Unfortunately, because of their experience and skills, they may be in greater demand and responsibilities may be heavier. Nutrition at this age, for both men and women, is even more urgent as one important step to a healthy old age.

Nutritive Status of Adults

The findings of the *Ten-State Nutrition Survey* were helpful in pinpointing nutritional problems of adults 17 to 59 years of age. Prevalence of deficient values in iron appeared most significant. Both female and male adults

from low-income-ratio states had a high prevalence of deficient values. White and Spanish-American adult females and males in the same income range had medium prevalence of deficient values in iron. Black and Spanish-American males and females in the high-income-ratio states had medium prevalence of deficiency values in iron; white males and females had a low prevalence of deficient values in iron. Spanish-American males and females in the low-income-ratio states had high prevalence of deficient values in vitamin A. Black males and females in both low- and high-income ratio states had low prevalence

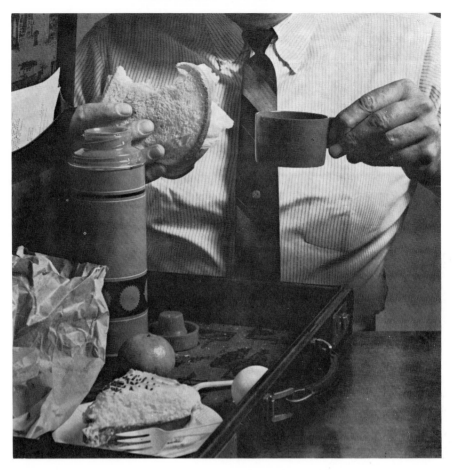

FIGURE 25–2. *Eating in a hurry can lead to nutritional problems. (Photo by permission of the Standard Register Company)*

of deficient values in vitamin A, and white females and males at both income levels had minimal deficiencies in vitamin A.

Only black and white males of low-income-ratio states had medium prevalence of deficient values in vitamin C. Black males and females in low-income-ratio states had medium prevalence of deficient values in riboflavin. Black females in both low- and high-income-ratio states had high prevalence of obesity. White females in both instances had a medium prevalence of obesity.[1] (See Table 2–2.)

---

[1] *Highlights, Ten-State Nutrition Survey, 1968–1970*, DHEW Publication No. (HSM) 72–8134, Center for Disease Control, Services and Mental Health Administration, U.S. Department of Health, Education, and Welfare, Atlanta, Ga., 1972.

In the HANES preliminary results, 49.52 per cent of the population indicated a consumption of less than 2000 kcalories daily. White persons above the poverty level had the highest kcaloric intake, while blacks in the lower-income group had the lowest intakes. A substantial proportion of the persons had low kcaloric intakes. Kcaloric intake will be related to activity and weight status in the final report.

Protein intakes were closely related to kcaloric intake. Mean protein intakes per 1000 kcalories showed little variation by race or income within most age groups. An exception was found in the group 18 to 44 years of age in which white males in the lower-income group had the highest mean intake, 42.22 g per 1000 kcalories. Another exception was found in the 45- to 59-year age group. Here white persons of both income groups reported less protein intake per 1000 kcalories, 38.48 and 42.30 g, respectively, than did blacks of either the lower or higher income group, 44.73 g per 1000 kcalories. Black adults had lower mean kcaloric intake than those of white adults; yet based on the protein intakes per 1000 kcalories, nutrient quality for black adults was higher. The mean protein intakes for whites under 45 years of age averaged about 80.19 g and ranged from 58.19 to 112.62 g; for blacks the average was 69.54 g and ranged from 52.30 to 99.31 g. Evaluating these findings with the 1974 recommended dietary allowance for protein, the intake of this nutrient was adequate except for the lowest range of blacks (52.30 g), which was slightly low.

Mean nutrient intakes for calcium and vitamin A were above the standard for most age, income, and race groups. Black females in the 18- to 44-year age group had mean calcium intakes below the standards, and mean vitamin A intakes were below standard for white females of childbearing age in the lower-income group. The higher kcaloric intakes of whites accounted for higher calcium intakes, yet the mean calcium intakes per 1000 kcalories were fairly comparable among all groups.

The mean vitamin A intakes per 1000 kcalories, in contrast, varied considerably in several age groups, between whites and blacks by income level. The ratio was higher in both income groups for blacks than for whites at ages 18 to 44 for females and males. The mean vitamin C intakes were higher for blacks than whites in the lower-income group for ages 18 to 44. The differences in vitamin A and vitamin C intakes between groups were more related to nutrient density than to total food consumed. About 73 per cent of the white females 18 to 44 years old in the low-income groups had intakes of vitamins A and C below standards.

Males 18 to 44 years old for both race and income groups had mean iron intakes that exceeded standards. For females 18 to 44 years of age for both race and income groups, the cumulative percentage distribution data showed that an average of about 95 per cent of

the group had iron intakes less than the standards. Blacks and white females on the lower-income group 45 to 59 years old did not meet the iron standards. Mean iron intakes per 1000 kcalories were higher for blacks in most age and income groups than whites.[2]

Nutritional problems were indicated in a national nutrition survey in Canada.[3] The group surveyed were young adult men and women (20 to 39 years) and middle-aged men and women (40 to 64 years) in the general population and 40- to 54-year-old Indians and Eskimos. Findings indicated that more than half the adult population was overweight. The problem exists for both sexes and for many age groups. Risks from obesity were most prevalent between 65 and 87 per cent of women over 40 years of age, for Indian men and women in the general population, and for Eskimos of both sexes. The kcaloric intake was 3200 kcalories for young adult men and 1900 kcalories for young adult women, and 2400 and 1700 kcalories, respectively, for middle-aged men and women.

Diets consumed showed the overall protein intakes of women of all ages to be poorer than for men. For most of the young and middle-aged men the dietary protein intakes were adequate on the whole. Lower protein intakes were found among Indians and Eskimos.

A high prevalence of iron deficiency was found among 20 to 60 per cent of the women at risk levels and 15 to 35 per cent of the men. There was a greater lack of iron intake among Indians and Eskimos than in the general population. The myth that only childbearing women are susceptible to iron deficiency was negated by results found among the men. About one in five of the women of all ages had a calcium deficiency. Vitamin A intake fell short of desirable levels for a large number of adults, being more pronounced

[2] National Center for Health Statistics, *Preliminary Findings, First Health and Nutrition Examination Survey, United States, 1971–1972,* DHEW Publication No. (HRA) 74-1291-1, Health Resources Administration, U.S. Department of Health, Education, and Welfare, Rockville, Md., 1974, pp. 1–25.

[3] Report by Nutrition Canada, *National Survey,* Department of National Health and Welfare, Ottawa, 1973, pp. 76–83.

among women than men. No clear-cut deficiency of vitamin C was found in the general population, but mild to moderate vitamin C deficiency was found among small numbers of Indian men. Eskimos had the highest clinical signs of a deficiency of this vitamin. Clinical signs of a thiamin deficiency were found in an appreciable proportion of adults in the general population and among Indians but none among Eskimos. Dietary intakes of riboflavin indicated less than adequate amounts for many adults, less frequently for men than for women. Niacin intakes in relation to kcalories were within or near adequate levels. No clinical evidence was found of thyroid enlargement among Eskimos and little among Indians. Moderate thyroid enlargement was observed with significant frequency among the general population, especially among women.

More research is needed to determine the nutritional status of adults. The three surveys cited here indicate instances of overnutrition and undernutrition of kcalories, leading to overweight, and lack of kcalories leading to a deficiency of important nutrients. Iron deficiencies even among men is the most serious concern. Low-income groups had vitamin A deficiencies. Except in certain segments of populations, there is less concern about protein, vitamin C, riboflavin, and niacin, but in certain areas iodine deficiencies are a matter of concern, especially among women.

Influences on Adult Nutrition

Education

In the *Ten-State Nutrition Survey* a correlation was found between educational attainment, that is the number of years of school completed, of the person usually responsible for the buying and preparation of the family's food and the nutritional status of children under the age of 17. As the homemaker's educational level increased, the evidence of nutritional inadequacies in the children decreased.[4] Among adults there was also a positive relationship in the *Ten-State Nutrition Survey* between the number of years of school completed by the individual and his

[4] *Ten-State Nutrition Survey,* op. cit., p. 10.

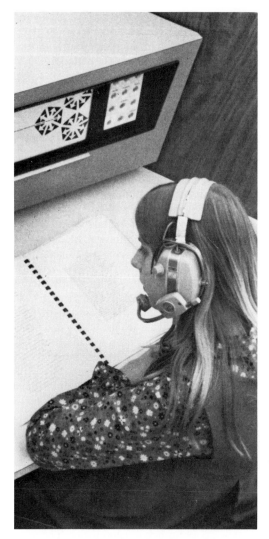

FIGURE 25–3. *There is a correlation between educational attainment and nutritional status.* (A T & T)

or her nutritional status. The effect is not so clear-cut because educational status is associated with other factors, such as income status, so it is not possible to identify these findings as the specific effect of education. Eppright and others[5] studied the correlation

[5] Ercel, Eppright, Hazel M. Fox, Beth A. Fryer, Glenna H. Lamkin, and Virginia M. Vivian, "Nutrition Knowledge and Attitudes of Mothers," *Journal of Home Economics,* Vol. 62, No. 4 (April 1970), pp. 327–332.

of a nutrition knowledge test and an attitude scale to the nutritional status of preschool children. Education of the mother was relatively highly correlated with nutrition knowledge and certain favorable attitudes, such as traditional concepts about the relationship between nutrition and well-being of children. Education was more highly related than income to dietary components. One recommendation of the study was to urge a focus not only on nutrition facts in nutrition education but on their application under various conditions of living.

Stress and the Nutrition of Adults

Stress implies that environmental factors burden the psychological adaptations of the body. Nutrition and stress interact in numerous ways.[6] The nutritional status of an individual affects his adaptation to stress and stress may alter nutritional requirements. If a person is well nourished, there seems to be some indication that tension can be handled with greater ease.

Reaction to psychological stress is highly individual depending upon genetic equipment, basic individual needs and longings, perception of the stress situation, life experiences, early conditioning influences, and cultural pressures. In addition, patterns of adaptation to different types of stress vary from individual to individual. For these reasons, research studies are difficult. Another personal variation is the susceptibility of various body organs and systems to tension.

Wolf and Goodell[7] cite studies that stressful experiences are associated with high blood cholesterol, which has been implicated as a risk factor in predisposition to coronary heart disease. Friedman[8] indicated a tendency to high triglycerides and cholesterol and other metabolic disturbances during stress. The majority of these studies showed a positive relationship between one or more behavioral variables and heart disease. One implication of these research endeavors is the possible bearing of social and psychological factors in future epidemiological studies of coronary heart disease.

Environmental stress, such as heat, cold, noise, and other disturbances, is important to consider in relation to nutritive requirements. Edman[9] in his review of nutrition and climate emphasized the importance of shivering, muscle tension, and the rise in metabolic rate in the complexities of maintaining thermal equilibrium in cold climates. Body fatness and excellent nutritional status are related to individual performance in the cold.

Because of increased sweating, water balance must be considered in an examination of the stress of heat. In addition, the loss of sodium, potassium, iron, chloride, sulfur, calcium, nitrogen, and other elements can become risk factors. The consumption of low-protein diets in tropical areas is serious in light of estimated losses of 20 to 30 per cent of protein during sweating, according to Mitchell and Edman.[10] There appears to be little evidence that extra vitamins are required. Energy requirements must be increased for individuals living and working in a hot desert climate in comparison to those who work in temperate zones.

Nutrition and Oral Contraceptives

Considerable scientific attention has been given to quantitative nutritional-metabolic changes that are produced in oral contraceptive users. More than 50 such metabolic changes have been recorded. In view of the success of oral contraceptives for women of childbearing age, their use will continue and

[6] "Some Interactions Between Nutrition and Stress," *Dairy Council Digest*, Vol. 42, No. 3 (May–June 1971), pp. 13–16.

[7] S. Wolf and H. Goodell, *Harold G. Wolff's Stress and Disease*, Charles C Thomas, Springfield, Ill., 1968.

[8] M. Friedman, S. O. Byers, R. H. Roseman, and F. R. Elevitch, "Coronary-prone Individuals (Type A Behavior Pattern); Some Biochemical Characteristics," *Journal of the American Medical Association*, Vol. 212 (May 4, 1970), p. 1030.

[9] M. Edman, "Nutrition and Climate," in S. Licht (ed.), *Medical Climatology*, Elizabeth Licht, Publisher, New Haven, Conn., 1964, pp. 553–556.

[10] E. Mitchell and M. Edman, "Nutritional Significance of the Dermal Losses of Nutrients in Man, Particularly of Nitrogen and Minerals," *American Journal of Clinical Nutrition*, Vol. 10, No. 9 (October 1962), p. 163.

increase. The challenge is to minimize the adverse effects of the drug–metabolism interaction.

Highlights of some of the important nutrient-metabolism effects will be discussed here. Tryptophan metabolism has been affected in approximately 80 per cent of users tested. An increased amount of metabolic intermediates, such as xanthurenic acid, of the trytophan–niacin pathway are excreted. Controlled intake of additional vitamin B_6 normalizes this metabolic derangement, according to Luhby and others.[11] McLeroy[12] and co-workers found that oral contraceptives reduced considerably the concentration of ascorbic acid as measured in leucocytes of healthy, sexually mature women. Hodges[13] cites other nutritional problems of oral contraceptive users. There is some impairment of carbohydrate metabolism and a substantial rise in triglyceride levels.

On the positive side, oral contraceptives have a beneficial effect on iron metabolism owing to an increased ability to absorb iron from the gastrointestinal tract and by lessening the amount of blood lost during menstruation. There may be a slight or substantial benefit in terms of nitrogen balance depending upon the type of contraceptive used. Oral contraceptives do not appear to deteriorate calcium metabolism. Research is under way on the effect on other nutrients.

Risk Factors

Middle-aged adults may be beset by certain degenerative diseases in which nutritional status may be one of the factors. Overconsumption of kcalories from food choices that are unwise and underexercise in a sedentary life may lead to excessive weight, which in turn may trigger a predisposition to atherosclerosis, hypertension, diabetes, coronary heart disease, and other diseases. A significant commitment to the prevention of these diseases has not been a goal of many adults or the nation's system of health care. These diseases exact high death rates and have become a major affliction of our society, according to McGandy and Mayer.[14]

Common aspects of these diseases are that the etiology is still uncertain, all are circulatory in nature or related, all are amenable to a course of treatment (the earlier started, the better) in which diet is important, and research indicates an interrelatedness that is not distinguishable. Treatment of one improves the others. Obesity is associated with all the diseases. Changes in lifestyle and diet in early stages of the diseases result in a favorable response.

Work and Nutrition

Work is an important aspect of the life of almost all adults. Studies of nutrition and work are concerned with the influences, stresses, and activities of various types of work so that nutritional requirements may be adapted accordingly, as indicated by Shils.[15] Changes in dietary intake have been studied to determine the effect on performance during work.

Durnin and Passmore[16] have established a grading system of energy expenditure in industrial work or occupational activities. The energy expenditure for light work is 2.0 to

[11] A. Leonard Luhby, Myron Brin, Myron Gordon, Patricia Davis, Maureen Murphy, and Herbert Spiegel, "Vitamin B_6 Metabolism in Users of Oral Contraceptive Agents. 1. Abnormal Urinary Xanthurenic Acid Excretion and Its Correction by Pyridoxine," *American Journal of Clinical Nutrition*, Vol. 24, No. 6 (June 1971), pp. 684–693.

[12] Vera Joyce McLeroy and Harold Eugene Schendel, "Influence of Oral Contraceptives on Ascorbic Acid Concentrations on Healthy, Sexually Mature Women," *American Journal of Clinical Nutrition*, Vol. 26, No. 2 (February 1973), pp. 191–196.

[13] Robert E. Hodges, "Nutrition and the 'Pill,' " *Journal of the American Dietetic Association*, Vol. 59, No. 3 (September 1971), pp. 212–217.

[14] Robert B. McGandy and Jean Mayer, "Atherosclerotic Disease, Diabetes, and Hypertension: Background Considerations," in Jean Mayer (ed.), *U.S. Nutrition Policies in the Seventies*, W. H. Freeman, San Francisco, 1973, Chap. 4.

[15] Maurice E. Shils, "Food and Nutrition Relating to Work and Environmental Stress," in Robert S. Goodhart and Maurice E. Shils (eds.), *Modern Nutrition in Health and Disease*, Lea & Febiger, Philadelphia, 1973, Chap. 26.

[16] J. V. G. A. Durnin and R. Passmore, *Energy, Work and Leisure*, Heinemann Educational Books, London, 1967, Chap. 4.

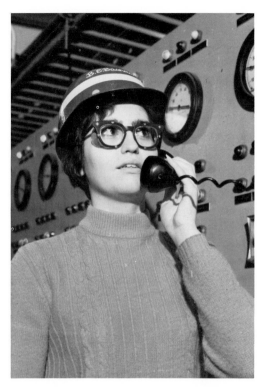

FIGURE 25–4. *The type of work an adult does is an important factor in determining nutritional needs as well as the influence of stresses and strain of the job. (Bethlehem Steel)*

4.9 kcal per min per 65 kg for men and 1.5 to 3.4 kcal per min per 55 kg for women. Energy expenditure increases through moderate, heavy, very heavy, to unduly heavy work, which requires 12.5 kcal per min per 65 kg for men and 9.5 kcal per min per 55 kg for women. Large amounts of energy are expended by some workers in heavy industry, but office work or other activities requiring mental activity, in contrast, require little extra energy. Typing 30 words per minute on an electrical typewriter requires 1.4 kcal per min. Household tasks such as sewing, range from 1.4 to 1.8 kcal per min for a 55-kg woman and a 65-kg man, respectively; scrubbing floors or furniture polishing ranges from 4.0 kcal per min for a 55-kg woman to 5.0 kcal per min for a 65-kg man.

The effect on work of actual food shortages reveals that psychological, physiological, and some psychomotor changes develop sooner or later, whereas intellectual functioning shows less deterioration. No proof has been found, according to Shils,[17] that frequent feedings increase the physiological capacity to do work. Working with little or no breakfast has been found by Tuttle[18] and co-workers to have adverse effects on maximum work output.

Correa[19] calls attention to the influence of present nutritional conditions on current working capacity. Few attempts have been made to research this problem. The working capacity of individuals in the working force of some countries is much lower than the potential because of nutritional deficiencies. This in turn has a profound effect on economic development. People do not work at their best when they are inadequately nourished. Not only are personal economic resources diluted, but social and human development may be affected.

Alcohol and Nutrition

Bebb[20] and others studied the nutritive content of the usual diet of men on a monthly 3-day diet record for 1 year. Individuals showed a wide range in kcaloric intake but intake was considered reasonable in comparison to other studies. Thiamin and riboflavin were above the two thirds of the recommended daily allowances. Allowances for phosphorus, niacin, and iron were met. Eighty-five per cent of the group met 100 per cent of the allowance recommended for ascorbic acid. Most subjects in the study met their calcium requirement, although a few were as much as 50 per cent below the calcium recommendation. Sixty-three per cent of the men in group 1 (execu-

[17] Shils, op. cit., pp. 713–716.

[18] W. W. Tuttle, Kate Daum, L. Myers, and C. Martin, "Effect of Omitting Breakfast on Physiologic Response of Men," *Journal of the American Dietetic Association*, Vol. 26, No. 6 (June 1950), p. 332.

[19] Hector Correa, "The Measured Influence of Nutrition on Personal and Social Development," *Newsletter*, March 1974, League for International Food Education, Washington, D.C., pp. 3–4.

[20] Helen T. Bebb, Harold B. Houser, Jelia C. Witschi, and Arthur S. Littell, "Nutritive Content of the Usual Diets of Eighty-two Men," *Journal of the American Dietetic Association*, Vol. 61, No. 4 (October 1972), pp. 407–415.

tives or management positions) met the recommendation for vitamin A and 61 per cent in group 2 (professionals and executives in a community physical fitness program) had adequate amounts in their diets. Protein was above recommended allowances. All but four of the men reported alcoholic beverages on half or more of the days of the study. Nine men reported alcohol consumption every day. The mean kcaloric intake per day from alcohol was 250 kcalories per day in group 1 and 70 kcalories daily for group 2. Considering only drinking days, group 1 men averaged 318 kcalories from alcohol and group 2 averaged 199 kcalories. It is important to consider the contribution of kcalories from alcohol in dietary studies. Depending upon the amount of alcohol consumed, a risk factor for liver disease and other conditions must be considered with this age group.

Handicapped Adults

There are millions of handicapped adults in America. The disability may have arisen as a result of an accident, birth defects, crippling diseases, heart trouble, mental disturbance, or other sources. Special attention may need to be given to the nutrition of these persons for several reasons. First, it is important that they enjoy the best of health so that they meet life

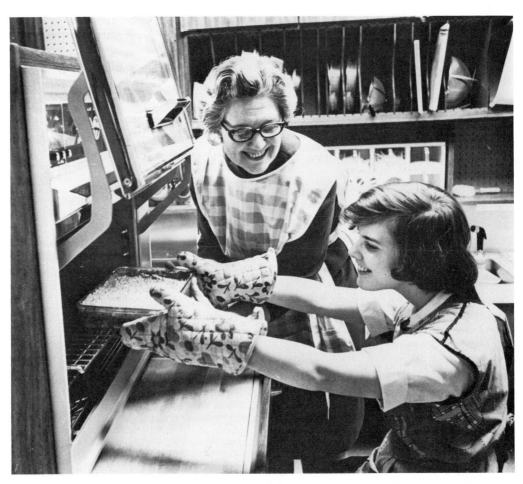

FIGURE 25–5. *A young handicapped adult learns to prepare food for her family in spite of limitations.* (USDA)

with greater stability. Second, many of them are very inactive owing to their disability, so kcalories need to be reduced. This may mean selecting foods very carefully so that nutrients are well represented in low kcaloric foods. In addition, an adult may be limited in the types of food preparation that can be undertaken. Personal diets and the diets of families may have to be adjusted accordingly.

Since some of these persons have limited contacts with the outside world, each meal may be an occasion and hold special interest. An effort should be made to have low kcaloric, nutritious food prepared and to serve it as attractively as possible. Doing so may be a decided morale-building factor.

Rusk[21] describes vividly the problems in food preparation for persons with physical limitations who are unable to unwrap a package, to cut meat, or to turn the knobs or push the buttons of an electrical appliance. Such

difficulties can contribute to the potential for an inadequate diet. Marketing for food may be even more of a hurdle. The Institute for Rehabilitation Medicine at New York University has studied the problems of the handicapped homemaker for many years and the obstacles to be overcome. The results have been gratifying to many patients. Wang and Bricker[22] have been successful in teaching blind homemakers to be more independent in their activities.

These and many other influences affect the nutrition of adults. Throughout this rather long span of life, the importance of good eating habits cannot be overemphasized. People should realize that maintaining a nutritious diet is like planning a sound financial program for old age. The benefits can be enormous.

[21] Howard A. Rusk, "Nutrition in the Fourth Phase of Medical Care," *Nutrition Today*, Vol. 5, No. 3 (Autumn 1970), pp. 24–31.

[22] Virginia Li Wang and A. June Bricker, "A Team Approach to Teaching Blind Homemakers: Home Economist as a Member of the Health Team," *American Journal of Public Health*, Vol. 60, No. 10 (October 1970), pp. 1910–1915.

SELECTED REFERENCES

Birch, Herbert G., and Joan Dye Gussow, *Disadvantaged Children, Health, Nutrition, and School Failure*, Harcourt Brace Jovanovich, Inc., New York, 1970.

Consumer and Food Economics Research Division, Agricultural Research Division, *Food for the Family with Young Children*, Home and Garden Bulletin No. 5, U.S. Government Printing Office, Washington, D.C., 1970.

———, *Food for the Young Couple*, Home and Garden Bulletin No. 85, U.S. Government Printing Office, Washington, D.C., 1971.

Food and Nutrition Board, *Recommended Dietary Allowances*, 8th ed., National Academy of Sciences—National Research Council, Washington, D.C., 1974.

Gifft, Helen H., Marjorie B. Washton, and Gail G. Harrison, *Nutrition, Behavior, and Change*, Prentice-Hall, Inc., Englewood Cliffs, N.J., 1972, Chapters 1, 4, and 5.

Lowenberg, Miriam E., E. Neige Todhunter, Eva D. Wilson, Jane R. Savage, and James L. Lubawski, *Food and Man*, John Wiley & Sons, Inc., New York, 1974.

Weight, Height, and Selected Body Dimensions of Adults, PHS Publication No. 1000, U.S. Department of Health, Education, and Welfare, Washington, D.C., 1965.

26

Nutrition for Older Americans

Any discussion of nutrition and aging must be based on the recognition that aging is a process beginning at conception and continuing until death, according to Watkin.[1] Any national policy on nutrition and aging must be based on this concept and programs planned accordingly.

Americans, on the whole, evade thought about old age; consequently, the literature about nutrition and the aged is thin. De Beauvoir[2] agrees by stating that society looks upon old age as a kind of shameful secret that is unseemly to mention. Unfortunately, many old people are condemned to live a life of poverty, loneliness, and despair. These factors along with others have a powerful impact on the nutritional status of the elderly.

What Is Old?

Old age is probably the greatest challenge that an individual faces. The body ages as minutes and heartbeats tick away, but individual differences in the rate of aging are great.

Aging is defined by Shock[3] as a developmental sequence of all living processes as they change with the passage of time. Gerontology is the scientific study of these processes, with special emphasis on the impairment of the performance capacity of an individual's cells and organs. Geriatrics is the aspect of medicine concerned with the treatment and prevention of diseases of older persons.

Watkin[4] cites aging as an area marked by limited productivity in thinking, investigation, education, and implementation. Definitive studies have been difficult because of the long life span of man. More effort has been expended on the harassments of the aged from disease and disabilities than on other aspects of the aging process. Many factors determine the health and longevity of people. Individuals have little or no control over their heredity; certain public health measures may determine the quality of air and water and exposure to biological pathogens. Other factors

[1] Donald M. Watkin, "The Aged," in Jean Mayer (ed.), *U.S. Policies in the Seventies*, W. H. Freeman, San Francisco, 1973, p. 53.

[2] Simone de Beauvoir, *The Coming of Age*, G. P. Putnam's New York, 1972, p. 1.

[3] N. W. Shock, "Some Biochemical Aspects of Aging," *Nutrition News*, Vol. 26, No. 3 (October 1963), pp. 1–12.

[4] Watkin, op. cit. pp. 55–56.

356

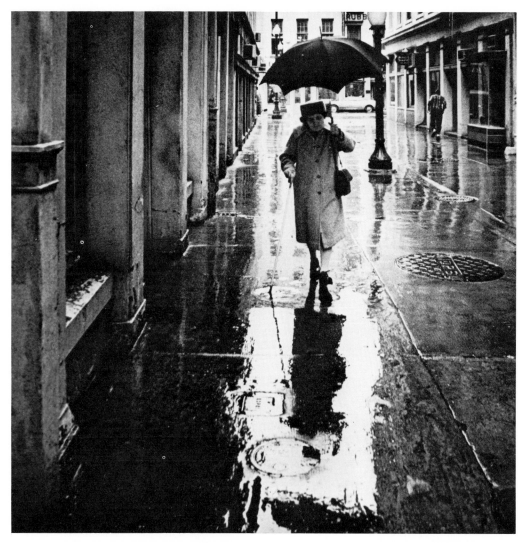

FIGURE 26-1. *Many old people are condemned to a life of poverty, loneliness, and despair.* (*Department of Labor*)

are subject to personal control, such as food, physical activity, and smoking.[5]

Growth and atrophy are processes that are present in the human body at all times. During youth, growth is decidedly in the ascension, whereas atrophy is most prominent in the aged. However, the rate of atrophy varies with

each individual, depending on his nutrition, mental health, heredity, the seriousness of any diseases and infections, fatigue, and general health. Old age is said to be related to three aging clocks—biological, psychological, and sociological.

Profile of the Aged

In the United States there are over 20 million persons in the age group over 65. Fifty-five per cent are females and 45 per cent are

[5] E. D. Schlenker, J. S. Feurig, L. H. Stone, M. A. Ohlson, and O. Mickelson, "Nutrition and Health of Older People," *American Journal of Clinical Nutrition*, Vol. 26, No. 10 (October 1973), pp. 1111-1119.

males. This age is the customary time for businesses to retire persons and, unfortunately, skills and knowledge acquired over a long period of time are usually discarded. Society almost ignores the aged and seems to expect them to accept this period before death.[6]

Physiological Changes in Aging

The primary factor in the process of aging, according to Watkin,[7] is cell death—that is, a specific cell within a specific organ system in the body dies and is replaced by some form of acellular material. Evidence is that the total body water is correlated with the actual number of living, nonfat cells in the organism. The water content of cells remains remarkably constant throughout the entire age span but the total body water decreases with age. Although the water content of the cell remains constant, the total intracellular water decreases with age and serves as an index of functioning cell mass, according to Shock.[8] Other supporting data are that the basal metabolic rate decreases with age, another reflection of fewer live cells.

Another proof of cell deterioration is related to the discrete functions of the kidney. There is a decrease in functioning units, or nephrons, because of the death of cells. Similarly, a study of brain tissue from a specified area of the cerebral cortex reveals a decrease in cells in the aging. Still unsolved is the reason for the death of cells.

Cell death leads to gradual deficiency in organ functioning. The heart in the elderly, for example, has a reduction of its reserve capacities so that the organ not only works harder than normal to meet a stress condition but also takes a longer recovery time. This loss of efficiency is most characteristic of highly specialized cells in the aged. Neural or endocrine breakdowns, which disrupt these essential regulatory mechanisms of the body, may occur.

Shock also states that certain cells, such as in the skin, hair, lining of the gastrointestinal tract, and liver, retain the capacity to divide and reproduce while other cells, such as muscle and nerve cells, lose this capacity. In addition to cell loss, there is cell impairment in aging tissues; for example, some of the enzymes associated with energy transformation reduce their activity with age.

The genetic makeup of an individual may be an important factor in determining longevity. Watkin[9] suggests that adults in late maturity years enjoying good nutritional status, intellect, health, and having resistance to disease and disabilities may well have an elite genetic endowment.

The problem of dentition, according to Sebrell, is a serious factor.[10] A high percentage of the elderly have lost their own teeth and the quality of dentures varies considerably. Many have never learned to masticate well with false teeth; hence, they avoid nutritious foods that may present a problem of chewing or cause mouth discomfort.

The senses of smell and taste are less acute, so food is less appetizing. A less sensitive sense of smell may inhibit the flow of saliva and other digestive juices. Elderly people do not enjoy the odor and taste of delicious foods as much as formerly. Faulty eyesight may complicate eating.

Psychological Changes in Aging

That functional changes in psychological processes are a product of physiological decline is an interesting hypothesis in the opinion of Kuypers.[11] The assumption underlying this position is that the rate of growth and development of the body correlates with the

[6] James E. Montgomery, "Magna Carta of the Aged," *Journal of Home Economics,* Vol. 65, No. 4 (April 1973), p. 7.

[7] Donald Watkin, "The Process of Aging," *Proceedings of the Seventh Annual Nutrition Institute of the Food and Nutrition Council of Greater New York* (mimeographed), May 11, 1967, pp. 4–8

[8] Nathan W. Shock, "Physiologic Aspects of Aging," *Journal of the American Dietetic Association,* Vol. 56, No. 6 (June 1970), pp. 491–496.

[9] Watkin, op. cit., p. 56.

[10] Henry Sebrell, Jr., "It's Not Age That Interferes with Nutrition of the Elderly," *Nutrition Today,* Vol. 1, No. 2 (June 1966), pp. 15–18.

[11] Joseph A. Kuypers, "Changeability of Life-Style and Personality in Old Age," *Gerontologist,* Vol. 12, No. 4 (Winter 1972), pp. 336–342.

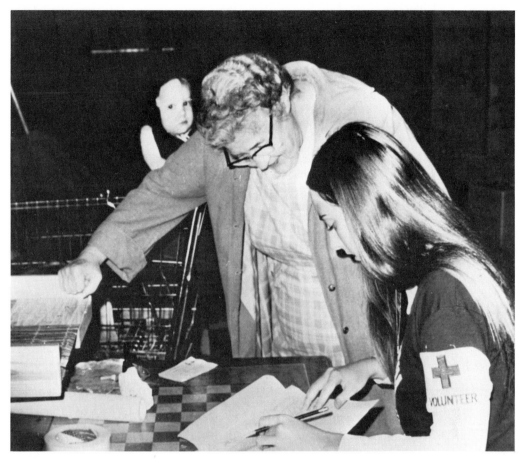

FIGURE 26–2. *Older persons often need help. Here a young woman is helping an older American to fill out her Food Stamp application.* (USDA)

ordering of psychological processes and role interpretation and performance.

Longitudinal studies of life-cycle movement are very limited in the study of old age because of expense and time. Riley and Foner[12] in a review of the literature on personality research on the aged found evidence of a number of single personality dimensions that changed in later maturity, such as greater rigidity, restraint, cautiousness, passivity, and emotionality. These psychological changes have an influence in the attitude of the elderly toward their food.

Weinberg[13] believes that food is not only necessary for nourishment but is an important symbol of certain psychological aspects of life, such as social interchange, evidence of love, and the meaning of pleasure. Weinberg further states that to an older person what he eats may be less important than with whom he eats.

The evidence of old age—gray hair, declining strength and muscle tone, wrinkles and impaired hearing—have a psychological impact at the upper levels of this age group. Retirement, unless planned, may bring about

[12] Martha White Riley and Anne Foner (eds.), *Aging and Society,* Vol. 1, *An Inventory of Research Findings,* Russell Sage Foundation, New York, 1968, pp. 12–15.

[13] Jack Weinberg, "Psychologic Implications of the Nutritional Needs of the Elderly," *Journal of the American Dietetic Association,* Vol. 60, No. 4 (April 1972), pp. 293–296.

a feeling of aimlessness and of being un-wanted. Income is usually cut drastically. Moving to another home, the death of a friend or a spouse, all require adjustments. The rate of psychological aging depends on the degree to which an individual accepts change.

Many of the aged show some signs of diffi-culty in thinking, in calculating, in remember-ing, and similar functions. Coupled with these mental impairments is an anxiety generated by these inabilities to function, according to Turner.[14] The "search for aid"—someone to help them—is crucial in the life of aged per-sons. The older person who retains his faculties and is active is indeed fortunate.

Economic and Social Conditions

Senior citizens are probably the single most economically deprived group in our nation. Most older Americans have problems of in-come, housing, transportation, clothing, and lifestyle, all of which are interrelated. The problems vary in intensity from individual to individual and will be influenced to an extent by where a person is in the spectrum of old age, which ranges from 65 to over 100 years of age.

More than one fourth of all older Ameri-cans are living below the poverty level and consequently are extremely limited in their choice of lifestyles. This restricted income limits the purchase of nutritious food, food preparation facilities, and other amenities of life.[15] Many of the elderly who do not live at the poverty level have only 50 per cent of the income of the younger segment of the population. The ravages of inflation are felt keenly by the aged with their fixed incomes. Researchers and policy makers label eco-nomics the most serious problem of this seg-ment of the population.

Sources of income for the aged population

in the United States come from Social Se-curity, public assistance, wages and salaries, pensions from former employers, children, and from rent, dividends, inheritance, interest, and annuities.[16] The aged who have been in poverty prior to old age depend largely upon Social Security and public assistance for in-come. Although Social Security offers con-siderable stability, changes often occur in public assistance and other forms of income. Assistance from children is frequently condi-tional and undependable. Many anxieties are engendered about money for living.

Older persons suffer from more health prob-lems than any age group and, according to the 1971 White House Conference on Aging, one third to one half of them can be traced to inadequate nutrition. Riley and Foner[17] found that over 75 per cent of the population 65 years and over suffered from at least one chronic ailment, about half reported two or more, and one third reported three or more. In Project FIND[18] the results indicated that the 97 per cent of the aged poor reported one or more symptoms.

The lack of transportation facilities inter-feres with the mobility of the aged and creates serious restrictions, such as in shopping for food, clothing, and other items, in par-taking of community activities, and in par-ticipating in other morale-building experi-ences. Only 40 per cent of persons over 65 have driving licenses, and many older persons have to depend upon public transportation that is often inconvenient, expensive, or non-existent.

Kreps[19] offers a number of insights about the lifestyles of the aged. Taste in old age reflects taste held during youth and middle

[14] Helen Turner, "Eating as Behavior," *Proceed-ings of the Seventh Annual Nutrition Institute of the Food and Nutrition Council of Greater New York* (mimeographed), May 11, 1967, pp. 71–72.

[15] "Selection Recommendations on Income," 1971 *White House Conference on Aging*, U.S. Government Printing Office, Washington, D.C., 1972, pp. 1, 12.

[16] Jack Ossofsky et al., *The Golden Years, a Tarnished Myth*, A Report for the Office of Eco-nomic Opportunity by the National Council on Aging on the Results of Project FIND, National Council on the Aging, Washington, D.C., 1970, pp. 40–42.

[17] Riley and Foner, op. cit., p. 205.

[18] Ossofsky et al., op. cit., p. 53.

[19] Juanita Kreps, "Lifestyle," in "A Colloquy on Growing Old in America," *American Association of University Women Journal*, Vol. 65, No. 8 (April 1972), pp. 24–25.

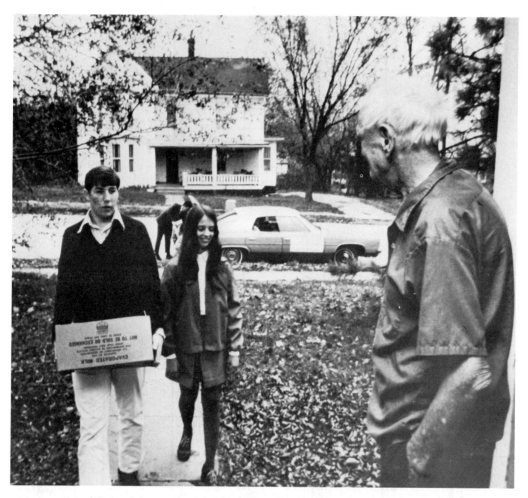

FIGURE 26–3. *Many oldsters are restricted in shopping because of health and other problems. Here high school student volunteers bring groceries to an elderly man.* (USDA)

age. There is little if any change in attitude, personality, or perspective. Change will reflect characteristics such as inquisitiveness, innovativeness, and interest and excitement in new experiences. Limitations to new opportunities for the aged, however, are real, such as travel, making new friends, and social interaction, because of limited income, health problems, habitual patterns of living, or disinterest. Lifestyle in any period of life including old age is determined to a degree by the status that society imposes upon the individual.

Nutritional Needs of Older Persons

The recommended daily dietary allowances[20] in Table 26–1 for persons 51 years and over indicate the basis for an adequate diet.

Lower kcaloric requirement of older adults demands special attention. When activity decreases, it is very easy to gain weight if interest in food remains high. The intake of high

[20] Food and Nutrition Board, *Recommended Dietary Allowances*, 8th ed., National Academy of Sciences—National Research Council, Washington, D.C., 1974.

TABLE 26–1

Recommended Daily Dietary Allowances for Men and Women Aged 51 and Over, Revised 1974

Designed for the maintenance of good nutrition of practically all healthy people in the United States

	MALES	FEMALES
Weight, kg (lb)	70 (154)	58 (128)
Height, cm (in.)	172 (69)	162 (65)
Kcalories	2400	1800
Protein, g	56	46
Fat-soluble vitamins		
Vitamin A activity, IU	5000	4000
Vitamin D, IU	—	—
Vitamin E activity, IU	15	12
Water-soluble vitamins		
Ascorbic acid, mg	45	45
Folacin, μg	400	400
Niacin, mg	16	12
Riboflavin, mg	1.5	1.1
Thiamin, mg	1.2	1.0
Vitamin B_6, mg	2.0	2.0
Vitamin B_{12}, μg	3.0	3.0
Minerals		
Calcium, mg	800	800
Phosphorus, mg	800	800
Iodine, μg	110	80
Iron, mg	10	10
Magnesium, mg	350	300
Zinc, mg	15	15

SOURCE: Food and Nutrition Board, *Recommended Dietary Allowances*, 8th ed., National Academy of Sciences—National Research Council, Washington, D.C., 1974.

kcaloric foods may need to be restricted. Checking on food habits for indulgence in second helpings and in frequent snacking may uncover the source of surplus kcalories. On the other hand, there is the possibility that in the later years interest in food may diminish and kcalories may be inadequate. In this instance, frequent small feedings and the inclusion of some high kcaloric foods may be necessary. The weight of an individual will reflect the adequacy of his kcalories.

For the protein requirement, it is important that animal proteins, such as those in milk, meat, eggs, and cheese, supplement the proteins found in vegetables and cereals. Some studies revealed an insufficient protein intake in older women. This lack can have serious repercussions if the person must undergo an operation or suffers from a bone injury, because healing is prolonged. Too little protein in the daily diet may also cause an older person to become easily fatigued and more susceptible to infections. However, recommendations for a higher protein intake, which are frequent, are unwarranted. The few experiments conducted in this area do not indicate any need for an increase of protein for this age group. The emphasis should be on the adequacy and on the quality of protein.

The calcium intake at this age is often very

low. Many older people are not convinced of the importance of milk and thus suffer from a calcium deficiency.

Older persons often suffer from nutritional anemias, which would indicate a lack of iron, protein, or certain vitamins. An emphasis on green vegetables, whole-grain and enriched cereals, and meat, especially liver, is recommended.

A number of studies have indicated that adequate vitamins in the diet produce general vigor and vitality. Yet mild vitamin deficiencies are not uncommon among older people. For example, a smooth red tongue and possible digestive disturbances or skin changes may be signs of a slight niacin deficiency. In these cases, physicians may prescribe additional vitamins. Some geriatricians have found that therapeutic doses of water-soluble vitamins may be needed to correct long-standing vitamin deficiencies, which are sometimes found in older people.

Again, an adequate diet will head off vitamin and mineral deficiencies. The daily diet should be checked for the presence of a fresh fruit or vegetable, green and yellow vegetables, milk, eggs, meat, and whole-grain or enriched cereals.

Many scientists emphasize the importance of water in the diet of older persons, for the functioning of kidneys decreases as one grows old. Water is important in carrying away wastes excreted by the kidneys, and it is easier for them to function with a diluted urine. Constipation is often an ailment in later life and drinking water may alleviate this also.

Nutritional Status of Older Persons

Dietary surveys of older persons provide useful information on the kind and amount of food consumed, food habits, eating patterns, and the frequency of use of specific foods, according to Todhunter.[21] By calculation of the nutrient content of the diets there is evidence of the nutritional status of the indi-

viduals studied. Comparatively few studies have been made of the older age group. In the *Ten-State Nutrition Survey*[22] persons over 60 years of age showed general undernutrition, which was not restricted to the very poor or to any single ethnic group. (See Table 2–2.) The preliminary findings of diet and biochemical tests in the *First Health and Nutrition Examination Survey*[23] are that 21 per cent of the white and 36 per cent of the black adults aged 60 and over in the lower-income group had intakes of less than 1000 kcalories. For the same ages in the income group above poverty 16 per cent of the white adults had intakes of 1000 kcalories or less, and 18 per cent of the black adults. Mean protein intake per 1000 kcalories showed little or no variation by race or income, indicating that protein consumption was closely related to total kcaloric intake for the group aged 60 and over. The same pattern was evident in calcium intake in relation to kcaloric intake. At both income levels the mean calcium values were consistently higher for whites than for blacks but the difference was because of a higher kcaloric intake among whites.

The mean ratios for vitamin A and vitamin C intakes per 1000 kcalories in both income groups for blacks were higher than for whites in the 60-and-over age group. The nutrient density of the food consumed rather than the total kcaloric intake accounted for these differences. In the lower-income group both blacks and whites of this age level had mean iron intakes that did not meet the standard established. In the income group above poverty level, whites and blacks either approached or were above the standard for iron.

[21] E. Neige Todhunter, *Nutrition, Background, Issues*, White House Conference on Aging, March 1971, U.S. Government Printing Office, Washington, D.C., 1971, pp. 14–17.

[22] *Highlights, Ten-State Nutrition Survey, 1968–1970*, DHEW Publication No. (HSM) 72–8134, Center for Disease Control, Health Services and Mental Health Administration, U.S. Department of Health, Education, and Welfare, Atlanta, Ga., 1972, p. 10.

[23] National Center for Health Statistics, *Preliminary Findings, First Health and Nutrition Examination Survey, United States, 1971–1972*, DHEW Publication No. (HRA) 74–1291–1, Health Resources Administration, Public Health Service, U.S. Department of Health, Education, and Welfare, Rockville, Md., January 1974, pp. 6–18.

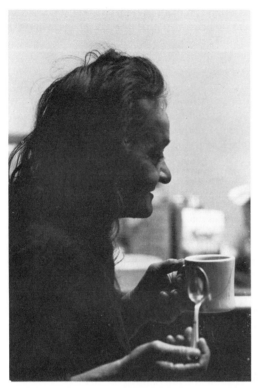

FIGURE 26–4. A malnourished, homeless woman comes to SOME (So Others Might Eat), a program in Washington, D.C. that has a soup kitchen for persons on "skid row." (USDA)

Schlenker and others[24] reviewed the research literature related to the nutrition and health of older people. Evidence has been presented that nutritional adequacy in early life is related to health and well-being in later life. Low hemoglobin in later stages of life was associated with a higher incidence of respiratory disease. Low vitamin A in the diet was related to increased incidence of nervous, circulatory, and respiratory disorders. Low thiamin intake was associated with diseases of the nervous and circulatory systems.

Elderly persons, 65 to 90 years of age, who complained of fatigue were administered vita-min B_{12}. The symptom disappeared in 89 per cent of the participants in the study. When the vitamin was replaced with a placebo, the symptom reappeared. Osteoporosis is a common disability in later life caused by a demineralization of the bone. The magnitude of the loss of mineral is greater in females than in males. The cause of this condition is unknown. It is suggested that leanness in humans will enhance longevity. The kind and amount of dietary fat may influence the length of life, particularly the development of atherosclerosis and cardiovascular disease. All in all, studies reveal that nutrition makes a significant contribution to health and longevity of older Americans.

A study of the food habits of older persons living at home by LeBovit[25] indicated that calcium and ascorbic acid shortages were most frequent. About one fourth of the households had diets that furnished less than two thirds of the 1963 recommended allowances for one or more of eight nutrients. Over one third of the households were using vitamin preparations. Most of them spent food money comparable to the U.S. Department of Agriculture low-cost food plan and had diets meeting two thirds of the recommended allowances. The poorest diets were found among the oldest homemakers, those over 75 years of age, and among those with the lowest incomes, under $1,000 for one-person households and under $2,000 for two-person households. Health problems had no relation to the nutritive quality of the diets. Persons trying to lose weight usually made poor food choices.

Daily Food Requirements for Older Persons

The nutrients required for an adequate diet can be translated into a variety of foods for appetizing meals by following "A Daily Food Guide."[26] This blueprint will serve as a guide for meals eaten at home or away from

[24] E. D. Schlenker, J. S. Feurig, L. H. Stone, and O. Mickelson, "Nutrition and the Health of Older People," American Journal of Clinical Nutrition, Vol. 26, No. 10 (October 1973), pp. 1111–1119.

[25] Corrinne LeBovit, "The Food of Older Persons Living at Home," Journal of the American Dietetic Association, Vol. 46, No. 4 (April 1965), pp. 285–289.

[26] Mable A. Walker and Mary M. Hill, Food Guide for Older Folks, U.S. Government Printing Office, Washington, D. C., 1972, pp. 1–7.

home. Everyday the older person should plan to incorporate the following foods into the diet:

MILK GROUP

Foods included in this group are fluid whole, skim, low-fat, evaporated, and dry milk and buttermilk. Milk alternatives for calcium content are discussed in Chapter 16. Two or more cups of milk (488 g or 0.48 liters) daily or the equivalent in a milk alternate are recommended.

VEGETABLE—FRUIT GROUP

All vegetables and fruits are included in this group. See Chapter 29 for additional information.

Four or more daily servings of vegetables and fruit are recommended, as follows: one serving as a source of vitamin C, one serving at least every other day of a source of vitamin A, and two or more servings of any vegetable or fruit, including those that are valuable for vitamin C and vitamin A. Count as one serving ½ cup (approximately 75 g) of vegetables or fruit, or a portion as ordinarily served, such as a medium apple, banana, orange, or potato, half a medium grapefruit or cantaloupe, or the juice of one lemon. See Chapter 29.

MEAT GROUP

Foods included in this group are beef, veal, lamb, pork, organ meats such as liver, heart, and kidney; poultry and eggs; fish and shellfish; and meat alternates—dry beans, dry peas, lentils, and peanut butter. Choose two or more servings every day. Count as a serving 2 to 3 oz (16 to 23 g without bone) of lean cooked meat, poultry, or fish. Equivalent in protein to 2 oz of meat are 2 eggs (limit to 3 or 4 per week), 1 cup (250 to 260 g) of cooked beans, dry peas, or lentils, or 4 tablespoons (64 g) of peanut butter.

BREAD—CEREAL GROUP

Foods included in this group are all breads and cereals that are whole grain, enriched, or restored. Check labels carefully. Specifically, the group includes breads, cooked cereals, ready-to-eat cereals, cornmeal, crackers, flour, grits, macaroni, spaghetti, noodles, rice, rolled oats, parboiled rice and wheat, and quick breads and other baked goods if made with whole-grain or enriched flour. Choose four servings every day. If no cereals are chosen, have one extra serving of breads or baked goods. Count as one serving 1 slice of bread (23 g), 1 oz (28 g) ready-to-eat cereal, or ½ to ¾ cup (118 to 177 g) of cooked cereal, cornmeal, grits, macaroni, noodles, rice, or spaghetti.

To round out meals and to meet energy needs, other foods not specified may be included, such as sugars, butter, margarine, and other fats. Some vegetable oil containing unsaturated fatty acids is recommended.

These foods may be included in a variety of meal patterns that are most suitable to the individuals concerned. According to studies of the U.S. Department of Agriculture, three meals a day comprised the most frequent meal pattern of persons 65 years and older. About 40 per cent ate more than three meals. Men ate more substantial breakfasts than women. Fifty per cent of the men but only 30 per cent of the women ate eggs and meat (usually bacon or both). Hot or cold cereal was the main breakfast item of almost as many men as women. About two thirds of both men and women ate bread for breakfast. Doughnuts, sweet rolls, and such were chosen by only 5 per cent of the men and 3 per cent of the women. Fruit, usually citrus, was consumed by 39 per cent of the women and 33 per cent of the men. Milk was used on cereal, as a beverage, or in coffee.

The midday meal, particularly for men, tended to be the most substantial meal of the day. Half of the elderly eat the larger meal at noon and about one third ate around 4 P.M. Seventy per cent of the men and 60 per cent of the women included meat in this meal with cheese and eggs as meat alternates. Potatoes were the most popular vegetable. Breads were included if potatoes were omitted. Desserts were eaten more often in the evening, although more than half the midday meals included fruit, milk dessert, or a bakery product other than bread.[27]

---

[27] "Meal Patterns of the Elderly," *Journal of the American Dietetic Association*, Vol. 63, No. 2 (August 1973), p. 129.

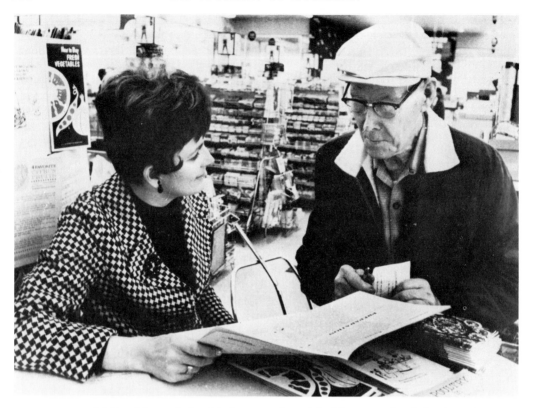

FIGURE 26–5.   *Many of the elderly are malnourished because of a lack of nutri- tion knowledge. Here a USDA extension worker helps an elderly man in a grocery store to plan nutritious meals for himself.*

Shopping for food presents problems to older Americans because of a lack of trans- portation and of disabilities that may limit the kind and amount of shopping. Sherman and Brittan[28] made a study of the food- shopping habits of an elderly urban popula- tion. The demise of the corner grocery store or the local drugstore affected the accessibility of such basic necessities as food and medications for the elderly. In addition, the curtailment of transportation routes and frequency of service and the high cost of taxis and other forms of individualized service were deterrents. Other influences such as poverty, aloneness, distance of shopping centers, having to walk to shop, carrying groceries, crossing busy streets, and

[28] Edith M. Sherman and Margaret R. Brittan, "Contemporary Food Gatherers," *Gerontologist,* Vol. 13, No. 3, Part 1 (Autumn 1973), pp. 358– 364.

enduring bad weather were apparent. This research pointed up the sizable effect of the patterns of merger and relocation of food stores upon many aging citizens whose shop- ping habits must be altered if food is to be secured. They walk, if possible, operate their own cars, or impose on friends, relatives, or neighbors to transport them to shopping centers.

The researchers suggest that there is a need for research and standard setting concerning the adequacy of food budgets as they relate to such factors as type of food store used, de- livery charges, transportation costs, and family size. One recommendation is the development of adequate social services to meet the spe- cialized problems of shopping for food by the elderly.

Another influence on the selection of food for the daily diet is food habits. The cultural, ethnic, or religious backgrounds persist and must be accommodated in the buying and preparation of foods. Lack of nutrition knowledge may prevent the aged from having adequate diets. This ignorance makes them especially susceptible to the wiles of food faddists and quacks, especially if vitality, cures, and other come-ons are emphasized. Sometimes these older Americans buy their food at health stores at high prices which many of them can ill afford.

Adaptation to the Family Diet

It is better for both the family and the older person if meal adjustments can be kept to a minimum, but some changes may be necessary. Owing to digestive difficulties or for other reasons, some older persons prefer to have their dinner at noon and a light supper at night. The time of meals may need to be changed. An older person may sleep later in the morning and prefer to have breakfast in a more leisurely manner. This change in mealtime has some disadvantages in that morale and appetite may be better if the oldster is up and eating with the rest of the family. Also, the preparation of an additional meal is an extra chore to a busy homemaker unless the older family member is capable of doing this himself.

If he or she has trouble with his or her teeth, meat and other protein foods may need to be ground or chopped. The strained and chopped fruits and vegetables prepared for infants can be used in many ways. For example, these fruits can be used as sauces for milk desserts or combined with tapioca or rice. The vegetables can be served in place of whole vegetables or added to ground meat. Sometimes these foods can be planned in such a way that they are a part of the family's diet. Although not an infant food, frenched string beans are an example of a vegetable that can be purchased either canned or frozen for the entire family. When the elderly have difficulty in chewing, they may lapse into the bad habit of omitting meat and vegetables and leaning on carbohydrate foods that are easier to masticate. In these cases, egg and milk beverages, fruit juices, and strained fruit and vegetables should be included in the daily diet.

If a person of this age seems to have little appetite, it is important that the food be tastily prepared and that it look attractive. Small servings with a provision for second helpings may be better than overwhelmingly large servings. Several small meals a day—five, for example—might be preferred. Adding dried skim milk or an egg to milk drinks and puddings, or using the concentrated evaporated or dried milk, will increase the nutrients in the diet for the light eater.

The elderly usually enjoy snacks. The snack should be light. Milk, milk drinks, fruit and vegetable juices with a cracker or two are advisable. A light snack before going to bed may be enjoyed.

The attitude of the entire family toward the eating habits of an older member is most important. The attitude should be positive, uncomplaining, and helpful. Everything should be done to make him feel that he is a part of the family, not someone who is an added responsibility. The whole atmosphere of family living will benefit from this decision.

Tips for Oldsters Preparing Meals for Themselves

To prepare meals for one person is costly and sometimes difficult. A man who lives alone may not have the necessary skills for preparing his own food. A woman may lose interest in planning and cooking her own meals.

To shop for one person is not easy. Packages that are practical for one or two servings may be difficult to find and often expensive, although many more foods are now appearing in small packages. Even "specials" may require too much effort to find and again the quantity may be too large. The market may be far away or difficult to reach, especially if the weather is unpleasant.

Here are a few suggestions that may be helpful:

1. Plan carefully. Follow recipes when necessary so that food is well prepared and not wasted. Try new dishes occasionally.

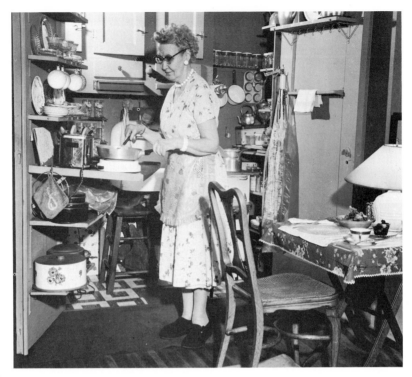

FIGURE 26–6. *An older person with limited space and facilities prepares her food efficiently. (Courtesy The Peabody Home, Bronx, N.Y.)*

2. Allow sufficient time to prepare the meal. Use shortcuts to save time and energy. Mixes—ready prepared or home prepared—and other prepared or partially prepared food will make fewer demands on one's energy.
3. Plan one-dish meals or a main dish that is especially liked.

The ingenious person can plan with a few pieces of equipment. A double boiler has the advantage of cooking two items at once, such as cooking a green vegetable in the bottom while a creamed meat or fish is heating in the top. A steam cooker with several compartments is even more useful. A heavy skillet or a Dutch oven is practical, too. A potato baker can be used as an oven on one burner to heat frozen meals, to bake casseroles, apples, or custards, and to heat rolls. Cooking a meal in steps, that is, cooking main dish first, then beverage, or hot dessert, is another way of using one

burner effectively. If one's budget is more liberal or if no burner is available, an electric skillet or saucepan has many possibilities.

Home-Delivered Meals

Many volunteers and community organizations in the nation have made home-delivered meals, popularly known as Meals on Wheels, possible for the elderly.[29] Recipients are the incapacitated elderly who are poor and have difficulty in preparing their own meals. One hot meal is delivered 5 or more days a week. Some plans include food for a cold supper. Paying for meals with food stamps has been possible in some areas.

Many factors must be considered in the

---

[29] Virginia Knauer, "Portable Meals Contribute to Nutrition Education Efforts," *Journal of Nutrition Education*, Vol. 3, No. 2 (Fall 1971), pp. 59–61.

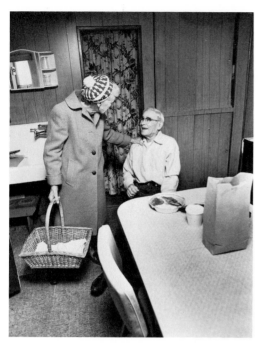

FIGURE 26–7. *Home delivered meals by volunteers are highly beneficial.* (USDA)

planning of these meals.[30] One third of the daily nutritive recommended allowances serves as a guide for the selection of foods for each meal. Depending upon the group served, allowances are usually made for difficulty in chewing. Meat is usually ground and vegetables like spinach are chopped. Potatoes are whipped or mashed. Foods are unseasoned if many of the elderly are on a low sodium diet. Food likes and dislikes as reflected in the entire group may be recognized in the planning.

In addition to making an excellent contribution nutritionwise to the daily diet, the encouragement of the volunteers who deliver the meals to eat all the food brought to the participant is helpful. A visitor from the outside world who is interested and cheerful has many positive psychological effects. Many of the aged benefiting from Meals on Wheels improve in health to the degree that they are able to participate in meals offered at a senior

or community center or in one of the federal government feeding programs. (See Chapter 23.)

The nutrient contribution of home-delivered meals was surveyed by Joering.[31] Findings indicated adequate protein, calcium, iron, vitamin A, and riboflavin. Approximately 75 per cent of the recommended dietary allowances for thiamin were met, 97 per cent of the niacin, and approximately 60 per cent of the ascorbic acid.

Simko and Babich[32] in a study sponsored by the Administration on Aging, Social and Rehabilitation Service have made over 300 inquiries to agencies in the United States and in other nations to secure information about studies and surveys, program development, legislation, volunteers, procedures, types of programs, and other aspects of this service, as related to home-delivered meals for the elderly.

The Older Person Who Eats Away from Home

Eating out may present a problem, for some older persons find it difficult to walk the required distance to an eating establishment. In addition, eating out can be expensive. Restaurant food is often priced out of reach for older persons. Fast food eating places have limited fare.

When a person eats away from home, he should keep in mind all his daily requirements. A list kept in a pocket or purse or in his room may serve as a reminder, because it is so easy to omit essentials. It may be necessary to make definite plans for apportioning the essential foods among the meals or snack times each day.

Not only is there a problem in finding a

[30] Carol Brent McLaughlin, "Meals on Wheels Reach Baltimore's Elderly," *Food and Nutrition*, Vol. 3, No. 1 (February 1973), pp. 2–4.

[31] Elizabeth Joering, "Nutrient Contribution of a Meals Program for Senior Citizens," *Journal of the American Dietetic Association*, Vol. 59, No. 2 (August 1971), pp. 129–132.

[32] Margaret D. Simko and Kathleen S. Babich, *Home-Delivered Meals*, A Selected Annotated Bibliography, Administration on Aging, Social and Rehabilitation Service, Department of Health, Education, and Welfare, Washington, D.C., 1974.

suitable place to eat, but eating alone may be equally serious. Finding agreeable companions may provide as much of a challenge as finding good inexpensive food.

Eating in Institutions

The multitude of problems facing a food service department in an institution for the elderly is complicated by the factor of food acceptance. Obviously, food is wasted unless eaten. This acceptance of food varies widely, but the problem is lessened when the food is prepared and served attractively. Attention must be given whenever possible to ethnic food preferences.

In those institutions where inmates can be up and about, they may eat in dining rooms. When mealtime is considered as a social hour, eating problems usually diminish. Also, when inmates participate in the planning of menus and service, the morale tends to be higher. In some homes, even if patients do not care for food, they are encouraged to sit at the table and socialize. While they sit there, their appetites often return and they are willing to eat.

Skipping breakfasts may be a problem in institutions. Many older persons claim that they cannot sleep at night and wish to sleep late in the morning rather than eat breakfast. This practice should be discouraged if possible because it is difficult to get in the day's dietary requirements when a meal is skipped. To help meet this situation, some institutions allow a 1-hour period for breakfast.

Patients who are bedfast may present another problem, especially if their interest in food is low. Small, frequent meals, attractively served, may be a stimulus.

Henriksen and Cate[33] compared the nutrient content of food with the amount of food actually consumed by patients in a nursing home. Results indicated the highest levels of actual consumption of iron and vitamin A while lowest intake levels occurred with kcalories, calcium, ascorbic acid, and riboflavin.

Joering[34] investigated the nutrient contribution of a senior center meal. Findings indicated that the average daily nutrient intake was greater for all nutrients when the center-prepared meal was included. The percentage of recommended daily allowances was adequate for protein, iron, vitamin A, and niacin; calcium and thiamin were met at approximately the 90 per cent level and riboflavin at approximately the 97 per cent level. Calculations were based on the average nutritive intake of all subjects in all centers surveyed.

---

[33] Betty Henriksen and Helen D. Cate, "Nutrient Content of Food Served vs. Food Eaten in Nursing Homes," *Journal of the American Dietetic Association*, Vol. 59, No. 2 (August 1971), pp. 126–129.

[34] Joering, op. cit., p. 131.

SELECTED REFERENCES

Brogdon, Helen G., and Betty B. Alford, "Food Preferences in Relation to Dietary Intake and Adequacy in a Nursing Home Population," *Gerontologist*, Vol. 13, No. 3 (Autumn 1973), pp. 355–357.

de Beauvoir, Simone, *The Coming of Age*, G. P. Putnam's Sons, New York, 1972.

Exton-Smith, A. N., "Nutritional Needs of the Elderly," in Dorothy Hollingsworth and Margaret Russell, *Nutritional Problems in a Changing World*, John Wiley & Sons, Inc., New York, 1973.

Fitch, William C., and Jack Ossofsky, *The Golden Years, a Tarnished Myth*, The Project FIND, National Council on the Aging, Washington, D.C., 1970.

Knauer, Virginia, "Portable Meals Contribute to Nutrition Education Efforts," *Journal of Nutrition Education*, Vol. 3, No. 2 (Fall 1971), pp. 59–61.

Mann, George V., "Relationship of Age to Nutrient Requirements," *American Journal of Clinical Nutrition*, Vol. 26, No. 10 (October 1973), pp. 1096–1097.

Montgomery, James E., "Magna Carta of the Aged," *Journal of Home Economics*, Vol. 65, No. 4 (April 1973), pp. 6–13.

Pelcovits, Jeanette, "Nutrition for Older Americans," *Journal of the American Dietetic Association*, Vol. 58, No. 1 (January 1971), pp. 17–21.

———, "Nutrition to Meet the Human Needs of Older Americans," *Journal of the American Dietetic Association*, Vol. 60, No. 4 (April 1972), pp. 297–300.

Schlenker, E. D., J. S. Feurig, L. H. Stone, M. A. Ohlson, and O. Mickelsen, "Nutrition and Health of Older People," *American Journal of Clinical Nutrition*, Vol. 26, No. 10 (October 1973), pp. 1111–1119.

Sherman, Edith M., and Margaret B. Brittan, "Contemporary Food Gatherers —A Study of Food Shopping Habits of an Elderly Urban Population," *Gerontologist*, Vol. 13, No. 3, Part 1 (August 1973), pp. 358–364.

Sherwood, Sylvia, "Sociology of Food and Eating, Implications for Action for the Elderly," *American Journal of Clinical Nutrition*, Vol. 26, No. 10 (October 1973), pp. 1108–1110.

Simko, Margaret, and Karen Colitz, *Nutrition and Aging*, a Selected Annotated Bibliography, DHEW Publication No. (SRS) 73–20237, Administration on Aging, U.S. Department of Health, Education, and Welfare, Washington, D.C., 1973.

Todhunter, E. Neige, *Nutrition, Background Issues*, 1971 White House Conference on Aging, U.S. Government Printing Office, Washington, D.C., 1971.

Troll, Lillian E., "Eating and Aging," *Journal of the American Dietetics Association*, Vol. 59, No. 5 (November 1971), pp. 456–459.

Walker, Mary A., and Mary M. Hill, *Food Guide for Older Folks*, U.S. Department of Agriculture, Home and Garden Bulletin No. 17, U.S. Government Printing Office, Washington, D.C., 1972.

Watkin, Donald M., "The Aged," in Jean Mayer (ed.), *U.S. Nutrition Policies in the Seventies*, W. H. Freeman and Company, San Francisco, 1973, Chapter 6.

———, "Nutrition and Aging in Technically Underdeveloped Societies," in Miloslav Rechcigl, Jr. (ed.), *Food, Nutrition and Health*, Vol. 16, S. Karger, Basel, 1973, pp. 46–58.

———, "Nutrition for the Aging and the Aged," in Robert S. Goodhart and Maurice E. Shils (eds.), *Modern Nutrition in Health and Disease*, Lea & Febiger, Philadelphia, 1973, Chapter 25.

Wells, Charles E., "Nutrition Programs Under the Older Americans Act," *American Journal of Clinical Nutrition*, Vol. 26, No. 10 (October 1973), pp. 1127–1132.

27

Nutrition in Pregnancy and Lactation

In the records of history, note has been made of the diets of pregnant women. Some foods were regarded as essential and others were restricted or prohibited.[1] Among primitive tribes, for example, pregnant Kikuyu women had a virtual monopoly on green leaves thereby enhancing the vitamin and iron content of their diets. During the Chou dynasty (1155 B.C.) pregnant women were warned about the quantity of meat consumed. Gifts of pigs feet boiled in mild acid until the bones were soft were brought to pregnant Chinese women as a delicacy but also contributed to their calcium and phosphorus intake.

Preliminary Considerations

Maternal nutrition should be considered as making a contribution to the well-being of the mother and child in the frame of reference that pregnancy is a normal and not a patho-

logical state of health. Hillman and Goodhart[2] indicate a number of reasons for the controversial, contradictory, and unfounded beliefs attached to maternal and fetal nutriture.

Factors such as parental age, birth rank, and birth interval have not been considered in some research and their impact is not well defined. The effects of changing food patterns, genetics, socioeconomic status, advances in food technology, dietary excesses, psychological stress, the use of drugs, smoking, and other factors make it difficult to untangle all these effects, for example, of malnutrition in contrast to other health factors and social problems. The availability of education to the pregnant woman and her interest in health matters are pertinent. Research has been stifled by ethical, moral, and legal limitations for the protection of the interests of the child and his parents, especially his mother. Although research has been performed on preg-

[1] Emma Seifrit, "Changes in Beliefs and Food Practices in Pregnancy," *Journal of the American Dietetic Association*, Vol. 39, No. 5 (November 1961), pp. 455–466.

[2] Robert W. Hillman and Robert S. Goodhart, "Nutrition in Pregnancy," in Robert S. Goodhart and Maurice E. Shils (eds.), *Modern Nutrition in Health and Disease*, Lea & Febiger, Philadelphia, 1973, Chap. 23.

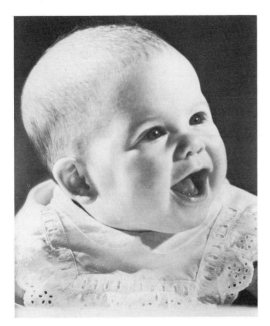

FIGURE 27–1. *A nutritious prenatal diet may be reflected in a happy, healthy baby.* (*Gerber Products Company*)

nant animals, the results cannot always be readily extrapolated to humans.

Importance of Nutrition in Preconception Stage

Nutrition is important not only at the onset and throughout pregnancy but long before conception. In fact, the reproductive capacity itself may reflect the adequacy of an individual's diet. Any dietary deficiency affects fertility because the whole organism is involved. All girls concerned with producing vigorous and healthy babies should practice good nutrition throughout their lives.

Studies made at Harvard University[3] concluded that a mother's nutritional state at the onset of pregnancy is an important factor in determining the condition of the infant at birth. This fact highlights the great need for education so that women will understand the

importance of good nutrition for a successful pregnancy.

A lifetime diet exerts more influence on the course of pregnancy than the diet consumed during gestation. The preconceptual nutritional status of future mothers, whether before or between pregnancies, is vitally important to mother and child, according to McGanity.[4] The food habits and beliefs of the pregnant woman's mother and even her grandmother can be strong influences on the preconceptual dietary and the dietary during pregnancy. Hughes[5] contends that all evidences of dietary deficiencies should be eliminated before onset of pregnancy.

Nutrition During Pregnancy

Research

Research has contributed information through records of large populations that varied in socioeconomic and health status, as well as other factors. Studies in England during World War II are noteworthy. The controlled and improved diet of the period plus special priority had a positive effect on pregnant women in spite of other adversities. Data from hospital and clinic records of supervised patients were another source of information. The classic Burke study[6] used pregnant women mostly of a middle-income group. A record was made of their diet, they were given periodic examinations, and the entire course of each pregnancy was carefully observed. The baby was thoroughly examined at birth, and reexamined periodically to 1 year of age.

The outcome of each pregnancy was classified as "good," "regular," or "poor." There was a striking difference among mothers on different kinds of diet. The positive relation between the mother's diet and the outcome of pregnancy was clearly demonstrated. The

[3] Bertha S. Burke, "Nutritional Studies During Pregnancy," *American Journal of Obstetrics and Gynecology,* Vol. 46, No. 1 (January 1943), pp. 38–52.

[4] William J. McGanity, "Obstetric and Nutritional Problems," *Proceedings of the Western Hemisphere Congress, 1965,* American Medical Association, Chicago, 1966, pp. 199–200.

[5] E. C. Hughes, "Nutrition and Fetal Growth," *Journal of the American Dietetic Association,* Vol. 31, No. 3 (September 1955), p. 783.

[6] Burke et al., op. cit., pp. 38–52.

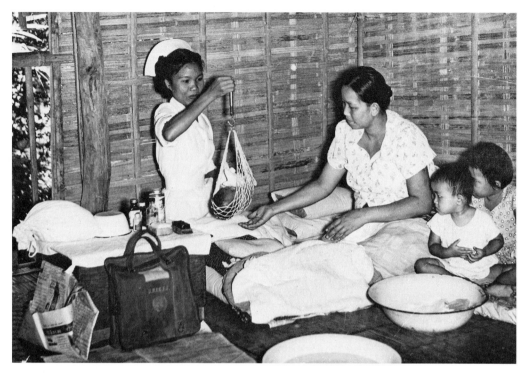

FIGURE 27–2. *Maternal nutrition is one factor in birth weight of an infant.* (UNICEF)

general condition, both mental and physical, of mothers who had a good diet, was found to be superior, and their babies were also in excellent condition. For mothers who were on a poor diet, the incidence of complications in pregnancies, such as miscarriage, premature birth, stillbirth, toxemia, and infections in the mother, was greatly increased. In addition, the condition of the babies was very poor.

In this study it was found that there was considerable difference in the birth weight and birth length of infants in the different dietary categories, those in the excellent category being heavier and longer. This finding leads to the conclusion that the fetus suffers considerably more than was originally believed when the mother is malnourished. Mothers who had excellent or good diets were more likely to be able to nurse their babies and provide a better quality of mother's milk.

Controlled studies of patients receiving prescribed diets, supplements, or both were another source of research into the role of nutrition in pregnancy. Most of these studies revealed a favorable influence of good nutrition. In some studies less favorable results were indicated especially when there was excessive intake of the recommended dietary allowances or of vitamin supplementation. Many researchers believe that all the variables have not been included. This may require improved research techniques to provide solid answers to many vexing questions.[7]

Maternal nutrition has been indicated as one factor in low birth weight, according to McGanity.[8] Infant birth weight appears to be correlated more closely with maternal weight and height at the time of conception than with weight gain of the woman in pregnancy. Low birth weight does not imply that only

[7] Committee on Maternal Nutrition, Food and Nutrition Board, *Maternal Nutrition and the Course of Pregnancy*, National Academy of Sciences—National Research Council, Washington, D.C., 1970, pp. 3–7.

[8] McGanity, op. cit., pp. 200–201.

large babies are desirable. Some investigators have found that babies with birth weights above average often fare as badly as those of low birth weight. More valid indexes may be birth length and duration of gestation, but birth weight is more simply determined so its adoption as an index has been encouraged. Criteria need to be developed.

The weight gain of a pregnant woman has been reexamined. Adequate kcalories, particularly for the woman of low socioeconomic status, is advocated by some authorities. Women of a more affluent status are warned about placing themselves on a reducing diet while pregnant. Jacobson[9] recommends a pregnancy weight gain of 25 to 30 pounds with particular attention to dietary needs and intakes. This weight gain is not a license to indulge. Extenuating circumstances may have to be considered in the weight gain of some pregnant women.

Bruch[10] indicates that the condition and attitude of the mother will influence the condition of the offspring. For that reason pregnant women are urged to be in optimal condition both mentally and physically to have well-developed babies.

Jelliffe[11] also emphasizes that there is a vital interdependence between the health of the mother, fetus, and infant. An inadequate diet for women, especially during pregnancy and lactation, is not only directly important for the fetus but can lead to cumulative nutritive deprivation with each succeeding pregnancy, which, in turn, may lead to increased maternal and perinatal mortality and disease.

There continues to be considerable conjecture about the exact mechanism in which maternal nutritional deprivation influences fetal growth, but there seems little doubt that

if the maternal organism is severely malnourished the outcome of the pregnancy will be less than satisfactory.[12] However, intrauterine growth failure may be influenced by other factors, such as socioeconomic status, some drugs, use of tobacco, and placental or fetal abnormalities.[13] Cellular growth patterns vary among organs. Dietary restriction is most harmful if coincidental with the most rapid cell growth. The need is crucial for more research in these areas.

The relationship of malnutrition to poor outcomes of pregnancy needs greater understanding, according to Jacobson and Mills.[14] The health needs of pregnant and lactating women will not be met until action takes place, such as a national nutrition policy for maternal health. These needs cannot be considered in isolation without recognition of the vicious cycle that malnourished mothers produce malnourished children who in turn become malnourished mothers. Close interrelationships exist between mother, family, and the total society.

Nourishment of the Fetus

Nutrition of the fetus is facilitated through the placenta. Its primary function is to store and to transport nutrients from the mother to the fetus and to make provision for the metabolic end products of the fetus to be returned to the mother's bloodstream. Little is known about how these functions are carried out. Most of the nitrogen reaches the fetus in the form of amino acids. Concentration of calcium and phosphorus are higher in fetal than in maternal blood. Carbohydrate is delivered in the form of glucose from which the fetus derives energy and makes its own glycogen and fat. There is some evidence that the maternal level of glucose influences fetal

[9] Howard N. Jacobson, "Nutrition and Pregnancy," *Journal of the American Dietetic Association,* Vol. 60, No. 1 (January 1972), p. 27.

[10] Comments of Hilde Bruch in a talk at the Annual Meeting of the American Dietetic Association on October 25, 1973, reviewed in the *Journal of the American Dietetic Association,* Vol. 64, No. 1 (January 1974), p. 98.

[11] D. B. Jelliffe, "Nutrition in Early Childhood," in Miloslav Rechcigl, Jr. (ed.), *Food, Nutrition and Health,* Vol. 16, S. Karger, Basel, 1973, p. 2.

[12] "Maternal Dietary Supplementation and Infant Birth Weight," *Nutrition Reviews,* Vol. 31, No. 2 (February 1973), p. 47.

[13] "Maternal Dietary Supplementation and Infant Birth Weight," *Nutrition Reviews,* Vol. 32, No. 6 (June 1973), p. 179.

[14] Howard N. Jacobson and Susan H. Mills, "Pregnant and Lactating Women," in Jean Mayer (ed.), *U.S. Nutrition Policies in the Seventies,* W. H. Freeman, San Francisco, 1973, Chap. 2.

growth. As in other areas, more research is needed. There are inherent difficulties in conducting research on pregnant women.[15]

There is a need for additional research in defining the causes and consequences of malnutrition in the fetus. The study of cell growth is challenging. There are three recognizable stages of growth. In the first, growth occurs predominantly by an increase in the number of cells, and second, by an increase in the number and size of the cells; finally, there is an emphasis on the increase in size of cell but hardly any in number. It has already been determined that the transition from one stage of growth to the next varies with the species of animal and with specific organs. This knowledge will provide the means for determining when nutritional deficiencies may be most critical.

Nutrients Needed During Pregnancy

The quality of the infant's skeleton and teeth and his condition in general are influenced considerably by the pregnant woman's diet. All the recommended dietary allowances (Table 27–1) of the National Research Council for pregnancy assume that her nutritional state is good at the onset of pregnancy. In other words, no allowances are made for any existing dietary deficiencies. It must also be borne in mind that these recommendations are for the average woman and that adjustments may have to be made. A physician can help to make these adjustments.

It is very important for a woman to be of somewhat normal weight at the time of conception. If she is underweight or overweight, she becomes much more of an obstetrical risk. It is extremely difficult to gain or to lose extra weight during pregnancy.

The energy requirement of pregnant women will vary considerably, depending on body weight, activity, and other factors. It is wise for the woman and her doctor to make some estimate of her weight gain during this period

[15] Working Group, "Relation of Nutrition to Fetal Growth and Development," in Committee on Maternal Nutrition, Food and Nutrition Board, *Maternal Nutrition and the Course of Pregnancy*, National Academy of Sciences—National Research Council, Washington, D.C., 1970, Chap. 5.

TABLE 27–1

Recommended Daily Dietary Allowances for Pregnancy and Lactation, Revised 1974

Designed for the maintenance of good nutrition of practically all healthy people in the United States

	PREG-NANCY	LACTA-TION
Kcalories	+300	+500
Protein, g	+30	+20
Fat-soluble vitamins		
Vitamin A activity, IU	5000	6000
Vitamin D, IU	400	400
Vitamin E activity, IU	15	15
Water-soluble vitamins		
Ascorbic acid, mg	60	80
Folacin, μg	800	600
Niacin, mg	+2	+4
Riboflavin, mg	+0.3	+0.5
Thiamin, mg	+0.3	+0.3
Vitamin B_6, mg	2.5	2.5
Vitamin B_{12}, μg	4.0	4.0
Minerals		
Calcium, mg	1200	1200
Phosphorus, mg	1200	1200
Iodine, μg	125	150
Iron, mg	18+	18
Magnesium, mg	450	450
Zinc, mg	20	25

SOURCE: Food and Nutrition Board, *Recommended Dietary Allowances*, 8th ed., National Academy of Sciences—National Research Council, Washington, D.C., 1974.

and the times when this gain will take place.

When the energy intake is adequate, protein is spared and there is less likelihood of a protein deficiency. Little argument can be advanced about whether the energy requirement should come from fats or carbohydrates. Both are needed. Concentrated carbohydrates, of course, usually carry few extra nutrients, and fats are needed for the source of certain fat-soluble vitamins and essential fatty acids. Since fats contain more kcalories than carbohydrates, a pregnant woman who is concerned about her weight may have to watch the amount and kind of fat she is eating.

Protein is needed for building tissues of the baby and for the enlargement of maternal tissues. The requirements are influenced by the quality of the protein, the total energy intake, and the protein status of the woman as she entered pregnancy. There should be an emphasis on foods of animal origin and consequently of high-quality proteins, such as meat, poultry, milk, eggs, cheese, and fish. These foods supply the essential amino acids in high concentration. The protein quality of cereal grains and vegetables is not as favorable, but they do supplement the total proteins of the diet and cannot be ignored. According to the recommended dietary allowances, the pregnant woman should have 30 additional g of protein daily.

Of all the nutrients, calcium is particularly important for normal development of the child, for the formation of his bones and teeth, and for the health of both the child and the mother. Extreme cases of calcium deficiency may cause osteomalacia and deformity in childbearing women. Yet calcium is the nutrient commonly lacking in the diet of pregnant women, possibly because it is not distributed widely in foods. Milk and milk products are the chief source, and when they are neglected in the diet, a calcium deficiency will result.

For the proper utilization of calcium, vitamin D is required. Phosphorus and magnesium are also needed.

The amount of iron found in the body of the infant at birth depends materially on maternal intake during pregnancy. Since his diet for the first few months after birth is inclined to be low in iron, it is extremely important that the baby be well provided for iron storage during fetal growth. Otherwise there is a risk of an iron deficiency after birth.

The need for iron for the fetus and the mother reaches a peak during the last 16 to 20 weeks of gestation. In the mother, there is a lag in return to normal hemoglobin concentration for many weeks after the delivery of her baby. This lag indicates the large amount of iron required for pregnancy and the serious consequences if a woman has frequent pregnancies because the possibility of anemia is even greater. According to Cook and Finch,[16] a large segment of the female population lacks adequate iron stores—so essential if the needs of pregnancy are to be met. It has been suggested that a diet nutritionally adequate in all other respects may be inadequate in iron and some form of fortification of this mineral in the diet may be a necessary step. This nutrient is often the most serious lack in the diet of the pregnant woman.

The recommended daily dietary allowance advises 18+ mg of iron daily. Some pregnant women encounter difficulty in utilizing iron, and in these special cases it may be necessary to increase this amount. Again, this should be on the advice of a physician. It is wise for the pregnant woman to avoid anemia, which results from a shortage of iron, for it will cause fatigue and other undesirable symptoms.

Because of the stress of pregnancy, the need for iodine is increased. The allowance is increased to 125 μg. If a mother develops goiter, the possibility is greater that her child will be equally affected. The adolescent mother may be especially susceptible if her storage of iodine is limited.

Vitamins need to be increased during the period of pregnancy. Each one has a unique contribution to make. The vitamin A allowance is increased to 5000 IU. One third of this vitamin A allowance should come from animal sources and two thirds may come from carotene, which is found in fruits and vegetables.

The thiamin allowance is increased 0.3 mg. It is wise to remember that this allowance is related to the energy allowance and should be adjusted accordingly. Niacin is increased 2 mg. Niacin, of course, is closely associated with the amino acid tryptophan, so it is important that the protein allowance be adequately met. Ascorbic acid is increased to 60 mg. This vitamin is frequently lacking in the diet during pregnancy, so it is particularly important that a deficiency does not occur. The

---

[16] J. D. Cook and Clement A. Finch, "Human Iron Requirements," *Proceedings of the Western Hemisphere Nutrition Congress II—1968*, American Medical Association, Chicago, 1969, pp. 174–176.

allowance for riboflavin is increased 0.3 mg. Vitamin D allowance is 400 IU.

Vitamin E is increased to 15 IU.; folacin is doubled to 800 µg because it is important to normal fetal growth and in the prevention of anemia; vitamin B₆ is raised to 2.5 mg; and vitamin B₁₂ is increased to 4 µg to provide adequate amounts for both mother and fetus.

Adolescent Pregnancy

One of every ten girls becomes a mother while still of school age, according to Howard.[17] Sexual maturation occurs earlier at 12½ to 13 years of age and the increasing number of girls entering childbearing years presents a challenge. These young mothers come from a wide variety of backgrounds. Studies indicate that they cannot be differentiated by psychological testing or other means from nonpregnant students.

Pregnant adolescents under 17 years of age cannot be considered psychologically, physically, or socially mature. Growth continues under the age of 17 years so greater nutritional requirements are necessary in relation to body size than for an adult woman. The additional demands of pregnancy may interfere with growth and development and increase the risk in pregnancy. The psychological impact of pregnancy on the adolescent girl and her child may be even more detrimental than the biological risks. The fact that adolescents are the least well nourished members of a family add other problems.[18]

A disportionately large number of infants of low birth weight are born to these young mothers. Death rates for both white and non-white infants born to mothers under 15 years of age are much higher than those born to older mothers. Not only are prematurity rates higher but adolescent pregnancies are more likely to be complicated by toxemia, anemia, and difficulties in labor and delivery. Jacobson[19] notes a growing awareness of the kinds of health and nutrition problems and of the needs of the pregnant school girl, as well as a growing concern for the dimensions of the problem and the implications for society.

Studies of nutritional adequacy of the diets of pregnant and nonpregnant girls have been made. Seiler and Fox[20] discovered that diet quality, nutrition knowledge, and family relations were interrelated among nonpregnant girls but not pregnant adolescents. Nonpregnant girls were better adjusted psychologically. Pregnant girls scored higher in only one category—adjustment to reality. Nutritionwise, iron and vitamin A were least adequately supplied by foods eaten by 50 per cent or more of both pregnant and nonpregnant girls. Nonpregnant adolescents showed higher values for energy, calcium, and B vitamins. The pregnant group received more iron, vitamin A, and ascorbic acid.

In a study at the University of Nebraska Medical Center reported by Mulcahy[21] the findings indicated that diets without supplements of pregnant girls, 15 years and younger, fell short in all respects of nutritional adequacy, except protein. Van de Mark and Wright[22] studied the dietary intake and blood findings of pregnant and nonpregnant adolescents. Results indicated that the diet and blood findings fell in a range below accepted standards for both groups. Folic acid intakes for pregnant girls were about one third less than recommended levels. A deficiency of

[17] Marion Howard, "Teen-Age Parents," *Today's Education*, Vol. 62, No. 1 (February 1973), pp. 39–78.

[18] Committee on Maternal Nutrition, Food and Nutrition Board, "Relation of Nutrition to Pregnancy in Adolescence," in *Maternal Nutrition and the Course of Pregnancy*, National Academy of Sciences—National Research Council, Washington, D.C., 1970, Chap. 6.

[19] Howard N. Jacobson, "Pregnancy in School Age Girls," *Food and Nutrition News*, Vol. 41, No. 8 (May 1970), pp. 1–4.

[20] Jo Ann Seiler and Hazel M. Fox, "Adolescent Pregnancy: Association of Dietary and Obstetric Factors," *Home Economics Research Journal*, Vol. 1, No. 3 (March 1973), pp. 188–194.

[21] Mary Jo Mulcahy, "Nutrition in a Maternity and Infant Care Project," *Journal of Nutrition Education*, Vol. 2, No. 3 (Winter 1971), pp. 99–101.

[22] Mildred S. Van de Mark and Audrey Clever Wright, "Hemoglobin and Folate Levels of Pregnant Teen-agers," *Journal of the American Dietetic Association*, Vol. 61, No. 5 (November 1972), pp. 511–515.

folic acid may be a far more common cause of nutritional megaloblastic anemia than is a deficiency of vitamin B_{12}. This condition may be especially serious during pregnancy when the folate requirement increases. Further research is needed on nutritional requirements in different stages of adolescent growth and development and the relation to pregnancy. Better methods of assessing the nutritional status of pregnant adolescents would be helpful. An exploration of educational possibilities for this age group is critical to help alleviate this serious problem.

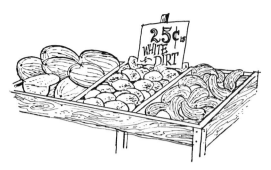

FIGURE 27–3. *White dirt (clay) may be purchased in some markets.*

Pica Practices

For centuries there have been records of pregnant women eating clay and starch. In recent years researchers have reported the continued existence of these unusual practices, particularly in Southern communities. When residents of the South move to the North, many of them retain this dietary habit. The motivation to eat these substances appears to be deep-seated and quite unyielding to change. According to Edwards and others,[23] eating these substances is not linked to weight control or to the influence of quacks. There does not seem to be any single motive. Some women are superstitious and believe that their babies will not be normal unless clay is eaten. Others believe that clay or starch produces feelings of relaxation, pleasure, and appetite stimulation, according to Edwards and others.[24] In some instances starch supplies kcalories in a diet that is low in energy value.

In a research study of Edwards and others involving clay- and starch-eating pregnant women and suitable controls, the results indicated that there may be an appetite stimulation due to pica because the control women consumed fewer kcalories. Protein, calcium, and iron were low, on the whole, in both

groups, but the clay eaters indicated mild anemia. In a study of their offspring, there were no differences in birth weight, length, head and chest size, or length of gestation. Infants born to control women, however, had a higher rating than the infants of mothers in the clay and cornstarch groups. Further study is needed to determine if iron and calcium are available from clay and if these substances do fulfill any physiological or psychological needs.

Gardner[25] noted in her study of the incidence of pica practices among female drug addicts that pica practices were not confined solely to the period of pregnancy; a number of subjects had been pica practitioners since childhood. Their mothers and grandmothers in some instances reflected similar pica practices.

Foods Needed During Pregnancy

The recommended dietary allowances must be translated into foods for the everyday diet.

One of the most important foods, milk, is necessary for adequate calcium as well as for other nutrients. Whole milk contains calcium, phosphorus, and magnesium in a favorable ratio for utilization. When calcium is taken in the form of concentrate, the minerals phosphorus and magnesium are not provided, and the body may suffer. Milk also contributes fat, high-quality proteins, and some of the other essential nutrients. Vitamin D milk will

[23] Cecile H. Edwards et al., "Clay and Cornstarch-Eating Women," *Journal of the American Dietetic Association,* Vol. 35, No. 8 (August 1959), pp. 810–815.

[24] Cecile H. Edwards et al., "Effect of Clay and Cornstarch Intake on Women and Their Infants," *Journal of the American Dietetic Association,* Vol. 44, No. 2 (February 1964), pp. 109–115.

[25] Jean Gardner, "The Incidence of Pica Practice Among Pregnant Female Drug Addicts," a research project in the author's class during summer 1972.

contribute a great deal toward the requirement for that vitamin. Milk may be used as a beverage, in custards or other milk puddings, in soups, in sauces, and in other ways. With a little ingenuity, it is very easy for a pregnant woman to include 3 or more cups of milk daily in her diet.

At least 2 quarts of liquid a day are necessary. These may take the form of soups, fruit juices, water, milk, and the like.

As protein is so important for a pregnant woman, it is well to include at least 6 oz of meat or fish daily. This does not mean that expensive meats are required. The nutritive value of meat does not vary according to the part of the carcass from which it is taken. Meats may be varied—lean pork, beef, veal, lamb, mutton, or poultry. Organ meats are generally inexpensive and very nutritious. Fish and seafood of all kinds provide a high-quality protein. A substitute for meat may be cheese like cottage cheese and cheddar cheese. One egg three or four times a week is recommended. Occasionally dried beans or peas may be substituted. Their iron and B vitamin contribution is invaluable. However, it is advisable to include generous amounts of milk, cheese, or other high-quality proteins with their use. The protein content of the diet is important.

There should be at least two or more servings of vegetables daily, with one of them raw. One serving should be a dark-green, leafy, or deep-yellow vegetable to provide an adequate amount of vitamin A. Vegetables may be used in salads and soups, served as accompaniments to the main dish, in casseroles, or in other ways.

At least two servings of fruit should be eaten daily, with an emphasis upon citrus fruits; otherwise it is very difficult to get an adequate amount of vitamin C. Citrus fruits such as orange or grapefruit may be served in the form of juice or as a fresh, frozen, or canned fruit. Other fruits, particularly fresh ones, contribute some ascorbic acid as well as other nutrients.

There should be four to five servings each day of cereal and bread products, either whole grain or enriched. Bread may be varied for the different meals. If hot breads, such as biscuits or muffins, or other types of bread

are included, the flour should be enriched. These types of bread often add considerable extra kcalories and so need to be watched, particularly if ingredients such as nuts are added. Breakfast cereals may be either hot or cold. A great variety is available; hence they need not become a monotonous item of the diet.

Some butter or margarine should be included in the diet each day. This fat might be used on bread, to flavor vegetables, or in other ways.

Other foods may be added to the diet to meet the energy requirement. Burke, however, admonishes the pregnant woman that it takes approximately 2000 kcalories of very carefully selected foods to meet this increased need for nutrients other than kcalories. This may mean that the choice of foods during this period is not as free as at other times because highly nutritious foods must be emphasized. It may be necessary to use iodized salt. In addition, the pregnant woman needs to watch her weight, so she will have to plan accordingly.

Meal Planning for a Pregnant Woman's Diet

A pregnant woman should not feel that she is on a special diet. Her food should be much like that of the rest of the family. In fact, her family may profit from improved nutrition during this period. The emphasis should be on simply prepared, wholesome food served attractively so that eating will be a pleasure. Mealtime should be enjoyable because the mental health of a pregnant woman is as important as her physical health. The father can help by eating wholesome food with enjoyment.

Furthermore, the pregnant woman should arrange her marketing and meal preparation carefully so that she has the extra time needed to make plans for the new baby.

The Daily Food Guide can serve as a blueprint for planning meals. Adequate amounts of the four food groups should be represented in the daily diet. (See Chapter 29 for suggestions about planning meals.)

For the woman who needs to watch her weight, such foods as mayonnaise, gravy, fat meats, doughnuts, pies, cakes, pastries, candies, soft drinks, nuts, popcorn, and alcoholic

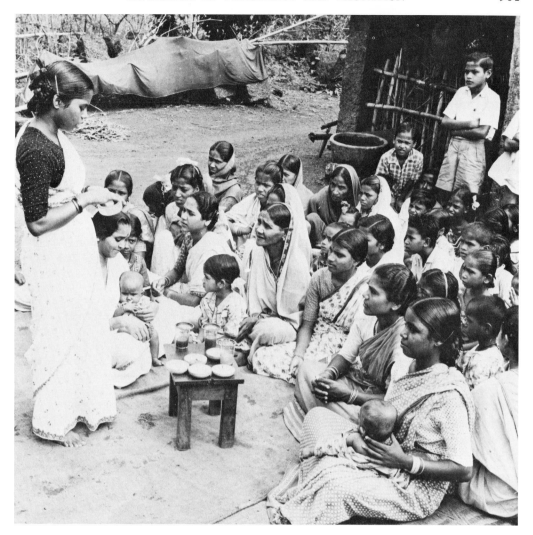

FIGURE 27–4. *A young Indian home economist teaches mothers how to improve their own and their children's diets.* (UNICEF Photo by Jack Ling)

beverages may need to be eliminated or reduced. Some pregnant women have increased appetites, and greater emphasis may have to be placed on nutritious low-calorie foods.

If a woman needs to gain weight, extra butter, bread, and other concentrated foods may be added, or jam or preserves may be added to the breakfast menu. The main meal may be eaten at noon instead of at night. Instead of having only one in-between feeding, she may like to have several during the day and reduce the amount of food in the other three meals accordingly. At all. times, it is necessary to bear in mind which foods are absolutely essential to have in the diet and which ones are optional.

Pregnant women should guard against any faddish or fallacious ideas about food in connection with pregnancy. Most of these ideas are old wives' tales and do not have any scientific merit. The ungrounded theories that certain foods will mark a baby or that milk should be eliminated from the diet are ridiculous and should be ignored. Some women indulge themselves in certain food cravings. If such a craving does occur, it is still important that the diet contain all essential nutrients. Most of this craving is of a psychological basis.

Undernutrition

Martin[26] states that maternal malnutrition, in addition to causing increased infant mortality, results in significantly increased intellectual deficit and learning problems. Ten per cent of pregnancies in the United States result in undergrown children.

Nutrition During Lactation

Nutritive Needs

According to the recommended allowances, the requirements of the lactating mother are the highest of any period in a woman's life. The allowances, however, must be adjusted to the needs of the particular individual. See Table 27–1 for the recommended daily dietary allowances for nutrients for lactation.

Importance of Food During Lactation

The health and welfare of a baby continue to depend on his mother's health if she nurses him. The quality and amount of the mother's food must be of such a nature as to provide not only her own needs, but also those of a fast-growing infant. Authorities tell us that no other food is equal to that of human milk for child nutrition. If a mother has maintained adequate nutrition during pregnancy, she should have little difficulty in nursing her baby.

The mother needs to include in her diet 1 quart of milk; adequate servings of dark-green, deep-yellow, and leafy vegetables; citrus fruits; whole-grain cereals and breads; adequate proteins in the form of meat, milk, eggs, and fish; and at least 1 tablespoon of margarine or butter. Frequent use of liver and other organ meats is highly recommended. Regular use of iodized salt is also advocated.

These diets may not meet the recommended dietary allowances for kcalories. Kcalories may be obtained easily from additional amounts of the foods listed in the table or from other foods that appeal to the individual.

Psychological Aspects of Lactation

In studies of breast feeding, success appeared to be closely correlated to a mother's attitudes toward breast feeding. Mothers with positive attitudes gave more milk and were more successful than mothers with negative feelings. Feelings of aversion toward breast feeding had a similar derogatory effect. Maternal interest and attitude fostered desirable breast feeding because there was a greater concern about the welfare of the infant, according to the researchers. The success or failure of previous breast-feeding experience, as well as labor experiences, had a strong impact on a mother's interest in breast feeding as well as aptitude for it. Women who breast feed also seem to be calm, more independent, and more

---

[26] Harold P. Martin in a speech at the annual meeting of the American Dietetic Association on October 25, 1973, in Denver, Colo., reviewed in *Journal of the American Dietetic Association,* Vol. 64, No. 1 (January 1974), p. 96, 98.

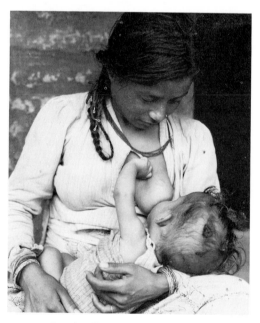

FIGURE 27–5. *Positive psychological benefits for mother and infant result from successful breast feeding. (UNICEF Photo by Jack Ling)*

affectionate. The behavior of the baby is an important consideration. If the baby has difficulty in sucking, this may prove to be discouraging to the mother.

Importance of Good Health Habits to Successful Lactation

Although nutrition is a critical factor in the well-being of a lactating mother, other health habits are also important. She obviously needs sufficient rest, but sometimes the new responsibilities of motherhood make it difficult for her to find the time. However, the mother, the baby, and the family will generally suffer if a mother does not have adequate sleep and rest periods during the day. In addition, it is important to have enough relaxation. This may be some time away from the baby, taking walks in the fresh air, or planning for other interests which do not deal directly with the baby. It is also wise for a mother to remember that other members of the family demand consideration and that all her attention cannot be centered on the young infant. This involves careful planning, but dividends will certainly be forthcoming when a mother gives first concern to her health.

Nutrition during pregnancy and lactation demands even more attention than usual because not only is the mother's health involved but also that of her child.

SELECTED REFERENCES

Bartholomew, Mary Jo, and Frances E. Poston, "Effect of Food Taboos on Prenatal Nutrition," *Journal of Nutrition Education*, Vol. 2, No. 1 (Summer 1970), pp. 15–17.

Beal, Virginia A., "Nutritional Studies During Pregnancy. Changes in Intake of Calories, Carbohydrate, Fat, Protein, and Calcium," *Journal of the American Dietetic Association*, Vol. 58, No. 4 (April 1971), pp. 312–320.

———, "Nutritional Studies During Pregnancy, Dietary Intake, Maternal Weight Gain, and Size of Infant, II," *Journal of the American Dietetic Association*, Vol. 58, No. 4 (April 1971), pp. 321–326.

"Cellular Development of the Human Fetus and Maternal Poverty," *Nutrition Reviews*, Vol. 20, No. 11 (November 1971), pp. 243–244.

Chopra, Joginder G., R. Camacho, John Kevany, and A. M. Thomson, "Maternal Nutrition and Family Planning," *American Journal of Clinical Nutrition*, Vol. 23, No. 8 (August 1970), pp. 1043–1058.

Committee on Maternal Nutrition, Food and Nutrition Board, *Maternal Nutrition and the Course of Pregnancy*, National Academy of Sciences—National Research Council, Washington, D.C., 1970.

"Fetal Growth and Maternal Nutrition," *Nutrition Reviews*, Vol. 39, No. 10 (October 1972), pp. 226–229.

Harrill, Inez, Lucille Lynch, and Dolores Shipman, "Nutritive Value of Foods Selected During Pregnancy," *Journal of the American Dietetic Association*, Vol. 63, No. 2 (August 1973), pp. 164–167.

Hillman, Robert W., and Robert S. Goodhart, "Nutrition in Pregnancy," in Robert S. Goodhart and Maurice E. Shils (eds.), *Modern Nutrition in Health and Disease*, Lea & Febiger, Philadelphia, 1973, Chapter 23.

Jacobson, Howard N., "Nutrition and Pregnancy," *Journal of the American Dietetic Association*, Vol. 60, No. 1 (January 1972), pp. 26–29.

————, "Pregnancy in School Age Girls," *Food and Nutrition News*, Vol. 41, No. 8, Part 1 (May 1970), pp. 1, 4.

————, "Pregnant and Lactating Women," in Jean Mayer (ed.), *U.S. Nutrition Policies in the Seventies*, W. H. Freeman and Company, San Francisco, 1973, Chapter 2.

McGanity, William J., "Obstetric and Nutritional Problems," in *Proceedings of the Western Hemisphere Nutrition Congress*, 1965, American Medical Association, Chicago, 1966, pp. 199–200.

Oppel, Wallace C., and Anite B. Royston, "Teen-age Births: Some Social, Psychological, and Physical Sequelae," *American Journal of Public Health*, Vol. 61, No. 4 (April 1971), pp. 751–756.

Seifrit, Emma, "Changes in Beliefs and Food Practices in Pregnancy," *Journal of the American Dietetic Association*, Vol. 39, No. 5 (November 1961), pp. 455–466.

Shank, Robert E., "A Chink in Our Armour," *Nutrition Today*, Vol. 5, No. 2 (Summer 1970), pp. 2–11.

"Smoking, Pregnancy, and Development of Offspring," *Nutrition Reviews*, Vol. 31, No. 5 (May 1973), pp. 143–145.

Swallow, Kathleen A., Lydia W. Mussenden, Veronica A. Robinson, and Annemarie F. Crocetti, "Tools for Evaluation of Diets of Pregnant Women," *Journal of Nutrition Education*, Vol. 3, No. 1 (Summer 1971), pp. 34–35.

Thomson, A. M., and F. E. Hytten, "Nutrition During Pregnancy," in Miloslav Rechcigl, Jr. (ed.), *Food, Nutrition and Health*, Vol. 16, S. Karger, Basel, 1973, pp. 22–45.

Webb, Ryland E., John A. Ballweg, and William Fougere, "Child Spacing as a Component of Nutrition Education Programs," *Journal of Nutrition Education*, Vol. 4, No. 3 (Summer 1972), pp. 97–99.

Weigley, Emma Seifrit, "The Pregnant Adolescent," *Journal of the American Dietetic Association*, Vol. 66, No. 6 (June 1975), pp. 588–592.

28

Contributions
of Foods

A knowledge of the nutrients found in food groups will facilitate the selection of an optimal diet. Food composition tables are an important tool in realizing this objective. These tables are a significant milestone in the study of nutrition for they reflect man's search for nutritive values in foods, according to Watt.[1]

History of Food Composition Tables

The first food composition table in the United States was the U.S. Department of Agriculture Experiment Station Bulletin No. 28, *Chemical Composition of American Food Materials*, compiled by W. O. Atwater and co-workers in 1896. Data about protein, fat, carbohydrate, ash, water, and refuse were listed in percentages and evaluated as maximum, minimum, or average. This bulletin was revised in 1899 and 1906. To enlarge upon these data, three specialized circulars, *Composition of Beef*, *Proximate Composition of Fresh Fruits*, and *Proximate Composition of Fresh Vegetables*, were issued from 1926 to 1931.

In 1940, Circular 549, *Proximate Composition of American Food Materials*, was published. The data from the three specialized publications, plus revised data from other food groups, were included. Active concern about minerals and vitamins led to the publication of Miscellaneous Publication 572, *Tables of Food Composition in Terms of Eleven Nutrients*, issued in 1945. The information was still limited, for only 275 food items were listed, mostly in raw or unprepared form. Few canned foods or ready-to-eat foods were included.

An enlarged and more comprehensive table, Agriculture Handbook No. 8, *Composition of Foods—Raw, Processed, Prepared*, was issued in 1950. Items numbered 751 and for the first time included an analysis of some frozen foods. A revision of this bulletin was published in 1963 and included 2,483 food items. Data are provided about kcalories, water, protein, fat, total carbohydrate, fiber, and ash; vitamins—thiamin, riboflavin, niacin, ascorbic acid, and vitamin A; and minerals—calcium, phosphorus, iron, sodium, and potassium.

These tables are not static but are constantly evolving as new research produces ad-

---

[1] Bernice K. Watt, "Implications of Food Composition Tables," *Nutrition News*, Vol. 27, No. 2 (April 1964), pp. 1, 4.

ditional information. Nutrients are sometimes added in the main tables or in supplemental tables at other times when limited data are available. The most recent handbook has supplementary tables, for example, for the content of oleic, linoleic, and total saturated fatty acids in 422 foods, cholesterol in 35 foods, and magnesium in 444 foods.

Instead of a simple listing of foods that is often based on the analysis of a single sample, the latest tables have representative values that consider the diversity of geographical origin and other factors, states Watt. In addition to primary forms, which are always studied first, potatoes, for example, there are examples of products derived from the primary forms. Reports of food analyses are assembled and studied from scientific and technical literature, special reports and unpublished data from laboratories of government, industry, scientific organizations, and colleges and universities of the world. These, in turn, are evaluated for soundness and significance, according to Watt, and the data are interpreted in terms most suitable for the intended reader. Consequently, some of the figures cited in a food composition table may represent hundreds of analyses. The shift to greater use of prepared or partially prepared foods has compounded the omissions and incomplete data in tables of composition for manufactured products.[2]

Consideration must be given to such variations as season, geographic differences, effect of harvesting, handling, processing, packaging, storage, as well as home food-preparation practices and service, and other factors. These tables are indispensable to a long list of workers who deal with the many aspects of the improvement of the nutritional status of man, and also to the individual interested in his nutritional status.

One way to a better understanding of the nutritive values of foods is to discuss them from the standpoint of food groups. Authori-

ties have divided foods into groups in various ways. The shorter the list of categories, the less discriminating can be the analysis, but the easier it is to remember. The longer the list of categories, the easier it is to highlight specific values. For purposes of this discussion, foods will be divided into the following groups:

1. Milk and milk products, including cheese.
2. Vegetables and fruits, legumes, and nuts.
3. Cereals and breads.
4. Meat, fish, poultry, and eggs.
5. Miscellaneous foods; beverages, sugars, fats, and oils.

Each group will be discussed from the standpoint of the foods to be included in it, the major nutritive contributions of the entire group, a comparison of food values within the group, and the effect of storage, processing, and preservation.

Use of Food Composition Tables

Tables of food composition are valuable guides. This practical information cannot be regarded, however, as having high accuracy; the tables are dependable in the selection of foods that are excellent sources of specific nutrients and as indexes of the adequacy of an individual's diet. Certain factors will cause variations in nutrient content, such as season, variety, breed, number of analyses, methods of analyses, processing techniques, part of the food analyzed, storage, food preparation, and other factors.

The Nutrient Data Bank

The upsurge of interest in the nutritive values of foods and nutrition labeling, as regulated by the Food and Drug Administration, has stimulated the analysis of products of the food industry. To handle this wealth of data, a computerized Nutrient Data Bank (NDB) has been established in the U.S. Department of Agriculture (USDA), as described by Watt and co-workers, to serve as an international repository for data submitted by in-

---

[2] Bernice K. Watt, Susan E. Gerhardt, Elizabeth W. Murphy, and Ritva R. Butrum, "Food Composition Tables for the 70's," *Journal of American Dietetic Association*, Vol. 64, No. 3 (March 1974), pp. 257–261.

dustry, experiment stations, government contracts and grants, and from literature searches. Data on the nutrient values of foods, including beverages and ingredients will be brought together in a central place. All nutrients will be included—those for which amounts are recommended and many of those that are considered essential but for which there are no recommendations. The advantages of the NDB are that food composition information is handled on an increased scope, the input of data and related information is vastly accelerated, and there is allowance for computerized input and withdrawal of data and the classification and coding of food items.

The NDB has triggered a number of changes. Certain canned foods have been reanalyzed using newer survey methods. The nutritive values of new varieties of fruits and vegetables have replaced older varieties used in older data. New research on the nutritional analysis of poultry, legumes, and ethnic foods has been encouraged. Tables of amino acids,

fatty acids, and trace minerals in foods have been added to the NDB operations.

Milk and Milk Products

From the earliest days of civilization, milk has been used as an important food by man. It ranks first among most nutritionists, physicians, dietitians, nurses, scientists, and public health officials as the number one basic food group. Of the total food consumed by civilians, according to preliminary 1974 data, the following nutrients were furnished by dairy products, excluding butter: 11.1 per cent of the food energy; 22.5 per cent of the protein; 12.4 per cent of the fat; 6.6 per cent of the carbohydrate; 75.7 per cent of the calcium; 36.1 per cent of the phosphorus; 2.3 per cent of the iron; 21.6 per cent of the magnesium; 12.9 per cent of vitamin A value; 9.0 per cent of the thiamin; 41.0 per cent of the riboflavin; 1.6 per cent of the niacin; 10.2 per cent of the vitamin B_6; 20.5 per cent of the vitamin B_{12};

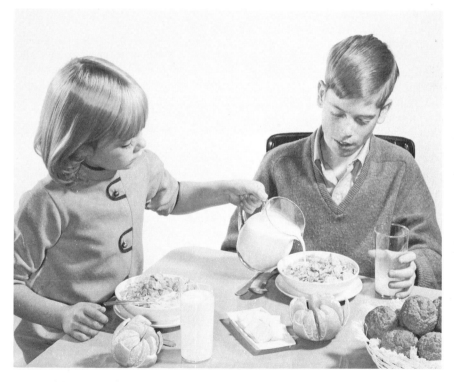

FIGURE 28–1. *Milk is the single most nutritious food in the diet at any age.* (*Cereal Institute, Inc.*)

and 4.0 per cent of the ascorbic acid.[3] (See Table 30–6.) Milk is often referred to as "Nature's most nearly perfect food."

Composition of Milk

Milk is an oil-in-water emulsion stabilized by complex phospholipids and proteins adsorbed on the surface of the fat globule. The calcium and phosphorus show highly significant relations to casein, one of the milk proteins. Both magnesium and citric acid tend to decrease as the casein content increases, and magnesium correlates inversely to calcium content. The lipids in milk contribute to palatability and satiety as well as to nutritive value. They are found in the fat globules and the adsorbed surrounding membrane, but small amounts are also found in the milk serum. Triglycerides of the fat globules form the bulk of the milk lipids—about 98 per cent of their total weight. Phospholipids constitute about 1 per cent of the total lipids and are complex substances containing phosphorus and nitrogen along with fatty acids. Small amounts of diglycerides, monoglycerides, free fatty acids, and sterols comprise the remainder of the fat content.

The proteins of milk include casein, lactalbumin, lactoglobulin, and a number of other simple proteins. The carbohydrates are lactose (the main carbohydrate) and traces of glucose, galactose, glucosamines, and others. The major minerals in milk are potassium, calcium, chlorine, phosphorus, sodium, magnesium, iron, and iodine.[4] Minor mineral elements in milk are aluminum, boron, bromine, chromium, cobalt, copper, selenium, manganese, molybdenum, nickel, and zinc. The fat-soluble vitamins present are vitamin A, vitamin D (in fortified milk), vitamin E, and vitamin K. The water-soluble vitamins are thiamin, riboflavin, niacin, pantothenic acid, vitamin B_6 (pyridoxine), folic acid, biotin, vitamin B_{12}, vitamin C, and choline.

---

[3] *National Food Situation*, Economic Research Service, U.S. Department of Agriculture, Washington, D.C., November 1974, p. 28.

[4] G. Icey Macy, J. H. Kelly, and R. E. Sloan, *The Composition of Milks*, Publication No. 254, National Academy of Sciences—National Research Council, Washington, D.C., 1963.

Major Nutritive Contributions of Milk and Milk Products

Milk forms an excellent base for planning an individual or family dietary. Most authorities agree that milk is the single most important food in the diet.

The greatest contribution of milk from the nutritive standpoint is calcium, which is very poorly distributed among other foods. It is therefore imperative that some kind of milk product be included in the diet every day to be assured of meeting the calcium requirement. When calcium needs are not met by food, the body must resort to drawing calcium from the bones of the body.

The amount of iron present in milk is low, but the quality is excellent and in a readily soluble form. Often the iron in milk is more completely absorbed than from foods that are richer in this mineral. The iodine content of milk is variable, depending on the feed and water of the cow. Milk is only a fair source of magnesium. It is high in phosphorus and low in copper.

The protein in milk is of an unusually high quality. Since it is particularly high in the amino acids lysine and tryptophan, it is noted for its ability to complement the protein value of breads and cereals, in which these amino acids are either lacking or very low. Milk protein is also very easily digested and does not putrefy as readily as some of the other animal proteins.

All known vitamins are present in milk in varying degree. Milk is best known for its contribution of vitamin A and riboflavin. It is especially rich in riboflavin. It also has a fair amount of thiamin. It is low in vitamin C owing to pasteurization or other processing and is especially low in niacin content. It is a good source of vitamin B_6 (pyridoxine), vitamin B_{12} (cobalamin), and folacin, but a fair source of vitamin E. The vitamin D content is low as milk is produced and will vary, depending on fortification.

The kcaloric value of milk cannot be ignored. Three glasses a day, for example, will contribute 500 kcalories to the diet. See Table 28–1 for nutrients in milk.

TABLE 28–1

Nutrients in Whole Milk

NUTRIENT	AMOUNT IN 1 QT (976 g)	AMOUNT IN ONE 8-oz GLASS (244 g)
Food energy, kcalories	640	160
Protein, g	36	9.0
Calcium, g	1.15	0.29
Phosphorus, mg	924	231
Iron, mg	0.4	0.1
Iodine, μg	348	87
Zinc, mg	4.46	1.12
Vitamin A, IU	1400	350
Thiamin, mg	0.29	0.27
Riboflavin, mg	1.64	0.41
Niacin, mg	0.08	0.02
Ascorbic acid, mg	8	2
Vitamin D, IU[a]	400	100
Vitamin B6, mg	0.4	0.1
Folic acid, μg	60	15
Vitamin B12	0.4	0.1

SOURCE: Bernice D. Watt and Annabel L. Merrill, *Composition of Foods*, Agriculture Handbook No. 8, Consumer and Food Economics Research Division, Agriculture Research Service, U.S. Department of Agriculture, Washington, D.C., 1963, p. 39; and "Composition and Nutritive Value of Dairy Foods," *Dairy Council Digest*, Vol. 42, No. 1 (January–February 1971), pp. 1–4.
[a] Applies only to vitamin D milk.

Comparison of Food Values Among Milk and Milk Products

Whole pasteurized milk, homogenized milk, reconstituted whole evaporated milk, and dried whole milk may be substituted for one another with the assurance that the food value is the same. Skimmed or nonfat pasteurized milk and reconstituted skimmed evaporated or dried skimmed milk are also equal to one another in food value and can be substituted in the diet with assurance. Skim milk has had most of the fat removed; thus it is lower in kcalories and also lower in vitamin A content unless fortified. Fortunately, the calcium content remains the same.[5]

[5] "Composition and Nutritive Value of Dairy Foods," *Dairy Council Digest*, Vol. 42, No. 1 (January–February 1971), pp. 1–4.

Whole pasteurized, skimmed pasteurized, whole evaporated, skimmed evaporated, or other types of milk may be fortified with about 400 USP units of vitamin D per quart.

Condensed milk is similar to evaporated milk but has sugar added before evaporation. Purchased condensed milk contains 42 per cent sugar. In the home it is generally used for the preparation of desserts, and commercially it is used by bakers in the preparation of candy, ice cream, and desserts. The very high percentage of sugar added dilutes other nutrients to such an extent that condensed milk cannot meet the requirements as adequately as whole milk does.

Yogurt is a cultured milk. Whole milk is used as a base and one or more types of bacteria are added. The action of this bacteria produces a consistency very much like that of baked custard. Yogurt has the nutritional value of whole milk unless the method of preparation alters it. In some cases, the nutrients are somewhat higher because part of the water has evaporated in the process. Yogurt may be made from skim milk. And sometimes jelly, jam, prune whip, or some kind of fruit is added. These additions alter the proportions of nutrients in a serving. The amount of calcium, for example, is reduced.

Cream is grouped according to the concentration of fat. Light or coffee cream contains 18 to 20 per cent fat, medium cream has 30 to 36 per cent fat, and heavy or whipping cream contains about 36 to 40 per cent fat. There is no difference in nutritive value between sweet and sour cream. Cultured sour cream is usually the 20 per cent cream to which a lactic acid culture has been added. Whipped cream is usually made from 40 per cent cream. Cream is commonly used in coffee, in desserts, and as whipped cream for a garnish. Half and half is generally used on cereals and on desserts. Seldom do we drink cream as we would milk. If we were to substitute cream for milk, we would not obtain as many nutrients nor as much of them (except fat and vitamin A).

Filled and imitation milks are in no sense a nutritional replacement for milk. Filled milk is a product made by combining fats and oils other than milk fat with milk solids,

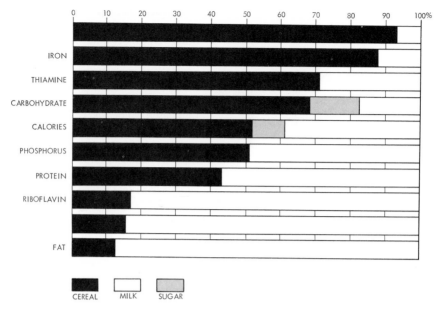

FIGURE 28–2. *Nutritional supplementation of cereal and milk. The 100 per cent equals total of nutrients common to both (plus sugar), and the bars indicate the percentage distribution of nutrients. (Cereal Institute, Inc.)*

TABLE 28–2

Comparison of Kcaloric and Fat Content of Dairy Products and Nondairy Products

PRODUCT	WEIGHT (g)	KCALORIES PER TABLESPOON	FAT PER TABLESPOON (g)
Heavy cream, whipped	8	27	3
Whipped topping			
From aerosol	4	10	1
From mix	4	10	1
Frozen	4	10	1
Coffee cream	15	30	1
Coffee lighteners			
Powdered (1 tsp)	2	10	1
Liquid (frozen)	15	20	2
Imitation sour cream (made with nonfat dry milk)	12	20	2

SOURCE: Consumer and Food Economics Research Division, Agricultural Research Service, *Nutritive Value of Foods*, Home and Garden Bulletin No. 72, U.S. Department of Agriculture, Washington, D.C., 1970, pp. 7–8.

which results in a product resembling milk. In one type, fluid skim milk may or may not be combined with additional skim milk solids and a vegetable fat to simulate milk. A second type basically contains water, nonfat dry milk, vegetable fat, and an additional source of protein, such as soy protein or sodium caseinate.

Because of a lack of information about their actual composition or nutrient analysis, it is not possible to make comprehensive comparisons with whole milk. The imitation milks may be low in calcium. One of the serious features of these milks is the great diversity in nutritive values; hence, they cannot be depended on as a group to supply certain nutrients. Imitation milks appear to fare less well than the filled milks. They do not compare favorably with whole milk in calcium and phosphorus content, total protein, and essential amino acids, and are practically devoid of riboflavin.

A number of nondairy products are on the market that are designed to resemble dairy products. Examples are whipped toppings for whipped cream, coffee lighteners, or imitation sour cream. These nondairy products are made with vegetable fats and cannot be recommended for low-fat or fat-restricted diets that call for polyunsaturated fats instead of saturated fats. Although the products do not contain butter or cream, they are usually made with saturated fats such as coconut oil or partially hydrogenated oils. Care must be exercised in the use of these products for individuals who are allergic to milk. Powdered whipped toppings mixes are made with whole milk and imitation sour cream may be made with nonfat dry milk. The labels of these products must be carefully checked for ingredients. Table 28–2 gives information about kcaloric and fat content of dairy products and nondairy products.

Cheeses

Cheeses vary in nutritive value according to the kind of milk used, the amount of moisture present, and the preparation of the cheese. In some cases, other foods are added to the cheese. The kind of milk used in the preparation of cheese depends on the part of the world where the cheese is made. In America, most of our cheese is made from cow's milk, whereas in other parts of the world sheep or goat's milk or the milk of other domestic animals is used. Either whole or skim milk is used in the preparation of cheese. Whole-milk cheese naturally has a higher fat content; therefore, the kcalories will be greater and the vitamin A content will be higher.

The amount of moisture in cheese will have an effect on its nutritive value. The harder the cheese, the higher the number of kcalories, and the greater the concentration of most other nutrients. Softer cheeses, such as cottage cheese, have considerable moisture.

Processed cheese consists of a blend of new and aged natural cheese that has been melted and pasteurized. In these cheeses there is no rind or waste, and the cheese melts smoothly without becoming stringy. The nutritive value of processed cheese depends on the kind of cheeses that it contains. The greatest variation among processed cheeses would be due to the

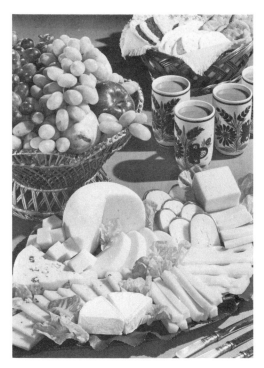

FIGURE 28–3. *Cheeses vary in nutritive value according to milk used, preparation, amount of moisture, and additions.* (National Dairy Council)

TABLE 28–3

Nutritive Value in Certain Types of Cheese

(1-oz or 30-g portions)

	KCALO-RIES	PRO-TEIN (g)	CAL-CIUM (mg)	IRON (mg)	VITA-MIN A (IU)	THIA-MIN (mg)
Camembert	85	5.0	30	0.1	290	0.01
Cheddar	113	7.1	206	0.3	400	0.01
Cottage	27	5.5	27	0.1	10	0.01
Cream	106	2.6	19	0.1	410	Trace
Limburger	97	6.0	167	0.2	360	0.02
Parmesan	112	10.2	329	0.1	300	0.01
Processed cheddar	105	6.6	191	0.3	370	Trace
Swiss	105	7.9	262	0.3	310	Trace

	RIBO-FLAVIN (mg)	NIACIN (mg)	ASCOR-BIC ACID (mg)	PHOS-PHORUS (mg)	MAG-NESIUM (mg)
Camembert	0.21	0.3	0	52	0.2
Cheddar	0.12	Trace	0	34	13
Cottage	0.09	Trace	0	43	—
Cream	0.06	Trace	0	23	—
Limburger	0.14	Trace	0	110	13
Parmesan	0.21	0.1	0	219	26
Processed cheddar	0.12	Trace	0	198	13
Swiss	0.11	Trace	0	158	12

SOURCE: Bernice K. Watt and Annabel L. Merrill, *Composition of Foods*, Agriculture Handbook No. 8, Consumer and Food Economics Research Division, Agricultural Research Service, U.S. Department of Agriculture, Washington, D.C., 1963.

amount of fat and moisture present. The higher the fat content, the higher the kcalories; also, the less moisture, the higher the kcalories.

There are many cheese foods or spreads available that contain added cream, nonfat dry milk solids, and other ingredients, such as bacon, olives, or pimentoes. These spreads have a soft texture and are high in moisture content. When nonfat dry milk solids are added, the nutritive value is increased accordingly. The addition of fat increases the kcalories.

An examination of Table 28–3 will give information about the nutritive value of various types of cheese. It is important that individuals do not assume that all cheeses have the same food value because there is considerable difference among them. However, as a group they do contribute materially to the protein and calcium content of the diet. And since most cheeses are quite concentrated, they also add to the kcaloric value of the diet.

In examining this table, it is interesting to note that cottage cheese and cream cheese, as well as Camembert, do not contribute as much calcium as the other cheeses, although many people eat large quantities of cottage cheese with the idea that it will compensate for the milk they did not drink. Cottage cheese is an excellent source of protein but is not so valuable for calcium. Parmesan cheese, because it is very dry, contains the most calcium for its weight. Since cheddar and Swiss cheese are used in large amounts by Americans, it is gratifying to note the large amount of nutrients that they contribute. By measure, 1 oz (30 g) of cheese is approximately 1 cubic inch.

Buttermilk varies according to the type of preparation. When butter is made from either sweet or sour cream, buttermilk is the by-product. The number of kcalories will vary, depending on the amount of fat remaining. If most of the fat is removed, the product is similar in nutritive value to skim milk.

Another type of buttermilk is cultured buttermilk. This is made by adding bacteria to either skim milk, partially skim milk, reconstituted soluble dry skim milk, fortified skim milk, or churned buttermilk. The nutritive value of these different types of buttermilk will vary again depending on the butterfat content. This generally ranges from 0.1 to 1.5 per cent. The type of buttermilk one drinks is important because the kcaloric and vitamin A content vary considerably.

Chocolate milk is made from whole milk that has a chocolate syrup added. Many mothers are unaware that a beverage called chocolate drink has skim milk as a base and consequently lacks vitamin A unless fortified. The chocolate syrup merely adds additional kcalories in the form of the chocolate and sugar.

Vegetables and Fruits, Legumes and Nuts

Historically, people living in humid temperate and tropical zones incorporated vegetables and fruits into their daily diet. They discovered that it was healthful to eat roots, stems, leaves, fruits, and seeds of certain indigenous plants, vines, shrubs, and trees. There is a greater diversity in nutritional composition of this food group than in any of the four main food groups. The nutritive contribution of fruits and vegetables depends on con-

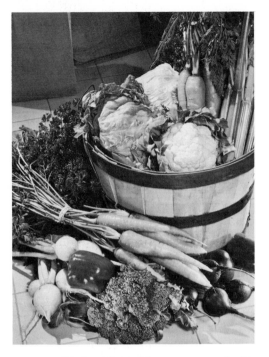

FIGURE 28–4. *Vegetables are a valuable source of minerals and vitamins.* (Western Growers Association)

sumer purchasing power, market availability, conservation of nutritive values in handling, processing, and preparing the food, food habits, and the variety of these foods consumed.

Major Nutritive Contributions of Vegetables and Fruits

One striking fact about the fruit–vegetable group is that the edible portion of fresh raw foods has low kcaloric values. Generally, a 100-g portion does not exceed 100 kcalories and often is only 50 kcalories. Foods highest in kcalories are the immature seeds, such as peas and lima beans, starchy roots, tubers such as potatoes and sweet potatoes, and fruits like bananas. Avocado is an exception (around 160 kcalories per 100-g portion), because of fat content, a nutrient found in small amounts in most of these foods.

This food group tends to be low in protein values, except for green leaf and immature seed products. Not only is the quantity higher in green leaves and immature seeds, but there is also an improved quality, because of superior amino acid composition. Generally, fruits and vegetables need to be supplemented with animal proteins that have a higher biological protein value.

Foods in this group are a rich source of certain minerals. The green-colored parts of plants, especially the leaves, are an excellent source of iron. Beet greens are an outstanding example. Other excellent sources of iron are dandelion greens, kale, chard, spinach, and broccoli. A ½-cup (100-g) serving of chopped broccoli will contribute approximately 40 per cent of the recommended daily allowance of iron for an 18-year-old girl or boy. Obviously, these green vegetables cannot be considered as the sole source for iron, but because of the quantities consumed they can make a very valuable contribution.

Vegetables are also a good source of calcium, ranking second to milk. This does not mean, however, that they are a rich source, but because of the amount included in the daily diet, they make an appreciable contribution. Vegetables that contain oxalic acid, like spinach, beet greens, chard, and lamb's quarters, present a problem because the acid interferes with the utilization of calcium in the body (see Chapter 16 for an explanation of oxalic acid). They are only a fair source of magnesium. Foods grown in iodine-rich soil make a contribution to the iodine requirement.

Although they are not rich sources, some fruits do contribute calcium and iron. Orange juice is a fair source of calcium, although it does not begin to compare with milk. Prunes contain some iron.

Two characteristics of vegetables have an important effect on their nutritive value: color and the part of the plant that is eaten, such as leaves and stems, fruit, flowers, seeds, and roots. Leaves and stems, such as lettuce, asparagus, and kale, are rich sources of vitamin A, iron, and ascorbic acid and low in kcalories. Roots and legumes are higher in kcalories if mature and furnish other nutrients, which vary according to color, amount of fiber and water, and other factors. Vegetables that are fruits will vary in kcalories depending upon the amount of water and carbohydrate they contain. One cup of cooked diced summer squash, for example, yields 30 kcalories but one cup of winter squash has 130 kcalories. Winter squash has a high value in vitamin A and contributes to ascorbic acid and calcium requirements. This is true of tomatoes, peppers and pumpkin—other vegetables that are fruits. Deep-yellow and dark-green vegetables have a superior contribution to make to the daily diet, particularly to its vitamin A value.

The vitamin C value of citrus fruits is high, whether the fruit or juice is canned, frozen, or fresh (Table 28–4). A few juices like pineapple juice are sometimes reinforced with vitamin C. Although tomatoes are generally classified as a vegetable, botanically they are a fruit and will be considered in this section. Frozen peaches have ascorbic acid added to keep the fruit from darkening, so the nutritive value is enriched.

Vegetables Rich in Vitamin A

Asparagus, green	Lettuce, Boston, bib
Beans, lima	Greens—beet, dandelion,
Beans, string	mustard, turnip
Broccoli	Okra
Brussels sprouts	Parsley
Cabbage, green	Pepper, green or red
Carrots	Pumpkin
Chard	Romaine
Chicory	Rutabagas
Collards	Spinach
Endive, curly	Squash, yellow
Escarole	Sweet potato
Kale	Yams
Lamb's quarters	

It is interesting to note that even among the fruits generally considered very rich in vitamin C there is some difference. This is notable, for example, in the difference between lemon juice and lime juice. If tomato juice is substituted for orange juice, it is important to remember that three times as much must be served to get the same amount of vitamin C. Prune or other fruit juices should not be substituted for citrus fruit juices. Many people are surprised at the large amount of vitamin C that fresh strawberries contain.

In some parts of the world, people have found a native fruit high in vitamin C. In

TABLE 28–4

Amounts of Various Fruits That Will Supply 45 Milligrams of Ascorbic Acid

FOODS	WEIGHT (g)	AMOUNT
Cantaloupe (medium-sized)	260	⅓ melon
Grapefruit juice, canned, unsweetened	123	½ cup
Grapefruit, fresh	241	½ medium
Lemon juice, fresh	122	½ cup
Lime juice, fresh	138	9 tbs
Orange, fresh	120	⅔ orange (2⅝-in. diameter)
Orange juice, fresh	83	⅓ cup
Pineapple juice, canned	498	2 cups
Raspberries, fresh	184	1½ cups
Strawberries, fresh, capped	44	½ cup
Tangerine juice, canned, sweetened	187	¾ cup

SOURCE: Consumer and Food Economics Research Division, Agricultural Research Service, *Nutritive Value of Foods*, Home and Garden Bulletin No. 72, U.S. Department of Agriculture, Washington, D.C., 1970, pp. 20–22.

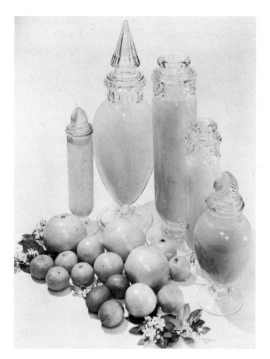

FIGURE 28–5. *Citrus fruits (oranges, lemons, and grapefruit) are an excellent source of ascorbic acid. (Florida Citrus Commission)*

Puerto Rico, for example, the acerola cherry has been found to be extremely rich. In tropical countries where large amounts of mangoes are eaten, this fruit will contribute considerably to the vitamin C of the diet. One medium mango contains 55 mg of ascorbic acid. It is assumed, of course, that these fruits will be eaten fresh.

A number of vegetables are quite rich in vitamin C but they do not contribute as much as citrus fruits. Two or three servings of these vegetables will supply as much vitamin C as a serving of citrus fruit, but they must be eaten raw. However, cooked tomatoes retain most of their vitamin C value. And the large amount of cooked potatoes in some diets makes a valuable contribution to vitamin C. When a potato famine occurred in Ireland, it was generally accompanied by an outbreak of scurvy. The pot liquor from the cooking of greens is another good source of vitamin C.

Other vegetables are not particularly outstanding in regard to minerals and vitamins, but because of the quantity consumed they do add materially to the day's quota. These vegetables also add variety to the diet.

The kinds of vegetables eaten will vary from section to section of the country. However, with present-day transportation and storage facilities, a variety of vegetables is fairly common throughout the country.

Vegetables contribute a little less than half of the vitamin A value to the diet of the American but do not require half its food budget, for they are comparatively inexpensive foods. Vegetables, including tomatoes, also contribute approximately one fourth of the vitamin C of the American diet. This is an appreciable addition to that supplied by the citrus fruits.

Vegetables Rich in Vitamin C

Broccoli	Greens—beet, dandelion,
Cabbage, green	mustard, turnip
Tomatoes	Salad greens
White potatoes	Green peppers

Among the yellow vegetables, the carrot is one of the best sources of vitamin A; one whole carrot (5½ by 1 inch) contains approximately an adult's daily allowance. Other examples of yellow vegetables are sweet potatoes, yellow squash, and yams.

When green vegetables are selected for salads, it is well to consider vitamin A value. A serving of three leaves of escarole, for example, can contribute as much as one half of a young man's (12 to 22 years of age) daily allowance of vitamin A, whereas ½ cup of finely shredded cabbage in salad may contribute only 4 per cent and Chinese cabbage about 5 per cent. However, it must be remembered that cabbage is an inexpensive source of vitamin C. Iceberg lettuce offers little vitamin A.

Parsley and the leaves of watercress are notable for vitamin A. When the entire plant of broccoli is used, the vitamin A contribution is superior, but generally only the stalks and buds are used and the twigs and leaves are discarded. The leaves contribute two thirds as much in vitamin A value, so this practice should be discouraged.

Several fruits have some vitamin A. One of them is prunes. Four medium prunes, uncooked, for example will yield 440 IU of vitamin A. One half of a raw cantaloupe, medium-sized, will yield 6540 IU of vitamin A. Three raw apricots will yield almost 2890 IU. And one wedge of watermelon (4 by 8 inches) will yield 2510 IU of vitamin A.

The green leafy vegetables and immature seeds tend to be higher in B vitamins than the stems, fruits, or underground portions. The unique contribution of green leafy vegetables is ascorbic acid and vitamin A. Among the vegetables, the concentration of ascorbic acid is highest in the cabbage family, sometimes referred to as the Brassica family.

Roots, according to Epstein,[6] are responsible for securing minerals from the complex system of soil and water in which they thrive. This is the only natural way for minerals to become available in food for man.

The root vegetable, actually a tuber, most frequently eaten in the American diet is pota-

[6] Emanuel Epstein, "Roots," *Scientific American*, Vol. 228, No. 5 (May 1973), pp. 48–58.

toes. White potatoes are consumed in larger amounts than sweet potatoes, but sweet potatoes and yams are favorite foods in the South. These vegetables are an economical source of various nutrients. A 100-g baked white potato and a sweet potato of the same size yield 90 and 140 kcalories, respectively. Both contain a small amount of relatively good quality protein and make an excellent contribution of iron, thiamin, niacin, and ascorbic acid to the diet. White potatoes have only a trace of vitamin A, but the 100-g sweet potato yields 8100 IU.

Beets, parsnips, turnips, and rutabagas are other root vegetables. Cooked turnips, parsnips, and rutabagas are good sources of vitamin C, zinc, and calcium. These raw root vegetables are delicious if shredded or diced and added to a tossed salad and the vitamin C contribution is enhanced. Their use should be encouraged.

Fiber Content of Fruits and Vegetables

All fruits and vegetables contain considerable fiber. The amount will depend on the portion of the plant. For example, tubers like potatoes have little, whereas celery stalks and apple skins contain a considerable amount. Fiber, whatever the amount, does contribute to good intestinal hygiene. Cooking will soften the fiber.

Nutritive Values of Additions to Fruits and Vegetables

The nutritive content or value of vegetables is increased considerably by the additions generally made to vegetables before they are brought to the table. Seldom are they served plain. When butter or margarine is added, the vitamin A value is increased and the kcalories also. Other additions may be sauces such as Hollandaise, white, mushroom, or egg. Depending on the ingredients, these sauces again add to the food value. If milk has been used in the preparation of sauces, more calcium, protein, and vitamin A are added. Sometimes vegetables are combined with other foods like meats, fish, or poultry in casseroles or other types of dishes; this practice will increase the protein value. Cheese is another common addition to foods and, like milk, will increase the calcium, protein, and vitamin A value. Since cheese is rather high in fat, it will add to the kcaloric value, too. Fruits may have additions, such as sugar and salad dressing, that increase kcalories and dilute other nutrients.

Storage of Fruits and Vegetables

The storage of vegetables and fruits will have considerable effect on the maintenance of nutritive values. If they are kept for long periods of time, at high levels of temperature and in a dry atmosphere, the losses of vitamin C particularly are great. Fat-soluble vitamins degradate at high temperatures in the presence of oxygen, according to Labuza.[7] Storing at lower temperature reduces the rate of loss. In Chapter 29 information is given on the importance of preparation in conserving nutritive values of vegetables.

Processing and Preservation of Fruits and Vegetables

In the preparation of fruits and vegetables for canning or freezing, the mineral content may be affected. The salt added for seasoning, plus the absorption of salt whenever a sodium chloride brine or preservative is used in processing, may result in vegetables high in sodium.

Ascorbic acid is added sometimes in the canning of fruit nectars and in the freezing of such fruits as apricots and peaches. The nature of the packing medium will affect the kcaloric value. If only water is added, there is dilution; if sugar is added, depending on the concentration, there will be an increase in kcalories.

Little vitamin C is lost in fruits during freezing. In vegetables, the washing and blanching process may result in a loss of water-soluble vitamins and some trace minerals. The temperature at which frozen vegetables are maintained has an effect on vitamin C value. Frozen beans, cauliflower, broccoli, and spinach lose only a small amount of vitamin C over a year's period if the temperature is maintained at −20°F. When stored at 0°F

they lose from one half to three fourths of the total vitamin content, and even greater losses occur when these vegetables are stored at higher temperatures. Frozen orange juice, owing to its acid content, maintains vitamin C content very well even if stored at 32°F for a year, losing only 5 per cent.

Some loss of vitamins occurs during canning, but the extent of the loss has been reduced by the improvement of processing techniques. These include the expulsion of air before sealing, the use of a shorter time of higher temperatures for processing, and agitation of can contents during the canning period. The temperature when stored has an effect on vitamin loss—the higher the temperature, the greater the loss. The most heat-labile vitamins are ascorbic acid, thiamin, vitamin D, and pantothenic acid, according to Lund.[8] Fat-soluble vitamins are generally less heat labile than water-soluble vitamins. A cool storage place is recommended.

An examination of Table 28–5 reveals the significant contribution of nutrients to the diet by the fruit–vegetable group. The kcaloric contribution is only 11.5 per cent of the total kcalories of all foods, yet of the total food nutrients available for civilian consumption in 1974, fruits and vegetables are responsible for 91.35 per cent of ascorbic acid, 48.05 per cent of vitamin A, 23.7 per cent of thiamin, and 23.3 per cent of niacin.

Legumes and Seeds

Legumes are often considered the "poor man's meat." However, Americans do not consume as large a quantity of this vegetable food as might be desirable considering the fact that they are inexpensive, on the whole. Some of the more common legumes are listed below:

Peas	Dried Beans
Whole	Kidney
Split	Navy
Green	Pinto
Yellow	Mexican
Chick	Lima
Lentils	Soy

[7] T. P. Labuza, "Effects of Dehydration and Storage," *Food Technology*, Vol. 27, No. 1 (January 1973), pp. 20–26, 51.

[8] D. B. Lund, "Effects of Heat Processing," *Food Technology*, Vol. 27, No. 1 (January 1973), pp. 16–18.

TABLE 28–5

Percentage Contribution of Fruit–Vegetable Food Group to Total Nutrient Supplies Available for Civilian Consumption According to Preliminary 1974 Data

NUTRIENT	CITRUS FRUITS	OTHER FRUITS	POTATOES AND SWEET POTATOES	DARK-GREEN AND DEEP-YELLOW VEGETABLES	OTHER VEGETABLES INCLUDING TOMATOES	DRY BEANS, PEAS, NUTS, SOYA FLOUR
Kcalories	0.9	2.2	2.7	0.3	2.5	3.4
Protein	0.5	0.6	2.4	0.5	3.3	5.4
Fat	0.1	0.2	0.1	0.05	0.4	4.0
Carbohydrate	1.9	4.7	5.3	0.5	4.7	2.2
Calcium	0.9	1.2	0.9	1.6	4.9	2.8
Phosphorus	0.7	1.1	3.9	0.7	5.0	6.2
Iron	0.8	3.3	4.4	1.6	9.0	6.4
Magnesium	2.2	3.9	7.1	2.1	10.4	11.7
Vitamin A	1.5	5.5	5.3	21.2	15.5	0.05
Thiamin	2.8	1.8	6.2	0.9	6.9	5.7
Riboflavin	0.5	1.5	1.7	1.1	4.5	2.0
Niacin	0.9	1.7	7.1	0.7	6.1	7.6
Vitamin B_6	1.2	5.5	11.2	1.7	9.2	4.3
Vitamin B_{12}	0	0	0	0	0	0
Ascorbic acid	26.3	11.4	18.0	8.3	27.6	0.05

SOURCE: *National Food Situation*, Economic Research Service, U.S. Department of Agriculture, Washington, D.C., November 1974, p. 28.

Legumes find their way to Americans tables in a variety of ways. They may be served boiled and seasoned with bacon or salt pork. Often they are the principal ingredients in a thick soup. At other times they might be used in a casserole dish. Tomatoes, onions, cheese, and other ingredients are often added. An American favorite is chili con carne, which uses the kidney bean. Baked beans are a tradition in the New England states and are used widely elsewhere, too. Mashed beans are served for breakfast in some areas of Latin America.

The nutritive contributions of legumes are many. They are quite high in energy value and compare very favorably with cereals. Thiamin content is good but not as high as that of whole-grain cereals. One of the most valuable contributions is protein. In most instances, the protein is of an incomplete quality, but they have about twice as much as cereals. Although the protein is incomplete, when it is combined with other proteins, particularly animal proteins like milk, cheese, meat, or eggs, it is indeed very valuable. Legumes may also be combined with the proteins of flour. In a combination of baked beans and brown bread, or split pea soup and croutons, the proteins help to supplement each other.

Legumes are an excellent source of iron. One cup of cooked red kidney beans is equal to one third of the daily iron requirements for a young woman 19 to 22 years of age. Legumes are a good source of zinc and magnesium.

Legumes are devoid of vitamin C. However, in many areas of the world, beans such as soybeans are sprouted, and these sprouts are found to be a very rich source of vitamin C. Legumes are a good source of niacin, and when combined with meat or other foods containing niacin, an excellent dietary contribution is made.

The United States produces more than 70 per cent of the world's crop of soybeans. Soybeans are used largely for human and animal food, but have many industrial uses as well. Although the greatest use is in the Orient, according to Heiser,[9] soybeans are being increasingly used for protein enrichment and as a meat substitute in many parts of the world.

Soybeans outrank all other legumes in protein content—38 per cent, almost double that found in cereals. All essential amino acids are in good supply, except for methionine and tryptophan, according to Wolf.[10] The high lysine content makes soy protein a useful complement to cereal proteins that are deficient in this amino acid. The 20 per cent fat content is in the form of high-quality soybean oil used in margarines, salad dressing, shortenings, and as cooking oil. In addition, soybeans are an excellent source of vitamin A, thiamin, phosphorus, potassium, calcium, iron, niacin, and riboflavin.

Many food products have been developed from soybeans, according to Keys and Keys.[11] Examples are bean sprouts, bean curd, fermented bean pastes (*miso*), soy sauce, soyflour, and soy milk. The soybean curd that resembles a white cheese in appearance is called *tofu* and is often fed to Chinese and Japanese children. The fermented bean paste, highly important in Japan, consists of cooked soybeans, yeast, and salt, which is allowed to ferment for 2 weeks or much longer. The rate of fermentation is controlled by the amount of salt. Soy milk is available for children and individuals with allergies. The immature green bean may be shelled and cooked, but the texture remains firm and nut-like, not soft as are other beans. Textured soybean protein is especially valuable for use as a meat substitute for those individuals whose meat intake has been restricted for religious or health reasons. This textured protein helps to reduce the family meat bill when combined in meat loaf or other ground meat dishes.

Seeds

With the high interest in natural foods and vegetarianism, more seeds are being consumed. Sunflower seeds, a favorite, were analyzed for nutritive value by Texas A&M University scientists.[12] The average proved to be 27.2 per cent protein, 50.7 per cent fat, and 10.7 per cent fiber. In addition, sunflower kernels are a good source of the B complex vitamins and contain high levels of carotenes. Calcium, phosphorus, and iron were found in good supply. Sunflower meal with a protein content of 56.8 per cent has many possibilities for incorporation into everyday foods.

Nuts

Nuts have played a practical role in the lives of people for hundreds of years. One of America's contributions is the peanut, also called groundnut, groundpea, goober, pender, and other names. The peanut is actually a legume, not a nut. China and Japan lead the world in peanut production; the United States ranks only fifth, but peanuts are put to far more uses than in any other part of the world, according to Heiser.[13]

The protein content of peanuts is 26 per cent, not as rich as soybeans. Peanuts also yield an oil that is used for margarines, salad dressings, and as a cooking oil. The large consumption of peanut butter contributes generously to the protein, sodium, potassium, phosphorus, thiamin, iron, riboflavin, and niacin content of the diet. All the essential amino acids are available in peanuts, but as in soybeans methioine and tryptophan are in shorter supply.

Sesame seeds may be added to other foods. All of the amino acids are present, but phenylalanine and leucine are in appreciable amounts. The fat content is high and so consequently are kcalories. These seeds have a superior content of phosphorus and niacin and

[9] Charles B. Heiser, Jr., *Seed to Civilization*, W. H. Freeman, San Francisco, 1973, Chap. 6.

[10] W. J. Wolf, "What Is Soy Protein?" *Food Technology*, Vol. 26, No. 5 (May 1972), pp. 44–54.

[11] Margaret Keys and Ancel Keys, *The Benevolent Bean*, Noonday Press, New York, 1972, pp. 167–177.

[12] L. M. Huffman, B. J. Brunnett, and E. E. Burns, "Sunflower as Food," *Journal of the American Dietetic Association*, Vol. 63, No. 5 (November 1973), p. 552. (Abstracted from *League for International Food Newsletter*, March 1973.)

[13] Heiser, op. cit., pp. 127–131.

a good amount of thiamin, riboflavin, and calcium.

Coconut is added to some combinations of foods enjoyed by vegetarians and natural food adherents. Coconut is rather high in kcalories because of the fat content, with considerable saturated fatty acids, and in potassium and phosphorus content; this nut also has a fair amount of iron and vitamin C and small amounts of thiamin, niacin, riboflavin, and all the essential amino acids, but not in adequate amounts.

Americans have not eaten nuts in as large a quantity as people in other parts of the world have. Here nuts are considered as a kind of adjunct to be eaten as a snack, or while attending a sports event, or as an important ingredient in desserts. The trend to natural foods and vegetarian diets has increased the use of nuts in the diet. Often they are combined with other foods such as cereals, vegetables, or dried fruit. The fact that nuts are very nutritious has received little credit.

Major Nutritive Contributions of Nuts

Because of their high fat and low moisture content, nuts are a concentrated food and consequently high in kcalories. Most of the common ones will yield 150 to 200 kcalories per ounce. However, chestnuts, which have much more starch than fat in them, are not

nearly so high. It takes almost three times the quantity to produce the same number of kcalories.

The protein found in nuts such as almonds and pecans is complete, but Americans eat so few that we do not think of them as contributing to our protein requirement.

In regard to minerals, the contribution is small, partly because kcalories are so high in proportion to other nutrients. Nuts do contribute some iron and some calcium to the diet. They are very poor in vitamin A and do not contribute any vitamin C. They are a fair source of thiamin, and some nuts also have a fair amount of riboflavin and niacin. Since they are so high in fat and in kcalories, they should be combined with low kcaloric foods like fruits and vegetables.

Comparison of Nutritive Values of Common Nuts

Nuts vary somewhat in kcaloric value. Pecans, for example, have about 200 kcalories in comparison to cashew nuts, which have about 165 kcalories per ¼ cup. Chestnuts, as has been previously mentioned, are comparatively much lower in kcalories. Cashew nuts are exceptionally high in iron, almonds are a good source of calcium, and pecans and Brazil nuts are good sources of zinc. Almonds appear to be the best source of riboflavin in nuts.

TABLE 28–6

Nutritive Value of Shelled Nuts

(1-cup portions)

NUTRIENT	ALMONDS	COCONUT	CASHEWS	PEANUTS	PECANS	WALNUTS, ENGLISH
Kcalories	850	450	785	840	740	650
Protein, g	26	25	24	37	10	15
Calcium, mg	332	17	53	107	79	83
Iron, mg	6.7	2.2	53	3.0	2.6	2.1
Thiamin, mg	0.34	0.7	0.6	0.46	0.93	0.48
Riboflavin, mg	1.31	0.3	0.35	0.46	0.14	0.13
Niacin, mg	5.0	0.7	2.5	24.7	1.0	1.2
Vitamin A, IU	0	0	140	0	140	0

SOURCE: Consumer and Food Economics Research Division, Agricultural Research Service, *Nutritive Value of Foods*, Home and Garden Bulletin No. 72, U.S. Department of Agriculture, Washington, D.C., 1970, pp. 12–13.

A comparison of the nutritive values of 1 cup of each of six common nuts is shown in Table 28–6.

Being such a concentrated food, nuts may interfere with digestion unless they are chewed well or have been chopped into fine particles. It is difficult for digestive juices to penetrate the particles of nuts if they are in large pieces. This is another argument for not eating nuts in the casual manner we do, but considering them as a substantial food in the diet. Since they do have a contribution to make to our daily nutrition, it might be wise to encourage greater use of them.

Cereals and Breads

Cereals and bread constitute the most important food of people around the world. Cereals are generally made into some kind of bread, although approximately half the people in the world eat rice,[14] which may or may not be made into a bread. Americans also eat breakfast cereals that are shredded, flaked, popped, coated, or in other forms. These foods find their way to the table for practically every meal that people eat. Even snacks often have cereal products as their base.

World Consumption of Cereals and Breads

The predominant cereal varies from one area of the world to another. Furthermore, it is supplemented by other cereals and foods. Rice[15] is usually the staple food in the Far East and in Latin America, but other grains and wheat predominate in large parts of India and Pakistan. In parts of Indonesia and the Philippines, maize and starch roots are the main staples of the dietary. Maize is the main cereal consumed in Central America, as baked cakes or bread called tortillas and as porridge, and in southeast Africa, as doughy balls called kenke or in gruel or paste. Barley, other coarse grains, and millets are characteristically associated with the poor man's diet in many areas. These cereals have a high consumption in many countries of Africa. The Near Eastern countries emphasize bread made from maize or wheat, although some barley and millet products are also included.

North African countries, like other Mediterranean countries, utilize the cereal product called couscous in place of bread. Couscous is a coarse cereal produced from wheat middlings, a by-product of flour milling. It is cooked somewhat like rice, according to Perl.[15] Barley is also used in this part of the world. In the savannah areas of Africa, millets and sorghum predominate, followed by maize. In West and Central Africa, the consumption of cassava, yams, and cocoyams is high. Rice is the main cereal in the West African coastal areas. The pattern is diverse in East Africa, where maize is usually the chief cereal and plantains are popular.

In Latin America rice is prized along with beans and bananas. Wheat predominates in most of the plains areas of South America. In the tropical coasts and plains, rice is widely grown, whereas cassava is important in Brazil and Paraguay.

Dietary patterns are constantly undergoing change. As diets become more varied, there may be a shift among the various staple foods. Millets, sorghum, and barley rate the lowest preference, whereas wheat and rice are highly prized. When incomes improve and choices are greater, people tend to ascend this scale of preference and modify their diets accordingly. In some instances, the traditional staples may not be discarded but the preferred cereals are merely added.

Thus geographic and social factors influence the type of cereal that is used. A cereal can become such an important part of the culture of a people that it is difficult to change this particular food habit. When cereal products from another part of the world are introduced into a section, there may be considerable resentment. One example that is cited is that homemakers in Pakistan do not care to have the American wheat used in the preparation of chapouti, a flat, thin bread made from wheat which they use for soaking up gravy or

---

[14] M. Pekkarinen, "World Food Consumption Patterns," in Miloslav Rechcigl, Jr. (ed.), Man, Food, and Nutrition, CRC Press, Cleveland, 1973, pp. 16–20.

[15] Lila Perl, Rice, Spice and Bitter Oranges, World Publishing, New York, 1967.

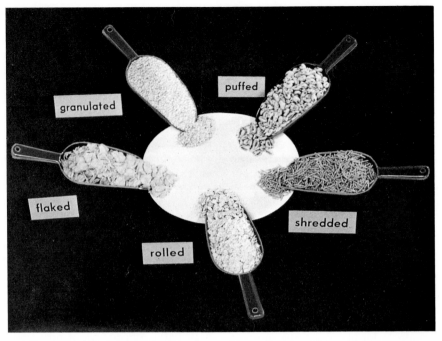

FIGURE 28–6. *Breakfast cereals are prepared in many ways. (Cereal Institute, Inc.)*

the juices of a chicken curry. The American wheat has a much higher protein content than the wheat to which they have been accustomed and the character of the *chapouti* is consequently changed materially, much to the irritation of the Pakistanis. Similarly, as we have noted, someone who comes to America from the Far East is quite disconcerted by the lack of rice in our diet.

Types of Cereals

Cereal foods made from wheat, rice, oats, rye, corn, or buckwheat may be listed in the following categories:

BREADS   Made of flour from whole grains, part of grains, or enriched.

BREAD-LIKE PRODUCTS   Muffins, coffee cakes, crackers, rolls, biscuits, pancakes, waffles, doughnuts, and such.

CEREAL   Dry or cooked, made from whole grain, part of the grain, or enriched.

FLOUR   Made from whole grain, part of the grain, or enriched; grains may be rice, corn, rye, wheat, buckwheat.

CEREAL PRODUCTS   Macaroni, noodles, spaghetti; made from whole grain, part of the grain, or enriched flour.

Major Nutritive Contributions of Cereals

Since cereals are a major article of the diet of the people of the world, it is important that we examine their nutritive contributions. The preparation of the grain has a great influence on its nutritive value. Is the whole grain used, is only a part of the grain used, or has the food been enriched? When a part or all of the bran coats are removed, as in the case of polished rice or white flour, the nutritive value is greatly reduced because the iron, phosphorus, magnesium, protein, vitamin B_6, and thiamin are lost—unless the product is enriched later. Also, bran contains considerable bulk for regulatory purposes. The germ is very frequently removed because it becomes rancid rather readily and bad flavors develop. However, when it is removed a very rich source of thiamin and vitamin E is lost. The endosperm is composed largely of starch and also has some protein. This part generally remains because it keeps well and because many cultures demand flours or cereal products that are white. There is a trend, especially among the young, for unrefined cereals.

In America, for instance, people are opposed to eating whole-wheat bread. One explanation is that dark bread is associated with the peasant classes and has unconscious status symbolism. In examining labels of breads, flours, and cereal products, it is well to determine what percentage of the grain remains because this does have a decided effect upon the nutritive quality. Is it 50 per cent whole wheat, for example, or 80 per cent whole wheat, or as in the case of shredded wheat, is it 100 per cent whole wheat?

The main contribution of cereals and breads is energy. These foods are very bland in flavor, are inexpensive, and easily prepared. For these reasons, they are readily incorporated into the daily diet. If the cereals are not too refined or are enriched, they are an excellent source of iron, vitamin B_6, thiamin, niacin, riboflavin, and a fair source of folacin. And when milk is added to the diet, the calcium content, as well as riboflavin, is increased. One pound of cereal will yield from 1600 to 1800 kcalories. One pound of bread will yield approximately 1200 kcalories, slightly less than cereals because there is more moisture in bread. Enriched cereals are an excellent source of iron, thiamin, riboflavin, and niacin.

The protein value of cereals depends on the portion of the whole grain that remains. Each cereal contains a number of proteins that vary somewhat in their nutritive value. The proteins of the highest quality are found in the outer layers of the seed and around the embryo or germ, but milling generally removes them. Although the proteins of cereals are inadequate in some of the essential amino acids, when combined with milk they are utilized very effectively. The bread–cereal group contributes about 18 per cent of the protein available in the national diet.

The nutritive value of rice depends on the extent to which it has been milled as well as the preparation. Rice may be brown, converted, polished, or enriched, and it may be found in dry or cooked breakfast cereals and flours as well.

Brown rice has been milled so that the hull has been removed but nearly all the bran has been retained. Since much of the bran is present, brown rice is a relatively rich source of thiamin, vitamin B_6, riboflavin, niacin, iron, and protein. The quality of protein is not high, but when used with a small amount of milk, it is well supplemented and utilized.

Converted rice is found in our markets and used by many. It is prepared by an American adaptation of a process that originated in India. The rice is placed in large cylinders, the air removed, hot water introduced, and the rice steeped under pressure for several hours. The hulls are then removed and the rice kernels are polished in the usual manner. This rice retains some of its bran coat, which makes it richer in protein, vitamins, and minerals. Thus converted rice is richer in nutrients than polished white rice.

When white rice has been enriched, it is an excellent source of the B vitamins and iron, but otherwise its only contribution is kcalories. All the nutritive value except kcalories has been removed in the milling process.

Wheat is the cereal most widely used in America and in certain other parts of the world. More study and attention have been devoted to it than to any of the other cereals. It is used largely for breads or flour in this country, with the highest portion going into white flour and white bread. Depending on the degree of milling—or whether the cereal has been enriched—wheat may be an excellent source of iron and the B vitamins.

Of the other grains, rye is largely used for bread flour and is very popular in central Europe. It is used to make pumpernickel and other breads. Barley is found as pearl barley and barley flour and is generally devoid of bran and germ, so it yields only kcalories. Corn is very popular in certain parts of this country, particularly in the South, and in Mexico and Latin American countries. It contains as much thiamin as wheat but only one fourth as much niacin. Oats, which are used primarily as a breakfast food in this country, are particularly rich in thiamin, magnesium, and iron. Buckwheat is actually a grass. It has only limited use as buckwheat flour for pancakes, or it is sometimes made into groats and dry cereal.

There are many types of breads. Some of the most common are cracked wheat, French, Italian, raisin, rye, white, whole wheat, soybean, wheat germ, natural grain or organic, Boston brown, and fruit-and-nut breads. Some breads contain a variety of flours. Their nutritive value varies considerably, depending on the ingredients added, if any, and on the degree to which the flour has been milled.

Bread-like products such as biscuits, muffins and other quick breads depend for their nutritive value on the kind of flour used as well as any other ingredients that are added. The value will also vary according to the amount of sugar added. If the product is very sweet, the nutritive density has been diluted because only kcalories have been increased. Sometimes other ingredients like eggs, milk, dried fruits, or nuts have been added, which will contribute nutrients. The foods accompanying these bread-like products sometimes increase the nutritive value. Take waffles, for example; any butter or margarine added will contribute both kcalories and vitamin A, whereas syrup contributes only kcalories. If the waffles are eaten with a creamed meat or some other sauce, the nutritive value will depend upon the ingredients added. There is a minor trend to baking more bread and bread products in the home because of high food prices. However, most breads consumed in America are baked in a bakery.

The consumption of breakfast cereals has unfortunately declined in our country. They are consumed largely by preschool and elementary school children and by some adults, especially older persons. Part of this decline is due to the fact that adults are very kcalorie conscious. Many natural-food advocates consume rather large amounts of cereal for a more concentrated source of kcalories as well as other reasons.

The contribution of a breakfast cereal will depend largely on the type of cereal. If the cereal has been only slightly refined, or not refined, in the milling, the nutritive value is much greater. In the case of shredded wheat, puffed wheat, and some of the rolled oats, the nutritive value is quite high. Some cereals are made from refined grains, such as cream of wheat, farina, and puffed rice. This type of cereal is usually enriched.

Besides the enrichment program, there is a considerable trend today to making other additions. For example, some dry cereals have been reinforced with protein—largely in the form of lysine, one of the essential amino acids.

The trend to sugar-coated cereals should be discouraged. The sugar merely adds kcalories to the cereal and does not contribute any of the valuable nutrients badly needed by growing boys and girls as well as adults. This type of cereal appeals to the sweet tooth and dilutes the day's diet of some of its nutrient density.

Foods, such as fruits, added to dry or cooked cereals are important. Cereals are also further enhanced, nutritionally, when they are eaten with milk.

The question, "Is there any difference in nutritive value between cooked and dry cereals?" often arises. Mothers frequently have the impression that the cooked cereal is much more nutritious than the dry one. This again depends entirely on the type of cereal—some dried cereals are even more nutritious than some cooked cereals.

Macaroni, spaghetti, and other pastas are cereal products that are very popular in this country as well as in some others. This group of foods is generally enriched. They are also often combined with very nutritious ingredients, such as cheese, tomatoes, meat, other vegetables, fish, and poultry. The eggs, cheese, and meats contribute materially to the protein value and supplement the inadequate proteins of the pastas.

There are other products made of cereals, such as crackers, pretzels, Zwieback, and cocktail tidbits. Again, the ingredients will largely determine the nutritive value. If flour is the main ingredient and if it is enriched, some protein, B vitamins, and iron will be included. The crackers may have other ingredients, usually seasoning agents, which may or may not

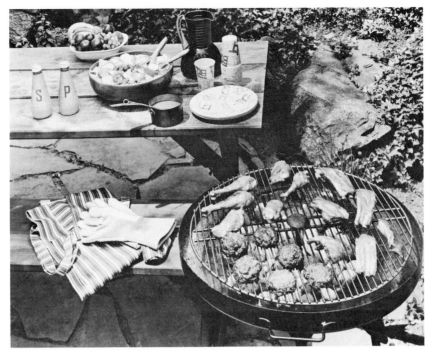

FIGURE 28–7. *Meat is an important source of protein.* (*Plate, Cup and Container Institute*)

be nutritious. They may be eaten with nutritious spreads, which will enhance their nutritive value. Tapioca, a cereal-like product used in desserts and as a thickening agent, largely contributes kcalories.

Although cereals are not consumed in as large quantities as they were at one time, they continue to play a very important role in the American diet. (See Table 30–6.) It is the sincere hope of nutrition experts that people will be interested in using many types of cereal. Just as a varied diet tends to greater assurance of adequacy, so does a variety of cereals. The custom of relying on only one cereal, and in many cases a refined one at that, has created many difficult feeding problems throughout the world.

Meat, Fish, Poultry, and Eggs

Meat is one of America's favorite foods. The consumption of meat is higher in de-

veloped countries than in developing countries.[16] Less meat is consumed than formerly because of high food prices reflecting inflation, recession, and food shortages in most of the world. The high cost of meat production is a frequent topic of discussion. Possible means of changing food habits and developing inexpensive forms of protein are being explored. With a lower protein allowance in the recommended allowance, smaller servings of meat are encouraged.

The kind of meat that is favored varies from one region of the country to the other. Beef and pork seem to head the list. And the use of poultry has increased tremendously. People along the seacoasts eat a fair amount of fish and shellfish, whereas in the interior near lakes and rivers, some freshwater fish are eaten. However, fish is used to a much lesser extent than either meat or poultry.

---

[16] Pekkarinen, op. cit., pp. 26–28.

TABLE 28–7

Contribution of Meat (Including Pork Fat Cuts), Poultry, and Fish to Nutrient Supplies Available for Civilian Consumption

NUTRIENT	PERCENTAGE
Kcalories	19.9
Protein	41.2
Fat	34.2
Carbohydrate	0.1
Calcium	3.5
Phosphorus	25.9
Iron	29.3
Magnesium	13.6
Vitamin A value	22.2
Thiamin	27.7
Riboflavin	24.2
Niacin	45.7
Vitamin B_6	45.6
Vitamin B_{12}	68.9
Ascorbic acid	1.1

SOURCE: *National Food Situation*, Economic Research Service, U.S. Department of Agriculture, Washington, D.C., November 1974, p. 28.

Major Nutritive Contributions of Meat, Fish, and Poultry

Meat, fish, and poultry are our greatest sources of complete protein in the diet. Meat proteins are adequate for both maintenance and growth and will do much to supplement incomplete proteins in the diet. Variables such as the amount of fat, connective tissue, and bone will have an effect upon the nutrients per pound or other measure of weight. As the fat increases, other nutrients are diluted. In other words, the leaner the meat, the higher the protein value.

Meat is also very rich in phosphorus and magnesium, but deficient in calcium, which is found in the discarded bones. Meat is also an excellent source of iron, but the iron content depends on the protein content. If the meat is high in fat, the iron content will naturally be less. Meat is a good source of niacin, riboflavin, and vitamins B_6 and B_{12}, but there is practically no vitamin A except in liver. There is also very little vitamin C, except in the or-

gans, and here the vitamin C may be lost during cooking. See Table 28–7.

Comparison of Nutritive Values Within the Meat, Fish, and Poultry Group

The higher the fat content, the greater the energy value of meat. Individuals who watch kcaloric intake should concentrate on lean meats. The cut of meat has no influence on its nutritive value. In other words, the nutrients found in chuck are as adequate as those found in porterhouse steak. Meat is considered one of the richest sources of iron; organ meats, however, have a much higher quantity than muscle meats. And shellfish are especially high in iron, particularly oysters and clams—a 3½-oz (60-g) serving of fresh oysters or clams will yield approximately one third of the day's iron allowance for an 18-year-old male or female. Oysters are an excellent source of vitamin A, zinc, and calcium and are a good source of niacin.

The dark meat of chicken and of certain fish contains more iron and more fat than the white meat. Most saltwater fish and shellfish are an excellent source of iodine. Of the foods in this group, pork is particularly rich in thiamin, and the others contain only fair amounts. Most of these foods are good sources of niacin and vitamins B_6 and B_{12}.

Organ meats, unfortunately, are seldom found in American diets, but their nutritive

TABLE 28–8

Iron Content of Cooked Liver

(100-g Portions)

	IRON (mg)
Chicken	8.5
Beef	8.8
Calf	14.2
Lamb	17.9
Pork	29.1

SOURCE: *Composition of Foods*, Agriculture Handbook No. 8, U.S. Department of Agriculture, Washington, D.C., 1963.

TABLE 28–9

Comparison of Nutritive Values of Hamburger (Cooked) and Selected Cold Cuts

(3-oz servings; 90 g)

NUTRIENT	HAMBURGER Lean	HAMBURGER Regular	BOILED HAM	LIVERWURST (Smoked)	BOLOGNA	SALAMI (dry)
Kcalories	185	245	203	292	277	390
Protein, g	23	21	17	13	10	21
Fat, g	10	17	15	22	24	33
Calcium, mg	10	9	9	9	7	12
Phosphorus, mg	163	133	97	220	115	254
Iron, mg	3.0	2.7	2.4	5.4	1.7	3
Vitamin A, IU	20	30	0	5895	0	—
Thiamin, mg	0.8	0.7	0.37	0.13	1.4	0.3
Riboflavin, mg	0.2	0.18	0.14	1.3	0.2	0.21
Niacin, mg	5.1	4.6	2.3	7.2	2.4	4.5

SOURCE: Consumer and Food Economics Research Division, Agricultural Research Service, *Nutritive Value of Foods,* Home and Garden Bulletin No. 72, U.S. Department of Agriculture, Washington, D.C., 1970, pp. 9–11; and Bernice K. Watt and Annabel L. Merrill, *Composition of Foods,* Agriculture Handbook No. 8, Consumer and Food Economics Research Division, Agricultural Research Service, U.S. Department of Agriculture, Washington, D.C., 1963.

value should be recognized. Kidney and liver are somewhat alike in their nutritive offerings, although liver is perhaps superior. It is especially rich in iron, vitamin A, riboflavin, and niacin. In the selection of liver, there may be some concern about which type will give the largest amount of iron. Table 28–8 shows the iron in cooked liver.

Heart, although a very nutritious kind of meat, is more representative of muscle meat nutritionally than it is of the organ meats.

Cold cuts or luncheon meats compare favorably in nutritive value with fresh meats. Liver sausage must contain not less than 30 per cent liver by weight, according to government laws. Liver paste and spread must contain at least 50 per cent liver. The amount of water in these cold cuts is limited to 10 per cent, and the amount of cereals, starchy flours, and dried milk products can be up to 3½ per cent by weight. Table 28–9 compares the nutritive value of some common cold cuts with that of hamburger.

A number of "meatless meats" are found on the market now. (These foods are also referred to as engineered foods, synthetics, soy-

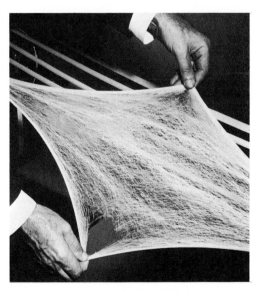

FIGURE 28–8. *Textured soy protein is the basis for meatless meat. (General Mills, Inc.)*

protein fiber foods, mock meats, food of the loom, prefab meats, and edible spun protein.) They are made from soybeans, wheat, yeast extracts, and other nonanimal proteins. Al-

Some Types of Meat, Fish, and Poultry

MEAT	FISH	POULTRY
Beef	Freshwater	Chicken
Lamb	Saltwater	Duck
Mutton	Shellfish	Goose
Pork (except bacon	Clams	Turkey
and fatback)	Crabs	Pheasant
Veal	Oysters	Quail
Organ meats	Lobsters	Guinea fowl
Liver	Shrimp	Squab
Heart	Scallops	
Kidney		
Tongue		
Tripe		
Sweetbreads		
Luncheon meats		
Opossum		
Muskrat		
Rabbit		
Venison		

though the process is secret and complicated, in general, the protein is processed and spun into fine silk-like threads. These filaments are combined, textured, and treated with synthetic colors, flavors, amino acids, minerals, and vitamins. This man-made protein can be adjusted for tenderness, amount of fat or amino acids, or the quantity of cholesterol. In color and flavor meatless meats may simulate bacon, beef, chicken, turkey, ham, or other products. The nutritive value will depend somewhat on the ingredients and the quality of protein used. In view of the world's protein shortage, these meatless meats can make a valuable contribution.

There is quite an array from which to choose in selecting meats, fish, or poultry for daily meals. The important foods to be considered are listed below.

In examining this long list of potentials for choice in selecting a dish for the family, Americans should have little difficulty in fulfilling their desire for meat.

Eggs

Eggs are generally considered a breakfast food, but find their way into other meals and many dishes. The number of eggs to include in the diet each week is three to four.

Major Nutritive Contributions of Eggs

Eggs are very similar to meat in their nutritive value. Two eggs are equal to one 2-oz serving of meat in protein value and are often utilized as a substitute. The protein in egg is very adequate, both in the white and in the yolk, and is one of the important sources of protein for growing children. The egg white, besides being an excellent source of protein, is also a rich source of riboflavin.

The yolk is the storage house of nutrients. It is one of the best food sources of vitamin A, and a good source of vitamins E, B_6, and B_{12}. It contains some thiamin and riboflavin, but no vitamin C. There is a trace of niacin, and, as foods go, the yolk is rich in vitamin D. However, egg yolk should not be considered a substitute for fish-liver oils. Eggs are a rather poor source of calcium, for most of the calcium is in the shell, which is not eaten, but they are rich in iron. As a source of energy, eggs are not high. One contributes approximately 80 kcalories.

There is no difference in nutritive value of eggs from different breeds of chicken, nor is the color of the shell an indication. They may vary in nutritive value at various seasons, depending on the food given to the hen. Eggs are an excellent reinforcement for the iron found in milk. The most serious delimitation of eggs is the high cholesterol content.

Miscellaneous Foods

Beverages

Beverages are associated with mealtimes, social occasions, or rest periods. Not only are they an important part of regular meals, but they are also consumed in large quantities between meals. Following is a list of some of the most common ones:

Coffee	Carbonated beverages
Cocoa	Other types of soft drinks
Chocolate	Fruit flavored drinks
Decaffeinated coffee	Alcoholic beverages
Coffee substitutes	Broth
Tea	

Beverages, on the whole, add little nutritive value to the diet, but they do contribute water, which is very necessary for health. And sometimes additions are made to them that do add to nutritive value.

Coffee is the popular American beverage. In itself, it has no nutrients; but when cream and sugar are added, kcalories are contributed to the diet. If a great deal of coffee is consumed with cream and sugar, the kcalories can be substantial. Coffee does have a stimulant, caffein, which proves to be very refreshing to many. Some people, however, have to avoid coffee because of the undesirable effects of this stimulant. For these people, certain coffee substitutes or decaffeinated coffee is often used. Many Americans have a cup of coffee at the end of dinner and skip dessert. This is a desirable practice for those who need to watch their weight.

Tea is popular with many people but not so much in America as in other parts of the world. It contains a stimulant known as theine. Sometimes slices of fruit, fruit juices, sugar, and spices are added. A teaspoon of sugar or small amounts of fruit juice will contribute only a few kcalories. However, tea is seldom drunk by itself; people generally eat cakes, bread and butter, or other foods with considerable kcalories.

Children and young adults frequently consume large amounts of cocoa and chocolate. Chocolate is exceptionally high in fat, containing not less than 50 per cent fat as purchased. It consequently lends itself to a very rich drink, particularly if it is sweetened and topped with whipped cream as it so often is. Cocoa has much less fat, only 22 per cent, and can be made into a very nutritious drink if milk is used instead of water. Both chocolate and cocoa contain starch in addition to the fat, and have small amounts of protein and minerals.

Many of the carbonated beverages and other types of soft drinks are merely water or carbonated water with flavorings. One measuring cup of these beverages contains from 80 to 100 kcalories. This energy value comes from sugar. They do not contain other nutrients unless that fact is indicated on the bottle.

There are two very decided dangers in drinking large quantities of these beverages. First, individuals may be mistaken about their nutritive contribution and, particularly in the case of fruit-flavored drinks, believe that they are actually deriving the same benefit as if they were using fruit juices. In reality, they have only the flavor or such a minute amount of fruit juice that the nutritive contribution is negligible. Another danger in the case of growing children is that these drinks are often substituted for milk, which is a very vital part of the diet. In addition, some research substantiates the idea that these beverages can be very deleterious to the teeth. There is quite a trend today to low kcaloric or non-kcaloric carbonated beverages. Authorities are raising a question about the amount and kind of artificial sweeteners that are not injurious to health.

TABLE 28–10

Kcaloric Values of Some Alcoholic Beverages

BEVERAGE	KCALORIES
Beer (12-oz or 360 cc bottle)	170
Brandy (cordial, approx. 4 oz or 120 cc)	60
Eggnog (4-oz or 120 cc punch cup)	338
Gin (1½ oz or 45 cc)	120
Rum (1½ oz or 45 cc)	135
Whiskey (1½ oz or 45 cc)	130
Wine, California white (4 oz or 120 cc)	90

Alcoholic beverages supply little to the diet but kcalories. Occasionally slices of fruit or fruit juices are added and some vitamin C and kcalories may be contributed as a result. From the values given in Table 28–10, it is obvious that alcoholic beverages can contribute considerable kcalories to the diet, particularly if more than one drink is consumed.

Another food, which is actually consumed as a beverage, is broth. It has little or no nutritive value, but the meat extracts do tend to stimulate appetite. Broth may have tomato, clam, or other juices added. When tomato juice is used, the vitamin C and vitamin A contents of the diet are enhanced.

It must be borne in mind that these beverages tend to refresh people, add fluid to the diet, or stimulate. Their use is often focused around social situations and for that reason may influence meals that follow.

Sugars

Americans have a sweet tooth and eat large amounts of candy and similar products. Sugar is also added to foods such as beverages and cereals. It is almost essential to desserts like cookies, cakes, pie, ice cream, and puddings, which are dear to Americans. Sugar does add to the palatability of food. The sugar habit, particularly among children, can be quickly acquired and should be discouraged.

Molasses, honey, maple and other table syrups are included with sugars. The most commonly consumed sugar, of course, is white sugar.

MAJOR NUTRITIVE CONTRIBUTION Sugar is primarily a source of fuel. Since such a large amount is consumed, it does tend to dilute other nutrients to an alarming degree. When 100 kcalories of sugar, for example, are added to 100 kcalories of fruit, the other nutrients in that particular dish have been cut in half. This is a rather dramatic way of looking at the role of sugar in our diet. The only sugar that does have some nutrients is molasses, which has calcium and iron. However, it would be necessary to have 10 tablespoons of molasses to equal the calcium found in 1 pint of milk. (The fallacies associated with blackstrap molasses are discussed in Chapter 33.) The role of sugar in relation to dental health is discussed in Chapter 19.

Fats and Oils

Americans are not consistent about the way fat in included in their meals. An individual may carefully cut away the fat on a serving of meat, and yet during the same meal may have a generous amount of salad dressing, whipped cream on dessert, or some kind of rich pastry.

Fat contributes palatability and appetite appeal to the diet. It also has high energy value.

Many types of fats are used in the daily diet. The following list gives a quick overview of some of the major ones.

Some Common Fats and Oils

FATS	OILS
Butter	Olive
Margarine	Peanut
Bacon fat	Soybean
Fatback	Safflower
Chicken fat	Corn
	Cottonseed
	Fish
	Salad dressings

Ethnic groups in different regions of the world have certain preferences in fats. Italians, for example, use a great deal of olive oil. We in the United States have learned to use large amounts of margarine to replace butter.

MAJOR NUTRITIVE CONTRIBUTIONS Fats and oils are very highly concentrated foods, a fact that must be borne in mind in planning the daily diet, for the main contribution of fat is kcalories. One tablespoon of butter or margarine, for example, will yield 100 kcalories. Some fats carry certain important nutrients such as vitamins A and D. Vitamin A is found in butter and in enriched margarine, and there is a trace of vitamin A in some of the oils but the contribution is negligible. Fish-liver oils are noted for their vitamin A and vitamin D value. These oils are given primarily to growing children for vitamin D.

Some fats also contain the essential fatty acid (see Chapter 6). Many Americans are interested in the saturated or polyunsaturated acid content of the fats they consume. Fats such as bacon fat or fatback largely contribute kcalories and flavor to foods in the daily diet.

Food Adjuncts

Although Americans are not noted for their gourmet taste as much as certain other people in the world—for example, the French—they are inclined to add many flavorings, spices, and the like to their foods to enhance flavor and to make them more palatable. Below is a list of some of the most common food adjuncts used in the diet today.

Catsup
Extracts—lemon, orange, etc.
Flakes—celery, parsley, onion, pepper
Garlic, fresh
Mustard
Paprika
Pickles
Powders—garlic, onion, chile, curry
Saffron
Salt
Seasoned salts—onion, garlic, celery
Spices and herbs
    Allspice
    Anise
    Basil
    Cardamon
    Cinnamon
    Cloves
    Dill
    Ginger
    Mace
    Marjoram
    Nutmeg
    Oregano
    Rosemary
    Sage
    Savory

Tarragon
Thyme
Tumeric
Seeds—celery, caraway, fennel, poppy, sesame, dill
Sauces—chili, Worcestershire
Horseradish
Pepper—red, black, cayenne, white
Sweeteners, noncaloric
Vanilla
Vinegar—wine, cider

Most of these food adjuncts have no nutritive value. Exceptions are catsup, which has tomatoes as a base and has sugar added. Large amounts of catsup can add materially to the day's kcalories. One tablespoon has 17 kcalories. Chili sauce is similar in kcaloric value to catsup. Pepper, mustard, and cinnamon are excellent sources of zinc.

These adjuncts do add to nutrition in an oblique way in that they make food more interesting and more appetizing, and consequently people may enjoy food to a greater extent. But doctoring foods with large amounts of spices and other condiments is to be discouraged.

SELECTED REFERENCES

Heiser, Charles B., Jr., *Seed to Civilization*, W. H. Freeman and Company, San Francisco, 1973.
Home and Garden Bulletins, U.S. Department of Agriculture, Washington, D.C.:
    HG 118, Beef and Lamb in Family Meals
    HG 150, Cereals and Pasta in Family Meals
    HG 112, Cheese in Family Meals
    HG 103, Eggs in Family Meals
    HG 125, Fruit in Family Meals
    HG 127, Milk in Family Meals
    HG 176, Nuts in Family Meals
    HG 110, Poultry in Family Meals
    HG 105, Vegetables in Family Meals
Kon, S. K., *Milk and Milk Products in Human Nutrition*, FAO Nutritional Studies, No. 27, Food and Agricultural Organization of the United Nations, Rome, 1972.

Rechcigl, Miloslav, Jr. (ed.), *Man, Food, and Nutrition*, CRC Press, Cleveland, 1973.

Stillings, Bruce R., and Mary H. Thompson, *Seafoods for Health*, National Oceanic and Atmospheric Administration, National Marine Fisheries Service, U.S. Department of Commerce, Washington, D.C., 1971.

Watt, Bernice K., Susan E. Gerhardt, Elizabeth W. Murphy, and Ritva R. Butrum, "Food Composition Tables for the 70's," *Journal of the American Dietetic Association*, Vol. 64, No. 3 (March 1974), pp. 257–261.

Zook, Elizabeth Gates, "Mineral Composition of Fruits," *Journal of the American Dietetic Association*, Vol. 52, No. 3 (March 1968), pp. 218–224.

29

Planning the Daily Diet According to Lifestyle

Social pressures have played havoc with a nutritious diet for many Americans. Breakfast is practically extinct. Individuals may lunch away from home. With a juggling of schedules, some families do well to have dinner together several times a week. Snacking or the consumption of many meals are other alternatives. Many variations occur because of differences in lifestyles.

Lifestyles

The broad spectrum of lifestyles emerging in this country have a powerful impact on how and what is eaten. Reeder[1] contends that lifestyles reflect social systems. Some of the most influential social systems are family, friendship groups, job, sports and hobby interest, other recreation groups, housing groups, and sometimes political or religious groups. From these special systems and others not listed, an individual will select his or her own set of systems in which participation may vary from

substantial in some to minor in others. A lifestyle represents a configuration of beliefs, values, attitudes, disbeliefs, and social action related to standards and goals that are unique to that person. Examination of the social systems that are rejected are also reflected in lifestyles. Food patterns mirror ways of living. Some examples that may be oversimplified are given here. A professional baseball player may have strong feelings about the influence of food on his ability to play. This does not imply that he automatically selects an adequate diet; he may succumb to faddish diets that give great promises but the lifestyle tends to emphasize food for health. A family that is moving upward on the economic scale may try to eat like the rich. A vegetarian may be reflecting the philosophy of a group affiliation. Certain social influences have an impact upon the way people eat.

Social Influences

The world in which America lives has a strong impact on the manner in which individuals plan their daily diet. Large supermarkets with over 8,000 items and small fruit and vegetable, fish, and other specialty mar-

[1] William W. Reeder, "The Attitudes, Values, and Life Styles of Youth," *Proceedings of the National Nutrition Conference*, Miscellaneous Publication No. 1254, U.S. Department of Agriculture, Washington, D.C., 1973, pp. 3–17.

413

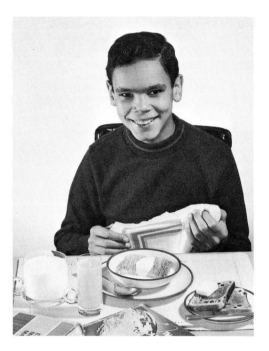

FIGURE 29–1. *Breakfasts are practically extinct for adults. (Cereal Institute Inc.)*

kets make decisions about what is to be eaten difficult. The cost of food because of food shortages, inflation, and other reasons has changed eating habits, such as a decreased consumption of meat. Static incomes of many citizens have made this situation a critical problem. More meals are eaten away from home[2]—at school, fast-food places, company cafeterias, drive-ins, restaurants, and other eating establishments. Changes have been made in the food supply, such as more prepared foods, partially prepared food, convenience foods, frozen or liquid meals, and engineered foods, such as spun protein. Further enrichment of foods has taken place, such as increased iron.[3] Americans have become more sophisticated about food and wine. Cooking schools in the community or as adult educa-

tion courses, chefs and gourmets on the mass media, a vast array of cookbooks, men cooking, cheese- and wine-tasting parties, exposure to foods of other countries through increased travel, and an effort made by many to find a restaurant with unusual food and service are only a few indications of this wider interest in food.

Food industries through research and development departments are rapidly increasing the number of mass-produced foods, some in the form of meals, that consumers may buy. Home-prepared foods are being replaced by these factory foods, except for natural-food advocates and for some individuals who have made a hobby of certain home-prepared foods. Food product analogs will increase and join the ranks of the convenience and substituted foods, according to Hansen.[4] One concern is that little assessment has been taken of the degree to which these technological foods take the place of the nutrients in the traditional foods that were formerly in the grocery cart.

Income is another social influence on what people eat. The static incomes of certain segments of the population, such as the elderly, have created serious problems and nutritional status has suffered. Naturally there are more restrictions among the poor on the amount of money that can be spent on food. Many middle-class families are shopping more carefully and doing without certain luxuries. One's income implies ways of life that may or may not be characteristics of economic level.

An increase in the number of working women, especially wives and mothers, has brought many changes to lifestyles. A large group of women, for example, consider convenience foods a necessity. Greater family participation in food preparation and management has emerged. The advent of the women's liberation movement has lead to less sharply defined sex roles in preparing food. There is little evidence about what these changes have done to nutritional status. The work not only of women but of men has many

[2] Faye Kinder, *Meal Management*, 2nd ed., Macmillan, New York, 1973, pp. 1–4.

[3] Ruth L. Huenemann, *Proceedings of National Nutrition Conference*, Miscellaneous Publication No. 1254, U.S. Department of Agriculture, Washington, D.C., 1973, pp. 41–42.

[4] R. Gaurth Hansen, "An Index to Food Quality," *Nutrition Reviews*, Vol. 31, No. 1 (January 1973), pp. 1–7.

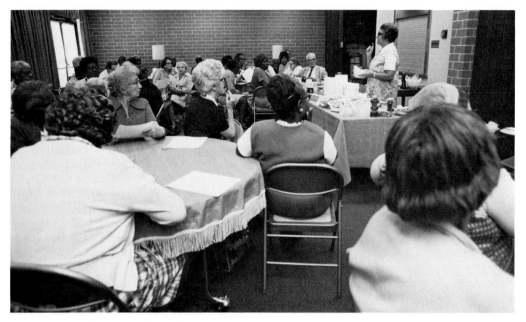

FIGURE 29–2. *Adult education courses have stimulated a wider interest in food.* (USDA)

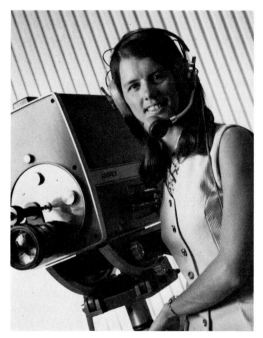

FIGURE 29–3. *Working women have influenced changes in lifestyles.* (*Bethlehem Steel*)

influences on the amount and kind, as well as timing, of food eaten. The energy crisis has triggered scrutiny of the kind and amount of fuel used in preparing food. Cooking on the top of an electric range, for example, will consume more fuel than if food is prepared in an electrical appliance such as an electric frypan. It is interesting to contemplate possible changes in food patterns because of this limitation.

Education of the homemaker or the person responsible for family meals has an impact on the nutritional status of the family. Young and others[5] reported that the level of educational attainment appeared to be consistently related to adequate performance in family

[5] Charlotte M. Young, Kathleen Heresford, and Betty Greer Waldner, "What the Homemaker Knows About Nutrition, 1. Description of Studies in Rochester and Syracuse, New York; 2. Level of Nutritional Knowledge; 3. Relation of Knowledge to Practice; 4. Her Food Problems, Shopping Habits, and Sources of Information," *Journal of the American Dietetic Association*, Vol. 32, Nos. 3–5: March 1956, pp. 214–222; (April 1956, pp. 321–326; May 1956, pp. 429–434.

feeding. The effect of income level was considerably less consistent and of smaller magnitude. The actual performance of the homemaker in feeding her family was considerably better than her theoretical knowledge of what to feed them. However, the food groups about which the homemaker's knowledge was the weakest were the most poorly used, such as citrus fruits, tomatoes, and cabbage; green, leafy, and yellow vegetables; and milk, cheese, and ice cream.

Factors Influencing Planning

For each individual and in each family, a unique set of influences affects the way dietary intake is planned. First, there is the emotional attitude—a concern about nutritious food. Another facet is knowledge about nutrition. These two components do much to assure good nutrition.

Cultural influences cannot be disregarded. The religion, the nationality background, and past or present regional influences are important. Fast days, feast days, family celebrations, patriotic or other holidays, and family likes and dislikes in food must all be considered.

The composition of the family is another possible influence. Is it a young couple? Are there a number of small children? Are there teen-agers in the family? Do older relatives, such as grandparents, reside in the home? Do workmen, such as helpers on a farm, eat with the family? Is it a single person or several unrelated persons sharing a home or an apartment? Is it a commune of 20 persons? The situation and the number of persons involved as well as their lifestyle must be taken into consideration. The amounts and types of foods to be served, as well as the preparations needed, will influence meal planning. Some modification of the diet for illness or chronic conditions, such as allergies, may be required (see Chapter 32).

Where the family, individual, or group eats is important. All meals are not eaten in the home. The trend to outdoor eating and cooking increases each year. Eating out, especially, in fast-food restaurants, has become very popular.

The part of the country in which the family lives will also influence meal plans. Although food is distributed more widely than ever before, there are certain regional influences. A family living in California or Florida, for example, will have greater access to many semitropical fruits and vegetables, whereas a family living in the New England states may have more seafoods. Wherever an American family lives there will be some typical regional foods that will influence the planning of meals.

A working mother who must leave earlier in the morning than her children has a real problem in planning breakfast. The same situation may be true of other meals. When children come home to lunch and their mothers are away at work, there must be considerable planning on the part of both the children and the mother to meet this situation. A father or a mother may work at night and sleep in the daytime, and this, too, may cause very serious adjustment problems as far as family meals are concerned.

The values that people place upon food cannot be overlooked. Some families feel, for example, that certain foods must appear on the table at certain times. In some households, pancakes or waffles are always served for the Sunday breakfast. The kind of foods served for holidays is another example. Having a well-set table with plenty of food may be another value.

Time is one of the most important factors to be considered in planning meals. Surveys show that women are extremely interested in quick ways to prepare meals that are tasty and attractive. This objective demands careful analysis and planning of the time required for the various steps in meal preparation.

Effect on Nutritive Values of Certain Food Preparation Techniques

Even though homemakers have every intention of feeding their families nutritious meals, what is done during the preparation of the meal may seriously dilute nutritive values. Soaking food in water for long periods of time will dissolve water-soluble vitamins. Cubing, crushing, mashing, chopping, grinding, and blending foods exposes greater food surface to oxidation and vitamins may be lost. Foods requiring such processing should be prepared as close to the cooking or serving time as possible.

The practice of preparing food hours before serving means the loss of vitamins and less palatable food. Warming up food should be done quickly in order to retain as many vitamins as possible. Storing foods like meats, fresh green vegetables, and fruit juices in the refrigerator keeps loss of vitamins at a minimum.

Effect on Nutritive Value of Different Types of Cooking Methods

Cooking may improve the taste of food; it also softens fibers and connective tissue, and it may be a safeguard against disease-producing organisms. Therefore, when the person planning the family meal decides on the foods to be served, she must then plan on the best way of cooking those foods to retain their nutritive values.

Baking and roasting—cooking with dry heat —are considered among the best methods for the retention of nutritive values of food, particularly if cooked at the proper temperature and not overcooked. Broiling and pan broiling are other dry-heat cooking methods that tend to preserve nutrients to a high degree.

Boiling can be quite destructive of water-soluble vitamins, especially if the boiling is prolonged. Cooking in small amounts of water for short periods of time will alleviate the destruction to a greater degree. Braising consists of browning a food in a small amount of fat and completing the cooking by simmering in a small amount of water or other liquid. Fat- and water-soluble vitamins may be lost unless the cooking liquid is consumed. Steaming is the process of cooking in a perforated pan over boiling water. Nutritive values are retained very well if cooking is not prolonged.

Pan frying or sauteing is cooking food in a small amount of fat. If green or yellow vegetables are pan fried, some fat-soluble vitamins may be lost, particularly if the cooking is overdone. Meat, other vegetables, and rice or corn may be satisfactorily cooked in this manner

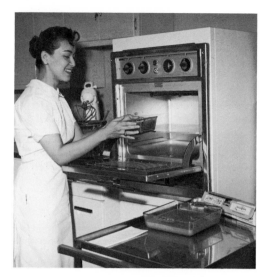

FIGURE 29–4.   *Electronic cookery retains nutritive values because it requires such a short period of cooking.* (Home Economic Department, New York University)

and nutritive values retained if the temperature is controlled and food is not overcooked. Deep-fat frying has somewhat the same effect on food nutrients as pan frying. The temperature is higher, but the cooking period is usually shorter.

Electronic cooking is done in a small oven or range by means of microwaves. The time of cooking is greatly reduced. Research indicates that nutritive values are well retained. Cooking foods in a pressure cooker compares favorably with other methods of cooking in regard to retention of nutrients. Because of the high temperature produced by raising the pressure, overcooking even for a short period of time has a greater impact on nutritive losses than overcooking by other methods.

Steps in Meal Planning

Appropriate Foods

Hill[6] suggests that the planner become familiar with the nutritive contribution of the

---

[6] Mary M. Hill, "Food Guides—Where Do We Go from Here?" *Nutrition Program News*, March–April 1973, pp. 1–8.

basic four food groups as background to planning. An overview of the groups with recommended amounts to consume, the foods included in a group, and their nutrient contributions, as outlined by Hill, are given here.

Milk and Milk Products

The foods included are fluid whole, evaporated and skim dry milk, and buttermilk; cottage cheese, cream cheese, and Cheddar-type natural or processed cheese; and ice cream. Some milk everyday is recommended for everyone. Recommended amounts are given below in terms of whole fluid milk:

	8-oz cup (240 cc)
Children under 9	2 to 3
Children 9 to 12	3 or more
Teen-agers	4 or more
Adults	2 or more
Pregnant women	3 or more
Nursing mothers	4 or more

Part or all of the milk may be fluid skim milk, buttermilk, evaporated milk, or dry milk. Cheese and ice cream may replace part of the milk. The amount required to replace a given quantity of milk is figured on the basis of calcium content. Common portions of various kinds of cheese and ice cream and their milk equivalents in calcium nutrient density are as follows:

1-inch cube of Cheddar-type cheese	= ½ cup of milk
½ cup of cottage cheese	= ⅓ cup of milk
2 tablespoons of cream cheese	= 1 tablespoon of milk
½ cup of ice cream or ice milk	= ⅓ cup of milk

NUTRIENT CONTRIBUTION   Milk is the leading source of calcium. It is almost impossible to meet allowances for calcium if milk is not included in the diet. This food group also contributes a good supply of phosphorus, magnesium, high-quality protein, vitamin B_6, and vitamin B_{12}. Milk and its products are excellent sources of riboflavin.

Fruits and Vegetables

All vegetables and fruits are included. This guide emphasizes those that are valuable as sources of vitamin C and vitamin A. Four or more servings every day are recommended, including one serving of a good source of vitamin C, or two servings of a fair source; one serving, at least every other day, of a good source of vitamin A. If the food chosen for vitamin C is also a good source of vitamin A, the additional serving of a vitamin A food may be omitted. The remaining one to three or more servings may be of any vegetable or fruit, including those that are valuable for vitamin C and vitamin A. Count the following as one serving: ½ cup of vegetable or fruit, or a portion as ordinarily served, such as one medium apple, banana, orange, or potato, half a medium grapefruit or cantaloupe, or the juice of one lemon.

Good sources of vitamin C are grapefruit or grapefruit juice, cantaloupes, guava, mangoes, papaya, raw strawberries, broccoli, brussels sprouts, green peppers, and sweet peppers.

Fair sources are honeydew melons, lemons, tangerines or tangerine juice, watermelons, asparagus tips, raw cabbage, cauliflower, collards, garden cress, kale, kohlrabi, mustard greens, potatoes and sweet potatoes cooked in the jacket, rutabagas, spinach, tomatoes or tomato juice, and turnip greens.

Good sources of vitamin A are liver, whole milk, fortified skim milk, butter, fortified margarine, cheese made with whole milk, dark-green and deep-yellow vegetables, and deep-yellow fruits.

NUTRIENT CONTRIBUTION   Fruits are relied on to furnish nearly all the vitamin C of the diet and over one half of the vitamin A that is needed. This food group is an excellent source of fiber.

Bread and Cereals

All breads and cereals that are whole grain, enriched, or restored are included; check labels to be sure. Specifically, this group includes breads, cooked cereals, ready-to-eat cereals, cornmeal, crackers, flour and grits, macaroni and spaghetti, noodles, rice, rolled oats, and quick breads and other baked goods, if made with whole-grain or enriched flour. Parboiled rice and wheat may also be included in this group. Four or more servings daily are recommended; if no cereals are used, have an extra serving of breads or baked goods. This will make at least five servings from this group daily. Count as one serving one slice of bread, 1 oz ready-to-eat cereal, ½ to ¾ cup of cooked cereal, cornmeal, grits, macaroni, noodles, rice, or spaghetti.

NUTRIENT CONTRIBUTION   The major contributions of this group are to iron, thiamin, riboflavin, niacin, protein, phosphorus, magnesium, and kcalorie allowances.

Meat or Alternatives

This group includes beef, veal, lamb, pork, variety meats such as liver, hearts, and kidneys; poultry and eggs; fish and shellfish; and as alternatives, dry beans, dry peas, lentils, nuts, peanuts, and peanut butter. Two or more servings every day are recommended. Count as one serving 2 to 3 oz (not including bone weight) cooked lean meat, poultry, or fish. As alternates for ½ serving of meat or fish, substitute one egg, ½ cup of cooked dry beans, dry peas, or lentils, or 2 tablespoons peanut butter.

NUTRIENT CONTRIBUTIONS   The most valuable contributions of this food group are to protein, niacin, vitamin B_6, and vitamin B_{12} allowances. Almost as valuable are the contributions to iron, phosphorus, thiamin, riboflavin, kcalories, and vitamin A allowances. Considerable input to the magnesium allowances is made.

Use of the Basic Four

Fortified with knowledge of the basic four food groups, the next step is to combine these foods to meet individual and family nutritive needs. One way to begin is to make a schedule of usual eating times and then to allocate representative foods of the basic four among the time slots in a manner that is compatible to food preferences, cost, availability of food, and other factors that have an impact on the way a person eats. Following is a menu that follows the guide and may represent a somewhat traditional lifestyle. Other foods usually have to be added to maintain weight.

A Day's Food Intake for an Adult

Based on specific amounts per serving as designated in daily food guide

BREAKFAST
Orange juice, ½ cup
Cold cereal, ½ cup
Milk for cereal, ½ cup
Whole-wheat or enriched toast, with butter or margarine and jam, 1 slice
Coffee

MIDMORNING SNACK
Small Danish
Cocoa with ½ cup of milk

LUNCH
Tunafish salad sandwich with lettuce and olive, 1
Milk, 1 cup
Apple, 1

DINNER
Baked ham, 3 oz
Baked sweet potato, 1 medium
String beans with onion, ½ cup
Tossed salad with salad dressing, ½ cup
Dinner roll and butter, 1
Pineapple sherbet, ½ cup
Coffee

BEDTIME SNACK
Crackers and peanut butter or cheese
Carbonated beverage

Making choices from a wide variety of foods and from all four food groups leads to a greater assurance of a nutritious diet. Energy needs can be evaluated according to weight of the individual. If a weight gain becomes obvious, food intake may have to be reduced. If the individual is still growing, it is sensible to cut back on the foods not included in the basic foods but in foods such as salad dressings, sugars, and the like. In contrast, if weight is being lost, more food is required. A checkup by a physician may be in order.

Evalation of the Nutritional Foundation of the Preceding Day's Diet for an Adult

MILK GROUP 2 SERVINGS	FRUIT–VEGETABLE GROUP 4 SERVINGS	MEAT OR ALTERNATIVES 2 SERVINGS	BREAD–CEREAL (ENRICHED) 4 SERVINGS
½ Cup on cereal	½ Cup orange juice	Tunafish (in sandwich)	½ Cup cold cereal
1 Cup at lunch	Baked sweet potato	3-oz Baked ham	1 Slice toast
½ Cup in cocoa	½ Cup string beans		2 Slices bread in sandwich
	1 Serving tossed green salad		

Foods That Provide Additional Nutrients and Kcalories in Preceding Adult Diets

FOODS FROM THE FOUR BASIC FOOD GROUPS	OTHER FOODS
Seconds from the basic foods: 1 Apple Lettuce and olive with sandwich Pineapple sherbet Crackers and peanut butter Milk in coffee Dinner roll	Butter or margarine on toast and roll Sugar in coffee Small danish Rest of cocoa Salad dressing in sandwich and salad Carbonated beverage

In the planning of the daily diet, individuals are encouraged to be as creative and flexible as possible. The servings indicated for each of the four basic food groups are minimal and extra amounts, if feasible and desired, may be included. An attempt should be made to have a balance among the basic four groups every time an individual eats. Make a habit of it. In this way, there is greater assurance of adequate nutrition. For the scientific-minded young person, actual calculation of nutrients may be the answer. Using a small calculator may be an incentive. Haphazard selection may lead to a choice of foods with low nutrient density. A challenge to a cosmopolitan attitude toward eating is offered—a willingness to try new foods, to be alert to new products or foods of other ethnic groups. Developing a taste for unfamiliar foods increases the variety of foods in the diet. Flexibility should be encouraged. Some families, individuals, or groups eat dinner in the morning and have breakfast at night. Others plan five or six small nutritious meals around their schedule. Meals may be at home or eaten out or a combination of both. Drinking breakfast is possible for folks in a hurry. Sensible use of vending machines may be helpful. The goal is to plan meals that are acceptable and satisfying to the person or persons who eat them and the development of food habits to the extent that the nutritive quality of foods are considered in all choices.

Effect of Lifestyles

It would be difficult to find two individuals or two families who consumed the same food each day. Even within a family, members eat more or less of certain foods and even ignore certain foods. Because it is impossible to describe the broad spectrum of lifestyle, several

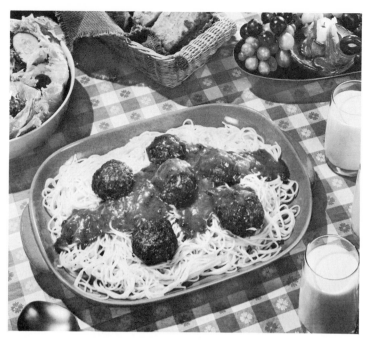

FIGURE 29–5. *A simple and nutritious dinner.* (*Lawry's Foods, Inc.*)

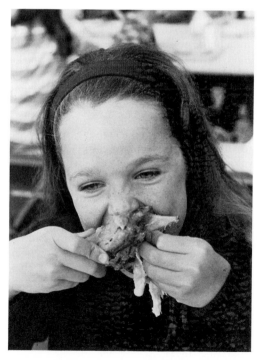

FIGURE 29–6. *Eating has become more casual.* (USDA)

examples have been selected for discussion. A daily menu for a somewhat traditional lifestyle has been analyzed previously in this chapter.

Vegetarians

At the present time there is a phenomenal upsurge of interest in vegetarianism in America, especially among the young adults. Many colleges have adapted menus especially for this group. Vegetarian restaurants have become quite popular. The number of vegetarians in the nation is uncertain, but there is an estimate of 6 million and the number is rapidly growing. Vegetarianism at one time was considered a bizarre idea but today it is widely acceptable.[7]

Individuals become vegetarians for a variety of reasons. Generally there is a single motivating force but it may be blended with other influences. The Trappist monks, for example,

[7] Lydia Sonnenberg, Kathleen Zolber, and U. D. Register, *Food for Us All, The Vegetarian Diet*, A Study Kit, American Dietetic Association, Chicago, 1973.

have practiced the use of this diet for many years because it was thought to be becoming to their simple mode of life. The Seventh Day Adventists have health and educational programs that encourage well-balanced vegetarian diets that include milk and eggs and are based on their interpretation of the Bible. Studies show that they have good health and longevity. Some of the Oriental religions believe in the transmigration of souls and the sacredness of animal life. Some of their eccentric food choices may be questionable for health purposes.

The new vegetarians, according to Erhard,[8] are identified as the initiators of a major movement underway in United States and Canada to revive vegetarianism as a way of eating. Sometimes it has not been recognized because attention was focused on the religions that are associated with these lifestyles. Erhard suggest that there may be millions who are following this regime and the commitment seems to be sincere. Their beliefs include the ideas that ethically the highest purpose in life is spiritual development, so all life is sacred; that the slaughtering of animals is degrading; that economically it takes less than 1 acre of land to produce food for a vegetarian diet but at least twice as much land for a meat-eating person's food; animal flesh contains toxins, bacteria, too much uric acid, and other undesirable ingredients; and, finally, the vegetarian way of eating is ecologically sound. A rebellion against additives, pesticides, manufactured foods, and other unnatural foods is evident. Health foods, organic foods, and natural foods in contrast are prized.

Some of the new vegetarians select foods for their spiritual value rather than their nutritive value. Exotic foods such as burdock root, adzuki beans, and brown rice are included in their diet. Selections are made in health stores from open bins of beans, pasta, grains, nuts, and seeds. These foods are usually much more expensive than regular supermarket fare although these markets also have special health food shelves. Spoilage is a problem. Cooking has become a ritual and the

kitchen an important place. A number of vegetarians have fled to rural areas, established communes, and produce much of their own food.

Johnson[9] studied the food habits of inhabitants of 10 communes in the Pacific Northwest and British Columbia. Judgments of desirable eating habits were made from observations and discussions during a short stay at each commune and are quantitative in nature only. The conviction on the whole that man should live as low on the food chain as possible was widely held, although one commune raised cattle for a livelihood. All groups had vegetable gardens, although about half of the communes had to supplement their production with outside purchases. Most used root cellars and canned and frozen food for off-harvest months. Only one community was strictly vegetarian; most groups had goats, cows, or some access to raw milk. Half of the groups raised chickens or ducks for egg production. Johnson concluded that at least six of the communes were successful in providing adequate nutrition for their participants. Three groups were inconsistent in their protein intake and one group appeared to be seriously deficient in their protein intake. Large amounts of vegetables, fruits, and fresh wholegrain bread were consumed. Breast-feeding of infants was universal. Little obesity was observed. Although a limited sample, this study gave some insight into food habits of members of various communes.

Horton[10] visited 43 communes from coast to coast and made interesting practical observations that might make excellent tentative hypotheses for further research in this area. A concern with food, the art of cooking, and the science of natural diet had high interest for the members of these communes. Vegetables were the focus of their diet, followed second in importance with grains. These simple ingredients were served in unusual combinations and flavors. Mexican, East Indian, Japanese, Chinese, Tibetan, Israelia, Turkish,

[8] Darla Erhard, "The New Vegetarians," *Nutrition Today*, Vol. 8, No. 6 (November–December 1973), pp. 4–12.

[9] Charley M. Johnson, "Nutrition and Contemporary Communal Living," *Journal of the American Dietetic Association*, Vol. 63, No. 3 (September 1973), pp. 275–276.

[10] Lucy Horton, *Country Commune Cooking*, Coward, McCann & Geoghegan, New York, 1972.

Armenian, North African, Ugandian, Italian, Danish, Swedish, Jewish, Hungarian, Russian, English, and American foods were represented among the various communes. Communes in the west adhere more strongly to vegetarianism than in the Middle West or the East. The rigors of winter in New England and the high country of the Southwest may make meat more appealing to commune members in those areas.

Suggested Vegetarian Menus and Analyses

A menu with the Hill[11] format and analysis for a lacto-ovo-vegetarian diet for an adult follows:

MORNING MEAL
Orange juice, 4 oz
Cooked oatmeal with dates ½ cup
Milk, ½ cup
Whole-wheat toast, 2 slices with 2 tablespoons peanut butter, and molasses or honey
Coffee (some prefer cereal-based beverage)

[11] Hill, op. cit., pp. 7–8.

MAIN MEAL (NOON OR EVENING)
Soyburger (meat analog)
Potato, boiled in skin, with sour cream
Broccoli, cooked, served with lemon
Shredded carrot and raisin salad with oil and vinegar
1 slice rye bread with margarine
Berry cobbler
Grape juice or coffee

LUNCH OR SUPPER
Goulash[a] with pinto beans and tomatoes, spaghetti, soy sauce oil, onions
Sliced tomatoes (1 medium tomato) with chopped egg salad dressing
Fruit cup, ½ cup, fruits in season
Bread and margarine (if needed)

SNACK
Milk, ½ cup combined with cereal-based beverage, nuts, and dried apricots (⅓ cup)

Note: This menu is appropriate also for a lacto-vegetarian diet without the chopped egg salad dressing.
[a] Recipe in Sonnenberg, Zolber, and Register, op. cit., p. 40.

Evaluation of the Nutritional Foundation of the Preceding Day's Lacto-ovo-vegetarian Diet for an Adult

MILK GROUP 2 SERVINGS	FRUIT–VEGETABLE GROUP 4 SERVINGS	MEAT AND ALTERNATES 2 SERVINGS	BREAD–CEREAL (ENRICHED) 4 SERVINGS
½ Cup on cereal 1 Cup for lunch or supper ½ Cup for snack	Orange juice, 4 oz Fruit cup, ½ cup Broccoli, ½ cup Sliced tomato, 1 medium	Soyburger, 1 Goulash (2 servings)	Oatmeal 2 Slices whole-wheat toast 1 Slice rye bread

Foods That Provide Additional Nutrients Plus Kcalories in Preceding Lacto-ovo-vegetarian Diet for an Adult

FOODS FROM THE FOUR BASIC FOOD GROUPS	OTHER FOODS
Seconds from the foundation foods: Dates in oatmeal Potato Berries in cobbler Grape juice Carrot and raisin salad Lemon on broccoli Nuts Dried apricots ⅓ Egg in salad dressing	Rest of cobbler Sour cream Salad dressing Bread at evening meal (if eaten) Molasses or honey Margarine Oil and vinegar

Evaluation of the Nutritional Foundation of the Following Day's Strict Vegetarian Diet for an Adult

MILK GROUP 2 SERVINGS	FRUIT–VEGETABLE GROUP 4 SERVINGS	MEAT AND ALTERNATES 2 SERVINGS	BREAD–CEREAL (ENRICHED) 4 SERVINGS
Fortified soy milk, midmorning, 1 cup Fortified soy milk, lunch or supper, 1 cup (Not a complete substitute Only one fourth as much calcium, one third as much riboflavin, and one half as much vitamin B$_{12}$[a] as cow's milk)	Orange juice, 4 oz Collards, ½ cup Fruit, 1 piece Apple and nut salad, 1 serving	Chick-peas Sunflower seeds	Granola, ½ cup Whole wheat bread, Potato–soy bread, 1 slice

[a] Sonnenberg, Zolber, and Register, op. cit., p. 43.

The items in this menu may be reallocated into other time slots to make fewer or more meals. Substitutions may be made with alternative foods within a basic four food group in keeping with food preferences.

A menu and analysis follows for a strict total or pure vegetarian diet without milk or eggs for an adult:

MORNING MEAL
Orange juice, 4 oz
Granola with ½ cup fortified soy milk

MIDMORNING
Potato–soy toast with margarine and jam, 1 slice
Fortified soy milk, 1 cup

MAIN MEAL
(noon or evening)
Chick-peas with rice (two 1-cup servings)
Collards, ½ cup
Apple and nut salad with French dressing
Date bread with margarine
Cereal-based beverage or fruit juice

LUNCH OR SUPPER
Split pea Soup, 1 cup
Peanut butter (2 tbs) and sliced cucumber sandwich on whole wheat, 2 slices
Tossed green salad with oil and vinegar
Fruit in season, 1 piece
Fortified soy milk, 1 cup

SNACK
Sunflower seeds, 3½ oz (100 g)

Foods That Provide Additional Nutrients in the Preceding Strict Vegetarian Diet for an Adult

FOODS FROM THE FOUR BASIC FOOD GROUPS	OTHER FOODS
Second servings of foundation foods: 2 Tbs peanut butter 1 Cup split pea soup ½ Cup fortified soy milk Cucumbers in sandwich Date bread Rice	Margarine French dressing Oil and vinegar Jam Cereal-based beverage or fruit juice

Nutritional Evaluation of Vegetarian Diets

There are a number of shortcomings in the pure vegetarian diet, according to Raper and Hill.[12] Vitamin B$_{12}$ is found only in animal sources so a vitamin preparation for a supplement may be necessary to provide this dietary need or foods fortified with vitamin B$_{12}$. Calcium is another nutrient of which there is a short supply because of a lack of milk. Great emphasis must be placed on certain dark-green vegetables—collards, dandelion greens, kale,

[12] Nancy R. Raper and Mary M. Hill, "Vegetarian Diets," *Nutrition Reviews*, Supplement (July 1974), pp. 29–33.

mustard greens, and turnip greens. One cup or 200 g of broccoli yields 206 mg of calcium; turnip greens, 490 mg; and the average of greens (dandelion, mustard, broccoli, Brussels sprouts, kale, and collards) is 305 mg of calcium, according to Sonnenberg, Zolber, and Register.[13] One cup of cow's milk contains 234 mg of calcium and 1 cup of soy milk contains 60 mg unless fortified. However, children, adolescents, and pregnant and lactating women should have milk if possible because of their greater need for this nutrient.

Adequate riboflavin is another problem without milk or meat in the diet. Green-leafy vegetables, asparagus, broccoli, Brussels sprouts, okra, and winter squash are good sources, but the amount of bulk to be eaten to acquire riboflavin and other nutrients may be difficult for an individual to handle, especially children. The quality of vegetable protein sources does not rate as highly as animal sources. Meat, milk, and eggs contain amino acids in the proportion as needed by the body. The assortment of amino acids in fruit, vegetables, and grains is not as good as in animal protein.

Supplementation of proteins requires a special knowledge, but is valuable. Generally speaking, combinations of legumes and cereals, such as beans and corn, beans with rice, and peanuts with wheat, are good. They do not have to be combined in the same dish but must be eaten at the same meal. Meat analogs made from textured vegetable protein, usually soybean, to resemble various meats will add variety to the diet but may not be equivalent to the meats they resemble in the quality of protein, vitamin, or mineral content. Some products contain egg white or nonfat dry milk, so individuals on a pure vegetarian diet must check the labels to determine this information. As in all diets, a wide variety of foods gives greater promise of an adequate diet.

Nutritional Status of Vegetarians

Individual total vegetarians from many populations of the world have maintained

seemingly excellent health according to the Committee on Nutritional Misinformation, Food and Nutrition Board.[14] If foods are carefully selected, diets can be nutritionally adequate. Harding and Stare[15] studied 200 subjects in three dietary groups: nonvegetarian, lacto-ovo-vegetarian, and total vegetarian. No evidence of deficiency was found and the nutrient intake of each group equaled or exceeded the recommended dietary allowances of the National Research Council, with the exception of vitamin B_{12} which was low in the total vegetarian diet. If the study had been continued longer, no doubt these subjects would have developed anemia, due to the lack of this vitamin. More attention must be given to the planning of the total vegetarian diet than if foods of animal origin are included. The risk becomes greater if dependence is placed on a single plant food, usually a cereal grain or starchy root crop. Special attention must be given to the amount and quality of protein, riboflavin, vitamin B_{12}, calcium, and possibly vitamin D.

Among the "new vegetarians" there is some evidence of malnutrition among infants, children, and pregnant and lactating women.[16] A knowledge of nutrition is lacking among many of the members of these groups so that they do not have competency in planning adequate diets. Dwyer[17] and others interviewed 100 urban American young adults who were vegetarians; none were Seventh Day Adventists. Red meat was universally avoided by all participants, poultry was usually the second avoid-

[13] Sonnenberg, Zolber, and Register, op. cit., p. 43.

[14] Committee on Nutritional Misinformation, Food and Nutrition Board, Division of Biological Sciences, Assembly of Life Sciences, *Vegetarian Diets*, National Academy of Sciences—National Research Council, Washington, D.C., May 1974.

[15] Mervyn G. Harding and Frederick J. Stare, "Nutritional Studies of Vegetarians," *Journal of Clinical Nutrition*, Vol. 2, No. 2 (March–April 1954), pp. 73–82.

[16] "A Starved Child of the New Vegetarians," *Nutrition Today*, Vol. 8, No. 6 (November–December 1973), pp. 10–12.

[17] Johanna T. Dwyer, Laura D. V. H. Mayer, Randy Frances Kandel, and Jean Mayer, "The New Vegetarians," *Journal of the American Dietetic Association*, Vol. 62, No. 5 (May 1973), pp. 503–509.

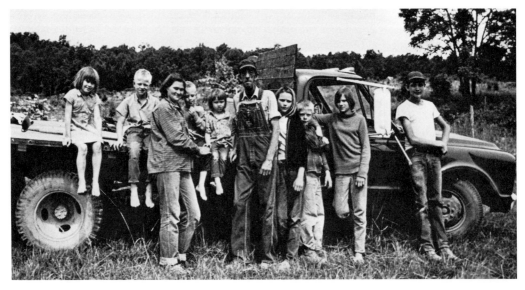

FIGURE 29–7. *Many needy families, such as these migrant workers, have to cope with the problem of planning for adequate food to meet their needs. (National Institute of Child Health, U.S. Department of Labor)*

ance, and fish and seafood were the third most commonly eliminated animal food. There was considerable difference among the subjects in their interpretation of vegetarianism. Weight loss was greater for men on this regime than for women, greater among the men with extreme animal food avoidances, and greatest if other nonanimal foods were also avoided. From their histories there was evidence of use of drugs, alcohol, or cigarettes. Being on a vegetarian diet encouraged some to drop the use of these substances. Variation among subjects ranged from semivegetarians who avoided only a few animal foods to vegans, who not only avoided all sources of animal foods but added other nonanimal foods to the list.

The Poor

Adults who are poor have to cope with the discouraging problem of providing adequate food. Their difficulty is compounded because these adults are often responsible for many children. Birch and Gussow[18] indicate that

low-income families with surviving children were almost two and a half times as likely to have six or more children than a high-income family. In addition to poverty incomes, folklore, ignorance about nutrition, and myths have a damaging influence on food choices. Poverty, however, is the basic factor that prompts inadequate diets. Some families consume limited, monotonous, and malnutrition-prone diets all of their lives, and their children continue the pattern when they establish their families.

The government has a number of nutrition and feeding programs as described in Chapter 23, but, unfortunately, all the needy are not reached. Education must be an integral part of these programs, as demonstrated by the success in the Expanded Food and Nutrition Programs of state extension services under the supervision of the U.S. Department of Agriculture. Target populations are the hard-to-reach rural and urban poor families. Paraprofessionals from the communities involved are employed as aides on the assumption that their backgrounds are more relevant to the

---

[18] Herbert G. Birch and Joan Dye Gussow, *Disadvantaged Children, Health, Nutrition, and* *School Failure*, Harcourt Brace Jovanovich, New York, 1970, pp. 85, 91, 150–152.

people served than most professionals.[19] Some nutrition programs have been sponsored by the Center for Disease Control of the Department of Health, Education, and Welfare in Atlanta, Georgia, for migrant families whose need for food and education is critical.[20]

A few pointers are given on the selection of foods from each of the basic four food groups.[21]

MILK GROUP

1. Nonfat dry milk and evaporated are the least expensive.
2. Cream is expensive so substitute whipped evaporated or nonfat dry milk. These foods are more nutritious.
3. Use less expensive cheese such as processed cheese.

MEAT GROUP

1. Dried beans and peas and peanut butter can be used in hearty dishes
2. Nutritive values of ground beef, liver, heart, and kidney are good, and cost is lower.
3. Locally caught fish, canned fish flakes (such as mackerel), and frozen fillets are often good buys.
4. Combine meat with macaroni, spaghetti, noodles, rice, legumes, or plentiful seasonal vegetables as extenders.

FRUIT AND VEGETABLE GROUP

1. Fresh vegetables that are plentiful and seasonal are usually the best buys.
2. Compare the cost of frozen spinach and other green vegetables with the price of fresh.
3. Cabbage, potatoes, and root vegetables are usually good buys.

4. Canned tomatoes may be a better buy and have higher vitamin C content than out-of-season tomatoes.
5. Canned greens, pumpkin, and green beans are often good buys.
6. Canned vegetables may cost less than frozen.
7. For most of the season frozen orange juice is cheaper than fresh.

BREADS AND CEREALS

1. Plain bread and rolls are cheaper than sweet and fancy-shaped varieties.
2. Buy enriched cereals and breads.
3. Day-old bread is a bargain.
4. Homemade bread and cookies are usually cheaper.

Special attention must be given to nutritious preparation and storage of food as well as the use of leftovers.

Drug Users

The use of drugs, a kind of social system, has an important influence on the lifestyle of some youth and adults as well as on their nutritional and health status. Washburn[22] states that malnutrition is prevalent among drug addicts, regardless of economic status, geographic location, religion, or ethnic background. Reasons cited for malnutrition were lack of proper food habits and inhibition by drugs of the central nervous system mechanisms that control appetite and hunger. A low-grade hypoglycemia is present, resulting in weight loss, anxiety, and irritability due to the stimulation or "euphoria" produced by drugs on the hypothalamic centers that regulate appetite. The frequent presence of liver disease (viral hepatitis) leads to the malfunctioning of trace elements that have been ingested with food. Progressive cell damage is the ultimate result. Some drugs may also increase nutritional needs.

The first step, according to Washburn, in the rehabilitation of an addict is to begin with

[19] Virginia Li Wang and Paul H. Ephross, "ENEP Evaluated," *Journal of Nutrition Education*, Vol. 2, No. 4 (Spring 1971), pp. 148–152.

[20] Lora Beth Larson and Donna M. Massoth, "A Nutrition Program for Texas Migrant Families," *Journal of Home Economics*, Vol. 65, No. 8 (November 1973), pp. 36–40.

[21] Evelyn B. Spindler, *Meal Planning*, Food and Nutrition, Supplemental Lessons for Training Extension Aides, Extension Service, U. S. Department of Agriculture, Washington, D.C., 1971.

[22] Alice B. Washburn, "Nutrition Counseling for Drug Addicts in Rehabilitation," *Journal of Nutrition Education*, Vol. 6, No. 1 (January–March 1974), pp. 13–15.

a diet containing adequate kcalories and nutrients to meet the recommended allowances. In-between nourishment is given to the addicts that are seriously debilitated. Drinking six to eight glasses of water daily is encouraged in addition to beverages served with meals. Nutrition education is valuable to addicts and helps to generate an interest in their own diet. This information is valuable when they return to society. Improved nutritional status is an important part of returning to health.

Another area related to the effect of drugs on nutrition are the drugs prescribed for ailments. Although little publicized, according to Roe,[23] the hazards of adverse side effects that interfere with the functioning of the body can be serious. Certain drugs are capable of producing nutritional deficiency diseases, decreased appetite, decreased absorption, increased excretion, or restricted utilization of certain nutrients. Amphetamines and similar stimulants may cause central depression of appetite, for example. Certain drugs form complexes with essential vitamins and are then excreted in the urine in amounts that may be sufficient to deplete body stores. This subject provides a challenge for further research and education for patients.

---

[23] Daphne A. Roe, "Nutritional Side Effects of Drugs," *Food and Nutrition News*, Vol. 45, No. 1 (October–November 1973), pp. 1, 4.

Other Lifestyles

There are many other styles of life that might be mentioned. The working wife or mother has an important management problem in planning nutritious meals, such as shopping for food, preparation, as well as juggling the food budget. Foods that may be used in other meals are helpful in cutting down preparation time. Securing the help of husband and children in these operations are other suggestions. Cutting down on the number of kinds of preparation for a meal, such as baking, broiling, and top-of-stove cooking all at the same time, saves energy and fuel.

The single person has the problem of finding foods that can be purchased in one- or two-serving packages. Eating alone may be boring, meals may be skipped, and consequently nutritional status is affected. "Pairing" of both sexes or opposite sexes or a group of individuals living together are lifestyles in which nutrition may not be considered important. The blending of food tastes and food preferences may be problems, as well as economic status. In all these situations, planning by the use of the basic four food groups is an excellent guide. Food intake should be evaluated regularly and adjustments made if necessary. Respect the importance of a plan, because no one is automatically well nourished.

SELECTED REFERENCES

Dwyer, Johanna T., Laura D. V. H. Mayer, Randy Francis Kandel, "Who Are They? The New Vegetarians?" *Journal of the American Dietetic Association*, Vol. 62, No. 5 (May 1973), pp. 503–509.

Erhard, Darla, "The New Vegetarians," Part One—Vegetarianism and Its Medical Consequences, *Nutrition Today*, Vol. 8, No. 6 (November–December 1973), pp. 4–12; Part Two—The Zen Macrobiotic and Other Cults Based on Vegetarianism, *Nutrition Today*, Vol. 9, No. 1 (January–February 1974), pp. 20–22.

———, "Nutrition Education for the 'Now' Generation," *Journal of Nutrition Education*, Vol. 2, No. 4 (Spring 1971), pp. 135–139.

Hansen, R. Gaurth, "An Index of Food Quality," *Nutrition Reviews*, Vol. 31, No. 1 (January 1973), pp. 1–7.

Hegsted, D. M., Philip L. White, and Robin Holab, "Nutrition Misinformation and Food Faddism," *Nutrition Reviews*, A Special Supplement (July 1974), entire issue.

Hill, Mary M., "Food Guides—Where Do We Go from Here?" *Nutrition Program News*, U.S. Department of Agriculture (March–April 1973), pp. 1–8.

Kinder, Faye, *Meal Management*, Macmillan Publishing Co., Inc., New York, 1973.

Leverton, Ruth M., "Nutritive Value of Organically Grown Foods," *Journal of the American Dietetic Association*, Vol. 62, No. 5 (May 1973), p. 501.

Lowenberg, Miriam E., "The Development of Food Patterns," *Journal of the American Dietetic Association*, Vol. 65, No. 3 (September 1974), pp. 263–268.

Marshall, William E., "Health Foods, Organic Foods, Natural Foods," *Food Technology*, Vol. 28, No. 2 (February 1974), pp. 50–51, 56.

Register, U. D., and L. M. Sonnenberg, "The Vegetarian Diet," *Journal of the American Dietetic Association*, Vol. 62, No. 3 (March 1973), pp. 253–261.

Shimoda, Naomi, "Observations of a Nutritionist in a Free Clinic," *Journal of the American Dietetic Association*, Vol. 63, No. 3 (September 1973), pp. 273–275.

Sonnenberg, Lydia, Kathleen Zolber, and U. D. Register, *Food for Us All, the Vegetarian Diet*, A Study Kit, The American Dietetics Association, Chicago, 1972.

Washburn, Alice B., "Nutrition Counseling for Drug Addicts in Rehabilitation," *Journal of Nutrition Education*, Vol. 6, No. 1 (January–March 1974), pp. 13–15.

Young, Charlotte M., "Effects of Frequency of Eating," *Food and Nutrition News*, Vol. 42, No. 8 (May 1971), pp. 1, 4.

30

Buying Food
for Good Nutrition

The buying of food has an important influence both on family health and on the family pocketbook. The amount of money spent, however, is no index to the food's nourishing qualities. A shopper must use considerable discrimination to select those foods that contribute the most nutrients to the daily diet and yet fulfill the many other requirements of the family's daily meals, such as likes, dislikes, or family traditions. The buying of food can be a bewildering and complex operation because shoppers have such a wide range of choice.

Impact of Social Changes
on Food Buying

There are a number of important trends that have contributed to changes in food-buying practices.[1] Changing lifestyles, such as more working women, greater emphasis on unisex roles, rather than strict adherence to masculine and feminine roles in food-marketing practices, and more meals eaten away from

home (many at fast-food places), are significant.

Americans who were accustomed to buying relatively inexpensive food in comparison to other countries have been beset with soaring prices. During 1973, according to U.S. Department of Agriculture data, food prices were boosted almost 20 per cent.[2] A significant change in food habits occurred because of these higher costs. Consumers turned to cheaper food. Buying became more selective. There was a decline in the buying of fresh meat, especially expensive beef cuts, and servings of meat became smaller. There was an increase in use of products such as spaghetti and macaroni.[3] The price of rice and beans, important food items in many low-income families, has risen even more sharply than many other foods. Some grocery items are taxed.

Food is no longer purchased solely in the traditional sense, such as a roasting chicken or fresh string beans, but frequently many services are built into the package, such as frozen

---

[1] David L. Call, "The Changing Food Market—Nutrition in a Revolution," *Journal of the American Dietetic Association*, Vol. 60, No. 5 (May 1972), pp. 384–388.

[2] "Why Grocery Bills Around the World Go Soaring," *U.S. News and World Report*, March 18, 1974, pp. 52–53.

[3] "Statistics Hint a Shift in Eating Habits," *The New York Times*, November 23, 1973, p. 18.

430

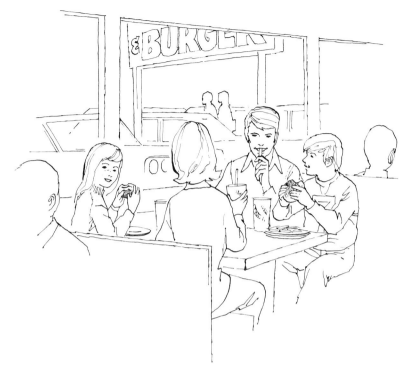

FIGURE 30–1. *More meals are eaten away from home.*

dinners, instant meals, brown and serve rolls, and a host of other conveniences. These services increase the food bill but the consumer may feel there are compensations.

Decisions must be made during food shopping from a wide variety of products. Factors such as quality, price, food value, eating enjoyment, and purpose must be considered in selection. Nutritional labeling, open dating, and unit pricing are helpful but the task is still formidable.

Nutrition and Other Aspects of Food Labeling

During the White House Conference on Food, Nutrition, and Health in December 1969, recommendations were made for increased nutrition information on food labeling. This culminated in the food-labeling regulations of the Food and Drug Administration, which were based on research studies and extensive discussions with members of the Food and Nutrition Board, the American Dietetic Association, the American Institute of Nutrition, and the American Home Economics Association. Six possible approaches to nutrition labeling were explored and finally reduced to three alternative labels. The results of public hearings and filed comments of the Food and Drug Administration were included. In the last stage five supermarket chains tested the labels.[4]

The two major purposes of nutrition labeling are (1) to improve nutritional information on food labels by the listing of nutrients through voluntary action by industry and (2) to make information on food labels more meaningful to the consumer through updating and improving past regulations of the Food and Drug Administration and through the presentation of new concepts in food labeling.

Nutrition labeling is voluntary for most

[4] Margaret L. Ross, "What's Happening to Food Labeling?" *Journal of the American Dietetic Association,* Vol. 64, No. 3 (March 1974), pp. 262–267.

foods. However, if a nutrient is added to any product, even to replace those lost in processing, or if a nutritional claim is made for this food in the labeling or in an advertisement, that product's label must have full nutrition labeling. For instance, if the label or advertisement makes any reference to kcalories, protein, fat, carbohydrate, vitamins, minerals, or use in dieting, the label must contain complete nutrition information. Foods that are normally sold as "enriched" or "fortified" would require nutrition labeling. Such foods are enriched flour or bread, fortified milk, fortified fruit juices, and diet foods.[5]

Regulations for nutrition labeling by the Food and Drug Administration require use of the following standard format: serving size or portion, for example, 1 oz of dry cereal or 1 cup of milk; servings per container, such as 4 servings for 1 quart of milk; kcaloric content or kcalories, expressed in the nearest 2-kcalorie increment up to and including 20 kcalories, in 5-kcalorie increments above 20 kcalories and up to and including 50 kcalories, and in 10-kcalorie increments above 50 kcalories; protein, carbohydrate, and fat to the nearest gram and the percentage of U.S. recommended dietary allowances (U.S. RDA). See Figure 30–1.

The U.S. RDA are based on the 1968 recommended dietary allowances for 1 day of the Food and Nutrition Board of the National Research Council by selecting the highest values for each nutrient for children over 4 years of age and adult males and females, exclusive of pregnancy and lactation. These same recommended dietary allowances were used for determing the U.S. RDA for infants and pregnant and lactating women. Table 30–1 lists the U.S. RDA for use in the labeling of foods, including foods that are also vitamin and mineral supplements. Note that the U.S. RDA for protein is 65 g for adults and 28 g for children under 4 years of age. However, if the protein efficiency ratio of the protein is equal or better than casein, U.S. RDA is 45 g for adults and 20 g for infants. See Table 30–2 for the percentage of the U.S. recommended daily al-

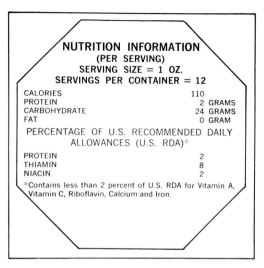

FIGURE 30–2. *Nutritional information on a label according to FDA regulations. (FDA Consumer Memo)*

lowance required to meet recommended dietary allowances for individuals by sex and age.

The lower part of the nutrition panel gives the percentages of the U.S. RDA of the mandatory nutrients, protein, vitamin A, vitamin C, thiamin, riboflavin, niacin, calcium, and iron.[6] Optional nutrients are vitamins D, E, B_6 and B_{12}, biotin, and pantothenic acid, folic acid, phosphorus, iodine, magnesium, zinc, and copper. These nutrients may be listed if they appear naturally in a food; listing is mandatory if any have been added to the food. If less than 2 per cent of the U.S. RDA of any of the nutrients is present, this may be indicated by a zero or an asterisk referring to another asterisk at the bottom of the panel followed by the statement "Contains less than 2 per cent of the U.S. RDA of these nutrients." If the food contains less than 2 per cent of the U.S. RDA of five or more of the eight mandatory nutrients, these need not be listed on the nutrition panel but a statement "Contains less than 2 per cent of the U.S. RDA of _____" and the list of the five or more nutrients is placed at the bottom of the nutrition panel.

Optional listings on the nutrition or in-

[5] *FDA Consumer Memo*, Public Health Service, Food and Drug Administration, U.S. Department of Health, Education, and Welfare, Washington, D.C., April 1973.

[6] "Food Labeling," *Dairy Council Digest*, Vol. 45, No. 2 (March–April 1974), pp. 7–12.

TABLE 30–1

U.S. Recommended Daily Allowances (U.S. RDA) for Use in Nutrition Labeling of Foods, Including Foods That Are Also Vitamin and Mineral Supplements

	ADULTS AND CHILDREN OVER 4 YEARS	INFANTS AND CHILDREN UNDER 4 YEARS
Protein	65 g[a]	28 g[a]
Vitamin A	5000 IU	2500 IU
Vitamin C	60 mg	40 mg
Thiamin	1.5 mg	0.7 mg
Riboflavin	1.7 mg	0.8 mg
Niacin	20 mg	9.0 mg
Calcium	1.0 g	0.8 g
Iron	18 mg	10 mg
Vitamin D	400 IU	400 IU
Vitamin E	30 IU	10 IU
Vitamin B_6	2.0 mg	0.7 mg
Folacin	0.4 mg	0.2 mg
Vitamin B_{12}	6 µg	3 µg
Phosphorus	1.0 g	0.8 g
Iodine	150 µg	70 µg
Magnesium	400 mg	200 mg
Zinc	15 mg	8.0 mg
Copper	2 mg	1.0 mg
Biotin	0.3 mg	0.15 mg
Pantothenic acid	10 mg	5 mg

SOURCE: "Nutrition Labels and U.S. RDA," *Facts from FDA*, DHEW Publication No. (FDA) 73–2042, Food and Drug Administration, Public Health Service, Department of Health, Education, and Welfare, Rockville, Md., 1973.

[a] If the protein efficiency ratio of protein is equal to or better than that of casein, U.S. RDA is 45 g for adults and 20 g for infants.

formation panels are the amount of sodium, fatty acids, or cholesterol in the food. This is helpful to individuals who have to restrict these substances on a physician's advice. Sodium is expressed in milligrams per 100 g. Cholesterol is stated in milligrams per serving or in milligrams per 100 g. The amounts of fats in grams per serving are listed in two categories: polyunsaturated and saturated. The total fat content as a percentage of the total calories in the foods should also be listed. If the cholesterol or fatty acid information is given, full nutrition information must also be provided and the label must contain the following statement: "Information on fat (and/or cholesterol) content is provided for individuals who, on the advice of a physician, are

modifying their total intake of fat (and/or cholesterol)." This is not to imply that the Food and Drug Administration is taking a position in the medical debate surrounding the role of fat in heart disease but is merely a service to consumers in their selection of food for fat-modified diets.

Regulations also include a standard of identity for supplements of vitamins and minerals that establishes criteria for a product to qualify for marketing as a dietary supplement. This category of products includes not only dietary supplements of vitamins and/or minerals prepared as tablets, capsules, wafers, or in liquid form, but also products in the form of conventional foods to which any nutrient has been added to the level of 50 per cent or

TABLE 30-2

Percentage of the U.S. Recommended Daily Allowance (Used in Nutrition Labeling) Needed to Meet the Recommended Dietary Allowance for Individuals by Age and Sex

ITEM	PRO-TEIN[a]	VITA-MIN A	VITA-MIN C (ascorbic acid)	B-VITAMINS			CAL-CIUM	IRON	FOOD ENERGY (calories)
				Thiamin	Riboflavin	Niacin[b]			
U.S. recommended daily allowance	100	100	100	100	100	100	100	100	—
Recommended dietary allowance:									
Years									
Child 4	46	50	67	53	53	28	80	56	1600
8	62	70	67	73	71	38	100	56	2200
Girl 14	85	100	83	80	82	40	130	100	2400
Boy 14	92	100	92	100	88	50	140	100	3000
Woman 25	85	100	92	67	88	32	80	100	2000
60	85	100	92	67	88	32	80	56	1700
Man 25	100	100	100	93	100	45	80	56	2800
60	100	100	100	80	100	35	80	56	2400

SOURCE: U.S. RDA, "Food Labeling," Federal Register, Vol. 38, No. 49, part II, March 14, 1973, and Recommended Dietary Allowances, 7th ed., Publication No. 1694, National Academy of Sciences—National Research Council, 1968. As quoted in Betty Peterkin, "Nutrition Labeling for the Consumer," Family Economics Review (Summer 1973), Table 1, p. 9.
[a] U.S. RDA of 65 g is used for this table. In labeling, a 45-g U.S. RDA is used for foods with high-quality protein such as milk, meat, and eggs.
[b] U.S. RDA is for preformed niacin only; RDA are for niacin equivalent—preformed niacin plus niacin equivalent from dietary tryptophan. In this table, one half the RDA was assumed to be from preformed niacin as occurs in the average U.S. diet.

NUTRITION INFORMATION
(PER SERVING)
SERVING SIZE = 8 OZ.
SERVINGS PER CONTAINER = 1

```
CALORIES  .....560     FAT  (PERCENT OF
PROTEIN  ....... 23 GM    CALORIES 53%) . 33 GM
CARBOHYDRATE . 43 GM      POLYUNSAT-
                           URATED*  ..  2 GM
                          SATURATED  ..  9 GM
                         CHOLESTEROL*
                         (20 MG/100 GM). 40 MG
                         SODIUM (365 MG/
                         100 GM)  .......830 MG
```

PERCENTAGE OF U.S. RECOMMENDED DAILY ALLOWANCES (U.S. RDA)

```
PROTEIN .............35   RIBOFLAVIN .........15
VITAMIN A ..........35    NIACIN .............25
VITAMIN C                 CALCIUM ............ 2
  (ASCORBIC ACID) ...10   IRON ...............25
THIAMIN (VITAMIN
  B₁) .............15
```

*Information on fat and cholesterol content is provided for individuals who, on the advice of a physician, are modifying their total dietary intake of fat and cholesterol.

FIGURE 30–3. *Nutritional information on a label about cholesterol, polyunsaturated and saturated fat, and sodium.* (FDA Consumer Memo)

more of the U.S. RDA per serving of any vitamin or mineral. These foods must comply both with the provisions established for dietary supplements and with nutritional labeling.

In general, if a product contains less than 50 per cent of the U.S. RDA for minerals and vitamins, it is not a dietary supplement and requires only nutrition labeling. If it contains 50 per cent to 150 per cent of the U.S. RDA, it is a dietary supplement and must meet the standard. If the product exceeds 150 per cent of the U.S. RDA, it cannot be sold as a food or as a dietary supplement but must be labeled and marketed as a drug.

There are certain exclusions from this category of products by the regulation. They are fabricated or conventional foods to which nutrients are added to a level less than 50 per cent of the U.S. RDA, food with nutrients restored to preprocessing levels or added so that the food is not nutritionally inferior to the food that it substitutes for and resembles, raw agricultural commodities, any food represented for use as the sole item of a meal or of a diet, foods the composition of which is defined by other statutes or regulations, other

standardized foods, and foods used under medical supervision. In addition, foods that are labeled dietary supplements must bear in their labeling the common name of the product plus a statement of the group (infants, children, adults, or pregnant/lactating women) for which it is intended. The label must include the list of nutrients, the percentages of U.S. RDA, and the natural or chemical form of each nutrient present. An expiration date must be given, if the product is subject to deterioration.[7]

Many foods do not have a listing of ingredients because they adhere to a standard of identity for that category of products. Many consumers were not familiar with the ingredients and expressed a desire to know them. Manufacturers, producers, and distributors are urged to disclose this information because the Food and Drug Administration does not have the statutory authority to require it.

Another regulation deals with common or unusual names for nonstandardized foods. The basic nature of the food or its characterizing properties or ingredients must be stated in accurate, simple, and direct terms. Common names, for example, have been established for such foods as seafood cocktail; crabmeat, in which the species of crab that may be included are identified; and diluted orange juice beverages in which the content of orange juice to the nearest 5 per cent must be stated along with a descriptive name (such as diluted orange juice).

Nutritional quality guidelines have been established for given classes of food. For example, for frozen heat-and-serve dinners there must be one or more sources of protein derived from meat, poultry, fish, cheese, or eggs. These sources, exclusive of gravies and sauces, must supply at least 70 per cent of the total protein in the dinner. Second, one or more vegetables or vegetable mixtures, other than potatoes, rice, or a cereal-based product, must be included. The third criterion is that the dinner contain rice, potatoes, or a cereal-based product. Table 30–3 indicates the quan-

[7] Nutrition Notes, "Nutrition Labeling 111," *Nutrition Reviews*, Vol. 31, No. 8 (August 1973), pp. 260–264.

TABLE 30–3

Nutritional Quality Guidelines for Heat-and-Serve Dinners

NUTRIENT	FOR EACH 100 KCALORIES OF THE TOTAL COMPONENTS	FOR THE TOTAL COMPONENTS
Protein, g	4.60	16.0
Vitamin A, IU	150.00	520.0
Thiamin, mg	0.05	0.2
Riboflavin, mg	0.06	0.2
Niacin, mg	0.99	3.4
Pantothenic acid, mg	0.32	1.1
Vitamin B_6, mg	0.15	1.1
Vitamin B_{12}, μg	0.33	1.1
Iron, mg	0.62	2.2

SOURCE: "Current and Useful Information from the Food and Drug Administration," *Facts from FDA*, DHEW Publication No. (FDA) 73–2036, Food and Drug Administration, Public Health Service, U.S. Department of Health, Education, and Welfare, Rockville, Md., 1973.

tities of nutrients for each 100 kcalories for the total of the three major components.

Shopping and Nutrition Labeling

A continuous education program on labeling appears imperative. Consumers may acquire a false sense of security of having an adequate diet if 100 per cent of each U.S. RDA of the eight mandatory nutrients is met, although additional nutrients are required which may or may not be listed on the label, such as vitamins B_6 and B_{12}, magnesium, zinc, folacin, phosphorus, and iodine—other recommended dietary allowances not included in the mandatory group.

If an individual emphasizes a high proportion of refined or fabricated foods in his daily diet, there may be other nutrient lacks. Certain nutrients, such as potassium, have not been included in the recommended dietary allowances. A human requirement has not been established for other nutrients. Fiber is not included in the U.S. RDA. Unidentified nutrients that may be present in refined foods will be missing. Through nutrition education, the importance of eating a wide variety of foods and depending upon whole foods such as milk, fruits, vegetables, eggs, whole-grain

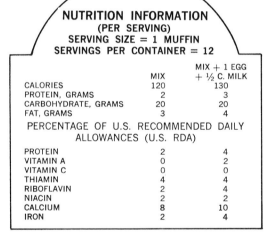

NUTRITION INFORMATION
(PER SERVING)
SERVING SIZE = 1 MUFFIN
SERVINGS PER CONTAINER = 12

	MIX	MIX + 1 EGG + ½ C. MILK
CALORIES	120	130
PROTEIN, GRAMS	2	3
CARBOHYDRATE, GRAMS	20	20
FAT, GRAMS	3	4

PERCENTAGE OF U.S. RECOMMENDED DAILY ALLOWANCES (U.S. RDA)

PROTEIN	2	4
VITAMIN A	0	2
VITAMIN C	0	0
THIAMIN	4	4
RIBOFLAVIN	2	4
NIACIN	2	2
CALCIUM	8	10
IRON	2	4

FIGURE 30–4. *Information on a label that is helpful to shoppers.* (FDA Consumer Memo)

cereals, and meat for basic nutritive needs should be highlighted.[8] See Table 30–4.

In 1959 an amendment was made to the Pure Food and Drug Law; it is known as the

---

[8] George M. Briggs, "Nutrition Education and the Food Labels," *Food and Nutrition News*, Vol. 44, No. 7 (April 1973), pp. 1, 4.

TABLE 30–4

Food Energy and Percentage of U.S. RDA for Eight Nutrients Provided by a Serving of Selected Foods[a]

FOOD[b]	SIZE OF SERVING (ready-to-eat)	FOOD ENERGY	PROTEIN	VITAMIN A	VITAMIN C (ascorbic acid)	B-VITAMINS			CALCIUM	IRON
						Thiamin	Riboflavin	Niacin[c]		
Milk, whole fluid	1 cup	160	20	6	4	4	25	—	30	—
Cheese, process cheddar	1 oz	110	15	6	0	—	8	—	20	—
Meat, poultry, fish (lean)	3 oz	220	50	15	—	10	15	25	—	15
Eggs	1 large	80	15	10	0	4	8	—	2	6
Dry beans	3/4 cup	230	20	2	6	10	4	6	15	20
Peanut butter	2 tbs	190	10	—	0	2	2	25	—	4
Bread, enriched	2 slices	140	6	—	—	8	6	6	4	6
Cereal, ready-to-eat[d]	1 oz	110	4	20	20	25	25	20	—	20
Citrus juice	1/2 cup	60	—	6	100	8	—	2	—	—
Other fruit, fruit juice	1/2 cup	60	—	6	15	2	2	2	—	4
Tomatoes, tomato juice	1/2 cup	25	—	20	35	4	2	4	—	4
Dark-green and deep-yellow vegetables	1/2 cup	45	4	140	40	6	6	4	6	6
Potatoes	medium	80	4	—	35	8	2	6	—	4
Other vegetables	1/2 cup	45	4	8	20	4	4	2	2	4
Butter, margarine	1 tbs	100	—	10	0	0	0	—	—	0
Sugar	2 tsp	25	—	0	0	0	0	0	0	—
Molasses	2 tbs	100	—	—	—	2	2	2	15	25

SOURCE: Betty Peterkin, "Nutrition Labeling for the Consumer," Family Economics Review, Summer 1973, Table 3, p. 11.
[a] Percentages expressed in increments as required by regulation for nutrition labeling ("Food Labeling," Federal Register, Vol. 38, No. 49, part II, March 14, 1973): 2 per cent increments up to and including 10 per cent level; 5 per cent increments above 10 per cent and up to and including the 50 per cent level, and 10 per cent increments above the 50 per cent level.
[b] "Nutritive Value of Foods," USDA, HG-72, was used as a basis for percentages for specific foods. Values for food groups are based on average selections of foods in the group by U.S. families.
[c] In addition, niacin equivalent from the amino acid, tryptophan, found principally in animal products, would contribute substantially toward meeting the body's need for this nutrient.
[d] Based on average of values on labels of 59 varieties of ready-to-eat cereals, February 1973.

Food Additives Amendment.[9] It requires that any new food additive must be tested for safety on animals and the results submitted to the Food and Drug Administration. Where animal experimentation is insufficient, the administration is required to resort to other means to determine whether the additive is harmful. Additives commonly used in food before January 1, 1958, and generally recognized as safe (GRAS) because of the experience based on such use are exempt from the law. In vegetable soup, for example, raw agricultural products, such as vegetables, could be classed as "GRAS substances." This means that a great many ingredients do not have to go through the declared procedures of the law.

It must be emphasized that there are many food additives that actually improve food and are very necessary—for example, certain minerals and vitamins in enriched foods. Sodium and calcium propionate are used in bread and in wrapped cheese to prevent mold. Lecithin is a vegetable emulsifier manufactured from soybeans that is used to make foods smoother and creamier. Other additives are used to improve food color, flavor, texture, and keeping qualities. Many packaged food products could not be produced without some food additive. Artificial sweeteners, added bulk, or other nonnutritive ingredients must be declared on the label.

Consumers have a genuine concern about the safety of the food that they eat. Additives are termed intentional as well as acceptable if any of the following purposes are served: improve or maintain nutritional value, enhance quality, reduce wastage, promote consumer acceptance, enhance keeping quality, increase availability of food, or facilitate preparation of food.[10] Additives should not be permitted unless employed in the best interests of the consumer.

Consideration must be given to the possibility of *toxicity* of an additive or the capacity of a substance to produce injury. A *hazard* implies probability of injury. Chemical and physical properties of an additive must be determined. Data from biological studies with laboratory animals should be studied with discrimination. To what extent can the evidence be translated to humans? The safety of the amount added to a food and the effects of accumulation must be considered. Virtual assurance that no injury will result must dominate decisions. When safe additives can be employed, the provision for a wholesome and adequate food supply is enhanced.

All meat and poultry shipped across state lines must be federally inspected by the Consumer and Marketing Service of the U.S. Department of Agriculture. The Wholesome Meat Act of 1967[11] standardizes state inspection programs through the assistance of the Department of Agriculture, so that state standards will equal federal standards. The labels on processed meat products must be accurate and give a true description of the product. All federally inspected prepackaged products will carry the circular mark of inspection, an assurance to the consumer of wholesomeness.

The Fair Packaging and Label Act of 1966 went into effect on July 1, 1968. This law provides for honest and informative material on the label. The net contents must be placed in the lower 30 per cent of the principal display plan, unless specifically exempted, so that the consumer can see what she is buying. Net contents must be stated in total ounces (if less than 4 pounds) followed by a separate declaration of pounds and ounces or decimal fractions of a pound. This facilitates comparison of prices.

Other Aspects of Label Protection

Specific points related to government requirements concerning labels[12] are as follows:

[9] *What Consumers Should Know about Food Additives*, Leaflet No. 10, U.S. Department of Health, Education, and Welfare, Washington, D.C., 1960.

[10] Special Report, "The Use of Chemicals in Food Production, Processing, Storage and Distribution," *Nutrition Reviews*, Vol. 31, No. 6 (June 1973), pp. 191–198.

[11] *Food and Home Notes*, Office of Information, U.S. Department of Agriculture, Washington, D.C., September 4–11, 1968.

[12] *Read the Label on Foods, Drugs, Devices, Cosmetics*, Miscellaneous Publication No. 3, Food and Drug Administration, U.S. Department of Health, Education, and Welfare, Washington, D.C., 1957.

1. The label must not use the name of another food. For example, peanut oil cannot be labeled olive oil.
2. It must be easily read and understood. For example, it should not have a name that is so unusual as to lack identity; maple syrup, for example, should not be labeled Vermont syrup.
3. Imitations must be prominently labeled.
4. Ingredients must be named in the order of their predominance in the food; for example, if a stew lists water first, then the container has more water than any other ingredient.
5. When the standards or definitions have been set by the government, the list of ingredients is not necessary.
6. Net contents must be noted in common units of measure. In the case of liquids, it must be a liquid measure and in the case of dry foods, such as fresh fruits and vegetables, it must be in terms of dry measure.
7. The container must not be misleading, that is, appear to be larger than it actually is, nor should other such illusions be used.
8. The label must give the name and place of business of the manufacturer, packager, or distributor. This gives the consumer an opportunity to know with whom he is dealing.
9. Any type of enrichment must be definitely stated in terms of units or milligrams or whatever measure is indicated for that nutrient, and it is inadequate to state "meets one third of the daily dietary requirements."

Guidelines for Food Shopping

The kind of store where the shopping is done is important. Delicatessens, small independent grocers who give credit, or specialty shops have much higher prices than self-service stores or supermarkets. Having groceries delivered adds to the cost.

The time available for meal preparation is assuming greater importance. As the number of working mothers increases and less time is spent at home, there will be a greater demand for convenience foods. In selecting them, it is important to compare their nutritive value, cost, and quality with that of home-prepared foods. Sometimes the lack of time causes shoppers to buy more expensive foods than they would otherwise.

The amount and kind of storage facilities are important. A spacious refrigerator, a large freezer, and adequate cupboards mean that food can be stored more readily. However, the

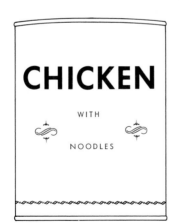
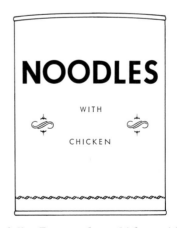

FIGURE 30–5. *Read the label carefully. Do you buy chicken with noodles or noodles with chicken? (Adapted from Food and Drug Administration drawing)*

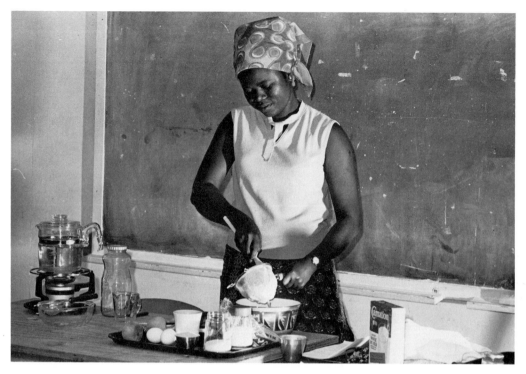

FIGURE 30–6. *Should a young mother prepare baby food at home or buy it? What are some determining factors?* (USDA)

homemaker must be familiar with the storage life of a food. Many are unaware of the fact that canned, frozen, and dried foods have definite time limits for use. Also, the ice cube compartment of a refrigerator is not as cold as a freezer, so frozen foods will not keep indefinitely. Nor should it be used to freeze foods.

Shopping skill cannot be underestimated. It means having a knowledge of quality, grades, best size of containers, brands, and the like. It also implies an ability to discriminate among the offerings. This may mean careful reading of the label, comparing different sizes of containers, a knowledge of the peak of season for certain foods, and how to compute the cost per serving of food.

Who does the shopping can make a great deal of difference. Today, the shopper is not always the woman of the family; many men shop, as well as children. Men are inclined to indulge in impulse buying more frequently than women. In some areas or upon some occasions an entire family may shop. Sometimes this can make for great convenience. A family may divide the market list into several lists and have each member buy certain items. Whoever is responsible for buying should be aware of food and money values so that the family dollar is wisely spent.

The home production of food may reduce the amount of money spent. Having a garden, freezing or canning foods that have been purchased at the height of the season, or preparing food at home rather than buying ready-prepared food are some examples of ways to reduce the budget, generally speaking. Home production depends, however, on the value that a homemaker places on her time.

Such a simple fact as a knowledge of the quantity of food can make a big difference. If more food is purchased and prepared than the family eats and there is little opportunity to use leftovers, food expenses will be increased considerably.

Balancing the cost of different foods for a

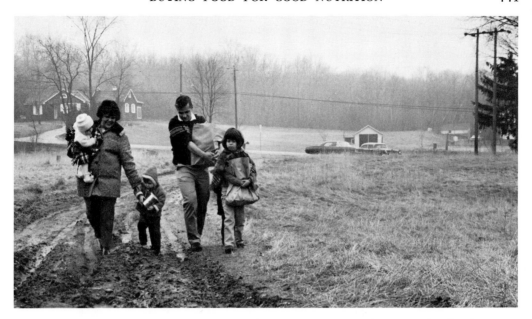

FIGURE 30–7. *Should shopping be a family affair or should one member be the expert? Some believe that there is more impulse buying if the father helps buy and that small children pressure for their favorite foods. Are there guidelines for a family to establish?*

meal is worthy of consideration. For example, if an expensive meat is purchased, it is wise to have less expensive vegetables and dessert. In this way, the cost of the meal can be distributed and the family can have an expensive meat occasionally. The same may be true for other foods in the meal.

Nutrition labeling may be used for information and related to the total nutrient needs of the day. The food with the highest U.S. RDA may not be suitable for the purpose; for example, buying foods high in vitamin C may be expensive when the vitamin C need is met with an adequate serving of orange juice.

Strong feelings about status foods may lead people to buy items that are not particularly nutritious but that they feel are important. An example is buying an imported cheese rather than a domestic cheese.

Selecting food appropriate to income may be necessary in times of inflation. Become familiar with the economic range of choices within a food group, such as dried milk in place of fresh milk in the milk group.

Buying in Food Groups

The Department of Agriculture food cost plans for different incomes (see Table 30–5) should be helpful.

For each food group, also, there is a table showing the average contribution of nutrients for civilians. See Table 30–6. The student of nutrition will find it interesting to consider the influence of changes in consumption on the nutritional status of the population.

Dairy Products

The contribution of dairy products to supplies of important nutrients should be noted. See Table 30–6.

The civilian per capita consumption per year for milk has decreased from 322 pounds in 1960 to 247 pounds in 1974. Consumption of condensed and evaporated milks have decreased from 13.7 pounds in 1960 to 5.3 pounds in 1974. Cheese consumption has increased from 8.3 pounds in 1960 to 14.5

TABLE 30-5

Cost of Food at Home

Estimated^a for 1974 food plans at three cost levels, October 1974, U.S. average

	COST FOR 1 WEEK			COST FOR 1 MONTH		
SEX–AGE GROUPS^b	Low-cost plan	Moderate-cost plan	Liberal plan	Low-cost plan	Moderate-cost plan	Liberal plan
	Families					
Family of 2						
20 to 54 years^b	$26.90	$33.60	$40.30	$116.60	$145.50	$174.40
55 years and over^b	23.90	29.40	35.20	103.30	127.60	152.20
Family of 4						
Preschool children^c	38.10	47.10	56.50	164.60	204.30	244.60
School children^d	46.10	57.30	68.70	199.30	248.50	297.50
	Individuals^e					
Child						
7 months to 1 year	5.20	6.30	7.40	22.40	27.30	32.20
1 to 2 years	6.20	7.50	9.00	26.70	32.70	38.90
3 to 5 years	7.40	9.10	10.90	31.90	39.30	47.20
6 to 8 years	9.60	11.90	14.30	41.50	51.60	61.80
9 to 11 years	12.00	14.90	17.80	51.80	64.60	77.20
Male						
12 to 14 years	12.80	15.90	19.00	55.30	68.70	82.20
15 to 19 years	14.00	17.50	21.00	60.90	75.70	90.80
20 to 54 years	13.60	17.00	20.50	58.80	73.80	88.70
55 years and over	11.90	14.70	17.70	51.60	63.90	76.60
Female						
12 to 19 years	11.30	14.00	16.60	49.10	60.50	72.00
20 to 54 years	10.90	13.50	16.10	47.20	58.50	69.80
55 years and over	9.80	12.00	14.30	42.30	52.10	61.80
Pregnant	13.40	16.50	19.60	58.30	71.50	85.00
Nursing	14.30	17.70	21.00	62.00	76.60	91.20

^a These estimates were computed from quantities of food plans presented in tables 1, 2, and 3. The costs of the food plans were first estimated by using the average price per pound of each food group paid by urban survey families at three selected food cost levels in 1965–1966. These prices were adjusted to current levels by use of *Retail Food Prices by Cities* released periodically by the Bureau of Labor Statistic.

^b Ten per cent added for family size adjustment.

^c Man and woman, 20 to 54 years; children, 1 to 2 and 3 to 5 years.

^d Man and woman, 20 to 54; child, 6 to 8 and boy 9 to 11 years.

^e The costs given are for individuals in a four-person family. For individuals in other sized families, the following adjustments are suggested: one person—add 20 per cent; two persons—add 10 per cent; three persons—add 5 per cent; five persons—subtract 5 per cent; six or more persons—subtract 10 per cent.

SOURCE: Betty Peterkin, "USDA Family Food Plans, 1974," *Family Economics Review*, Winter 1975, p. 11.

pounds in 1974. Ice cream consumption has decreased from 18.3 pounds in 1960 to 17.5 pounds in 1974.[13]

[13] Table 6, Economic Research Service, "Civilian Per Capita Consumption of Major Food Commodities (Primary Distribution Weight) and Civilian Population, Selected Years," *National Food Situation*, Economic Research Service, U.S. Department of Agriculture, Washington, D.C., February 1975, p. 16.

General Hints for Buying Dairy Products

A number of points might be considered in getting the best buy nutritionally in dairy products. Compare the cost of fresh, evaporated, and dried milk. Canned and dried milk may be used successfully in cooking and baking, or even for drinking, and can be used therefore to reduce food costs. Home delivery

TABLE 30–6

Contribution of Major Food Groups to Nutrient Supplies Available for Civilian Consumption, 1974 (Percentages[a])

FOOD GROUPS	FOOD ENERGY	PROTEIN	FAT	CARBOHYDRATE	CALCIUM	PHOSPHORUS	IRON	MAGNESIUM	VITAMIN A VALUE	THIAMIN	RIBOFLAVIN	NIACIN	VITAMIN B_6	VITAMIN B_{12}	ASCORBIC ACID
1974[b]															
Meat (including pork fat cuts), poultry and fish	20.2	41.5	34.7	0.1	3.5	26.2	29.1	13.7	21.5	28.1	24.5	45.6	45.8	69.7	1.0
Eggs	2.0	5.1	2.9	0.1	2.3	5.4	5.1	1.3	5.8	2.2	5.1	0.1	1.9	8.3	0
Dairy products, excluding butter	11.1	22.5	12.4	6.6	75.7	36.1	2.3	21.6	12.9	9.0	41.0	1.6	10.2	20.5	4.0
Fats and oils, including butter	17.8	0.1	42.6	c	0.4	0.2	0	0.4	8.1	0	0	0	0	0	0
Citrus fruits	0.9	0.5	0.1	1.9	0.9	0.7	0.8	2.2	1.5	2.8	0.5	0.9	1.2	0	26.3
Other fruits	2.2	0.6	0.2	4.7	1.2	1.1	3.3	3.9	5.5	1.8	1.5	1.7	5.5	0	11.4
Potatoes and sweet potatoes	2.7	2.4	0.1	5.3	0.9	3.9	4.4	7.1	5.3	6.2	1.7	7.1	11.2	0	18.0
Dark green and deep yellow vegetables	0.3	.5	c	.5	1.6	.7	1.6	2.1	21.2	0.9	1.1	0.7	1.7	0	8.3
Other vegetables, including tomatoes	2.5	3.3	.4	4.7	4.9	5.0	9.0	10.4	15.5	6.9	4.5	6.1	9.2	0	27.6
Dry beans and peas, nuts, soya flour	3.2	5.4	4.0	2.2	2.8	6.2	6.4	11.7	c	5.7	2.0	7.6	4.3	0	c
Flour and cereal products	19.2	17.8	1.3	34.8	3.3	12.5	28.2	17.9	0.4	36.3	17.4	24.0	8.9	1.5	0
Sugars and other sweeteners	17.3	c	0	38.4	1.5	.3	7.4	0.2	0	c	c	c	0	0	c
Miscellaneous[d]	0.7	.4	1.2	.6	1.0	1.8	2.4	7.6	2.3	0.1	0.7	4.8	0.1	0	3.5
Total[e]	100.0	100.0	100.0	100.0	100.0	100.0	100.0	100.0	100.0	100.0	100.0	100.0	100.0	100.0	100.0

source: Economic Research Service, *National Food Situation*, Table 11, U.S. Department of Agriculture, Washington, D.C., November 1974, p. 28. [a] Percentages for food groups are based on nutrient data included in totals in Table 4–1. [b] Preliminary. [c] Less than 0.05 percent. [d] Coffee and chocolate liquor equivalent of cocoa beans and fortification of products not assigned to a specific food group. [e] Components may not add to total due to rounding.

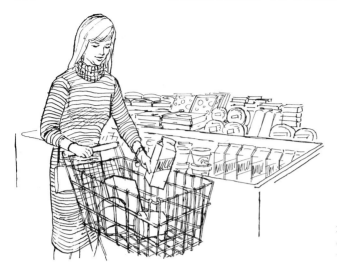

FIGURE 30–8. *Check labels of dairy products for the best buys, nutritionally.*

of dairy products increases the cost, for this is a service. Check the prices of milk in various-sized containers. If a large container, such as a 2-quart or 1-gallon size, can be utilized by the family, there is generally a saving. Similarly, it is usually cheaper to buy a quart container of milk than two pint containers of milk.

All fresh milk that reaches the consumer is pasteurized for health reasons. This process destroys many of the germs that are dangerous. Yogurt, because it is a cultured milk requiring additional handling and processing, is more expensive than fresh milk. Chocolate milk should be checked to see if it is made with skim or whole milk. The cost of buttermilk should also be compared with that of fresh or skim milk, depending on the type of buttermilk purchased.

Fresh milk is very perishable and should be stored in the coldest part of the refrigerator. Storage life of milk is only a few days, and it should not be kept longer. Evaporated milk, if unopened, can usually be kept for a period of 6 months.

CHEESE The nutritive value of cheese is not reflected in its price. Imported cheeses are generally more expensive than domestic. Compare the cost of a pound of cheese with that of a pound of meat. Cheese may serve as a substitute for meat. Determine whether cheese is made from whole milk, skim milk, or whether fat or other ingredients have been added. Cheese that is sliced, cubed, shredded, or grated will usually cost more than a wedge of cheese, since the price includes services. Fancy packages increase the price but not the nutritive value. Storage life of cheese is short once it is cut or the container opened.

ICE CREAM Compare the cost of ice cream in different containers and buy the size most suitable for family use. Large containers can be stored in a freezer. Consider nutritive contributions, such as those of fruit, nuts, or chocolate that may be added to ice cream. Look at the label for ingredients such as type of milk, cream, additional fat, or other additions.

See Table 30–6 for nutrient contribution as a food group.

Meat, Fish, and Poultry

Meat is one of the most expensive items in the family budget.

General Hints for Buying Meat, Fish, and Poultry

MEAT Special care should be taken in the purchase of meats so that the greatest return, from a nutritional standpoint, can be secured. This group of foods is very perishable and should be refrigerated. Use promptly. The consumer should select the kind of meat best suited for the use planned for it. Cuts for roasting and broiling are the most expensive because there are fewer of these cuts on each carcass, and yet there is the greatest demand for them. Skill in identifying cuts and the most desirable preparation for each are imperative. Quality in meat is highly variable and difficult to judge in small retail cuts.

One of the problems in buying meat is to determine the amount that should be purchased. Unless the cut has a large amount of

TABLE 30–7

Cost of 20 Grams of Protein from Meat, Poultry, and Fish[a]

RATING	FOOD	MARKET UNIT	PRICE PER UNIT (cents)	PART OF MARKET UNIT TO GIVE 20 G OF PROTEIN (%)	COST OF 20 G OF PROTEIN (cents)
1	Tuna, canned	6.5 oz	54	44	24
2	Sardines, canned	4 oz	26	94	24
3	Hamburger	1 lb	102	24	25
4	Beef liver	1 lb	103	24	25
5	Chicken breasts	1 lb	101	25	26
6	Pork, picnic	1 lb	89	32	29
7	Turkey, ready to cook	1 lb	84	35	30
8	Ham, whole	1 lb	124	29	36
9	Round, beef-steak	1 lb	177	22	39
10	Ocean perch, fillet, frozen	1 lb	112	36	40
11	Pork loin, roast	1 lb	123	33	41
12	Liverwurst	8 oz	75	60	45
13	Frankfurters	1 lb	125	36	45
14	Ham, canned	1 lb	189	24	45
15	Salami	8 oz	95	50	48
16	Sirloin, beef-steak	1 lb	173	28	49
17	Chuck, roast, beef, bone in	1 lb	139	35	49
18	Rib roast of beef	1 lb	156	33	51
19	Haddock, fillet, frozen	1 lb	148	35	52
20	Pork chops, center cut	1 lb	163	35	57
21	Bologna	8 oz	82	73	59
22	Pork sausage	1 lb	127	52	66
23	Porterhouse steak	1 lb	203	34	68
24	Veal cutlet	1 lb	330	21	71
25	Lamb chops, loin	1 lb	232	31	71
26	Bacon, sliced	1 lb	139	52	73

SOURCE: Adapted from *Costs of Meats and Meats Alternates*, Two Tables Devised by Food Economists of the U.S. Department of Agriculture, Agricultural Research Service, Washington, D.C., 1974.
[a] January 1974 prices.

bone and inedible material, ¼ pound per person is sufficient. Larger servings increase food costs. Therefore, consider the best buy on the basis of cost per serving. Except for such items as chopped meat and stew, the price per pound includes bone and gristle, which are not eaten. Sometimes cuts of meat like spareribs seem relatively inexpensive, but the amount of edible meat is small.

The consumption of beef, veal, and pork increased during 1974. Consumption of chicken has remained constant and turkey has increased slightly. The consumption of fish has decreased.[14]

One way to compare costs among meats is to compare costs on the basis of protein content. A 3-oz serving of cooked lean beef, lamb, veal, turkey, or fish provides 20 g of protein. In Table 30–7 the average prices (January 1974 prices) of a pound or other market unit to provide a 3-oz serving is listed, with the percentage of pound yield necessary to provide this size of serving. To figure a comparable cost, multiply the price by the part of pound or market unit indicated in the table.

The price of meat is not a criterion of its nutritive value. All cuts have the name nutritive value except the organ meats, which are more nutritious. Pork is richer in thiamin.

The round purple federal meat inspection stamp means that the meat was wholesome at the time of inspection. This is the government's way of protecting the consumer against diseased animals or meat that is unfit for consumption. This stamp also implies that the meat was processed under sanitary conditions and that there are no misleading labels. This meat inspection law governs the condition and the production of fresh, cured, smoked, canned, frozen, and other meat food products. Look for the meat inspection label on cans and packages as well as fresh meat.

As beef is the kind of meat most in demand, it is the most expensive, generally speaking. The thrifty shopper will therefore search for better buys, such as lamb, veal, and mutton cuts. At certain periods of the year, pork may be less expensive. Prices should be compared

[14] *National Food Situation*, February 1975, p. 16.

among fresh, frozen, and canned meat. From a nutritional standpoint, there is little or no difference. Sometimes canned meats have other ingredients such as cereal products added, so it is well to check the label.

POULTRY   Shoppers should compare the cost of fresh, frozen, or canned poultry, and also parts versus whole birds. Americans seem to prefer the fresh or the frozen types to the canned, but there are ways in which all three can be used to advantage in the diet. Check various types to see which one will save money. If the price per pound of roasting turkey is less than one and one third the price of a roasting chicken, the turkey is a better buy, for there will be more meat per dollar. Large turkeys as well as large chickens generally sell at a lower price per pound than the smaller birds, and have more meat per pound. Poultry is often a good buy in spite of the large proportion of bone to meat.

In buying poultry, the allowance per serving is generally ½ pound of ready-to-cook poultry. In the case of duck or certain other wild game, it may be necessary to increase this to ¾ pound per serving because there is less meat on these birds.

FISH   Compare the cost of fresh, frozen, and canned fish to see which is the best buy. The market styles for fresh fish are whole, drawn, pan-dressed, filets (portions cut from the backbone), or steaks from large fish. The shopper will need to determine the best buy for the type of preparation intended.

Shellfish and other types of seafood are very nutritious, and at certain seasons are good pocketbook stretchers. In most sections of the country, frozen fish sticks are a good buy.

As the purchase of this food group is such an important budget item, it is advisable for consumers to consider ways to make the best buy and, if possible, to consider possible substitutes from time to time. See Table 30–8 and compare the cost of selected meat alternates with the cost of meat in Table 30–7.

Eggs

The civilian per capita consumption of eggs has decreased from 344 eggs in 1960 to 285

TABLE 30–8

Cost of 20 Grams Protein from Meat Alternates[1a]

RATING	FOOD	MARKET UNIT	PRICE PER UNIT (cents)	PART OF MARKET UNIT TO GIVE 20 G OF PROTEIN (%)	COST OF 20 G OF PROTEIN (cents)
1	Peanut butter	12 oz	56	23	13
2	Dry beans	1 lb	57	24	14
3	Bean soup, canned	11.5 oz	20	96	19
4	Milk, whole fluid	Half-gallon	76	29	22
5	Eggs, large	Dozen	93	25	24
6	American processed cheese	8 oz	71	38	27

SOURCE: Adapted from *Costs of Meats and Meat Alternates*, Two Tables Devised by Food Economists of the U.S. Department of Agriculture, Agricultural Research Service, Washington, D.C., 1974.
  [a] January 1974 prices.

eggs in 1974. The high cholesterol content of eggs may account for some of this decrease.

General Hints for Buying Eggs

The size of eggs indicated on the carton is determined by the weight per dozen, which has been standardized by law. These weights are as follows:

SIZE	OUNCES PER DOZEN
Extra large	27 or more
Large	24 or more
Medium	21 or more
Small	18 or more

The size does not affect the quality or food value. The color of the shell does not affect quality or food value. The demand for white- or brown-shelled eggs is a matter of personal preference and does not indicate a knowledge of nutrition.

Grade AA and grade A eggs are generally used for table use. Grade B and grade C are perfectly satisfactory for most cooking purposes and can be much less expensive. Grade is not related to size but to quality. Eggs vary in price according to the season. Consumers will wish to watch egg prices. Here is a formula that might be used to determine which size of egg is the best buy: If the price of

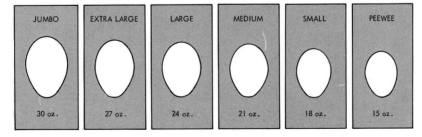

FIGURE 30–9. *Buy the size of egg best suited to the purpose. The six United States weight classes are shown above with the minimum weight per dozen for each size.* (USDA, redrawn)

medium eggs is seven eighths that of large eggs, the actual cost is the same for both sizes. Small or pullet eggs costs as much as large eggs if their price is three fourths as much as the large eggs.

Fats and Oils

The yearly per capita civilian consumption of fats and oils has gradually increased from 45.3 pounds per year in 1960 to 53.5 pounds in 1973.[15] Lard consumption has decreased, but there has been a fairly steady increase in the use of shortening (primarily fats made from hydrogenated vegetable oils) and other edible fats and oils.

In addition to the fats listed, homemakers often use chicken fat, bacon drippings, or other household fats.

There is a wide variation in the cost of the various fats used for household purposes, and the wise buyer will wish to make comparisons to find those that are best suited for her purposes. A few points that might be kept in mind are that butter and margarine compare favorably from a nutritive standpoint, but some consumers prefer butter because of the flavor even though the cost is higher. Another factor to consider is the saturated/unsaturated fatty acid content. Margarines usually have a higher concentration of unsaturated fatty acids than butter because they are made of oils—generally corn or cottonseed oil, but sometimes safflower or other oil—that are high in unsaturated fatty acids. The oils are partially hydrogenated to produce the desired consistency.

In buying butter or margarine, it is well to compare the difference in cost between quarter-pound and pound packages. Some homemakers feel that the advantage of having quarter-pound sticks compensates for the extra cost, for they are easy to use for measuring and can be prepared more easily for the table.

Dressings for salad vary in price and in nutritive value. Mayonnaise or mayonnaise dressing must contain vegetable oil of at least 55 per cent by weight and some acid ingredient, such as vinegar, lemon, or lime juice, an emulsifier, either egg or egg yolks, plus seasonings. Salad dressing has only 30 per cent vegetable oil by weight, contains egg yolks, an acid ingredient, and a starch paste. French dressing must contain at least 35 per cent vegetable oil by weight and the same types of acid as mayonnaise or salad dressing. Flavoring ingredients, such as tomato paste, ketchup, or spices, may be added as well as egg yolk, vegetable gum, or other emulsifiers. This fact will be stated on the label. Flavor preference and costs are the guides generally used by consumers. It is advisable to compare the cost of equal amounts of salad dressings by comparing the measure or the weights as indicated on the labels. Cost of home-prepared salad dressings may be compared with the commercially prepared. The saving may be considerable.

The cost of various brands of vegetable fat shortening should be compared by weight. Vegetable fats can generally be stored on the shelf for several months without becoming rancid, depending on the temperature. Margarine and butter do become rancid rapidly and should not be kept more than 1 week in the refrigerator.

There are regional differences in the type of fats used. Lard is very commonly used in rural areas, while bacon or fatback drippings are used in the South, especially for the seasoning of vegetables. Vegetable fats are widely used throughout the country.

Legumes

The available statistics on the civilian per capita consumption of legumes indicates a gradual decline from 7.3 pounds in 1960 to 7.0 pounds in 1974 for beans and a gradual increase for peanuts from 4.9 pounds in 1960 to 6.4 pounds in 1974.[16] Most of the dried beans on the American table are baked and canned with tomato sauce, pork, or other additions. The consumption of peanuts has steadily increased. Much of the peanut crop is utilized as peanut butter, a popular American food. Roasted salted peanuts are consumed as munchers during athletic events and mixed with nuts for cocktail accompaniments.

---

[15] Ibid.

[16] Ibid.

General Hints for Buying Legumes

Consumers will want to survey the market carefully for the best buy in legumes. Some general points are listed here. Compare the price of canned dried baked beans with dried beans in bags or packages. The cost of fuel and preparation time will need to be considered in comparing this cost. Compare prices among brands and also the cost of adding certain ingredients. Consider use of other legumes, such as peas of different varieties, lentils, and other varieties of beans.

Nuts

Nuts are seldom considered as a food by Americans, who use them largely for snacks. Nuts are being consumed in larger quantities especially by the young who are vegetarians. The valuable nutritive contribution should be examined in purchasing nuts.[17]

General Hints for Buying Nuts

Compare the cost of nuts in shelled, unshelled, bulk, packed tins, and cellophane bags. Here is the yield of some of the most common nuts:

VARIETY	CUPS, SHELLED, FROM 1 LB UNSHELLED	CUPS FROM 1 LB SHELLED
Almonds	1½	3½
Pecans	2¼	4
Peanuts (a legume)	2¼	3
Walnuts	1⅔	3

It may be wise to estimate the cost of certain services, such as chopping or salting nuts, in comparison to doing these operations at home.

Vegetables

The consumption of fresh vegetables has increased to 100.4 pounds for 1974, canned vegetables, excluding potatoes and sweet potatoes, to 54.3 pounds, and frozen vegetables, excluding potatoes, have increased steadily to 10.1 pounds.[18]

[17] Ibid.
[18] Ibid.

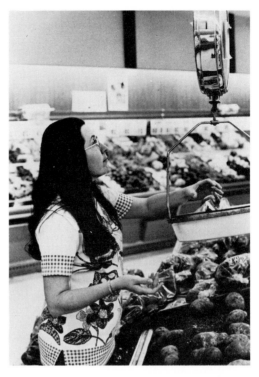

FIGURE 30–10. *Select vegetables carefully and weigh to estimate cost per serving.* (USDA)

General Hints for Buying Vegetables

The display of vegetables in supermarkets has undoubtedly had an effect on the variety in present-day menus. As vegetables are very perishable and flavor deteriorates, they should be used soon after being purchased. Some general suggestions to bear in mind in buying vegetables are given here.[19]

The size of a vegetable does not indicate quality or nutritive value. For example, oversized vegetables may be pithy, tasteless, or woody. Sometimes a small-sized vegetable is a better buy for the price. Select vegetables for the purpose intended. Tomatoes or celery, for example, that are going to be used in soups or stews do not have to be as attractive in appearance as they would for other purposes. Choose vegetables of somewhat the same size

[19] *How to Buy Fresh Vegetables,* Home and Garden Bulletin No. 143, Consumer and Marketing Service, U.S. Department of Agriculture, Washington, D.C., 1972.

so they will cook in the same length of time.

Vegetables should have a bright, fresh color, for the greenness or yellowishness of the vegetable is often an indication of the vitamin and mineral content. Select vegetables that have a good shape. Forked, rough, or deeply cracked ones are often very wasteful unless the price is so low that buying is warranted. Avoid root or tuberous vegetables that have sprouts. This condition deteriorates the vegetable. Fresh vegetables are the cheapest at the peak of the season.

Federal standards for grades require that the label be marked Grade A or Fancy, Grade B or Extra Standard, or Grace C or Standard. This grading takes into consideration color, texture, form, flavor, and similar aspects. Foods in all these grades are edible and nutritious but will vary in the factors mentioned. The use of the vegetable must be kept in mind. For example, if canned tomatoes are to be used for soup or stew, then grade C is perfectly desirable. Compare the cost per serving of the same vegetable in fresh, canned, or frozen form. Also compare the flavor and quality.

In the purchase of fresh vegetables, there is a great deal of variation in the number of servings per pound. Some have much more waste than others. The following might be helpful:

ONE POUND AS PURCHASED	SERVINGS
Lima beans in pod	2 to 3
Peas in pod	2 to 3
Onions	2 to 3
Potatoes	3 to 5
Asparagus	3 to 4
Broccoli	4 to 5
Cabbage	5 to 6
Beets	3
Spinach	4 to 5
Turnips	3 to 4
Carrots	3 to 4
String beans	6
Kale	5 to 6
Beet, mustard, and turnip tops	3 to 4
Eggplant	5 to 6
Summer squash	3 to 4
Hubbard squash	2 to 3

It is well to be familiar with the size and content of the most common cans used for vegetables. See Table 30–9. Strained and homogenized foods for infants, and chopped junior foods, come in small jars and cans suitable for the smaller servings used. The weight is given on the label. Meats, poultry, fish, and seafood are almost entirely advertised and sold under weight terminology.

Fruits

There have been some changes in the consumption of fresh fruit. Citrus fruits (fresh) have declined in per capita civilian consumption from 93.4 pounds in 1960 to 80.0 pounds in 1974; apples from 18.3 pounds in 1960 to 15.7 pounds (does not include apples that individuals consume from their own orchards); other fruits, excluding melons, from 41.4 pounds in 1960 to 35.5 pounds in 1974. The consumption of melons has decreased from 25.8 pounds to 19.1 pounds. Canned fruit has decreased from 22.6 pounds in 1960 to 21.3 pounds in 1974, and dried fruit dropped slightly from 3.1 pounds to 3.0 pounds. The use of canned fruit juice increased from 13 pounds in 1960 to 14.7 pounds in 1974, and frozen fruit, including juices, increased in consumption from 9.1 pounds in 1960 to 11.9 pounds in 1974.[20]

General Hints for Buying Fruits

As fruits are a very popular item in the American diet and there is such a wide variation from which to choose, the consumer should exercise care in making the wisest selection from a nutritive standpoint.[21] Some general suggestions are the following:

1. Compare the cost per serving of fresh, canned, or frozen fruit for the best buy.
2. Consider waste in the preparation of fruit. Fresh pineapple, for example, has considerable waste, which increases the cost per serving.

[20] National Food Situation, op. cit., p. 16.

[21] How to Buy Fresh Fruit, Home and Garden Bulletin No. 141, Consumer and Marketing Service, U.S. Department of Agriculture, Washington, D.C., October 1967.

3. When fruits are purchased in season they are much less expensive.

4. One rule in buying fruit is that the weight indicates the juiciness of fruit. This is particularly true of grapefruit and other citrus fruits.

5. Some citrus fruits may be bronze or russeted and still have plenty of juice as well as being edible and nutritious. Pears may also have a russeted appearance, which does not interfere with their flavor or nutritive value.

6. Dried fruits are graded according to size. The larger the size, the greater the cost per pound, generally speaking.

7. The consumer must realize that when fruits are canned in heavy syrup or preserved in some similar manner, she is paying for sugar; also, the nutrients have been diluted as a result of the sugar, but the kcalories increased. Some fruits have a limited growing area and for that reason are more expensive. Such fruits are avocado pears, figs, kumquats, pomegranates, and loganberries.

8. The grades for canned fruits are Grade A or Fancy, Grade B or Choice, and Grade C or Standard with criteria established for standards. Top quality

TABLE 30–9

Size and Content of Cans and Common Uses

INDUSTRY TERM	APPROXIMATE NET WEIGHT[a]	APPROXIMATE CUPS	PRODUCTS
8 ounce	8 oz	1	Fruits, vegetables, specialties[b]
Picnic	10½ to 12 oz	1¼	Condensed soups, small quantities of fruits, vegetables, meat and fish products, specialties[b]
12 oz (vacuum)	12 oz	1½	Used largely for vacuum-packed corn
No. 300	14 to 16 oz	1¾	Pork and beans, baked beans, meat products, cranberry sauce, blueberries, specialties[b]
No. 303	16 to 17 oz	2	Fruits, vegetables, meat products, ready-to-serve soups, specialties[b]
No. 2	1 lb 4 oz or 1 pt 2 fl oz	2½	Juices, ready-to-serve soups, specialties,[b] and a few fruits and vegetables
No. 2½	1 lb 13 oz	3½	Fruits, some vegetables (pumpkin, sauerkraut, spinach and other greens, tomatoes)
No. 3 Cyl.	3 lb 3 oz or 1 qt 14 fl oz	5¾	Fruit and vegetable juices, pork and beans, condensed soup and some vegetables for institutional use
No. 10	6½ lb to 7 lb 5 oz	12–13	Fruits, vegetables for restaurant and institutional use

SOURCE: Courtesy Consumer Service Division, National Canners Association.

[a] Check label.

[b] Specialties: usually a food combination such as macaroni, spaghetti, Spanish-style rice, Mexican-type foods, Chinese foods, tomato aspic, etc.

costs the most and usually has the best flavor. Grade C may have uneven or broken pieces but could be used in a baked fruit pudding or for other purposes where size and shape or general appearance are not so important.[22]

Cereals

There have been increases in the consumption of cornmeal and flour, wheat cereals (slight), and milled rice but a decrease in the consumption of wheat flour.[23]

General Hints for Buying Cereals

The principal cereal products are breakfast cereal, either hot or cold, and the various types of breads. Cereals also find their way into a wide variety of baked goods on the market and into spaghetti and macaroni products. A few suggestions for buying are the following:

1. The cost of various breads and cereals should be compared by the ounce as a good indication of the best buy or to estimate the cost per serving. Puffed cereals are more expensive than shredded or flaked varieties.
2. Frequently day-old bread is sold at a reduced price and may be used very satisfactorily for toast, sandwiches, and stuffings.
3. The label should be read very carefully, not only for breads but also for cereals, to determine nutritive value.
4. In comparing the cost among cooked cereals, there can be considerable variation in the type. Flaked cereals such as rolled oats double in quantity when cooked; granulated cereals such as farina increase five to six times; whole cereals such as rice increase about four times in volume.

---

[22] *How to Buy Food,* A Bilingual Consumer Aid, Stock Number 0100–1416, U.S. Department of Agriculture, Washington, D.C., 1971, pp. 3–17.

[23] *National Food Situation,* op. cit., p. 16.

5. Check to see if flour is enriched. This is applicable not only to all-purpose flour, but to cake flours and cake mixes, too.

Being Resourceful

If the price of a common food suddenly rises, or if the food is difficult to get, the wise consumer will learn how to make substitutions of equal nutritive value. For example, canned grapefruit can be used if fresh grapefruit or oranges are expensive; eggs and cheese might be substituted for meat and still provide the nutritive value. Substitute other salad greens when family preferences are dear.

Instead of making an inflexible menu plan, the homemaker might look for the best buys of the day in the market and then plan accordingly.

To be an expert shopper, every source of information must be utilized. Radio and television programs with marketing information often give best buys of the day. Similar programs may also give hints as to good buying procedures. Newspapers are an excellent source of information and afford a way of comparing prices among stores. Booklets on buying various foods may be obtained from the State Extension Service. Exchanging information with friends and neighbors often turns up good ideas. Keeping an eye open for new products on the shelves of the store may lead to interesting additions to the family diet. Magazines and lectures are other sources of information.

Food shoppers should consider themselves in the same role as an expert purchasing executive and should use all devices possible to make every dollar of the food budget go as far as possible. There can be a great deal of satisfaction in purchasing carefully, and savings can be used in furthering other family plans. There is indeed a challenge to save when one considers that a homemaker who purchases food for family meals spends a considerable sum each year.

SELECTED REFERENCES

Asam, Edward, and Louis P. Bucklin, "Nutrition Labeling for Canned Goods: A Study of Consumer Response," *Journal of Marketing*, Vol. 37, No. 4 (April 1973), pp. 32–37.

Bing, Franklin C., "More Comments on Nutritional Labeling," *Food and Nutrition News*, Vol. 44, No. 8–9 (May–June 1973), pp. 1, 4.

Briggs, George M., "Nutrition Education and the Food Labels," *Food and Nutrition News*, Vol. 44, No. 7 (April 1973), p. 1, 4.

Bryant, Shari, et al., *Your Food Dollar*, Household Finance Corporation, Chicago, 1972.

Damon, G. Edward, "Primer on Food Additives," *FDA Consumer*, May 1973, pp. 10–16.

Daniels, Richard W., "Handbook No. 8 and Nutrition Labeling," *Food Technology*, Vol. 28, No. 1 (January 1974), pp. 46–47, 60.

"Food Labeling," *Dairy Council Digest*, Vol. 45, No. 2 (March–April 1974), pp. 7–12.

Forbes, Allan L., "The Role of the Food and Drug Administration in the Nutritional Quality of Foods," *American Journal of Public Health*, Vol. 62, No. 9 (September 1972), pp. 1207–1215.

Hall, Richard L., "Food Additives," *Nutrition Today*, Vol. 8, No. 4 (July–August 1973), pp. 20–28.

Kermode, G. O., "Food Additives," *Scientific American*, Vol. 226, No. 3 (March 1972), pp. 15–21.

Keys to Quality, Food Buying Guides from USDA, Agricultural Marketing Service, U.S. Department of Agriculture, Washington, D.C., July 1972.

Kinder, Faye, *Meal Management*, Macmillan Publishing Co., Inc., New York, 1973, Chapters 2 and 4–11.

Linch, Paula Floyd, "New Labels Help Sell Nutrition," *Journal of Home Economics*, Vol. 64, No. 9 (December 1972), pp. 28–29.

Moore, Jerry L., and Pamela F. Wendt, "Nutrition Labeling—A Summary and Evaluation," *Journal of Nutrition Education*, Vol. 5, No. 2 (April–June 1973), pp. 121–125.

"Nutritional Quality and Food Product Development," *Nutrition Reviews*, Vol. 31, No. 7 (July 1973), pp. 226–227.

Secretariat of the Joint FAO/WHO Food Standards Programme, *List of Additives Evaluated for Their Safety-in-Use in Food*, Food and Agriculture Organization of the United Nations and World Health Organization, Rome, 1973.

The Real Facts About Food, Office of Communication, U.S. Department of Agriculture, Washington, D.C., 1974.

"The Use of Chemicals in Food Production, Processing, Storage and Distribution," *Nutrition Reviews*, Vol. 31, No. 6 (June 1973), pp. 191–198.

31

Snacks

Snacking is a way of life common not only to Americans but to most peoples of the world. The times for eating between meals may be different, and certainly the type of food consumed will vary from one part of the world to another. Hot tea in a glass, a carbonated beverage, chopped radishes and grated onions spread on black bread, a puffy Chinese doughnut, a small glass of wine, or an elaborate high tea may be characteristic of some of these in-between feedings found among different cultures.

From time immemorial, snacks have been of prime importance in people's lives. In the early days of our country, Indian runners carried small sacks of corn for munching. Caesar found that offering food was a good way to gather a crowd to hear his orations. Hospitality in feudal days was shown by offering food to guests. Today, the coffee break and the cocktail hour are ordinary occurrences in our daily lives.

Snacks Are Big Business

An estimated 96 per cent of all households in the United States made purchases from a list of 20 snack foods during 1971, according to Collins and Sanders.[1] These items were valued at $3.4 billion. Market projections for the future estimate growth at the rate of 6 per cent per year so that by the year 1977 the value may be approximately $5 billion. Snack foods in descending order of economic value were potato chips and corn chips, cookies, snack nuts, crackers, popcorn, pretzels, and puffed snacks.

Beverages consumed by Americans have reached an all-time high. This thirst has spawned a multimillion dollar industry that yearly grows more than 10 per cent in the United States and by some 15 per cent overseas, according to Nagle.[2] Statistically, during 1972 more than 30 gallons of soda (63 per cent of all sales are of the cola formula), 35.6 gallons of coffee, 25.3 gallons of milk, 19.6 gallons of beer (approximately 210 12-oz

---

[1] J. L. Collins and G. G. Sanders, "Deep-Fried Snack Food Prepared from Soybeans and Onion," *Food Technology*, Vol. 27, No. 5 (May 1973), pp. 46–54.

[2] James J. Nagle, "Soft Drinks, Beer or Iced Tea: They All Carry Taste of Profits for Industry," *The New York Times*, July 28, 1973, p. 31.

cans), 7.2 gallons of tea, 5 gallons of canned juices, 1.9 gallons of distilled spirits and 2.8 gallons of wine were consumed per adult.

Soft drinks sell best in the warm southern states with 31 per cent of the population consuming 38 per cent of the country's soda of the sweetened kinds instead of the nonkcaloric versions. The low-kcalorie, or diet, drinks sell best in the West with 15 per cent of the market and in the Northeast, which has 14 per cent of the market.

Reasons for Eating Snacks

The most important reason for eating snacks is probably the decrease in social significance of family meals, according to Breeling.[3] More meals are eaten away from home, many in hamburger drive-ins in which the meals selected may be short of sufficient servings of fruits and vegetables and a soft drink may replace milk. Family members eat fewer meals together so often less effort is spent in preparation. The breakfast and lunch meals have eroded significantly and have been replaced by some type of snack food.

Man's desire for companionship and sociability is obviously an important reason for a snack period. This is true of all ages. Whenever two or more people get together, sooner or later thoughts turn to food or drink. Going to the local hangout, stopping at a cocktail lounge, or going to the school or industry cafeteria are some of the means for satisfying this need for sociability.

The very social fabric of our culture highlights food. Even committee meetings demand service of a beverage and some kind of snack. When people are invited to homes, some kind of refreshment is usually offered. The evening snack has become a part of our cultural ways.

Snacks for teen-agers definitely have a social implication. The desire to be with others is unusually strong, and there are many occasions provided so that teen-agers can get together. Food eaten during this age is generally much larger in quantity than it is at other ages, since

[3] James L. Breeling, "Are We Snacking Our Way to Malnutrition," *Today's Health*, Vol. 48, No. 1 (January 1970), pp. 48–50.

these young folks are in the period of greatest growth and consequently are often hungry.

Many of their snacks are eaten at "pairing" time. Hungry friends at record sessions or postgame get-togethers will consume such foods as three-decker sandwiches, pizzas, hamburgers, hot dogs, chili, pickles, toast, buns, cake, cookies, or fruit. This informal type of party does much to foster friendships and also gives an opportunity to develop social poise, but little thought is given to the nutritive value of such pick-up fare. However, the number of kcalories and the nutrients that may be added cannot be ignored. Sometimes with this teen-age group there are special hangouts that they greatly admire, such as "Joe's Diner," the corner drugstore, or "Suzy's Shack."

Although social reasons are usually the main motivation for eating something between meals, hunger itself is often a factor. A lowered blood sugar, as has been indicated in Chapter 8, may be responsible for this. Or the mere habit of eating between meals may lead one to crave something to eat. Many people become extremely uncomfortable when they are hungry and are unable to concentrate on the task before them. This may occur when little or no breakfast has been eaten or lunch has been light.

Another reason for having snacks is that fatigue may be relieved. If the work of an individual is rather monotonous or nerve-racking, as is true of many jobs, then a break will provide a necessary rest period. Manufacturers have found that a short period of respite will eventually increase output.

All too often people eat for want of something to do. When they have to wait for a plane, train, or bus, they may eat something even if they are not hungry because they do not know what to do with their time. Just sheer boredom results in raiding the refrigerator at home or eating available snacks.

Not only have many Americans abandoned active sports for spectator sports, but they also eat while watching them. The concessions selling peanuts, candy bars, hot dogs, and beverages are quite a lucrative operation in our athletic coliseums.

The kind of foods in the markets will have

an effect on what people eat between meals. The foods that are advertised through the various media of communication also have an impact. If people become familiar with a new tasty snack, there may be a demand for it.

A person's age also has an influence on the reasons for eating snacks. The nutritive value of in-between feedings receives more emphasis during the early years of life than any other time. In the food given to very young children and preschool children, generally fruit juices, milk, and similar nutritious foods are emphasized. In-between feeding for youngsters of elementary school age may or may not have a nutritive emphasis. When parents are concerned about food youngsters eat, their concern may be reflected in the snacks. When there is a lack of supervision, however, youngsters are inclined to help themselves to whatever they find and the choice may or may not be nutritious. Children often bring their friends home after school. Refreshments may have been planned beforehand or they may have a "fix-it-yourself" kind of fare. Whatever the refrigerator or the kitchen shelves yield

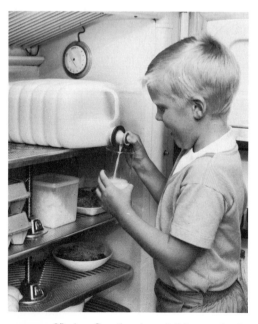

FIGURE 31–1. *Snacks for children of elementary school age should be nutritious and readily available. (Haskon, Inc.)*

will form the menu for this particular snack. However, although even small children enjoy preparing their own snacks, some guidance is necessary.

College students have made an institution of the coffee break. The Student Union building on a campus has become a center for the gathering of college youth. Sometimes establishments on the fringe of the campus also serve this purpose. Some students are known to feel so strongly about being able to get together with their crowd that they refuse to have a 10 o'clock class in their schedule. They may even select the same booths day after day and the same friends will gather there with them. Coffee and carbonated drinks are the favorite beverages.

Older individuals plan their snacks according to their occupation or interest at the moment. Business men and women have their coffee break. Almost everyone will take some time out for a snack. People, from force of habit, generally indulge in the kind of snack to which they have been accustomed. The time may be in midmorning, in the afternoon, bedtime, or all three. If they are in a locale where there are other people their age, they may gather together and share this snack period. It is not uncommon for friends to meet while shopping or on a business errand. They may wish to have a few social moments and have a snack someplace. Many a business conference is held over a cocktail or some other type of refreshment.

Light refreshments have often been used by businesses and institutions as a means of putting people in a receptive mood. For example, if a business is interested in introducing a new product to a group, it may be done at a meeting where refreshments are served. Conferences with advisory boards, with other groups of people, or between employers and employees, usually are more productive if some kind of food is eaten before the meeting.

When and What People Eat for Snacks

The hour of day determines the type of snack eaten. Sometimes the previous meal or the one following has an influence. A snack eaten in the middle of the morning may very

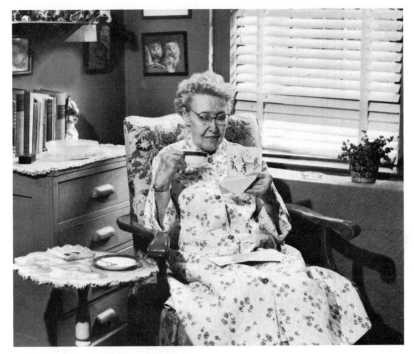

FIGURE 31–2. *An elderly woman has a snack while enjoying her mail.* (*Courtesy The Peabody Home, Bronx, N.Y.*)

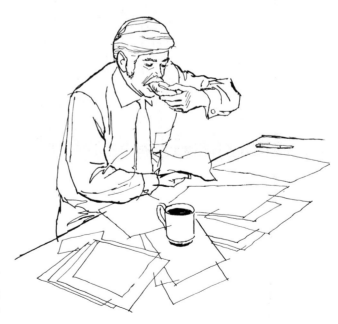

FIGURE 31–3. *Business men and women have coffee breaks.*

457

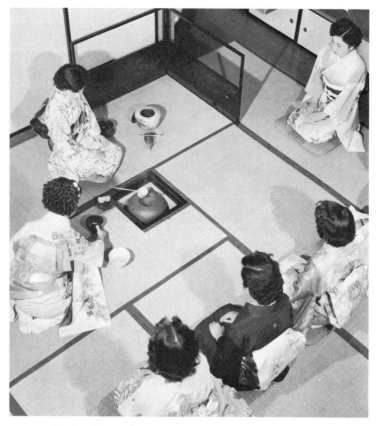

FIGURE 31–4. *Many Japanese enjoy a special tea service.* (*Japan Tourist Association*)

well have certain types of breakfast foods. Coffee is certainly the most popular beverage, and coffee cake or other breakfast types of breads are often served with it. Sometimes waffles or other hot breads are a part of this in-between feeding. If breakfast has been neglected, this midmorning snack may actually become a minimeal. In the home, for example, a mother frequently consumes some breakfast leftovers in the middle of the morning. In elementary schools, children are often given milk or fruit juice in the middle of the morning, particularly the younger children.

Snacks in the middle of the afternoon may again be dominated by beverages such as coffee, tea, or carbonated soft drinks. In warm weather, drinks with citrus fruits are common, particularly lemonade. Some form of frozen confection is also very popular for this type of

snack. Or sometimes pie or cake is eaten with the beverage. Children rush for some kind of food as soon as they come home from school. Adults may have a cocktail on their way home or before dinner at home.

Homemakers are often guilty of continuous nibbling, which may become quite an indulgence. A bite here or there may seem insignificant but can add up to a considerable number of kcalories. Here are the items that one homemaker ate between meals in one day:

> One-half slice of bacon left from breakfast.
>
> One brownie, sampled while baking in the morning.
>
> A pickled peach—the last in the jar— eaten while cleaning the refrigerator.
>
> One cup of coffee with a lump of sugar,

while reading the morning mail.

An apple—felt hungry for something around 2:30.

One fourth slice of bread and peanut butter—"Just had a taste with the children when they came home from school."

Four crackers and cheese and a glass of ginger ale with husband while watching TV.

These may have seemed like a mere nibble each time, yet they added considerable kcalories—approximately 400. For a person who may need to watch her weight, nibbling becomes a hazard.

One of the most popular times for nibbling is bedtime. Many persons believe that they sleep much better if they have something to eat before going to bed. A warm or hot beverage is somewhat relaxing and may help to induce sleep. Hot milk, cereal and milk, crackers and milk, soup, or fresh fruit are commonly served as bedtime snacks. Certainly foods that are very high in kcalories and rich desserts should be avoided at this time. These foods will tend to disturb sleep for some individuals. Bedtime snacks should be examined for nutritive values.

In different parts of the world, the type of food eaten at different hours has become strongly identified with certain customs. English people are very fond of their tea hour. This may range from a simple menu to an elaborate high tea. A high tea involves more of an assortment of food, and it forestalls hunger if dinner is to be very late in the evening. The hour is noted for a period of sociability. Friends and relatives may drop in and share this particular occasion with a family. Other countries have a similar social hour. The Japanese tea service is an important ritual.

The season of the year also has an influence on snacking. Although some feel that a hot beverage is desirable during warm weather, most people prefer cold drinks, particularly in America, where quantities of carbonated drinks, iced tea, iced coffee, and beverages made with ice cream are drunk. Cold weather and winter sports, especially, demand a much heartier type of food for snacks.

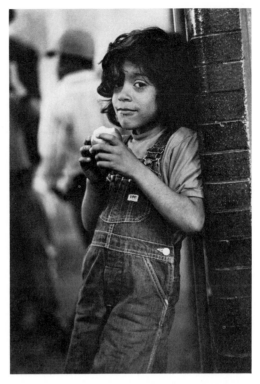

FIGURE 31–5. *A child enjoys an apple during a free period at school.* (UDSA)

Vending machines influence the choices that people make in their selection of snacks. The availability of these machines in bus and train stations, airports, institutions, offices, schools and colleges, and in many industries indicates the scope of their impact. Foods offered are usually of the type that can be easily handled and for which there is a demand. Major offerings are soft drinks, coffee, sandwiches, milk, ice cream, candy and other confections, and canned or frozen food that can be heated.

The foods available in the family refrigerator or on the cupboard shelves will determine the snacks consumed by family members. Mothers who bemoan the "junk foods" that their children eat may reverse this habit by paying attention to what is provided.

It must not be overlooked that snacks serve other purposes than nourishment. There are fun foods for the young, celebration foods, nostalgic foods, and cultural snacks that are an integral part of lifestyles. For the poor child, according to Blackburn,[4] soda pop and potato chips may be a treat, an opportunity to spend money that he seldom has, with a sense of freedom. What is eaten during the remainder of the day and what compensation these foods offer for these snack experiences is what counts.

Nutritive Contributions of Snacks

A large intake of snack foods of low nutritional density could reduce the nutritional variety furnished by the basic four food groups, according to Breeling.[5] Charges are made that the changes in food habits that have increased the use of snack foods may be partially responsible for low levels of iron, vitamin A, and vitamin C, as indicated in recent nutritional surveys.

Thomas and Call[6] made a nutritional analysis of foods eaten between meals by adolescents in the *Ten-State Nutrition Survey*. The mean nutrient intake per 100 kcalories from between-meal foods met or exceeded the 1968 RDA for protein, riboflavin, and ascorbic acid. Both males and females had vitamin A intakes that were below the RDA, but the mean vitamin A intake per 100 kcalories among males exceeded the RDA. The mean vitamin A intake per 100 kcalories for females represented 92 per cent of the RDA of 212 IU per 100 kcalories.

The calcium and iron content of in-between meals for males and females adolescents was below recommendations. The intake of calcium for males supplied about 89 per cent per 100 kcalories and the intake of females yielded about 74 per cent of the RDA for calcium per 100 kcalories. Males obtained about 86 per cent per 100 kcalories for iron,

and females received about 69 per cent per 100 kcalories of the U.S. RDA.

The authors conclude on the basis of their analysis that the nutrients supplied to these teen-agers rated well in a number of important nutrients. A number of implications are offered in regard to the speculation about fortifying snack foods with certain nutrients. No evidence is given that protein must be added. There appears little need for fortification of these foods with the B vitamins or vitamin C. Serious study is suggested for the problems of inadequate iron, calcium, and vitamin A. Nutrition education may be one answer.

Young and others[7] have done a series of research studies on the metabolic effects of frequent feeding. The study cited here was on young college men for a 15-week period in which metabolic tests were made to determine the effects of frequent feeding (1 to 6 meals a day) on body composition and nutrient absorption and utilization. Results indicated that no significant differences existed for men on six meals versus one meal in skinfold thicknesses, average nitrogen retention, percentage of fat intake excreted, and xylose absorption. Serum cholesterol was significantly higher on the one-meal per day regimen than on six meals. Subjective responses indicated that 60 per cent of the men had an overwhelming need to sleep after the one large meal per day and a like percentage commented on the distraction of extreme hunger during the day. In terms of preference for the number of meals, 40 per cent preferred one meal daily largely for reasons of convenience; 30 per cent preferred the six-meal pattern, primarily for reasons of comfort; the remaining 30 per cent were ambivalent.

A serious question has been raised about the effect of frequent eating on dental health. Incidence of dental caries would be determined to an extent by the type of food consumed. Foods with high sugar content and

[4] Mary L. Blackbrun, "Who Turns the Child Off to Nutrition?" *Journal of Nutrition Education*, Vol. 2, No. 2 (Fall 1970), pp. 45–47.

[5] Breeling, op. cit., p. 52.

[6] Jean A. Thomas and David L. Call, "Eating Between Meals—A Nutrition Problem Among Teenagers?" *Nutrition Reviews*, Vol. 31, No. 5 (May 1973), pp. 137–139.

[7] Charlotte M. Young, Louise Hutter, Sonia S. Scanlan, Catherine E. Rand, Leo Lutwak, and Vladimir Simko, "Metabolic Effects of Meal Frequency on Normal Young Men," *Journal of the American Dietetic Association*, Vol. 61, No. 4 (October 1972), pp. 391–398.

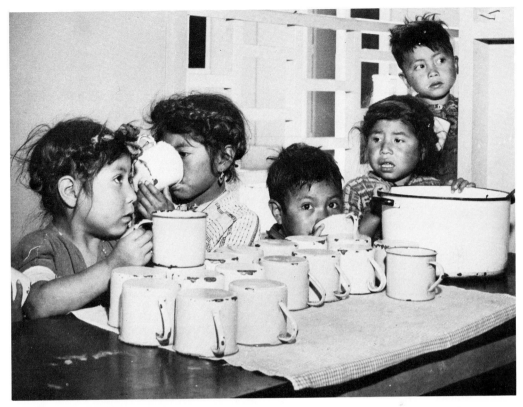

FIGURE 31-6. *Children in a Guatemalan village receive 2 servings of milk to guard them against malnutrition.* (UNICEF)

with properties of sticking to the teeth would be questionable selections.[8] Madsen contends that each time that these foods are eaten the possibility of dental caries is increased unless vigorous brushing and flossing are used as preventive measures. The slow and continued sipping, sucking, chewing, and nibbling make candy, sweet liquids, gum, sweet gelatine desserts, sherbets and the like, especially hazardous.

Suggestions for Snacks

Although individual preferences for in-between food will vary, an attempt to consider choices from the basic four food groups would enhance the nutritive quality of the diet. Some suggestions are offered in Table 30–1. Items from groups may be combined, such as crackers and cheese, cereal cookies and milk or fruit juice, frankfurters on a roll with raw vegetables or cole slaw, a milk shake and a cereal muncher, such as granola. Foods should be unsweetened.

Huenemann[9] and others discovered in their research on the eating practices of teen-agers that the snacks consumed did not always represent their preferences but rather what was

[8] Kenneth O. Madsen, "Frequency of Eating and Dental Health," *Food and Nutrition News,* Vol. 46, No. 4 (March–April 1975), pp. 1, 4.

[9] Ruth L. Huenemann, L. R. Shapiro, M. C. Hampton, and B. W. Mitchell, "Food and Eating Practices of Teenagers," *Journal of American Dietetic Association,* Vol. 53, No. 1 (July 1968), pp. 17–24.

TABLE 30–1

Snacks from the Basic Four

CEREALS	MILK	MEAT	FRUITS AND VEGETABLES
Dry cereals as munchers	Milk shakes or beverages	Hamburger	Raw carrots, celery, green pepper, cauliflower,
Cereal with milk	Use unsweetened carbonated	Soybean nuts	asparagus, and others kept
Crackers	beverages to	Frankfurters	in the refrigerator in a plastic
Small sandwiches	reconstitute	Cold cuts	bag for easy access
Bread sticks to stir soup	dried milk	Fish sticks	Fruit or vegetable juices served
Oatmeal cookies or cereal bars	Cheese cubes of many varieties	Peanut butter	cold or as soups
Pizza	Ice milk and	Egg rolls	Fresh fruit such as apples,
Angelfood cake	ice cream	Tacos	berries, melon, bananas,
Popcorn	Buttermilk	Nuts	plums, grapes
	Cottage cheese or other soft cheeses		Bean Dips

available. This evidence strengthens the need for planning this increasingly important aspect of daily nutrition.

Buying Snacks

Snack foods should be carefully selected. Ten or more per cent of the cost of food for a week may be due to the unwise addition of such snacks as doughnuts, corn chips, pretzels, or a pack of carbonated cola beverage. These foods are high in kcalories but offer only small amounts of other nutrients. Any tendency toward overweight will be encouraged if these foods are provided. Out of sight and out of mind may lead snackers to more nutritious fare. If individuals have strong preferences for some of these salty, fried, or sweet snack foods, perhaps they may be offered occasionally, depending upon the situation.

There are many ways to cut costs of snacks. Use dried milk powder that costs half as much as fluid milk and combine with fruit juices such as orange or pineapple juice, mashed banana, frozen fruit such as strawberries, or use with pudding mixes and substitute for individual snack pack cans in a carton. A low-cost muncher can be made from peanuts, pretzels, and unsugared ready-to eat cereals. Raisins,

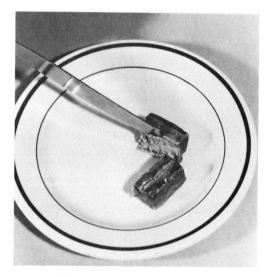

FIGURE 31–7. *Try a new food for a snack, such as Sufu, a Chinese cheese made from a soybean curd, known as Tofu.* (USDA)

prunes, figs, dates and other dried foods are inexpensive and nutritious. Some may be stuffed with peanut butter. Processed cheese costs less than natural American cheese. It can be quite a challenge to look at the supermarket shelves for unusual snacks that are cheap and contribute to your nutritive needs.

If time is more precious than money, look in the dairy cases and the frozen food sections for ideas. The health food section of a supermarket may have some suggestions, but watch the prices.

Be as vigilant when snacks are eaten out. Would fish and chips be cheaper than a hamburger, provided there was an equal preference for them? Study the menu for good buys.

SELECTED REFERENCES

Breeling, James L., "Are We Snacking Our Way to Malnutrition," *Today's Health,* Vol. 48, No. 1 (January 1970), pp. 48–50.

Huenemann, Ruth L., L. R. Shapiro, M. C. Hampton, and B. W. Mitchell, "Food Eating Practices of Teenagers," *Journal of the American Dietetic Association,* Vol. 53, No. 1 (July 1968), pp. 17–24.

Martin, Ethel Austin, *Nutrition in Action,* Holt, Rinehart and Winston, Inc., New York, 1971, pp. 297–303.

Murphy, Roger, and Ruth Hodgson Klein, "Shop for Snack Foods Carefully," *Focus on the Food Markets,* Cooperative Extension, New York State, Cornell University, State University of New York, U.S. Department of Agriculture, New York, September 6, 1971.

"Points of View, Pro and Con: Chips and Soda," *Journal of Nutrition Education,* Vol. 2, No. 4 (Spring 1971), p. 130.

Thomas, Jean A., and David L. Call, "Eating Between Meals—A Nutrition Problem for Teenagers?" *Nutrition Reviews,* Vol. 31, No. 5 (May 1973), pp. 137–139.

Young, Charlotte M., Louise F. Hutter, Sonia S. Scanlan, Catherine E. Rand, Leo Lutwak, and Vladimir Simko, "Metabolic Effects of Meal Frequency on Normal Young Men," *Journal of the American Dietetic Association,* Vol. 61, No. 4 (October 1972), pp. 391–398.

32

Modifications of the Diet

Almost everyone at some time or another has to make some modification of his daily eating habits because of illness. A cold, a digestive upset, or something more serious, such as high blood pressure, may force a change in eating. Often a person in such circumstances may plan his own diet based on hearsay, family tradition, or a neighbor's advice. This practice can be extremely dangerous. Only a physician is competent to prescribe a diet, and his directions should be carefully followed.

Ideas concerning food during illness have undergone a number of changes. At one time a person may have spoken of his "special" diet, which connoted that he was deprived of certain foods. The present emphasis is to provide an adequate diet whenever possible. According to the ailment, the diet may be modified (1) in consistency—such as liquid, strained, chopped, and the like; (2) in the method of preparation—such as avoiding fried or raw foods, or limiting certain kinds or amounts of seasonings; (3) in the amounts of certain nutrients—such as an increase or decrease; (4) in the omission of certain foods as in allergies; (5) in frequency of feeding; (6) in specific ratio of carbohydrate, fat, or pro-

tein; or (7) in combinations of these modifications. Diets are generally named by the modification—like a low-residue, high-iron, or liquid diet.

Diets a Physician May Prescribe

Often persons who are ill do not realize that the type of diet a physician prescribes is an important part of the total treatment for the illness. Any modification of the usual diet is planned by the physician to aid the person's recovery. A dietitian or nutritionist may explain the diet and the food permitted to the patient or family member.

A number of fallacious ideas are connected with eating during illness. People need not necessarily lose weight because they are sick. Pollack and Halpern[1] emphasize that "weight loss is not an inevitable result of disease or injury and can usually be minimized by sufficient attention to nutrition." This highlights the inaccuracy of the idea that it is not necessary to eat all the food that a doctor indicates.

[1] Herbert Pollack and Seymour Halpern, "Therapeutic Nutrition—A Review," *Nutritional Observatory*, Vol. 12, No. 3 (July 1951), pp. 14–17.

464

Granted that appetite may not be at par during illness, yet every effort should be made to consume the food so that other deficiencies will not complicate the situation. Not only must the diet be adhered to, but special attention must be given to the length of time for which the physician advises the diet. There may be an inclination to stop before the prescribed time or to continue on the diet long after the physician has recommended that it be discontinued. Any deviation from a physician's orders may result in serious malnutrition or other conditions.

The condition of the person on a modified diet must be considered. If the diet is associated with surgery, injury, or illness, there may be certain important restrictions in regard to allowable foods. In contrast, a person who is not ill but has to make adjustments because of loss of teeth, malformations of the jaw or mouth, or other problems may have to consider only the consistency of the food and should not be deprived of well-liked foods, such as apple pie, if they can be suitably prepared for consumption.

Liquid Diet

Sometimes the doctor orders a full liquid diet. This diet is characterized by foods that are liquid or will liquefy at body temperature and may be considered an adequate diet if it is planned to include all nutrients. It is different only in that the consistency is changed. It can be very palatable if prepared and served with ingenuity. (An electric blender is helpful in the preparation of food for this diet.) Plain milk may be flavored with vanilla, spices, coffee, honey, or molasses. Molasses will contribute iron to the diet, as well as some of the B vitamins. Proprietary liquid preparations are sometimes used for extra nutrients. Delicious drinks can be prepared from evaporated milk and diluted with fruit or vegetable juices instead of water, thus making a more nutritious beverage. Evaporated milk will not curdle as easily as plain milk when fruit juice is added, which is an advantage. As orange juice is a valuable source of vitamin C, the combination of evaporated milk and orange juice is a good one. Other fruit juices or combinations of fruit juices may be used equally effectively, like tomato or combination vegetable juices seasoned with celery salt.

The nutritive value of milk might be increased by the addition of malted milk, whole or skimmed dry milk, ice cream, mashed banana, egg, or cream. Eggs can be made into various types of eggnogs. If additional kcalories are required, the use of cream or "half and half" is desirable. If kcalories are to be reduced, it is wise to omit large amounts of these kcalorie-rich foods.

Cream soups make a valuable and interesting addition to liquid diets and are often welcomed because they are a hot food. Vegetables may be used in cream soups, but it is wise to strain all soup. If a family member is interested in preparing the cream soup at home in preference to the use of canned soups, milk or milk and cream may be added to strained baby foods for a very palatable cream soup. If kcalories are needed in the diet, then, in addition to cream, it is possible to add a spoon of butter or margarine to a bowl of cream soup for flavor as well as nutritive value. Dried brewer's yeast might be added to any of these beverages or soups for additional nutritive value.

Cereal can be introduced into a liquid diet in the form of a gruel. This dish has a higher proportion of water than the ordinary cooked cereal. Instead of water, milk or undiluted evaporated milk can be used. If kcalories need to be decreased, skimmed milk might be used. The cereal should be prepared so that it is of liquid consistency. Any type of cooked cereal can be used. After cooking, it is advisable to strain the cereal. It is especially important that the gruel be well seasoned with adequate salt. It should be served hot and be smooth in consistency. Possible additions to gruels are a slightly beaten whole egg, cream, egg yolk, butter, or a small amount of molasses.

Fruit is generally served as a fruit juice in a liquid diet. These juices might be enhanced by the addition of a little lemon or lime juice, sherbet, ice cream, cream, or a beaten egg. Other beverages that may be used are various carbonated drinks. When ice cream, cream, or dried skim milk is whipped into the drink, a very palatable beverage results. Unless otherwise directed, tea and coffee in moderation can be served. Cocoa is another possibility.

Persons on a liquid diet may need to be served six or eight times a day. It is wise to keep sugar at a minimum, for it does tend to cause gas if consumed in large quantities. Too many eggs will raise the cholesterol content of the diet. Large amounts of fat, such as cream or butter, may need to be guarded against, too, since in some individuals they may cause diarrhea. Serving foods in attractive dishes and at the correct temperature will do a great deal to induce the patient to consume his food.

In some cases a physician may prescribe a clear liquid diet. This is a very inadequate diet from a nutritional standpoint and is generally indicated for only a few days. The main contribution of this diet is fluids.

Liquids that may be included in this diet are clear or strained fruit and vegetable juices, gelatin, carbonated beverages, tea or coffee without cream or milk, and sugar. Fruit or vegetable juices may be made into ices providing they do not have milk or other ingredients added. And some physicians will permit beaten egg white to be included in either the ices or the gelatin dishes. Fat-free broth may be served hot or chilled, or it may be jellied and served as consomme. Some of these foods can be combined for variety, for example, broth and clear vegetable juice, or fruit juices and carbonated beverages.

Soft Diet

This diet is prescribed by the physician when a person has an injury or for some other reason cannot masticate food well. It may also be prescribed for cardiac cases to prevent any danger of choking on more difficult foods. And sometimes ill persons who are too weak to chew find a soft diet easier to handle. If the physician desires the diet to be low in residue as well, special care will have to be taken to select foods that are low in fiber, cellulose, and connective tissue.

The major change in food in this type of diet is its consistency. To produce a soft diet, it is necessary to cook, mash, chop, strain, or homogenize food. Since vitamins may be lost in these processes, it is wise to prepare the food as near serving time as possible.

Milk and milk products make an excellent nutritive contribution to a soft diet. However, highly seasoned cheeses are often prohibited by the physician although doctors sometimes permit some of the hard mild cheeses, particularly if they are melted and cooked with other foods—macaroni and cheese, for example. Fruits and vegetables are cooked, and skins and seeds are removed. Cooking softens those cells that are composed of cellulose and other types of carbohydrate. For low-fiber content, it may be necessary to strain or sieve the fruits or vegetables, a process known as pureeing. Vegetable purees are unpopular with many persons, so if the patient is not too ill and the doctor permits, cooked, tender, mild, young vegetables or vegetables of low fiber content, such as potatoes, asparagus, spinach, squash, pumpkin, or carrots that are boiled, steamed, creamed, made into a souffle, or escalloped, but not fried, may be served. Vegetables may be chopped, mashed, or diced. Skins and seeds should be removed. Fruit or vegetable juices are permitted. And certain doctors allow the use of some raw fruit such as peeled pears, peaches, apricots, and bananas, but the skin and seeds must be removed. Avocado filled with cottage cheese is pleasing. A more liberal use of fruits and vegetables is now being permitted on this diet to encourage patients to eat; the doctor's orders must be followed, however.

Strongly flavored vegetables like cabbage, Brussels sprouts, and onions are generally prohibited.

Breads and cereals should be of the refined, enriched type. Dry cereals without roughage, if well moistened with milk or cream and masticated thoroughly, can be used as well as cooked cereals.

Meats are included in this diet, although occasionally a doctor will prohibit or limit meat for certain patients. Beef, veal, lamb, and poultry are suggested. Meat should be tender with as little connective tissue as possible. It may be tenderized by long cooking for some cuts. Grinding, mincing, removing some of the connective tissue before cooking, or selecting cuts with a minimum amount of connective tissue are other suggestions. Also, if the doctor does not object, meat tenderizer is valuable for making tough cuts tender. Eggs, except fried eggs, are allowed on this type of diet.

Desserts should be simple; possibilities include milk puddings, rennets, ice cream, gelatin desserts, custards, fruit whips, plain cookies, and angelfood or sponge cake. Chocolate is restricted by some physicians. No nuts should be added to any of these desserts.

The type of beverage is generally not restricted on a soft diet. Thus individuals may have tea, coffee, cocoa, carbonated beverages, or cereal beverages.

A soft diet can provide both adequate nutrients and considerable variety. An examination of some of the family cookbooks may offer suggestions for preparing foods that are permitted. The diet may be made more interesting by the addition of certain spices. The ones usually permitted are cinnamon, sage, thyme, paprika, and allspice, whereas the following are usually prohibited: black pepper, chili pepper, mustard seed, cloves, and, in some instances, nutmeg.

Such items as jams, marmalade, or candy with fruit or nuts are not allowed. However, jelly and hard candy may be included.

Low-Fiber or Low-Residue Diet

Low-fiber or low-residue diets are characterized by a combination of liquid and solid foods that have had the cellulose and connective fiber removed to the degree recommended by the physician. The reduction of indigestible carbohydrates, like cellulose, and connective fiber, like that found in meats, may be done in several ways. Commercial processing like that done in the refinement of flour to make white bread is one example; cereals are refined, too. Another method is to remove as much fiber and cellulose as possible during the preparation of the food at home. Fruits and vegetables may be cooked and then strained or sieved. This is also done commercially, as in baby foods. Cooking fruits and vegetables will tenderize the cellulose and the fibers of meat, too.

Foods permitted on a low-fiber or low-residue diet are coffee, in limited amounts; tea; refined breads and cereals, such as cream of

wheat, farina, rice flakes, macaroni, noodles, rice, and cornmeal; and mild cheddar, cottage, or cream cheeses (avoid sharp cheeses). Desserts such as plain cake, custard, gelatin, ice cream without fruit or nuts, plain puddings and rennet and fats like butter, cream, margarine, or vegetable oils are included. Only strained fruit juices are permitted on a very low residue diet, but strained cooked fruits may be added if diet is moderated. Tender chopped or minced lean meat, fish, or poultry, white potato, and tomato juice are permitted. On a moderate-residue diet bland vegetables may be cooked and strained. Other acceptable foods are clear and low-fat soups; sweets, such as hard candies, honey, jelly, or syrup. Foods to be avoided are fruits, nuts, marmalade, preserves, or jams; popcorn, pickles, or excessive seasonings. Luncheon meats and sausage should be avoided, and the skin should be removed from poultry. Some doctors prohibit citrus fruits and juices.

A low-fiber diet requires considerable imagination to prevent it from becoming monotonous. The length of time for the diet may vary. If the diet is for a long period of time, it is particularly important that the food be interesting and nutritious.

Light Diet

A light diet serves as a transition from a soft to a regular diet or is used for other purposes indicated by the physician. This diet is not clear-cut and varies from doctor to doctor, but the general emphasis is on foods prepared in a simple manner. It usually includes cooked whole vegetables and fruits, with the exception of strong-flavored vegetables—onions, cabbage, or cauliflower—and vegetables that may cause gas, like baked beans; fruit and fruit juices; milk and milk products; whole meats, but not pork; simple desserts, but not rich ones like pies, cake, doughnuts, or pastries; refined cereals and breads. Some physicians will permit fresh oranges and lettuce and tomato. All fried foods and heavily spiced foods are to be avoided. Soups are generally clear or creamed and cannot be spiced. Concentrated sweets, such as jam, marmalade, or candy with fruit, are omitted, but nuts are allowed. Relishes and pickles are to be avoided. This diet actually involves only minor modifications of the regular diet.

Regular Diet

A regular diet is given to patients whose ailment does not interfere with the digestive system, such as a patient with a broken arm or leg. If the person cannot move around or if activity is curtailed in any way, the kcaloric content of the diet may need to be reduced. A regular diet would include all the foods that the family regularly has, but it is necessary to give special attention to food likes and dislikes in these circumstances because this type of diet acts as a kind of morale builder.

Other Modifications

Sometimes a doctor will ask the patient to modify his diet in other ways. It may be in terms of nutrients, that is, by either increasing or decreasing the nutrient for some particular reason. This change is indicated in specific amounts, such as 40 g of fat or 100 g of carbohydrate. These modifications vary greatly and consequently are explained very carefully by the physician. Special attention may need to be exercised, too, in preparation and marketing.

A low-sodium diet may be prescribed by a physician for a variety of conditions. The physician's order may indicate "no salt added" or amounts varying from 200 to 1000 mg of sodium daily, depending on the condition and its severity. This diet requires unusual vigilance because the sources of sodium, including common table salt, are many.

If the amount of sodium is seriously limited, it may be necessary to have low-sodium milk, which may be secured in powder or liquid form. Labels on commercial products made with milk must be checked carefully to determine if low-sodium products are available. These would include milk shakes, condensed milk, ice cream, sherbets, and cheeses. Sodium alginate may be added to some chocolate milk drinks or ice creams for a smooth texture.

Fresh and frozen fruit and fresh vegetables are permitted on most low-sodium diets. However, spinach, chard, dandelion greens, beet greens, celery, and sauerkraut may be limited by the physician's recommendations. Canned and frozen vegetables usually have salt added. Check the label. Look for "salt," "sodium," or "Na." Sodium hydroxide is used to soften the skins of some fruits, such as olives and vegetables. Glazed or crystallized fruit, some dried fruits, and maraschino cherries often have sodium sulfite added in the processing or as a preservative.

Depending on sodium limitations, the amount of meat may be controlled. All canned fish, such as herring, tuna, caviar, and dried cod, is usually restricted. Smoked and salty meats, such as ham and bacon, must be eliminated in most cases. Shellfish are particularly high in sodium content and must be omitted. Frozen fish fillets have salt added. Sometimes canned fish is prepared without salt. Luncheon meats, sausages, bologna, frankfurters, and smoked tongue must be included on the prohibited list.

Most commercial breads are on the restricted list. Unsalted crackers, Melba toast, and matzoth can be used instead, and some markets have low-sodium breads. Cooked cereals are confined to farina, grits, oatmeal, rolled wheat, and rice, which must be cooked without salt. Flour, macaroni, noodles, cornmeal, tapioca, cornstarch, and spaghetti are usually permitted. Puffed rice, puffed wheat, and shredded wheat are allowed. Quick-cooking cereals and enriched cereals, except those listed, have salt added. Pretzels, salted popcorn, and other munchers must be eliminated.

Fats and oils allowed are unsalted butter, margarine, cooking oils, lard or vegetable fat shortenings. Cream of various types, including sour cream, may be limited, because the sodium content is rather high. Sweet foods like syrup, honey, jam, marmalade, or jelly (look at label of last three for inclusion of salt) or homemade candy or candied fruits made without salt are allowed.

Items that are high in sodium are bouillon cubes; catsup; celery, garlic, and onion salts; chili sauce; pickles; relishes, soy sauce; meat tenderizers; monosodium glutamate, used to enhance flavors; mustard; and salted nuts. Salt may be added in the softening of water that is consumed.

A number of cookbooks with interesting recipes and menu suggestions for the individual on this restricted diet are available.

A physician may order a fat-controlled diet in which the level of saturated fats is low. Foods emphasized are skim milk, fish, poultry, vegetables, fruit, breads, cereals, sweets, cooking oils like corn, soybean, or cotton, and margarines made with polyunsaturated fats. Foods such as beef, lamb, pork, eggs, and other cholesterol-rich foods may be controlled as to amount allowed.

Some individuals erroneously believe that whipped and soft margarines have fewer kcalories. Others are unfamiliar with the foods that have saturated fats, such as butter, hydrogenated shortenings, cheeses, and whole milk. Individuals should not be swayed by information about fat in the diet gained through mass media but should follow the advice of a physician. The research in this field is very active and the answers are still tentative in certain areas. Only a physician is competent to make decisions about fat-controlled diets.

Seriousness of Severe Restrictions

Sometimes it may be necessary to live on a modified diet for a long period of time and, in some cases, even for a lifetime. This is true of people who have diabetes, for example. Careful consideration must be given to the food the doctor prescribes, not only for every meal but also for foods eaten between meals.

In diabetes there is a lack of insulin or hypoinsulinism that results in elevated blood sugar. Insulin to compensate for this lack is usually prescribed by the physician plus a diet. Although carefully estimated to distribute the carbohydrate somewhat evenly through the day as well as protein and fat, with careful planning the restrictions are not burdensome. A simplified plan, the Exchange List, assists a diabetic after instruction to plan his meals and snacks. Foods of comparable nutrient value are listed under the various food groups, such as milk, bread, meat, and vegetables into amounts equal to one exchange. For example, one slice of bread equals ½ cup of cooked cereal. The number of exchanges under each group are matched to meet the diet prescribed by the physician.

A disorder of carbohydrate metabolism that is almost opposite in effect is hyperinsulinism or hypoglycemia, which results in decreased blood sugar. Diets prescribed for such individuals generally include a reduction of carbohydrate because this nutrient further stimulates insulin secretion; an increase in protein is desirable because sugar from protein is released very slowly and there is no appreciable challenge to increased insulin secretion; and fat is increased to provide for adequate kcalories because of the reduction in carbohydrate. Between-meal feedings are recommended. The Exchange List may be used to plan the diet so that the carbohydrate, protein, and fat are as evenly distributed through the day as possible. Individuals with this condition cannot eat sweets, desserts, and even the bread exchanges may have to be eliminated for some persons.

A similar situation applies to those who have allergies. They must be conscious of all the possible sources of foods to which they are allergic. For example, if one is allergic to mustard, he must be very careful about the kind of salad dressings he eats, for many of the commercial types include it.

In the case of diets that either increase or decrease certain nutrients, such as a vitamin, mineral, carbohydrate, fat, or protein, a person must know the foods that contain these nutrients.

Whatever the modification of the diet, it is essential that the individual, his family, and his friends do everything to cooperate in helping him adhere to his diet. Failure to follow the diet will adversely affect his well-being.

Adapting the Family Diet

Occasionally a modified diet may create quite an upheaval in the family food buying and preparation. Whenever possible, the modified diet should be planned from the regular family diet. Consideration should be given to the foods eaten by the entire family with the idea of modifying these foods for the patient. In the case of a low-sodium diet, for example, the food may be cooked without salt and salt added later for the rest of the family. In the case of a low-residue diet, some dishes, such as the meat, can be served to everyone. Some-

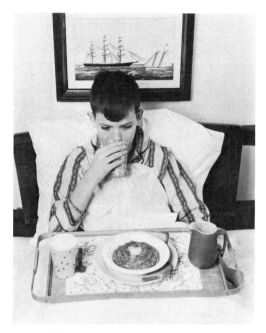

FIGURE 32–1. *The tray and its contents may have an important psychological effect on a sick person. (Plate, Cup and Container Institute)*

times the food can be served to the other members of the family in its natural state and strained or sieved for the patient. With a soft diet, some of the food eaten by the family can be mashed, minced, or mixed in a blender for the patient.

If labels do not give adequate information about a well-liked food, it is possible to write to the company to get additional information about the constituents of the food or its processing. Companies are generally very willing to give this information under these circumstances. The person whose diet is to be modified may become very interested in the preparation of certain foods on his own. This interest may increase the palatability of his diet and will also remove some of the responsibility from others.

Those who are responsible for the modified diet must have an appreciation of its contribution, for the modification has a very definite function. One must realize that this diet is an important part of the total therapy. Consequently, it is extremely important that there be a clear understanding of the type of modification required and what it involves. Furthermore, people must develop a keen sense of responsibility in adhering to the diet, for recovery will obviously be retarded if this is not done. It is also essential that all persons concerned realize that every effort must be made to provide adequate nutrients for the one on a diet. Personal likes and dislikes should be considered when possible; some limitations may be in order. Because of modifications, it is even more important for the person to eat all the foods he is permitted. With this thought in mind, it is also easier to modify the family diet in whatever way necessary so that the person on the diet will not feel that he is too different in his eating pattern.

Those who must remain on modified diets for an extended period of time may occasionally have to eat away from home. It is then very important that they be familiar with the foods that they are permitted to eat. With a little creative thinking it is quite possible to have almost any type of diet away from home. This applies not only while traveling or when eating meals out but also when one is a guest in someone's home. It may be necessary to select judiciously from the food served so that the diet will continue to be adequately modified. Above all, the patient should not develop a martyr complex but should make every effort to enjoy his food under these circumstances and to realize that he is doing what he should do to contribute to his well-being.

SELECTED REFERENCES

Anderson, Linnea, Marjorie V. Dibble, Helen S. Mitchell, and Henderika J. Rynbergen, *Nutrition in Nursing*, J. B. Lippincott Company, Philadelphia, 1972.

Goodhart, Robert S., and Maurice E. Shils (eds.), *Modern Nutrition in Health and Disease*, Lea & Febiger, Philadelphia, 1973.

Krause, Marie V., and Martha A. Hunscher, *Food, Nutrition, and Therapy*, W. B. Saunders Company, Philadelphia, 1972.

Nutrition Department, The Johns Hopkins Hospital, *Manual of Applied Nutrition*, The Johns Hopkins Press, Baltimore, 1973.

Robinson, Corrine H., *Normal and Therapeutic Nutrition*, Macmillan Publishing Co., Inc., New York, 1972.

Staff of the Department of Nutrition, University Hospitals, The University of Iowa, *Recent Advances in Therapeutic Diets*, Iowa State University Press, Ames, Iowa, 1973.

33

Food Fads, Foodlore, and Fallacies

Magical qualities have been attributed to certain foods since the earliest days of history. For example, the early Greeks compelled criminals to eat garlic to purify themselves of the crimes they had committed. The Egyptians fed garlic to the laborers who were building the pyramids so they would be endowed with strength. The Romans pressed the juice from artichoke hearts to use as a lotion to restore hair. Nero ate leeks several days each month to clear his voice. These ancient fallacies may seem silly today, but almost everyone harbors a few baseless ideas about the qualities of certain foods.

Definitions and Identification

A distinction must be made among fad, foodlore, fallacy, and fact. A fad is identified by a food or combination of foods that are declared to be beneficial or to serve as a cure-all. Fads are generally short-lived. They are intensely popular for a period of time until replaced by another fad. They originate with individuals who are untutored in nutrition.

Many fads have dominated the reducing scene from time to time. Foods faddish for cure-alls or for promoting health have been blackstrap molasses, yogurt, alfalfa tea, wheat germ, and raw sugar. In contrast, the elimination of certain foods or occasionally a combination of foods because they contain harmful ingredients, such as grapes causing polio or dried currants being poisonous, is another type of food faddism. However, experts have demonstrated again and again that an adequate diet does not rest on one food or even one combination of foods.

Foodlore deals with food notions whose origin is usually obscure but may have arisen from "old wives' tales," regional fables, or from family dictums. Some Southerners, for instance, may believe that hot biscuits are better for you than other types of bread. A mother in a family may firmly believe that all vegetables should be soaked in water before using. Her daughters may subscribe to the same belief, and so it may go from generation to generation. Sometimes these food ways are embellished as they pass from one family to the next.

Fallacies in regard to food are based on misrepresentation, misinterpretation, and misinformation. Some folks, for example, believe

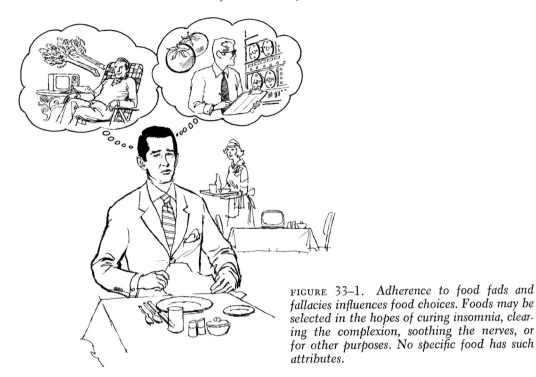

FIGURE 33–1. *Adherence to food fads and fallacies influences food choices. Foods may be selected in the hopes of curing insomnia, clearing the complexion, soothing the nerves, or for other purposes. No specific food has such attributes.*

that the only kind of sugar to be used is honey because it is a natural sugar. White sugar is not synthetic, and there is little difference in nutritive value between honey and sugar. Many people are thus misinformed about the true nutritive value of a food and are ignorant of the fact that specific curative qualities cannot be attributed to foods.

A nutrition fact implies a scientific basis. Facts about food emerge from the research and work of leading scientists and nutritionists. Their work in universities, research foundations, hospitals, government agencies, and laboratories in industry provides a background for making authoritative statements about what food will or will not do for us.

Food Faddism a Matter of Concern

The heightened interest and receptivity of the public in regard to nutrition and health have encouraged food faddism to flourish. The impact of mass media, the health-food industry, and the pursuit of fashionable patterns of food consumption are other important fac-

tors in the development of this public health problem.[1]

Many people are inclined to be amused at the antics of the food faddist. In reality, food faddism is a serious problem in the United States. Faddism has emerged as a billion-dollar business, and according to the Food and Drug Administration, is the most widespread kind of quackery in the United States. Rynearson[2] contends that nutrition quackery is not only misleading but also dangerous.

Quackery and food faddism become especially dangerous, according to Bruch,[3] when false promises prevent people from seeking the medical advice and treatment that might save their lives or alleviate their pain and suffering.

---

[1] "Food Faddism," *Dairy Council Digest,* Vol. 44, No. 1 (January–February 1973), pp. 1–4.

[2] Edward H. Rynearson, "Americans Love Hogwash," *Nutrition Reviews,* Supplement, July 1974, pp. 1–14.

[3] Hilde Bruch, "The Allure of Food Cults and Nutrition Quackery," *Journal of the American Dietetic Association,* Vol. 57, No. 4 (October 1970), pp. 316–320.

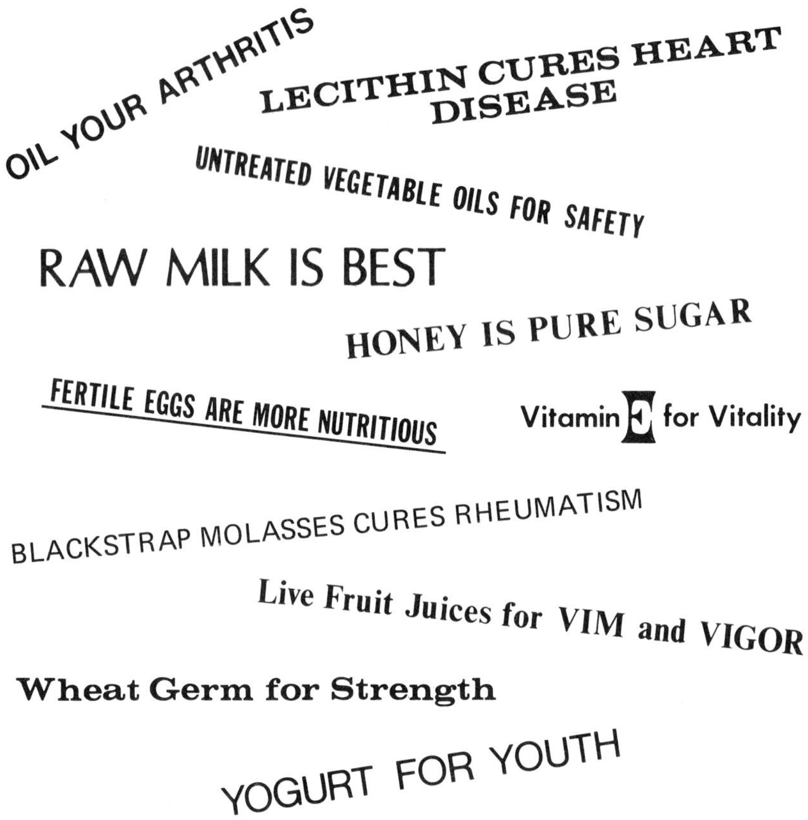

OIL YOUR ARTHRITIS

LECITHIN CURES HEART DISEASE

UNTREATED VEGETABLE OILS FOR SAFETY

RAW MILK IS BEST

HONEY IS PURE SUGAR

FERTILE EGGS ARE MORE NUTRITIOUS

Vitamin E for Vitality

BLACKSTRAP MOLASSES CURES RHEUMATISM

Live Fruit Juices for VIM and VIGOR

Wheat Germ for Strength

YOGURT FOR YOUTH

FIGURE 33–2. *Quackery slogans in nutrition.*

Not only the fatally ill seek help from these nostrums; many who are not physically ill but only insecure about the uncertainties of living, so that they become concerned about their health and their bodies, resort to fads. Those who suffer from ill-defined pains and aches are often the most susceptible. It may be easier to worry about their pains or their digestion than to meet the stresses and strains of everyday living. The high cost of foods that may be sold in special stores or by mail order can be ill afforded by many people and is another concern. Adherence to faddish diets or including only a few foods in the diet may lead to serious inadequacies of certain nutrients, as well as to giving a false sense of security.

Checklist on Information About Fads

Everyone should be concerned with his personal awareness of fads and fallacies. The fol-lowing checklist may provide some insights. Answer each question with a "yes" or "no." *Do you believe that—*

1. Onions will cure a cold?
2. Blackstrap molasses will cure rheumatism?
3. A pregnant woman must eat for two?
4. Milk is constipating?
5. Food cooked in aluminum causes cancer?
6. An apple a day will keep the doctor away?
7. Milk and fish eaten together are "murder"?
8. Tomato juice is too acid for the system?
9. Celery is a brain food?
10. Protein and starches should not be eaten at the same meal?
11. Only young children need milk?

12. Raw cucumbers without salt are poisonous?
13. Oysters increase sexual potency?
14. There is a difference between the nutritive value of white and brown eggs?
15. Popcorn will take the place of meat and milk?
16. Gelatin is one of the best sources of protein?
17. Diabetes is caused by eating too many sweets?
18. A good way to reduce is to skip breakfast?
19. Rice, plus a regular diet, cures high blood pressure?
20. Margarine is harder to digest than butter?

Each of these above questions is from a list of over 200 compiled by the American Dietetic Association.[4] A single "yes" means that a person is the victim of some degree of misinformation about foods. Even a record of all "no's" can mean that one nevertheless believes something fallacious that was not included on the list. Every "yes" is a danger signal. More than five "yes" answers is a serious matter.

Emergence of Misconceptions About Food

There are many sources of faddish food ways. Some of them originated through early superstitions. Primitive man believed that the qualities of the animal he ate would be transferred to him. He believed, for example, that if he ate a lion he would become fierce, and if he ate a snake he would be sly and mean. Even the organs denoted certain qualities; the heart of an animal would give courage; the liver promoted merciful attributes.

Beliefs about food are also associated with certain religious practices, regions of the country, nationalities, and with family traditions. Frequently, individuals will misinterpret the advice of a physician or a nutritionist or even misunderstand the claims of an advertisement.

Sheer ignorance is the reason for many silly ideas about food. The idea that eating food will change a condition of tension, discomfort, or pain has been engendered as an early experience in the lives of most everyone and enhances the potential use of fads.

A desire for a quick cure will lead many persons to eat a quantity of a certain food. An adolescent with a poor complexion, a man with arthritis, or a young woman who is overweight are good potentials for believing that a certain food or combination of foods will work miracles. They are easy prey for high-pressure salesmanship for health foods or for gadgets, such as a press for making vegetable juice. Others who appear to succumb to the promises of the quack are the poor and underprivileged, the elderly, the uneducated, the seekers of eternal youth or an improved self-image, or the idle rich.

Social pressure is another potent factor. The desire among adolescents for a clear complexion is so great that they may succumb to a faddish diet. In a similar manner, the advice of "old-timers" may be followed without examining it for fallacies. The origin of fads and fallacies is very complex and can be traced to many sources.

Fallacies About Certain Foods

The American Dietetic Association,[5] in a study of food misinformation, has divided the list into several categories. A few examples are cited for each category.

Fallacies Related to the Caloric Value of Food

1. Toast has fewer calories than bread. (*Fact*: Same number.)
2. Honey is not fattening. (*Fact*: 1 tablespoon is 50 kcalories.)
3. Dark bread contains fewer kcalories than white bread. (*Fact*: Approximately the same.)
4. Milk, potato, and bread are high in kcalories. (*Fact*: 1 glass (cup) of milk, 166 kcalories; 1 medium po-

---

[4] *Food Facts Talk Back*, American Dietetic Association, Chicago, 1957.

[5] Ibid.

tato, 100 kcalories; 1 slice of bread, 60 to 75 kcalories.)

5. Vegetable fats and oils can be used in any amount and are not fattening. (*Fact:* Same kcaloric value as animal fats and as well utilized.)

6. Sour cream contains fewer kcalories than sweet cream. (*Fact:* Same.)

7. High-protein foods have no kcalories. (*Fact:* Meat, cheese, or eggs have kcalories; for example, sirloin steak without bone has 86 kcalories per ounce.)

8. Homogenized milk contains no fat. (*Fact:* Cream does not come to the top because fat has been broken into tiny particles and is distributed throughout the milk.)

9. Water is fattening. (*Fact:* Water is free from kcalories.)

10. Uncolored soda pop contains no kcalories. (*Fact:* Ordinary carbonated beverages contain 85 to 100 kcalories per cup.)

Falacies Related to Specific Qualities of Food

1. Garlic cures high blood pressure.
2. Milk is constipating.
3. Beets build blood.
4. Fish is brain food.
5. Celery is good for the nerves.
6. Tomatoes clear the brain.
7. Onions cure insomnia.
8. Cucumbers are cooling.
9. Strawberries purify the blood.
10. Egg white injures the kidneys.

Since foods are broken down to nutrients in the process of digestion and metabolism, there is no basis for the idea that any one food has magical qualities either good or bad.

Fallacies Related to Combinations of Food

1. Milk and fish are poisonous together.
2. Proteins and starches should not be eaten at the same meal.
3. Milk and cherries are harmful.
4. Ice cream and lobster are dangerous together.

5. Coffee with cream is more harmful than black coffee.
6. Meat should not be eaten with milk.
7. Acid fruits should not be eaten with starches.
8. Milk and orange juice will explode in the stomach.

No experimental or clinical evidence shows that combining foods will have a poisonous effect. Many of these ideas originated in the days before refrigeration and other means of keeping food fresh. If two foods can be tolerated separately, there is reasonable assurance that they can be combined without harm.

Fads and Fallacies According to Age

One of the most common fallacies about milk is that adults do not need it, only children. The argument advanced is that adults are grown and have their teeth. Experimental evidence bears out the fact that for all ages milk provides certain essential nutrients that would be difficult to substitute in other foods. Another fallacy disturbing to adolescents is that the continued use of margarine will affect the development of secondary sex characteristics, such as the distribution of hair and the depth of voice. Sex characteristics are controlled principally by the secretions of endocrine glands and certainly cannot be attributed to the consumption of certain foods. Some people are silly enough to believe that no red meat should be eaten after 40. The need for adequate protein is present at all ages. Certain middle-aged women cling to the belief that age adds pounds, when actually they are overeating. Older people may be more susceptible to food fads, for they are interested in regaining youth or are anxious to cure some chronic ailment.

Food Notions in Pregnancy

It is unfortunate that some pregnant women adhere to erroneous beliefs about food. Some of the most common ones are as follows:

1. "Certain foods eaten during pregnancy mark the child." These accused foods vary from region to region and from

people to people. Strawberries, pepper, cornstarch, red clay, baking soda, and salmon are a few. (*False.*)

2. "A pregnant woman should indulge any cravings for certain foods because the body needs them." (*False.* Cravings for food have an emotional basis rather than a physiological need.)

3. "Green vegetables should not be eaten because the color might show up in the mother's milk." (*False.*)

4. "Fish and milk are poisonous if eaten during the first few weeks following childbirth." (*False.*)

5. "Cooked cabbage will taint a mother's milk." (*False.*)

6. "Sweet milk gives 'milk fever.'" (*False.*)

Other Myths

The results of a national study of health practices and opinions conducted for the Food and Drug Administration[6] revealed a large number of myths in connection to nutrition. Three fourths of the public believed that extra vitamins provided more pep and energy. One fifth agreed that certain diseases such as arthritis and cancer are caused, at least in part, by vitamin or mineral deficiencies. Twenty-six per cent, representing about 15 million adults, reported having used nutritional supplements (vitamins and/or minerals in pills or liquid tonics) without a physician's advice and expected actual observable results. About 10 per cent had eaten food advertised or labeled as "organic" or "natural," such as health stores sell. Nearly all the health-food users were acting without a physician's advice. A majority of them expected to be "helped" by the health food. About half the population of the United States has been concerned at some time about losing weight. One third agreed with fallacious concepts of weight control and about 6 per cent had followed one or more questionable reduction practices. Although some of the

practices were effective, most of them regained the weight lost.

The demographic characteristics of followers of questionable health practices change materially from one area to another, and generalizations for the total population cannot be made. It appeared that the majority of the population overstressed the relationship between health and diet or nutrition. Seventy-five per cent seemed to believe that actual observed cases of poor health were more often due to "not eating right" than any other cause. Very large numbers of people believe that almost anyone can gain noticeable improvement in vigor and energy by improving his diet or by using supplements.

Another myth is associated with the proportion of nutrients in a diet. Some athletes believe that large amounts of protein promote vigor and endurance. Other persons believe that large amounts of fat with small amounts of carbohydrate will aid in reduction of weight. Megadoses of vitamins and minerals are used for a host of reasons. None of these myths can be substantiated scientifically and may in fact be dangerous.

Health, Organic, and Natural Foods

Although there has been an interest in health foods for many years, the health-food movement has burgeoned from interest of youth in communes to socialites, according to Margolius.[7] This "back-to-nature" emphasis has emerged from a concern over and a resistance to the use of commercial fertilizers, pesticides, complicated food processing, orthodox medicine, deterioration of the environment, and the use of food additives. People want to know where and how food is grown and what happens to it in the body.

Authorities condemn the use of the word "health" or "healthful" in the sale of foods. The Food and Drug Administration says: The use of the word "health" in connection with foods constitutes a misbranding under the Food and Drug Act. The use of this word implies that these products have health-giving or

---

[6] Final Report, A *Study of Health Practices and Opinions*, Food and Drug Administration, Department of Health, Education, and Welfare, Washington, D.C., June 1972, pp. ii–v, xvii.

[7] Sidney Margolius, *Health Foods, Facts and Fakes*, Walker & Company, New York, 1973, Chap. 1.

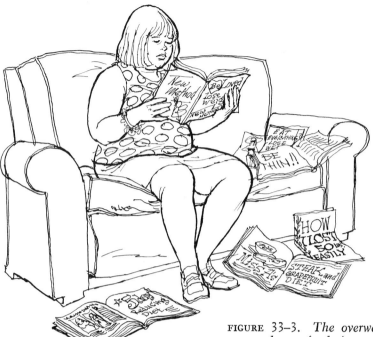

FIGURE 33-3. *The overweight are lured by many schemes for losing weight.*

curative properties, when, in general, they merely possess some of the nutritive qualities to be expected in any wholesome food product. The label claims on these products are such that the consumer is led to believe that our ordinary diet is sorely deficient in such vital substances as vitamins and minerals, and that these so-called health foods are absolutely necessary to conserve life and health.

This position of the Food and Drug Administration is further strengthened by the stand of the Council on Foods of the American Medical Association, which states:

The term "health" food and equivalent claims or statements to the effect that the food gives or assures health are vague, misinformative, and misleading. An adequate or complete diet and the recognized nutritional essentials established by the science of nutrition are necessary for health, but health depends on many other factors than those provided by such a diet, or nutritional essentials. No one food alone is essential for health. There are no health foods.

Health foods are frequently sold in special shops that promote foods for beauty or for the cure of various ailments. These shops can usually be identified by their name, and a look at their shelves shows "iodine-rich" tablets made from "sea greens," "unprocessed foods," and similar products with extravagant claims.

Many of these so-called "health" foods are concoctions of alfalfa, seaweed, salts, and other ingredients. Sometimes a single food such as yogurt, wheat germ, blackstrap molasses, stone-ground flour, brewer's yeast, or honey is packaged and given overrated qualifications. Some of these foods are sold in capsule or pill form. Some health foods contain many ingredients for which the nutrition need has not been demonstrated. One such product had 21 ingredients that are not essential to optimal human nutrition. There is both sense and nonsense to the health-food movement. From a positive standpoint, there is a greater awareness and concern in the nation about the accumulation of pesticides and chemicals in the soil and the increased use of additives in foods that has led to some changes, such as banning of cyclamates in soft drinks and of diethylstil-

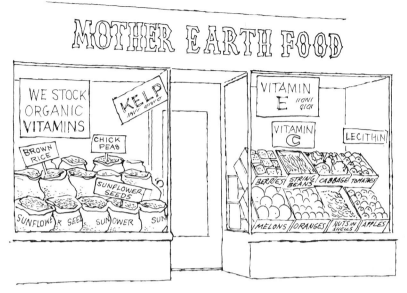

FIGURE 33–4. *Food purchased in a health food store is usually very expensive.*

bestrol (DES), a synthetic hormone-like substance added to cattle feeds. Both have been linked with cancer although some doubt has been expressed about the effect of the cyclamates. A trend to home-grown food and an interest in gardening has emerged. The use of fresh fruit and vegetables, nuts, dried fruits, seeds, legumes, whole-grain cereals, vegetable oils, cultured milks, and herbs has improved the diets of even non-health-food adherrents. Some of these foods are used as snacks. Adding the foods of other cultures, such as Chinese bean curd and fermented bean paste, millet from Far Eastern people, and seaweed from the Japanese, has added variety and interest to the diet.[8]

The taste of natural foods is claimed to be superior to supermarket fare. The use of humus, compost, and natural waste is praised by ecologists and agriculturists. The movement has heightened an interest in nutrition throughout the nation. Glyer[9] reports that

many health-food followers have effectively eliminated bad habits such as excess alcohol, smoking, and overeating. There is also a strong group identification through organizations, meetings, philosophy, and publications.

From a negative viewpoint the claim that organic foods are more nutritious than nonorganic foods is without scientific evidence. Such indications are not substantiated by the results of a 10-year research program at the Michigan State Experiment Station, a 25-year program at the U.S. Plant, Soil, and Nutrition Laboratory in Ithaca, New York, and a 34-year study on an experimental research farm in England.[10] Soil improvement can increase the size and yield of crops but not the composition of the plant in regard to major nutritional characteristics that are determined by the genes of the plant. Fertilizers may influence the mineral content, however. The iodine content of a plant will vary according to the iodine content of the soil. Both organic and inorganic nutrients must be in soluble

[8] Jean Hewitt, *The New York Times Natural Foods Cookbook*, Quadrangle Books, New York, 1971, p. 1.

[9] John Glyer, "Diet Healing: A Case Study in the Sociology of Health," *Journal of Nutrition Education*, Vol. 4, No. 4 (Fall 1972), pp. 163–166.

[10] A Scientific Status Summary by the Institute of Food Technologists' Expert Panel on Food Safety and Nutrition by the Committee on Public Information, "Organic Foods," *Food Technology*, Vol. 28, No. 1 (January 1974), pp. 71–72.

form to be utilized by the plant—organic fertilizers must be converted by microorganisms into their inorganic components such as potassium, phosphorus, and nitrogen.

The economic factor must be considered in a study of organic foods. Garbage compost provides nitrogen at a cost of $12 per pound, dried cow manure would supply nitrogen at $5 per pound, and the commercial chemical fertilizer would cost 7½ to 15 cents per pound. Likewise, a consumer pays almost twice as much for organic groceries as compared to similar nonorganic foods in a supermarket. Many people on low incomes purchase these high-priced foods and the quality of their diet may suffer; for example, smaller amounts of certain foods such as fruit may be purchased.

Beliefs about the miracle effect of these foods on health is grossly exaggerated. Nutritive intake is only one facet of the total health condition. In addition, false claims are made for longevity, sexual potency, beauty, and as cures of diseases such as arthritis and cancer. Many health-food adherents consume large amounts of vitamin capsules or tonics. This practice can be dangerous, particularly in the case of fat-soluble vitamins. Natural vitamins are boosted over synthetic vitamins. The potency and nutritional value are the same.

Porter[11] discloses other practices that have emerged in the boom for organic foods. Deceptive labeling, such as attaching "organic," "natural," or "nature's own" labels to nonorganic foods, is one. The statement has been made that more organic food is sold than grown. Dried fruit may be labeled "natural organic" when the fine print actually reveals preservatives. Diet-packed vegetables and fruit have been labeled as organic but actually are the same as all diet-packed foods. There is a lack of control of health-food stores so the customer has no way to discriminate between the organic and the nonorganic product.

Darden[12] discusses some of the health claims made for health foods. Wheat germ is a rich source of the B vitamins, vitamin E,

and protein that are lost in the refinement of cereals. Claims about this food for greater endurance of athletes, prevention of aging, muscular dystrophy, and heart disease are unfounded. Fertile eggs are considered more nutritious than nonfertile eggs by some promoters when the nutritive content is actually the same. Certified raw milk is no more nutritious than safe pasteurized milk, which is infinitely less expensive. Brewer's yeast is well supplied with amino acids, B vitamins, and minerals but is bitter in taste and somewhat unappetizing. Blackstrap molasses has been hailed as a health food for a long time and is advocated as a cure for a long list of diseases, which has not been authenticated, but the food does contain iron, calcium, and most of the B vitamins. The use of dessicated liver, a rich source of vitamin B_{12}, seems sensible only as a therapeutic agent. Lecithin, a natural emulsifier, is sold in capsule and powder form as an antidote for high cholesterol and heart disease without justification. Protein supplements come in pill and powder form and are sold to athletes and other active individuals in the belief that they need to replace protein lost during active exercise, a false belief.

In spite of the enthusiasm for health foods, advocates do not always get the necessary foods together to produce an adequate diet. Some ignorantly believe that a few health foods will provide all the health requirements. Erhard[13] in a study of vegetarian groups in the San Francisco area gained information that led her to believe that nutritional and medical deprivation existed, and there was a definite need for some clinical and/or biochemical appraisal to further varify this conclusion for educational and other purposes in working with these groups. Beliefs about food and nutrition held by health-food adherents must be regarded as congruent with and a part of their total belief structure, according to Wolff.[14] Attitudes about food are not isolated but are an expression of the total person.

[11] Sylvia Porter, "Organic Living: II," The New York Post, February 8, 1972, p. 34.

[12] Ellington Darden, "Sense and Nonsense About Health Foods," Journal of Home Economics, Vol. 64, No. 9 (December 1972), pp. 4–8.

[13] Darla Erhard, "Nutrition Education for the 'Now' Generation," Journal of Nutrition Education, Vol. 2, No. 4 (Spring 1971), pp. 135–139.

[14] Robert J. Wolff, "Who Eats for Health?" American Journal of Clinical Nutrition, Vol. 26, No. 4 (April 1973), pp. 438–445.

Science Versus the Medicine Man

Leverton[15] cites the fact that as knowledge of nutrition has increased, so have food quacks become more active. As people become aware of the importance of food, the charlatans capitalize on the opportunity to advance their own ideas. Legitimate medical research is often exploited by these promoters who cash in on new developments and attempt to utilize the information—often inaccurately—to boost the exaggerated claims of their products.

In the past, the pseudoscientists had to limit their audiences to a crowd on the street corner or to hawk their wares at a fair. With the advent of mass communications, the so-called "food specialist" gives misinformation on the air, in books and other literature, or in a series of lectures in large auditoriums. This faker is usually short on knowledge, but a clever salesman. He has a panacea for all ills and health problems, but his price is high. He appeals to emotions, fears, and hopes rather than to reason. It is disheartening to realize that millions of Americans support such faddism with enthusiasm.

The Danger of Half-Truths

Many of the faddists read published reports of reputable workers. They select isolated bits of information or take facts out of context and integrate these items into their own embellished story. One example is to distort the nutritional contribution of certain foods. Often this material is written so well that it sounds reasonable. Even the expert may have difficulty at times in recognizing these half-truths because they may be firmly enmeshed in scientific language. Moreover, in recent times a number of professional men and women have given lectures and written books that gave unsound information or faddish ideas. This situation has complicated nutrition education and the layman has a problem discriminating fact from fallacy and selecting reliable literature on nutrition.

Detection of Quackery

Burns and Gifft[16] suggest that individuals resort to intelligent skepticism and reliable sources of information to protect themselves so that supporters of food fads do not take advantage of them. Strong warnings are indicated when cure-all qualities are implied for a certain food or foods, when immediate or dramatic results are promised, or when claims for miraculous qualities are made. Equally strong warnings are implied if the product or service is being offered as a "secret remedy," if the sponsor claims that he is battling the medical profession, which is attempting to suppress his wonderful discovery, if the remedy is being sold from door to door by a self-styled "health advisor" or promoted in lectures from town to town, if the promotor shows "testimonials" of the wonderful miracles his product or service have performed for others, or if the product or service is good for a wide variety of illnesses.[17]

Other signs of quackery are promotion of the miracle diet or food in a sensational magazine, by a crusading organization of laymen, or if the promoter has products, literature, or a plan to sell. Watch for jargon that sounds scientific but is meaningless. High price is no guarantee of superior nutrition quality. Health promotors are in business to make a profit.

Where to Go for Reliable Information

The public can be protected against food fads and fallacies if people are willing to turn to qualified sources of information. Authorities in nutrition are most willing to give information when asked; the following are some sources:

1. Nutritionists in city, county, and state health offices or with social welfare agencies.
2. Professors of nutrition or biochemistry in colleges.

[15] Ruth M. Leverton, "Nutrition in Perspective," in *Proceedings of the National Nutrition Education Conference*, November 2–4, 1971, Miscellaneous Publication No. 1254, U.S. Department of Agriculture, Washington, D.C., 1973, pp. 77–81.

[16] Marjorie Burns and Helen Gifft, *Nutrition Sense and Nonsense*, Home Economics Extension Leaflet 5, New York State College of Human Ecology, Cornell University, Ithaca, N.Y., 1963.

[17] *Quackery*, FDA Consumer Memo, November 1971, p. 2.

3. Extension specialists and workers in experiment stations.
4. The family physician. Physicians receive a great deal of information from the American Medical Association about questionable material and products so they are informed about the latest fads.
5. The Federal Food and Drug Administration. This agency can be consulted about questionable labels on foods as well as practices related to food.
6. The Federal Trade Commission. This agency has jurisdiction over advertising, and doubtful statements heard on radio, seen on television, or read in newspapers or magazines may be referred to it.
7. Food editors of newspapers or magazines.
8. Home economics teachers.
9. Dietitians who are members of the American Dietetic Association.
10. Professional organizations that can give authentic information: the American Medical Association, the American Dental Association, the American Dietetic Association, the American Home Economics Association, Society for Nutrition Education, Nutrition Today Society, and the American Public Health Association.
11. The National Better Business Bureau and local Better Business Bureaus. The major function of these groups is the promotion of public confidence in responsible business. They are concerned about misrepresentations to the public, including advertising and other promotional endeavors involving health products.
12. State and local departments of health.

The truth should be sought whenever a person is skeptical. In this way the American public will become better informed about nutrition so that misinformation will be more difficult to dispense.

Undesirable Effects of Following Fads

A number of serious concerns arise as a result of food faddism. Following foolish diets or leaning on a certain food product often leads to malnutrition. A careful examination of most fad diets reveals glaring deficiencies. It is even more serious to depend on one source for nutrients.

The cost of buying faddish products or following such diets is great. Often this money is spent by individuals who can ill afford it. They buy expensive vitamin pills in place of milk, fruit, vegetables, and other rich sources of nutrients. The feeling of complacency from following a faker's advice about foods or diets can be dangerous.

Unwise food practices may imperil health, hamper the growth and development of children, delay needed medical attention, and actually deprive families of certain comforts and pleasures because they have spent their money foolishly on quackery.

Combatting Nutritional Quackery and Faddism

Combatting nutritional quackery is difficult, according to Henderson,[18] because indeterminate areas of scientific, legal, social, and moral issues are involved. Criteria for action are determined by the extent of nutritional inadequacy; economic effect, especially for the poor; or a threat to life or health. Questionable nutritional claims can be controlled by regulation or by education.

The activities of federal, state, or local regulatory agencies are confined to enforcements by law. The Food and Drug Administration and the Federal Trade Commission are examples. Education efforts by nutrition professionals can be directed to the consumer, producer, wholesaler, retailer, public health personnel, others concerned with health services, and to other educators. Sound information that is communicated with conviction is

[18] LaVell M. Henderson, "Programs to Combat Nutritional Quackery," *Journal of the American Dietetic Association*, Vol. 64, No. 4 (April 1974), pp. 372–375.

generally met with receptivity. The Extension Service has well-developed programs and literature in this area that have been highly effective. Professional efforts can be made through such organizations as the National Academy of Sciences, Engineering, and Medicine (nongovernmental), especially the Food and Nutrition Board and the Committee on Nutritional Misinformation of the National Academy of Sciences; the American Academy of Pediatrics Committee on Drugs and Nutrition; and the American Dietetic Association. Erhard[19] indicates that young food faddists and cultists reject professional help unless there is a sincere desire to meet them in the context of their particular needs. By working within their structure and systems, an effort has been made to work with George Oshsawa's successor in the Macrobiotic Foundation in the writing of new publications that appear to promote sounder nutritional diets. When the information comes from the foundation, followers of macrobiotics are more likely to respond than from other sources. Information is being disseminated through health-food store owners and commune newspapers. Many members of these groups are open to information presented in factual and readable form. The message by Erhard is go to the people who need nutrition education.

Schafer and Yetley[20] believe that food faddists use food as a means of meeting self-needs, such as an anti-establishment individual selecting a fad diet. "Patterning" is the stabilization of experiences in relation to beliefs about food. If a football player believes that meat is essential to his performance on the football field, he would feel threatened if he were denied meat in his diet. Sometimes a fad gives structure and stability to an individual who faces many uncertainties in life. In combatting faddism, nutritionists may wish to consider these concepts.

---

[19] Darla Erhard, participant of an individual discussion meeting on "How Can Food Faddism and Cultism Best Be Combatted," sponsored by the Council of Food and Nutrition of the American Medical Association in Chicago and reviewed in the *Journal of the American Dietetic Association*, Vol. 61, No. 2 (August 1972), p. 126.

[20] Robert Schafer and Elizabeth A. Yetley, "Social Psychology of Food Faddism," *Journal of the American Dietetic Association*, Vol. 66, No. 2 (February 1975), pp. 129–133.

SELECTED REFERENCES

Beeuwkes, Adelia M., "Characteristics of the Self-Styled Scientists," *Journal of the American Dietetic Association*, Vol. 32, No. 6 (June 1956), pp. 627–629.

Bruch, Hilde, "The Allure of Food Cults and Nutrition Quackery," *Journal of the American Dietetic Association*, Vol. 57, No. 4 (October 1970), pp. 316–320.

Carberry, James F., "Food Faddism Spurts as Young, Old People Shift to Organic Diets," *The Wall Street Journal*, January 21, 1971, pp. 1, 12.

Darden, Ellington, "Sense and Nonsense About Health Foods," *Journal of Home Economics*, Vol. 64, No. 9 (December 1972), pp. 4–8.

Erhard, Darla, "Nutrition Education for the 'Now' Generation," *Journal of Nutrition Education*, Vol. 2, No. 4 (Spring 1971), pp. 135–139.

Fleck, Henrietta, and Margaret Simko, "Combatting Nutrition Misinformations," *Forecast for Home Economics*, Vol. 17, No. 9 (May–June 1972), pp. 37, 56, 58.

Food Facts Talk Back, American Dietetic Association, Chicago, 1957.

"Food Faddism," *Dairy Council Digest*, Vol. 44, No. 1 (January–February 1973), pp. 1–4.

Margolius, Sidney, *Health Foods, Facts and Fakes*, Walker & Company, New York, 1973.

McCarthy, M. Ellen, and Jean H. Sabry, "Canadian University Students' Nutrition Misconceptions," *Journal of Nutrition Education*, Vol. 5, No. 3 (July–September 1973), pp. 193–196.

"Nutrition Misinformation and Food Faddism," *Nutrition Reviews*, A Special Supplement, July 1974.

Porter, Sylvia, "Organic Living: II," *The New York Post*, February 8, 1972, p. 34.

Rose, Mary Swartz, "Belief in Magic," *Journal of the American Dietetic Association*, Vol. 8, No. 4 (April 1933), p. 489.

A Scientific Status Summary by the Institute of Food Technologists' Expert Panel on Food Safety and Nutrition and the Committee on Public Information, "Organic Foods," *Food Technology*, Vol. 28, No. 1 (January 1974), pp. 71–74.

Seelig, R. A. "The 'Organic Food' Kick," *United Fresh Fruit and Vegetable Association June 1971 Supply Letter*, No. 53, p. 7.

Todhunter, E. Neige, "Food Habits, Food Faddism and Nutrition," in Miloslav, Rechcigl, Jr. (ed.), *Food, Nutrition and Health*, Vol. 16, S. Karger, Basel, 1973, pp. 287–317.

Trager, James, *Foodbook*, Grossman Publishers, New York, 1970, Chapter 10.

White, Hilda S., "Organic Foods—A Growing Phenomenon," *What's New in Home Economics*, Vol. 35, No. 6 (September 1971), pp. 53–55.

White, Philip L., "The Perfect Environment for Nonsense," *Nutrition News*, Vol. 36, No. 3 (October 1973), pp. 9–12.

Wilson, Mary Margaret, and Mina Lamb, "Food Beliefs as Related to Ecological Factors in Women," *Journal of Home Economics*, Vol. 60, No. 2 (February 1968), pp. 115–117.

Wolff, Robert., "Who Eats for Health?" *American Journal of Clinical Nutrition*, Vol. 26, No. 4 (April 1973), pp. 438–445.

34

Looking Ahead

Two engravings, "The Thin Kitchen" and "The Fat Kitchen," done by Pieter Brueghel the Elder in 1563 (see Figure 34–1) depict to a certain extent the status of nutrition in the world in its extremes. What will be the future?

Nutrition is no longer solely a personal matter but is beginning to have a strong social thrust. For some individuals, famine and food shortages may be remote, but people and nations have become so interdependent that each person may be faced with decisions about national and global nutrition. Malnutrition is an impediment to personal and national development in connection with economic, environmental, educational, and social opportunities.

It has been a rude awakening in the 1970's to realize that human economic activity depends on natural resources and processes of the earth, including the production of fresh water, land to till, energy fuels, minerals, and other raw materials. The earth's ability to absorb wastes is important, and no interference can be tolerated with the natural cycles of nitrogen and oxygen. This may mean a limit to the expansion of certain types of economic activity in light of ecological stress and scarce resources. All this has a direct or indirect rela-

tion on food resources for adequate nutrition for the peoples of the earth.[1]

Population and Hunger

Alarm is widespread over the ability of the world to feed itself. Although differences in race, religion, and economic conditions beset the world, a recognition of a basic common problem emerges: population.[2] Between 1900 and 1970 the world's population more than doubled, according to United Nations demographers, from 1.6 billion to 3.6 billion. The population today is rapidly approaching 4 billion, compounding at the rate of 2 per cent per year; two persons are born each second or 200,000 people every day, over 6 million a month, and about 74 million per year. In less than 35 years, unless growth is reduced, the population will have doubled.

The underdeveloped countries have about

[1] Harold G. Shane, "The Coming Global Famine," A Kappan Interview with Lester R. Brown, *Phi Delta Kappan*, Vol. 56, No. 1 (September 1974), pp. 34–38.

[2] Gladwin Hill, "Population Boom and Food Shortage: World Losing Fight for Vital Balance," *The New York Times*, August 14, 1974, pp. 35, 41.

485

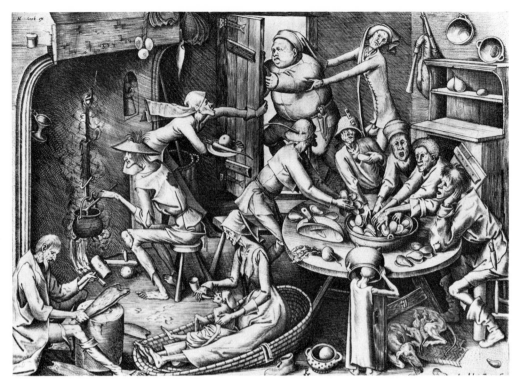

FIGURE 34–1. *"The Thin Kitchen" and "The Fat Kitchen" by Pieter Brueghel the Elder depict the extremes of human nutrition in the world.*

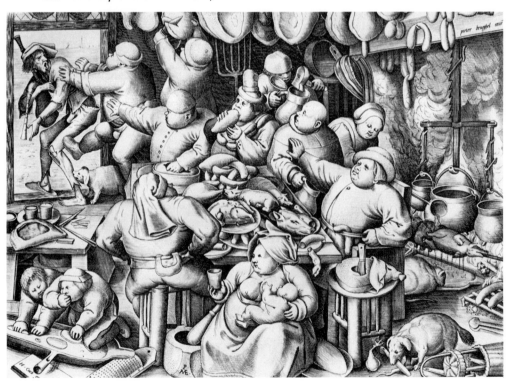

486

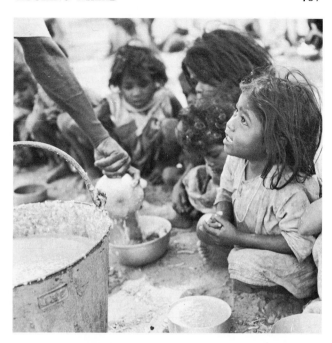

FIGURE 34–2. *Malnutrition is an impediment to personal and national development* (UNICEF)

two thirds of the world's population and the highest birth rates. For every birth in the developed countries there are five births in the underdeveloped countries. Numerically, the responsibility for growth appears to rest mainly with the developing countries. But the answer is not so simple. While the developed countries have about one third of the population, they consume 60 per cent of the total food energy produced in the world. Other basics of living are similarly disproportionate in many respects, according to Revelle.[3] Human beings can survive on much less than the optimum amount of food, although vitality, health, and ability to work and play are diminished accordingly. The effect of inadequate nutrition on children can be critical. If diets in developing countries can be improved, food requirements will increase. It has been demonstrated, however, that when this occurs birth rates begin to fall in time.

Family planning has been advocated as a means of limiting population. Although results have been observable, according to Hill, they have been disappointing. Sometimes efforts have been cut back because such programs were considered nonessential, when money became short, as in India. The only populous less-developed country that appears to have overcome the economic and logistical problems associated with such a program, is the People's Republic of China. Another reason for ineffectiveness of family planning is the high value placed on children by many families. In some countries there is an effort to have a minimum of two sons. Children seem to be a source of security. They provide the extra hands in the fields so vital to existence. More children are needed to replace the ones that die.

When there are crop shortages and inflation makes buying prohibitive, food is out of the reach of millions of poor people in the Third World, according to Power,[4] and starvation becomes imminent.

Food Production

World population has long since outstripped food supplies. Food reserves have declined by 10 million tons yearly to further

[3] Roger Revelle, "Food and Population," *Scientific American*, Vol. 231, No. 3 (September 1974), pp. 161–170.

[4] Jonathan Power, "Starvation in Living Color," *The New York Times*, October 2, 1974, p. 43.

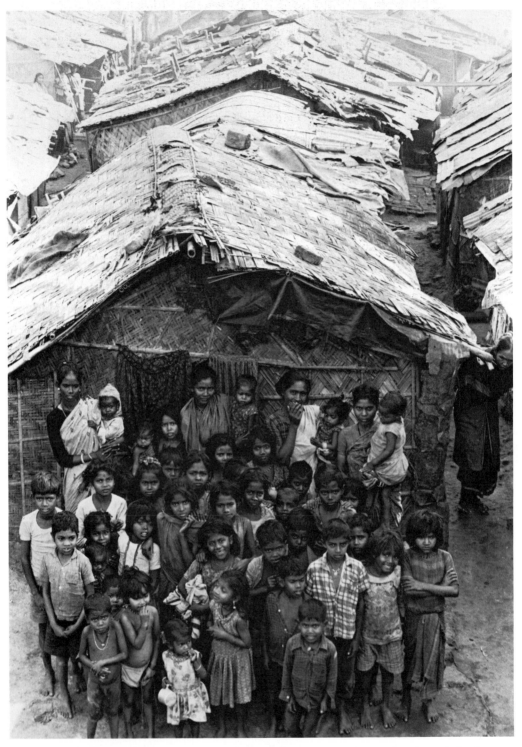

FIGURE 34–3. *Mothers and children in a slum area in Dacca that is typical of many large cities in the world representative of our population problem. (UNICEF Photo by Bernard Pierre Wolff)*

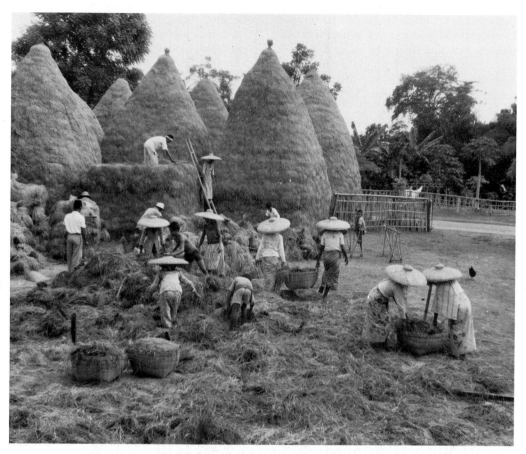

FIGURE 34–4. *Rice production in a West Java village is accelerated by modern farming methods.* (UNICEF Photo by Jack Ling)

complicate the situation. Half the world's people are chronically undernourished and every week more than 10,000 people die of starvation. With near-famine conditions in some parts of the world, the problem of an adequate food supply has been pushed to the forefront, according to Sullivan.[5]

Agricultural production is considered an important key to improved nutrition, according to Berg and Muscat.[6] Seldom, however, are agricultural policies centered on nutrition ob-

jectives, but rather on such areas as expanded exports, reduction of dependence on foreign suppliers for major staples, or production of raw materials for industry. A few considerations about agricultural production as related to nutritional status will be discussed here.

The amount of potentially arable land in the world is an important question in times of food shortages. In the United States, according to Quentin M. West, director of the U.S. Department of Agriculture's Economics Research Service, 25 million acres of unused land were put back into cultivation in 1973, and by 1985 27 million more acres will be added. West's projections suggest that this nation could meet nearly all the world's increased import demands for coarse grains

[5] Walter Sullivan, "Computer 'Model' of World Sought to Cope with the Food Shortage," *The New York Times*, August 10, 1974, pp. 31, 58.

[6] Alan Berg and Robert J. Muscat, *The Nutrition Factor*, The Brookings Institution, Washington, D.C., 1973, Chap. 5.

through 1985. Lester Brown of the Overseas Development Council is not so optimistic and predicts that starvation may strike millions or even tens of millions of people. Studies at the Brookings Institution using computer techniques predict severe global shortages will not occur until the year 2000.[7]

Revelle[8] indicates that the largest areas of available land for food crops are in Africa and South America. Outside of the humid tropics, 630 million hectares (1 hectare = 2.471 acres) with sufficient water remain uncultivated. It is estimated that North America and Australia have 300 million hectares for possible cultivation. Limitations for agricultural development in these areas are economic, institutional, social, and political constraints. Actually, the uncultivated potential is greater in area than the present cultivated land.

Increased production on the presently cultivated land has great potential, according to Robbins.[9] Estimates of increases in food production that could be reached with reasonable effort and without government intervention range up to 50 per cent of the present output. To achieve this end, additional land will have to be used, technological advances will continue, and a favorable economic climate, including attractive prices for farmers, must be assumed, with the greatest emphasis on the economic incentive for farmers.

Other suggestions are stepped-up irrigation and research, areas that have lagged. Present increases are impressive. Corn production has increased at a phenomenal rate, and soybean exports now bring in more money than all technological exports, such as computers or jet aircraft. In a similar manner, the production of milk and eggs has advanced. The average milk production of a cow in India is 600 pounds per year; in the United States it is 10,000 pounds per year. Research is under way for producing multiple births in cattle but has not been successful. Modernization of agriculture in underdeveloped countries is a tremendous challenge facing the world. This modernization should proceed more rapidly than population growth to be truly effective.

Food production has caused some ecological deterioration through possible excessive use of fertilizers and pesticides. Research is needed to maintain high production that minimizes environmental degeneration. The shortage of fertilizer, according to McElheny,[10] may intensify the possibility of famine. The three main fertilizers are nitrogen, phosphate, and potash. Curtailing the use of fertilizer for ornamental uses, such as on lawns, flower gardens, cemeteries, and golf greens, would release nearly 3 million tons a year. Fertilizer on nutrient-starved soils will produce yields nearly twice as large, such as are found in Asia, Africa, and Latin America, rather than in the United States. With high prices for food products, farmers in developed countries are also anxious to secure as much fertilizer as possible. Petroleum, one of the raw materials in fertilizers, has doubled and tripled in cost during the last few years and causes another complication. One promising practice, based on research, is the genetic "tailoring" of bacteria living in the soil or plant roots to do a better job of "fixing nitrogen" from the air, thus offering new supplies of nitrogen for food crops.

Climatic changes threaten to alter some of the estimates of world food production, according to Schmeck.[11] Many weather scientists anticipate greater variability in the earth's weather, and the world may even be on the verge of new patterns of adverse global climate, although there is no agreement among the experts in their predictions. Whatever the weather will be in the days ahead, all agree that climate can change the estimates of food crops drastically.

Kenyon[12] offers the challenge of examining

---

[7] Sullivan, op. cit., p. 31.

[8] Revelle, op. cit., pp. 168–169.

[9] William Robbins, "Farm Experts See a U.S. Opportunity to Lessen Hunger," The New York Times, August 25, 1974, pp. 1, 48.

[10] Victor K. McElheny, "Rising World Fertilizer Scarcity Threatens Famine for Millions," The New York Times, September 1, 1974, pp. 1, 34.

[11] Harold M. Schmeck, Jr., "Climate changes Endanger World's Food Output," The New York Times, August 8, 1974, pp. 35, 66.

[12] Richard L. Kenyon, "Science, Technology, and Food," Chemical and Engineering News, April 29, 1974, p. 4.

the best system for feeding people. The objective of the system is to transport protein and energy from the molecules of the earth, air, and water into the human body. It is a chemical process. Basic energy resources are almost infinitely beyond the energy delivered to human beings through nutrition. In contrast, a considerable portion of the scientific and technological effort applied to food problems continues to be directed to a technical modification of a relatively primitive and inefficient system. Because all foods are combinations of chemicals, the further development of synthetic foods may be an answer, but attitudes would have to be changed about these foods. Adequacy of knowledge about the nutrients to be incorporated into these synthetic foods may be questioned. Kenyon further recommends that an assessment and inventory of the material and scientific knowledge now available for making an attack on this basic problem of adequate food should be undertaken. This might avoid a world panic.

Economics and Nutrition

The rise in the cost of food is a disturbing problem, according to Brown and Eckholm.[13] World food prices began rising in 1972 and have increased steadily. Food prices rose more rapidly in the United States than in any other nation.[14] Wheat and rice prices tripled by 1974 and soybean prices more than doubled. Soaring food prices coupled with energy price increases have contributed to two-digit inflation that has affected the entire world in Brown and Eckholm's estimation. Recession, accompanied by high unemployment, has created other problems. Poor nations and the poor in more affluent countries are in a serious predicament nutritionwise, as well as in other areas of living. Many of the poor in developing countries, who usually spend 80 per cent

of their income on food, now find needed food has become unavailable to them.

Coupled with high prices is the concern that industrial nations have large herds of livestock that consume huge resources of grain that might be freed to feed the hungry. Serious consideration by Americans to the modification of their diets to lower the extravagant use of meat is urged. Brown[15] contends that this action is morally desirable and may prove helpful healthwise.

Popkin and Lidman[16] believe that limited food resources make economics an essential study from several viewpoints. Alternative uses of food resources must be determined for production and consumption. Allocation of these resources should be related to efficiency (most productive use of scarce resources) and equity (fairness and justice in distribution). Another economic facet is that adults and children who are well nourished are an economic asset to any nation.

Children of the World

Children are the first victims of population growth, inflation, inadequate nutrition and health services, and minimum education, according to LaBouisse.[17] The future of a community, a nation, or the world depends upon the health and vitality of children.

An examination of Figure 34–5 can be quite revealing about the location of the world's children and how their population will grow. There are many more children in less-developed regions and consequently subjected to the many problems of malnutrition and living than children in the more developed regions. Furthermore, projections for future populations indicate a continued increase in the less-developed areas.

A review of the conditions of children in Latin America will reveal these problems more

---

[13] Lester R. Brown and Erik P. Eckholm, "Grim Reaping: This Year the Whole World Is Short of Grain," *The New York Times*, September 15, 1974, p. 6, Sec. E.

[14] "Why Grocery Bills Around the World Go Soaring," *U.S. News and World Report*, March 18, 1974, pp. 52–53.

[15] Shane, op. cit., p. 37.

[16] Barry Popkin, and Russell Lidman, "Economics as an Aid to Nutritional Change," *American Journal of Clinical Nutrition*, Vol. 25, No. 3 (March 1972), pp. 331–334.

[17] Henry R. LaBouisse, "The Right to a Good Life," *UNICEF News*, Issue 78 (December 1973–January 1974), pp. 1–3.

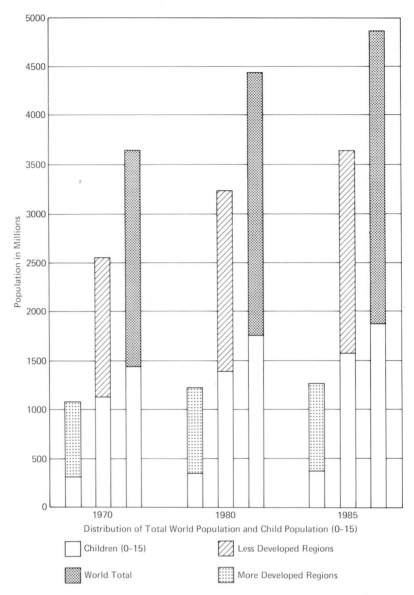

FIGURE 34–5. *Children are the first victims of population growth, especially in less developed countries.* (SOURCE: "Children in a Crowded World," UNICEF NEWS, Issue 78, December 1973/January 1974, p. 2.)

clearly.[18] About 1 million of the 2.5 million deaths occurring annually are children under 5 years of age. About 57 per cent of these

[18] Editorial, "Child of Latin America," *UNICEF News*, Issue 80, 1974/2.

deaths of children under 5 probably result from malnutrition as a primary or contributory cause. In some instances the percentage is close to 65 or 70. About 286 million inhabitants of Latin America—approximately 37 per cent of the people—do not have medi-

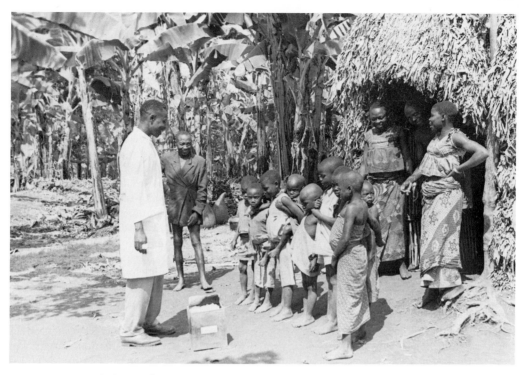

FIGURE 34–6. *Malnutrition is an increasingly serious problem in the world. Children in the Belgian Congo are being relieved of kwashiorkor by the distribution of fish meal biscuits. (WHO Photo by Paul Almasy) Note distended abdomens.*

cal care of any kind. The children in this group represent some 45 million children under 15 years of age. Problems will increase in the years ahead as the population grows. This figure is estimated to increase to 54 million by 1975, to 69 million by 1985, and to 77 million by 1990. The picture may look hopeless but actually many projects and programs in which the people themselves are involved are attempting to improve the living conditions through collective effort. All the needs of the child, the family, and the community are being scrutinized.

The nutritional status of the child in the United States is a complex problem, according to Fomon and Egan.[19] In 1970 there were

71 million persons less than 18 years of age. Of this number, 3.5 million were infants less than 1 year of age, more than 18 million were 1 to 5 years of age, 25 million from 6 to 11, and 24 million from 12 through 17. The nutritional needs for the children in this age range will be substantially different between younger and older children, between boys and girls, and between more rapidly and less rapidly growing children of the same age and sex.

Malnutrition is up sharply among the world's children, according to Nevin S. Scrimshaw as discussed by Schmeck.[20] Although genuine progress had been made during the last two decades in the malnutrition problem, there has been a sharp deterioration in recent

[19] Samuel J. Fomon and Mary C. Egan, "Infants, Children, and Adolescents," in Jean Mayer (ed.), *U.S. Nutrition Policies in the Seventies*, W. H. Freeman, San Francisco, 1973, Chap. 1.

[20] Harold M. Schmeck, Jr., "Malnutrition Is Up Sharply Among World's Children," *The New York Times*, October 6, 1974, pp. 1, 42.

times. The causes are inflation in food and energy costs, growth of the world population, and hazards of weather and the effect on food crops. Nations of high suffering are India, Pakistan, Bangladesh, the sub-Saharan countries of Africa, Indonesia, and parts of several countries in Latin America. Malnutrition in an adult can seriously affect health and productivity; in a child, the future is grim and often foreclosed.

Another dimension to this situation is the move of poor people from the land to urban areas because of inflation. In the city slums, work is scarce, and a government handout of food offers the only hope of survival. Many mothers try to find work and as a result do not breast feed their babies, which accentuates their malnutrition, for the substitute food is often diluted and offered in unsanitary conditions so that infection may be added to the complications.

There are a few notable exceptions to widespread malnutrition among children in many parts of the world. Chile has made significant progress against infant malnutrition by intensive programs of milk supplements to poor women and children, together with a large-scale public health education program. Maternal and infant mortality rates have been reduced. There is an opinion based on observations of nutritionists and experts in child care that the People's Republic of China has managed to provide food for its children and families.

Other influences on the status of child nutrition are the income level of the family, cultural patterns, parental education, attitude of parents toward children and their upbringing, access to health facilities, the establishment of food habits that are compatible with adequate nutrition, access to nutritious foods, and others. The feeding and nutrition programs outside of the home, such as in day-care centers, schools, and community facilities, are important. Frequent assessment of the nutritional status of children seems urgent. Optimal nutrition for each child will contribute to total health status and assist him or her in achieving a good life not only for himself or herself but for the nation. Children are our most precious asset.

National Nutrition Policy

The National Nutrition Consortium[21] representing the following major scientific and professional societies—the American Institute of Nutrition, the American Society for Clinical Nutrition, the American Dietetic Association, and the Institute of Food Technology—have developed a concise statement of guidelines for a national nutrition policy. This statement is to be used by the membership of these organizations to identify the many considerations for a sharp focus on effective short- and long-range governmental planning and the implementation of food and nutrition programs for the maintenance of national health and other responsibilities. Some of the major points of these guidelines are discussed here.

The major goals of a national nutrition policy should include (1) assurance of available food of high quality and safety to provide an adequate diet to every American in light of national and world food needs and during other emergencies, (2) provision of nutrition education for both health professionals and the general public that will promote maximal nutritional health, and (3) support of basic and applied research and education in foods and nutrition to solve important problems in the order of a discriminating priority.

Measures, objectives, and programs indicated in these goals are briefly described here. The establishment and expansion of nutrition programs in all geographical areas that are coordinated cooperatively with Health Care Centers, such as clinics, hospitals, and neighborhood centers, that are identified with good nutrition practices, and that are supervised by professional nutritionists should have high priority. Nutrition centers of excellence for diagnosis, treatment, research, and preparation of nutrition personnel should be included.

Nutrition education should be incorporated into all types of educational programs and through informal means, such as mass media, adult education, and agency programs for the

[21] The National Nutrition Consortium, Inc., "Guidelines for a National Nutrition Policy," Nutrition Reviews, Vol. 32, No. 5 (May 1974), pp. 153–157.

general public. All types of nutrition professionals and paraprofessionals, physicians, dentists, nurses, veterinarians, social workers, health educators, physical education teachers and all health-care personnel should be expertly prepared for nutrition-related responsibilities. Special attention should be given to education and assistance to the disadvantaged, such as migrant families and poor minority groups, as well as to high-risk groups such as the elderly, infants, and pregnant women.

Nutrition input is necessary in planning food production and distribution, not only in the United States but in the world. Nutrition professionals should participate in nutrition policy decisions at all levels of government. The establishment of an Officer of Nutrition or a National Nutrition Center is recommended; responsibilities and activities should include identification and coordination of food and nutrition programs in government agencies, nutrition surveillance of the quantity, quality, and safety of the food supply, continuing accumulation of information about food consumption and food composition. A nutrition information service would be helpful. Adequate resources for basic and applied research as related to the many ramifications of optimal nutrition and health are critical. Cooperative endeavors with international agencies concerned with nutrition should be encouraged.

International Food and Nutrition Policy

Development plans of many nations seldom include nutrition as a critical aspect. If mentioned, resources are seldom allocated and low priority is typical. Nutritionists cannot assume that malnutrition can be treated in isolation but rather as one facet of man's development. Often good nutrition is a prerequisite for the advancement of other factors, according to Berg and Muscat.[22]

There is an urgent need for making a strong case for the importance of nutrition. This will require discussion and sharing of concerns, issues, and possible rationales for placing nutrition in the mainstream of development, so it will receive the attention it deserves. Health and economic losses from malnutrition have often been emphasized, but the loss of leadership from potentially outstanding individuals must be considered. The restriction of a malnourished child's opportunity for social mobility is another serious consideration, for without adequate mental capacity combined with a sense of curiosity and mental energy, such opportunity is unlikely. All in all, the stress on nutrition in conjunction with other aspects of development is to generate a higher level of human well-being for the future. This is a problem of such magnitude that international policy seems imperative.

There is a complicated relationship between world and national food problems, as indicated by the panel on the international food situation, headed by D. Gale Johnson, chairman of the department of economics at the University of Chicago, and Peter G. Peterson, chairman of Lehman Brothers and former Secretary of Commerce, at the public hearings held by the Senate Select Committee on Nutrition and Human Needs as part of its National Nutrition Policy Study. The panel's recommendations plus recommendations of other students of the world's food problems stressed the following elements: (1) food reserve, (2) food aid, and (3) growth of individual productive capacity of each nation.[23]

There is an urgent need to ensure relief from food shortages, especially in times of famine or other crises. The economics of food reserves is a comparatively underdeveloped science because few data are available on the impact of varying sizes of reserves. Ideally, an internationally coordinated reserve system would be helpful.

Food aid can only be a short-term goal to be replaced with the results from long-range planning to solve this problem. There are serious questions about the use of food aid for political purposes.

Many areas of endeavor must be incorpo-

[22] Alan Berg and Robert Muscat, "Nutrition and Development," *American Journal of Clinical Nutrition,* Vol. 25, No. 2 (February 1972), pp. 186–209.

[23] Staff, *Report on Nutrition and the International Situation,* Select Committee on Nutrition and Human Needs, U.S. Senate, Washington, D.C., September 1974.

rated into increasing the productive capacity for food in all the countries of the world. The most important short-term step is the increase of fertilizer supplies. Other possibilities are studies in regard to crop rotation that alternates legumes with grains for fixation in the soil, increase in crop yields, proper cultivation procedures, and improved irrigation systems. The need for more funds for agricultural research is more critical now than ever.

SELECTED REFERENCES

Berg, Alan, and Robert Muscat, "Nutrition and Development: The View of the Planner," *American Journal of Clinical Nutrition*, Vol. 25, No. 2 (February 1972), pp. 186–209.

———, and portions with Robert J. Muscat, *The Nutrition Factor*, The Brookings Institution, Washington, D.C., 1973.

Blacken, Emma M., *National Nutrition Policy: Selected Papers on Technology, Agriculture Advances and Production*, A Working Paper, Select Committee on Nutrition and Human Needs, U.S. Senate, Washington, D.C., June 1974.

Brown, Lester R., *By Bread Alone*, Praeger Publishers, New York, 1974.

"Child of Latin America," UNICEF News, Issue 80, 1974/2.

"Children in a Crowded World," UNICEF News, Issue 78, December 1973–January 1974.

Goldsmith, Grace A., "For a National Nutrition Policy," *Nutrition Today*, Vol. 8, No. 4 (July–August 1973), pp. 32–35.

Harrer, J. George, "Nutrition and Numbers in the Third World," *Nutrition Reviews*, Vol. 32, No. 4 (April 1974), pp. 97–104.

Hegsted, D. Mark, "Food and Nutrition Policy—Now and in the Future," *Journal of the American Dietetic Association*, Vol. 64, No. 4 (April 1974), pp. 367–371.

Hollingsworth, Dorothy, and Margaret Russell, *Nutritional Problems in a Changing World*, John Wiley & Sons, Inc., New York, 1973.

"The Human Population," *Scientific American*, Vol. 231, No. 3 (September 1974). (Entire issue is on population; see "Food and Population," pp. 160–170).

King, Maurice, Felicity King, David Morley, Leslie Burgess, and Ann Burgess, *Nutrition for Developing Countries*, Oxford University Press, New York, 1972.

Mayer, Jean (ed.), *U.S. Nutrition Policies in the Seventies*, W. H. Freeman and Company, San Francisco, 1973.

Nichaman, Milton Z., "Developing a Nutritional Surveillance System," *Journal of the American Dietetic Association*, Vol. 63, No. 1 (July 1974), pp. 15–17.

Quimby, Freeman H., and Cynthia B. Chapman, *National Nutrition Policy: National Nutrition Policy Experiences*, A Working Paper, Select Committee on Nutrition and Human Needs, U.S. Senate, Washington, D.C., May 1974.

Shane, Harold G., "The Coming Global Famine," A Kappan Interview with Lester R. Brown, *Phi Delta Kappan*, Vol. 56, No. 1 (September 1974), pp. 34–38.

Staff, *Report on Nutrition and the International Situation*, Select Committee on Nutrition and Human Needs, U.S. Senate, Washington, D.C., September 1974.

"Symposium: World Food Supply," reported in *Food Technology*, Vol. 29, No. 8 (August 1975), pp. 54–66.

The National Nutrition Consortium, Inc., "Guidelines for a National Nutrition Policy," *Nutrition Reviews*, Vol. 32, No. 5 (May 1974), pp. 153–157.

Things to Come, The World Food Crisis—The Way Out, The United Nations World Food Conference, Food and Agriculture Organization of the United Nations, Rome, 1974.

APPENDIXES

Appendix A

Glossary[*]

Absorption. In physiology, absorption pertains to the uptake of nutrients, water, or other substances by stomach or intestinal walls following digestion of food. For example, glucose, a common simple sugar, is absorbed without change, but starches must be broken down into sugars before absorption can take place. In food processing, absorption may also refer to uptake of other substances by foods, such as absorption of fats by foods during cooking in deep fat, or absorption of water by cereals during cooking.

Adipose. Animal fat. Adipose is commonly used in describing the part of the body where fat is stored, which is adipose tissue.

Adolescence. The period of years between the beginning of puberty (when the reproductive organs become functionally active) and maturity.

Adrenal. Near the kidney. The adrenal glands are ductless glands near the upper end of the kidneys. Their secretions are essential for the maintenance of life.

Amino acid. Organic compounds of carbon, hydrogen, oxygen, and nitrogen. Each amino acid molecule contains one or more amino group ($-NH_2$) and at least one carboxyl group ($-COOH$). In addition, some amino acids (cystine and methionine) contain sulfur. Many amino acids linked together in some definite pattern form a molecule of protein.

Antioxidant. A substance capable of chemically protecting other substances against oxidation.

Arteriosclerosis. A thickening and hardening of the walls of the arteries and capillaries, which lead to loss of their elasticity.

Ascorbic acid. Another name for vitamin C.

Atherosclerosis. A degeneration of blood vessels caused by a deposit of fatty materials along the lining of the wall of the blood vessel. Cholesterol is one of these fatty materials.

Available. A nutrient is available to the body when it is in the form that can be absorbed from the digestive tract and then used for its intended function in the body.

Avidin. A protein material that can combine with the B vitamin, biotin, causing the vitamin to be unavailable to the body. Cooking renders avidin inactive.

Bacteria. Very small, one-celled organisms visible only under a microscope and widely distributed in the air, water, soil, and animal and plant tissues. They have some useful functions, such as in decaying of dead matter and in fermentation of fruit or vegetable juices—as in the making of sauerkraut. Many bacteria

---

[*] Selected from *Food, The Yearbook of Agriculture, 1959,* U.S. Department of Agriculture, Washington, D.C.

501

produce disease or cause harmful spoilage of foods.

Basal metabolism. The energy produced by an individual during physical, digestive, and emotional rest, measured directly by the heat evolved and indirectly by the oxygen consumed and carbon dioxide given off.

Bile. A thick green or yellow fluid formed in the liver, collected in the gall bladder, and emptied into the intestinal tract at intervals, particularly during the digestion of fats. It is a complex mixture containing salts of bile acids, which aid in digestion of fats, and cholesterol and other substances from different body sources. It carries cholesterol from the liver into the intestine for excretion or for reuse in digestion as needed.

Biological catalyst. A substance produced by living organisms that speeds up the rate of a chemical reaction but is not itself used up in the reaction. An enzyme.

Biological value. The biological value of a food protein is the efficiency with which that protein furnishes the proper proportions and amounts of the amino acids needed, at the time of synthesis of body proteins, by man or animals eating these foods. The more nearly a protein supplies the tissues with the necessary proportions and amounts of these amino acids, the higher is its biological value.

Biotin. One of the 10 recognized vitamins of the B complex. It is widely distributed in foods. It is needed in the diet of certain laboratory animals, such as the chick, rat, and mouse. A deficiency in man has never been observed under normal conditions.

Blanch. To preheat in boiling water or steam. Blanching is used to inactivate enzymes and shrink food for canning, freezing, and drying. Blanching also is used to aid in removal of skin from nuts, fruit, and some vegetables.

Bland. Mild flavored, not stimulating to the taste; smooth, soft textured.

Boiling point. The temperature at which the vapor pressure of a liquid equals the atmospheric pressure. At the boiling point, bubbles of vapor rise continually and break on the surface. The boiling temperature of pure water at sea level (barometer 30 inches) is 212°F. At high altitudes, the boiling point of water is lower because the atmospheric pressure is lower. At 5,000 feet above sea level, for example, the boiling point of water is 203°; at 10,000 feet it is 194°.

Buffer. A substance that can help a solution resist or counteract changes in free acid or alkali concentration. There are many buffers in the body.

Calcification. Process by which organic tissue becomes hardened by a deposit of calcium salts.

Calcium. A mineral element that is an essential constituent of bone and is essential for blood clotting, muscle tone, and nerve function.

Calorimeter. An instrument for measuring the heat change and the energy in any system.

Calorimetry. The science of measuring heat.

Carbohydrate. An important group of organic substances that contains carbon, hydrogen, and oxygen. The hydrogen and oxygen are present in the same proportion as in water (H_2O), and there is one molecule of water for every carbon. Starch and sugar are carbohydrates.

Carbon. The chemical element present in all substances designated as organic. These include proteins, carbohydrates, and fats. When a compound containing carbon combines with oxygen in the body, energy is liberated and carbon dioxide is formed. Compounds that do not contain carbon are classed as inorganic.

Carbon dioxide. A compound that is formed when carbon combines with oxygen. It leaves the body chiefly when air is exhaled from the lung.

Caries, dental. Tooth decay.

Carotene. A yellow compound of carbon and hydrogen that occurs in plants and is a form of vitamin A. Alpha, beta, and gamma carotenes may be converted into vitamin A in the body.

Cartilage. A special form of white connective tissue that is attached to the ends of bones that are either divided into joints or united by joints. It is more flexible but not so strong as bone. Cartilage is the first substance to form in growing bone; then calcium and phosphorus are deposited in the cartilage, thus changing it to bone.

Catabolism. The breaking down in the body of chemical compounds into simpler ones, usually accompanied by the production of heat.

Catalyst. A substance that speeds up the rate of a chemical reaction but is not itself used up in the reaction.

Cell. The structural and functional microscopic unit of plant and animal organisms.

Cellulose. A carbohydrate found in the woody part of plants and trees. It is converted to glucose on hydrolysis. Cellophane and cotton are almost pure cellulose.

Chemical additives. Substances added to foods to improve their flavor, color, texture, or keeping quality.

Cholesterol. The commonest member of the group of sterols; it is present in many foods and also can be made within the body.

Coagulation. The change from a fluid state to a thickened jelly, curd, or clot.

Coenzyme. A partner needed by some enzymes to accomplish a biochemical change.

Collagen. A protein that forms the chief constituent of the connective tissue, cartilage, tendon, bone, and skin. Collagen is changed to gelatin by the action of water and heat.

Colostrum. Milk secreted during the first week of lactation.

Combustion. The combination of substances with oxygen accompanied by the liberation of energy.

Culture (i.e., added to milk). Microorganisms, such as bacteria, molds, and yeasts, which are usually grown under controlled conditions. Specific cultures are used to produce many kinds of cheese and buttermilk and other fermented milks.

Decalcification. The withdrawal of calcium from the bones where it has been deposited. It may be caused by an inadequate supply of calcium in the diet so that calcium has to be taken from the bones to help meet the body's needs. It may be caused also by an imbalance in some of the hormone activity in the body.

Deficiency disease. A disease resulting from an inadequate dietary intake of something required nutritionally; most commonly refers to diseases resulting from dietary deficiencies of vitamins or trace elements.

Dehydration. The loss of water from the body.

Diet or dietary. The food consumed daily by an individual family or group of people with an emphasis on the nutrients included.

Digestion. In physiology, the breaking down of foods into simpler components in the alimentary or digestive tract. Foods may be digested by natural body enzymes in the stomach and intestines, or be broken down similarly by the chemist using chemicals and prepared enzymes, heat, or microorganisms. Proteins are digested to peptides and amino acids, fats to fatty acids and glycerol, carbohydrates to dextrins and sugars. Buttermilk is an example of a food partially digested by natural enzymes and microorganisms in the milk.

Edema. Swelling of a part of or the entire body due to the presence of an excess of water. Edema is most noticeable at the end of the day around the ankles, which increase in size. When the condition becomes severe, an impression remains for a few minutes where a finger was pressed against the skin.

Edible. A term applied to food that is fit to eat. It usually refers to food that is suitable for human consumption. The initials E.P. are used to denote the edible portion of a food—for example, a banana without its skin, a pork chop without the bone, a melon without its seeds and rind.

Element. Any one of the fundamental atoms of which all matter is composed.

Emulsification. A process of breaking up large particles or liquids into smaller ones, which remain suspended in another liquid. Emulsification may be done mechanically, as in the homogenization of ice cream mixtures. It may be hastened by chemicals, as by the use of acid and lecithin (from egg yolk) in emulsification of oil for mayonnaise. It may be accomplished naturally in body processes, as when bile salts emulsify fats during digestion.

Emulsify. To make into an emulsion. When small drops of one liquid are finely dispersed (distributed) in another liquid, an emulsion is formed. The drops are held in suspension by an emulsifying agent, which surrounds each drop and makes a coating around it.

Endemic. An endemic disease is one that occurs in low incidence but more or less constantly in a given population.

Endocrine. Secreting internally, or into the bloodstream, as endocrine glands, or glands of internal secretion.

Endogenous. Originating within or inside the cells or tissues.

Endosperm. The starchy portion within the kernel of wheat, corn, or other cereal, from which refined flour is produced after the germ and fibrous outer layers are removed.

Energy. Capacity to perform work.

Environmental. Pertaining to external influences.

Enzymatic. Related to that class of complex organic substances called enzymes, such as amylase and pepsin, that accelerate (catalyze) specific chemical reactions in plants and animals, as in digestion of foods.

Enzyme. One of a class of substances formed in living cells. It speeds up chemical reaction but does not change during the process.

Epidemic. A disease is epidemic when many

people in a region are attacked at the same time or when the disease is spreading rapidly.

Epithelial. Refers to those cells that form the outer layer of the skin, those that line all the portions of the body having contact with the external air (such as the eyes, ears, nose, throat, lungs), and those that are specialized for secretion as the liver, kidneys, and urinary and reproductive tract.

Ergosterol. A substance belonging to the class of sterols that is found chiefly in plants and animal tissue, yeasts, and molds. It is white and crystalline and similar in appearance to the material that candles are made of. On exposure to ultraviolet light it is converted to vitamin D_2

Excretion. The products of digestion and metabolism that are discarded from the body —feces from the intestinal tract and urine from the kidneys.

Exogenous. Originating from outside the cells or tissues.

Extrinsic factor. Literally, a constituent from outside; in nutrition, something obtained from food, commonly used to refer to vitamin B_{12} in relation to the disease known as pernicious anemia.

Factor. In nutrition, any chemical substance found in foods. A factor might be a vitamin, a mineral, or any other nutrient or nonnutrient. Usually it has some effect on growth or reproduction of animals. A factor may be "identified" or remain "unidentified." In arithmetic, factor is a value or ratio expressing the relationship between two items, such as liters of oxygen and the equivalent amount of oxygen in grams.

Fat. A glyceryl ester of fatty acids. Fats generally are substances of plant and animal origin. Fat may be in solid form, as butter, margarine, lard, or other shortening, or in liquid form, as the vegetable oils.

Fat soluble. Refers generally to substances that cannot be dissolved in water but can be in fats and oils, or in fat solvents. The fat-soluble vitamins are vitamins A, D, E, and K.

Fatty acid. Organic compound of carbon, hydrogen, and oxygen, which combines with glycerol to make a fat.

Ferment. To undergo chemical change brought about by the enzymes contained in certain microorganisms.

Flora (intestinal). The bacteria and other small organisms that are found in the intestinal contents.

Folacin. The name officially selected to re-

place the term folic acid, a vitamin of the B complex.

Folic acid. One of the vitamins of the B complex. Its official name is folacin; it is also known as pteroylglutamic acid. It is a bright-yellow compound needed in very small amounts in the diet of animals and man. A deficiency results in poor growth, anemia, and other blood disorders.

Fortify. To add one or more nutrients to a food so that it contains more of the nutrients than were present originally before processing. Milk is often fortified with vitamin D.

Galactose. A white crystalline sugar obtained from lactose (milk sugar) by hydrolysis.

Gamma globulin. A protein in the blood that forms antibodies.

Gastric. Pertaining to the stomach.

Gastrointestinal. Refers to the part of the digestive system made up of the stomach and the intestines.

Gingivitis. Inflammation of the gums of the jaws.

Glandular. Adjective of gland. A gland is an organ that makes and discharges a chemical substance that is used elsewhere in the body or eliminated.

Gluten. An elastic substance that gives adhesiveness to dough. It is formed when the proteins in flour, especially those in wheat flour, absorb water. Gluten assists in giving shape to the cooked product as it coagulates when heated.

Glycerol. Same as glycerin. Serves as the backbone radical or framework of the fat molecule, permitting attachment of three fatty acids. Glycerol is an alcohol containing three carbons and three hydroxy (—OH) groups; methyl, or wood, alcohol contains one carbon and one hydroxy group; ethyl, or grain, alcohol contains two carbons and one hydroxy group.

Heat labile. Changeable by heat; unstable to heat.

Heat-of-combustion values. The amount of heat produced (usually expressed as kcalories) when a unit weight of a substance is oxidized.

Hemoglobin. A protein in the blood that contains iron and carries oxygen from the lungs to the tissues.

Homogenized. Broken up into small particles of the same size. Homogenized milk has been treated to break the fat into such small globules that it will not rise to the top as cream.

Hemostatic. Steady biochemical states in

the body, maintained by physiological processes.

Hormone. A chemical substance that is produced in an organ called an endocrine gland and is transported by the blood or other body fluids to other cells. A hormone greatly influences the functions of some specific organ and of the body as a whole. Thyroxin is a hormone secreted by the thyroid gland. Insulin is a hormone secreted by the pancreas.

Hydrogen. The chemical element with the smallest atomic weight. Present in proteins, carbohydrates, fats, and water. Hydrogen makes up approximately 10 per cent of the human body.

Hydrogenation. The addition of hydrogen to any unsaturated compound. Oils are changed to solid fats by hydrogenation.

Hydrolysis. The splitting of a substance into the smaller units of which it is composed by the addition of the elements of water. For example, when starch is heated in water containing a small amount of acid or subjected to the action of digestive enzymes, the simpler sugar glucose is released.

Hypervitaminosis. The undesirable effects produced by taking an excess of a vitamin concentrate or pure vitamin.

Inactive. To suspend or terminate certain biological activities, such as by heat, irradiation, or other forms of energy.

Incidence. The frequency of occurrence of a situation or of a condition, like a disease.

Inedible. A substance that is not fit for food, such as poisonous nuts and plants. Tough skins, seeds, and decayed spots of fruits and vegetables and bones of meat are considered inedible parts because they are not suitable for human consumption.

Ingest. To eat or take in through the mouth.

Inorganic. A large group of chemical compounds that do not contain carbon.

Insulin. A chemical substance in the group of hormones that is secreted from special cells in the pancreas. It is essential for the normal utilization of sugar by the body. A lack of insulin results in the development of diabetes.

Intake. Substances or amounts of substances which are taken in by the body, for example, the intake of food.

Intestinal juices. The digestive juices secreted by the intestinal walls (in contrast to gastric juices secreted by the stomach walls) and pancreatic juices secreted by the pancreas. The intestinal juices contain enzymes, which complete the final stages in digestion of protein, fat, and carbohydrate.

Intestinal tract. The entire intestines, both small and large.

Intrinsic factor. A chemical substance in normal stomach juice. It is necessary for the absorption of vitamin B_{12} from the intestine.

Irradiation. To treat with ultraviolet rays from sunlight or an artificial source; to treat with X rays or other radioactive agent.

Irritability. A term usually applied to nerves. It refers to their ability to respond or react to a stimulus.

IU The abbreviation for international unit, the measure of the potency of vitamins A, D, and E.

Kcaloric. Pertaining to heat or energy; used in reference to the kcaloric value of a food, it means the heat or energy that can be obtained as muscular work and heat when the body uses or metabolizes that food.

Kcalorie. The unit by which heat is measured. It is defined in terms of the amount of heat required to raise the temperature of a specified amount of water 1 degree centigrade. A kcalorie is the amount of heat required to raise 1000 g (1 kg) of water from 14.5 to 15.5°C. The kcalorie is used exclusively in expressing the caloric value of foods and the calorie needs of humans and animals.

Labile. Easily destroyed.

Laboratory animals. Mice, rats, guinea pigs, dogs, and many other small animals that are used in laboratories as the subjects for scientific experiments.

Lactation. The secretion of milk or the period during which milk is formed.

Lactic acid. A compound formed in the chemical metabolic processes that accompany muscular activity; also a substance formed by the fermentation of lactose, the sugar in milk.

Lactose. A sugar that occurs in milk. It is a white, crystalline sugar that is less soluble and less sweet than ordinary cane sugar (sucrose).

Linoleic acid. One of the digestion products from certain fats, which is essential to body tissues.

Lipids. A broad term for fats and fat-like substances; characterized by the presence of one or more fatty acids. Lipids include fats, cholesterol, lecithins, phospholipids, and similar substances, which do not mix readily with water.

Lymph. A yellowish liquid that contains corpuscles and is present in the lymphatic vessels or channels of the body.

Lymphatic system. The tissue spaces, all the small and large lymphatic vessels, and the two large ducts or canals in the thorax.

Lysine. One of the amino acids essential to the nutrition of man and animals. It is of special dietary concern because it is one of the amino acids that is present at a relatively low level in some food proteins of plant origin.

Malformation. A deformity; an abnormal development or formation of a part of the body.

Mammary glands. The milk-secreting glands; the breasts.

Matrix. The intercellular framework of a tissue.

Maturation. The process of coming to full development, maturity, or adulthood.

Membrane. A thin, soft, pliable layer of animal or vegetable tissue.

Menstruation. The monthly discharge peculiar to women. It begins at the age of puberty and continues to menopause.

Metabolic. Refers to metabolism.

Metabolism. The sum of the chemical changes that go on in the body as food is made into body tissues, energy is produced, and body tissue is broken down. There are two parts to body metabolism.

Anabolism is constructive and includes building, maintaining, and repairing tissue.

Catabolism is destructive and includes changing or breaking down tissue or other materials in the body into simple substances for producing energy and for excretion.

Microbiological. Pertaining to microorganisms—that is, microscopic plants or animals. Refers usually to a method by which certain microorganisms are used to determine the amounts of a particular nutrient, like a vitamin or an amino acid, in a food. Such assays are possible because these microorganisms must have these vitamins and amino acids in order to grow. These determinations are called microbiological assays or analyses.

Microorganisms. Very small living beings. Bacteria, yeasts, and molds are microorganisms found in foods.

Molecule. A chemical combination of two or more atoms that form a specific substance. For example, the combination of an atom of sodium and an atom of chlorine makes a molecule of sodium chloride, or table salt. This is a comparatively simple molecule. There are also large, complex molecules, such as hemoglobin. Proteins and starches are examples of even larger and very complex molecules containing many atoms.

Mucosa. The mucous membrane that lines the passages and cavities of the body, as in the gastrointestinal tract.

Mucous membrane. A membrane lining the cavities and canals of the body that have contact with the air. It is kept moist by mucus secreted by special cells and glands. The eyes, ears, nose, throat, lungs, digestive tract, genitourinary, and reproductive tracts are lined with mucous membrane.

Musculature. The muscular apparatus of the body or any part of it.

Nitrogen. A chemical element essential to life. Plants can use nitrogen compounds direct from the soil, and nitrogen-fixing bacteria can use nitrogen directly from the air, but animals must have their nitrogen supplied by protein foods.

Nitrogenous. A substance containing nitrogen is referred to as nitrogenous. Proteins contain nitrogen, as do the amino acids, the chemical components of proteins. Protein-decomposition products containing nitrogen are called nitrogenous extractives. They are found in well-ripened meat and contribute to the flavor of meat.

Nonfat solids. The portion of milk remaining after the water and butterfat have been accounted for; nonfat-dried-milk solids.

NRC. An abbreviation for National Research Council; usually used when referred to the recommended dietary allowances.

Nutrient. A chemical compound with specific functions in the nourishment of the body, such as tryptophan, an amino acid; thiamin, a vitamin; or calcium, a mineral. The body depends on food for about 50 different nutrients.

Nutritionist. A professionally trained person who applies the science of nutrition and related subjects in research, teaching, or advisory services.

Nutriture (or nutritional status). The condition of physical health and well-being of the body as related to the consumption and utilization of food for growth, maintenance, and repair.

Nutriture, or nutritional status, may be appraised by such methods as clinical examinations with special attention to condition of the skin, eyes, mouth, tongue, gums, muscles; determination of overweight or underweight, often by measurement of the thickness of a skinfold; blood pressure and pulse rate; biochemical tests on the blood for various constituents associated with health; and tests of urine samples, with or without the administration of certain nutrients.

Obese. Fat; excessive overweight due to the presence of a surplus of body fat.

Organic. A large group of chemical compounds that contain carbon.

Organic acids. Acids containing only carbon, hydrogen, and oxygen. Among the best known are citric acid (in citrus fruits) and acetic acid (in vinegar).

Osmosis. The transfer of materials that takes place through a semipermeable membrane that separates two solutions, or between a solvent and a solution, that tends to equalize their concentrations. The walls of living cells are semipermeable membranes, and much of the activity of the cells depends on osmosis.

Osmotic pressure. The pressure exerted by the movement of a solvent through a semipermeable membrane into a more concentrated solution on the other side of the membrane. This pressure on the walls of the membrane is the driving force that causes diffusion of particles in solution to move from one place to another.

Ossification. The process of forming bone. Cartilage is made into bone by the process of ossification. The minerals calcium and phosphorus are deposited in the cartilage, changing it into bone.

Overweight. An excess of more than 10 per cent above the desirable weight.

Ovum. A female germ cell.

Oxidation. The removal of electrons, in the most general sense; may also mean the combining with oxygen or the removal of hydrogen.

Oxidative. Refers to the processes of oxidation.

Oxygen. One of the most plentiful chemical elements. Oxygen makes up 65 per cent of the human body. When other chemical substances combine with oxygen, energy is released.

Palatability. The quality characteristics (such as color, flavor, and texture) of a food product that makes an impression on the organs of touch, taste, smell, or sight and have significance in determining the acceptability of the food product to the user.

Pancreas. A glandular organ extending across the upper abdomen close to the liver. It secretes into the intestinal tract digestive

juices containing enzymes to act upon protein, fat, and carbohydrate. It also secretes directly into the blood the hormone insulin, which is essential for one stage in the oxidation of sugar to carbon dioxide and water. Adjective: pancreatic.

Permeable. Capable of being penetrated.

Phosphorylate. A chemical term that applies to the introduction of a phosphorus and oxygen group into a complex chemical compound.

Plaque. Tiny patches of unnatural formations on tissues such as on tooth surfaces and on inner arterial walls. The plaques, called atheroma, that are found in walls of arteries contain some lipids, usually cholesterol and oleic acid, and some connective or scar tissue of protein origin. Their formation is related to abnormal fat metabolism. They contribute to stiffening of blood vessel walls, closing of arteries, choking circulation, and ruptured arteries. They may be formed in coronary arteries of people of all ages but appear to be most prevalent in men 45 to 60 years of age engaged in light work or sedentary occupations.

Polyunsaturated fatty acids. A class of fatty acids that have more than one unsaturated linkage in the chain, each lacking two hydrogens. Saturated fatty acids have all the hydrogens the carbon chain can hold. Monounsaturated fatty acids have only one unsaturated linkage. Although there are many kinds of polyunsaturated fatty acids, linoleic appears to be the only one that the body cannot synthesize and that must be obtained from food sources.

Potent. Strong, powerful, efficacious.

Potential energy. Energy in chemical form, which may be released either as heat or muscular work when the substance is oxidized.

Preconceptional. Before pregnancy.

Precursor. Forerunner; something that precedes. In biochemistry, a compound that can be used by the body to form another compound.

Processing of foods. Subjecting them to various manufacturing procedures to change their characteristics. Processing includes canning, freezing, and dehydrating, so the foods can be stored; it includes changing the form of the food, such as making oil or flour from seeds and making pickles from cucumbers; it includes simply cooking foods, for example, baking bread.

Protein. One of a group of complex organic

compounds that contain nitrogen, carbon, hydrogen, and oxygen and are essential for life and growth. They are formed by various combinations of different amino acids.

Protoplasm. The essential protein substance of living cells upon which all the vital functions of nutrition, secretion, growth, and reproduction depend.

Provitamin A. Any of a number of substances, called carotenes, that occur in nature and can be converted into vitamin A in the body.

Puree. A smooth, pulpy food product from which the rough fiber has been removed by sieving or other means. Most baby foods are in the pureed form.

Pyridoxine. One of the B vitamins, commonly designated as vitamin B_6. Strictly speaking, vitamin B_6 includes a group of three vitamins of nutritional interest—pyridoxine, pyridoxamine, and pyridoxal.

Radioisotope. One of a broad class of elements capable of becoming radioactive and giving off atomic energy, such as is detectable with a Geiger counter. Some radioisotopes occur naturally; others are produced artificially. The word is synonymous with radioactive elements and includes tracer elements.

Reconstitute. To restore to the normal state, usually by adding water, such as reconstituting dry milk by adding water to make it fluid milk.

Reducing (chemical action). The taking up of oxygen from air and from other materials.

Rehydration. Soaking or cooking or using other procedures to make dehydrated foods take up the water they lost during drying.

Secretory. The formation of a secretion. Thus the salivary glands of the mouth secrete saliva and are secretory glands.

Specific gravity. The relation of the weight of a definite volume of a substance to the weight of an equal volume of water.

Stress. Intense strain. In medicine, any circumstance great enough to disrupt the normal, steady functioning of the body.

Subclinical disease. A disease, usually mild, that has no definite symptoms or signs which can be recognized by the usual visual or clinical means.

Substrate. A substance that is acted upon, as by an enzyme.

Sugar. Usually means cane sugar used as ordinary sugar. May also mean any simple carbohydrate with a sweet taste.

Syndrome. A medical term meaning a group of symptoms that occur together.

Synthesis. A coming together of two or more substances to form a new material.

Therapeutic. Refers to curing a disease.

Therapy. The medical treatment of disease.

Toxicity. The quality of a substance that makes it poisonous or toxic; sometimes refers to the degree of severity of the poison or the possibility of being poisonous.

Tracer element. A radioactive element used in biological and other research to trace the fate of a substance or follow stages in a chemical reaction, such as the pathway of metabolism of a nutrient or growth formations in plants or animals. Radioactive elements that have proved useful for tracer work in nutrition research are carbon 14, calcium 45, cobalt 60, strontium 90, and phosphorus 32. Carbon 14 is used widely in studies of fat and sugar metabolism and cholesterol formation.

Tryptophan. An amino acid that is essential for the nutrition of man and animals. It is frequently present in inadequate amounts in food protein of plant origin; when such foods are the sole diet, tryptophan is often one of the limiting amino acids for the synthesis of animal tissues.

Unsaturated fatty acid. A fatty acid that has a double bond between two carbon atoms at one or more places in the carbon chain. Hydrogen can be added at the site of the double bond. An unsaturated fat is one that contains an unsaturated fatty acid. A saturated fatty acid has no double bonds.

Urea. An end product of protein metabolism excreted in the urine.

Vascular. Full of vessels that contain a fluid. In physiology, the blood and lymph vessels in the body.

Vitamin. One of a group of substances that in relatively small amounts are essential for life and growth.

Water extract. Whatever can be removed or dissolved out of a substance with water. A substance like sugar is completely soluble in water, whereas when yeast is shaken up with water only a small portion of it goes into solution. What remains is insoluble and does not pass into the water extract.

Water soluble. Refers generally to substances that dissolve in water. Water-soluble vitamins are ascorbic acid, thiamin, riboflavin, niacin, folacin, vitamin B_6 and vitamin B_{12}.

Appendix B

Nutritive Value of Foods

Explanation of the Table

The table that follows on pages 512–534, from the U.S. Department of Agriculture, shows the food values in over 600 foods commonly used in this country.

FOODS LISTED   Foods are grouped under the following main headings: milk; eggs; meat, poultry, and fish; dry beans and peas, nuts; vegetables; fruits; grain products; fats; sugars; and miscellaneous items.

Most of the foods listed are in ready-to-eat form. Some are basic products widely used in food preparation, such as flour, fat, and cornmeal.

Weight in grams—rounded to the nearest whole gram—is shown for an approximate measure of each food as it is described; if inedible parts are included in the description, both measure and weight include these parts.

The approximate measure shown for each food is in cups, ounces, pounds, some other well-known unit, or a piece of certain size. Usually, the measure shown can be calculated to larger or smaller amounts by multiplying or dividing. Because the measures are approximate (some are rounded for convenient use), calculated nutritive values for larger quantities of some food items may be less representative than those calculated for smaller quantities.

The cup measure refers to the standard measuring cup of 8 fluid ounces or ½ liquid pint. The ounce refers to ⅟₁₆ of a pound avoirdupois, unless fluid ounce is indicated. The weight of a fluid ounce varies according to the food measured.

Factors in general use for converting from one measure to its equivalent in another measure include those shown below.

EQUIVALENTS BY VOLUME
(All measurements level)

1 quart	= 4 cups
1 cup	= 8 fluid ounces
	= ½ pint
	= 16 tablespoons
2 tablespoons	= 1 fluid ounce
1 tablespoon	= 3 teaspoons
1 pound regular butter or margarine	= 4 sticks
	= 2 cups
1 pound whipped butter or margarine	= 6 sticks
	= 2 8-ounce containers
	= 3 cups

EQUIVALENTS BY WEIGHT

1 pound (16 ounces)	= 453.6 grams
1 ounce	= 28.35 grams
3½ ounces	= 100 grams

FOOD VALUES Values are shown for protein, fat, fatty acids, total carbohydrates, two minerals—calcium and iron, and five vitamins—vitamin A, thiamin, riboflavin, niacin, and ascorbic acid (vitamin C). Kcalories are shown in the column headed "Food energy." The kcalorie is the unit of measure for the energy furnished the body by protein, fat, and carbohydrate.

These values can be used as the basis for comparing kinds and amounts of nutrient in different foods. For some foods, the values can be used in comparing different forms of the same food.

Water content is also shown in the table because the percentage of moisture present is needed for identification and comparison of many food items.

The values for food energy (kcalories) and nutrients shown in Table 1 are the amounts present in the edible part of the item, that is, in only that portion of the weight of the item customarily eaten—corn without cob, meat without bone, potatoes without skin, European-type grapes without seeds. If additional parts are eaten—the skin of the potato, for example—amounts of some nutrients obtained will be somewhat greater than those shown.

For many of the prepared items, values have been calculated from the ingredients in typical recipes. Examples of such items are biscuits, corn muffins, oyster stew, macaroni and cheese, custard, and a number of other dessert-type items.

For toast and for vegetables, values are without fat added, either during preparation or at the table. Values for the thiamin content of toast are about 20 per cent lower than for fresh bread; it was impossible to show this loss adequately because of the small amount of thiamin present in a slice of bread. Some destruction of vitamins in vegetables, especially of ascorbic acid, may occur when foods are cut or shredded. Such losses are variable, and no deduction for these losses has been made.

For meat, values are for meat as cooked, drained, and without drippings. For many cuts, two sets of values are shown: meat including the fat, and meat from which the fat has been trimmed off in the kitchen or on the plate.

A variety of manufactured items, such as some of the milk products, ready-to-eat breakfast cereals, imitation cream products, fruit drinks, and various mixes are included in Table 1. Frequently these foods are fortified with one or more nutrients. If nutrients are added, this information is on the label. Values shown for these foods are usually based on products from several manufacturers and may differ somewhat from the values provided by any one source.

Nutritive Values of the Edible Part of Foods*

[Dashes in the columns for nutrients show that no suitable value could be found although there is reason to believe that a measurable amount of the nutrient may be present]

Milk, Cheese, Cream, Imitation Cream; Related Products

	Food, Approximate Measure, and Weight (in grams) gm	Water per cent	Food Energy calories	Protein gm	Fat gm	Fatty Acids Satu-rated (total) gm	Unsaturated Oleic gm	Lin-oleic gm	Carbo-hy-drate gm	Cal-cium mg	Iron mg	Vita-min A Value I.U.	Thia-mine mg	Ribo-flavin mg	Niacin mg	Ascor-bic Acid mg
	Milk: Fluid:															
1	Whole, 3.5% fat 1 cup 244	87	160	9	9	5	3	Trace	12	288	0.1	350	0.07	0.41	0.2	2
2	Nonfat (skim) 1 cup 245	90	90	9	Trace	—	—	—	12	296	0.1	10	0.09	0.44	0.2	2
3	Partly skimmed, 2% nonfat milk solids added 1 cup 246	87	145	10	5	3	2	Trace	15	352	0.1	200	0.10	0.52	0.2	2
	Canned, concentrated, undiluted:															
4	Evaporated, unsweetened 1 cup 252	74	345	18	20	11	7	1	24	635	0.3	810	0.10	0.86	0.5	3
5	Condensed, sweetened 1 cup 306	27	980	25	27	15	9	1	166	802	0.3	1,100	0.24	1.16	0.6	3
	Dry, nonfat instant:															
6	Low-density (1 1/3 cups needed for reconstitution to 1 qt) 1 cup 68	4	245	24	Trace	—	—	—	35	879	0.4	120	0.24	1.21	0.6	5
7	High-density (7/8 cup needed for reconstitution to 1 qt) 1 cup 104	4	375	37	1	—	—	—	54	1,345	0.6	130	0.36	1.85	0.9	7
	Buttermilk:															
8	Fluid, cultured, made from skim milk 1 cup 245	90	90	9	Trace	—	—	—	12	296	0.1	10	0.10	0.44	0.2	2
9	Dried, packaged 1 cup 120	3	465	41	6	3	2	Trace	60	1,498	0.7	260	0.31	2.06	1.1	—
	Cheese: Natural: Blue or Roquefort type:															
10	Ounce 1 oz. 28	40	105	6	9	5	3	Trace	1	89	0.1	350	0.01	0.17	0.3	0
11	Cubic inch 1 cu. in. 17	40	65	4	5	3	2	Trace	Trace	54	0.1	210	0.01	0.11	0.2	0
12	Camembert, packaged in 4-oz pkg. with 3 wedges per pkg. 1 wedge 38	52	115	7	9	5	3	Trace	1	40	0.2	380	0.02	0.29	0.3	0
	Cheddar:															
13	Ounce 1 oz 28	37	115	7	9	5	3	Trace	1	213	0.3	370	0.01	0.13	Trace	0
14	Cubic inch 1 cu in 17	37	70	4	6	3	2	Trace	Trace	129	0.2	230	0.01	0.08	Trace	0
	Cottage, large or small curd: Creamed:															
15	Package of 12 oz, net wt. 1 pkg 340	78	360	46	14	8	5	Trace	10	320	1.0	580	0.10	0.85	0.3	0
16	Cup, curd pressed down 1 cup 245	78	260	33	10	6	3	Trace	7	230	0.7	420	0.07	0.61	0.2	0
	Uncreamed:															
17	Package of 12 oz net wt. 1 pkg 340	79	290	58	1	1	Trace	Trace	9	306	1.4	30	0.10	0.95	0.3	0
18	Cup, curd pressed down 1 cup 200	79	170	34	1	Trace	Trace	Trace	5	180	0.8	20	0.06	0.56	0.2	0

No.	Food	Measure	Weight (g)	Water (%)	Food energy (cal)	Protein (g)	Fat (g)	Saturated (g)	Unsaturated Oleic (g)	Unsaturated Linoleic (g)	Carbohydrate (g)	Calcium (mg)	Iron (mg)	Vitamin A (I.U.)	Thiamin (mg)	Riboflavin (mg)	Niacin (mg)	Ascorbic acid (mg)
	Cream:																	
19	Package of 8 oz, net wt.	1 pkg	227	51	850	18	86	48	28	3	5	141	0.5	3,500	0.05	0.54	0.2	0
20	Package of 3 oz, net wt.	1 pkg	85	51	320	7	32	18	11	1	2	53	0.2	1,310	0.02	0.20	0.1	0
21	Cubic inch	1 cu in	16	51	60	1	6	3	2	Trace	Trace	10	Trace	250	Trace	0.04	Trace	0
	Parmesan, grated:																	
22	Cup, pressed down	1 cup	140	17	655	60	43	24	14	1	5	1,893	0.7	1,760	0.03	1.22	0.3	0
23	Tablespoon	1 tbsp	5	17	25	2	2	1	1	Trace	Trace	68	Trace	60	Trace	0.04	Trace	0
24	Ounce	1 oz	28	17	130	12	9	5	3	Trace	1	383	0.1	360	0.01	0.25	0.1	0
	Swiss:																	
25	Ounce	1 oz	28	39	105	8	8	4	3	Trace	1	262	0.3	320	Trace	0.11	Trace	0
26	Cubic inch	1 cu in	15	39	55	4	4	2	1	Trace	Trace	139	0.1	170	Trace	0.06	Trace	0
	Pasteurized processed cheese: American:																	
27	Ounce	1 oz	28	40	105	7	9	5	3	Trace	1	198	0.3	350	0.01	0.12	Trace	0
28	Cubic inch	1 cu in	18	40	65	4	5	3	2	Trace	Trace	122	0.2	210	Trace	0.07	Trace	0
	Swiss:																	
29	Ounce	1 oz	28	40	100	8	8	4	3	Trace	1	251	0.3	310	Trace	0.11	Trace	0
30	Cubic inch	1 cu in	18	40	65	5	5	3	2	Trace	Trace	159	0.2	200	Trace	0.07	Trace	0
	Pasteurized process cheese food, American:																	
31	Tablespoon	1 tbsp	14	43	45	3	3	2	1	Trace	1	80	0.1	140	Trace	0.08	Trace	0
32	Cubic inch	1 cu in	18	43	60	4	4	2	1	Trace	1	100	0.1	170	Trace	0.10	Trace	0
33	Pasteurized process cheese spread, American	1 oz	28	49	80	6	6	3	2	Trace	2	160	0.2	250	Trace	0.15	Trace	0
	Cream:																	
34	Half-and-half (cream and milk)	1 cup	242	80	325	8	28	15	9	1	11	261	0.1	1,160	0.07	0.39	0.1	2
35		1 tbsp	15	80	20	1	2	1	1	Trace	1	16	Trace	70	Trace	0.02	Trace	Trace
36	Light, coffee or table	1 cup	240	72	505	7	49	27	16	1	10	245	0.1	2,020	0.07	0.36	0.1	2
37		1 tbsp	15	72	30	Trace	3	2	1	Trace	1	15	Trace	130	Trace	0.02	Trace	Trace
38	Sour	1 cup	230	72	485	7	47	26	16	1	10	235	0.1	1,930	0.07	0.35	0.1	2
39		1 tbsp	12	72	25	Trace	2	1	1	Trace	1	12	Trace	100	Trace	0.02	Trace	Trace
40	Whipped topping (pressurized)	1 cup	60	62	155	2	14	8	5	Trace	6	67	Trace	570	Trace	0.04	Trace	—
41		1 tbsp	3	62	10	Trace	1	Trace	Trace	Trace	Trace	3	—	30	—	Trace	—	—
	Whipping, unwhipped (volume about double when whipped):																	
42	Light	1 cup	239	62	715	5	75	41	25	2	9	203	0.1	3,060	0.05	0.29	0.1	2
43		1 tbsp	15	62	45	Trace	5	3	2	Trace	1	13	Trace	190	Trace	0.02	Trace	Trace
44	Heavy	1 cup	238	57	840	5	90	50	30	3	7	179	0.1	3,670	0.05	0.26	0.1	2
45		1 tbsp	15	57	55	Trace	6	3	2	Trace	1	11	Trace	230	Trace	0.02	Trace	Trace
	Imitation cream products (made with vegetable fat): Creamers:																	
46	Powdered	1 cup	94	2	505	4	33	31	1	1	52	21	0.6	[2]200	—	—	—	—
47		1 tsp	2	2	10	Trace	1	1	Trace	Trace	1	1	Trace	[2]Trace	—	—	—	—
48	Liquid (frozen)	1 cup	245	77	345	3	27	25	1	Trace	25	29	—	[2]100	0	0	0	—
49		1 tbsp	15	77	20	Trace	2	1	Trace	Trace	2	2	—	[2]10	0	0	0	—
50	Sour dressing (imitation sour cream) made with nonfat dry milk	1 cup	235	72	440	9	38	35	1	1	17	277	0.1	10	0.07	0.38	0.2	1
51		1 tbsp	12	72	20	Trace	2	2	Trace	Trace	1	14	Trace	Trace	Trace	Trace	Trace	Trace
	Whipped topping:																	
52	Pressurized	1 cup	70	61	190	1	17	15	Trace	Trace	9	5	—	[2]340	—	0	—	—
53		1 tbsp	4	61	10	Trace	1	1	Trace	Trace	Trace	Trace	—	[2]20	—	0	—	—

*Nutritive Value of Foods, Home and Garden Bulletin No. 72. U.S. Department of Agriculture, Washington, D.C., 1970.

[1] Value applies to unfortified product; value for fortified low-density product would be 1500 I.U. and the fortified high-density product would be 2290 I.U.

[2] Contributed largely from beta-carotene used for coloring.

	Food, Approximate Measure, and Weight (in grams)		gm	Water per cent	Food Energy calories	Protein gm	Fat gm	Satu-rated (total) gm	Unsaturated Oleic gm	Lin-oleic gm	Carbo-hy-drate gm	Cal-cium mg	Iron mg	Vita-min A Value I.U.	Thia-mine mg	Ribo-flavin mg	Niacin mg	Ascor-bic Acid mg
	Whipped topping (cont.)																	
54	Frozen	1 cup	75	52	230	1	20	18	Trace	0	15	5	—	2560	—	0	—	—
55		1 tbsp	4	52	10	Trace	1	1	Trace	0	1	Trace	—	230	—	0	—	—
56	Powdered, made with whole milk	1 cup	75	58	175	3	12	10	1	Trace	15	62	Trace	2330	0.02	0.08	0.1	Trace
57		1 tbsp	4	58	10	Trace	1	1	Trace	Trace	1	3	Trace	220	Trace	Trace	Trace	Trace
	Milk beverages:																	
58	Cocoa, homemade	1 cup	250	79	245	10	12	7	4	Trace	27	295	1.0	400	0.10	0.45	0.5	3
59	Chocolate-flavored drink made with skim milk and 2% added butterfat	1 cup	250	83	190	8	6	3	2	Trace	27	270	0.5	210	0.10	0.40	0.3	3
	Malted milk:																	
60	Dry powder, approx. 3 heaping teaspoons per ounce	1 oz	28	3	115	4	2	—	—	—	20	82	0.6	290	0.09	0.15	0.1	0
61	Beverage	1 cup	235	78	245	11	10	7	5	1	28	317	0.7	590	0.14	0.49	0.2	2
	Milk desserts:																	
62	Custard	1 cup	265	77	305	14	15	7	5	1	29	297	1.1	930	0.11	0.50	0.3	1
	Ice cream:																	
63	Regular (approx. 10% fat)	1/2 gal	1,064	63	2,055	48	113	62	37	3	221	1,553	0.5	4,680	0.43	2.23	1.1	11
64		1 cup	133	63	255	6	14	8	5	Trace	28	194	0.1	590	0.05	0.28	0.1	1
65		3-fl-oz cup	50	63	95	2	5	3	2	Trace	10	73	Trace	220	0.02	0.11	0.1	1
66	Rich (approx. 16% fat)	1/2 gal	1,188	63	2,635	31	191	105	63	6	214	927	0.2	7,840	0.24	1.31	1.2	12
67		1 cup	148	63	330	4	24	13	8	1	27	115	Trace	980	0.03	0.16	0.1	1
	Ice milk:																	
68	Hardened	1/2 gal	1,048	67	1,595	50	53	29	17	2	235	1,635	1.0	2,200	0.52	2.31	1.0	10
69		1 cup	131	67	200	6	7	4	2	Trace	29	204	0.1	280	0.07	0.29	0.1	1
70	Soft-serve	1 cup	175	67	265	8	9	5	3	Trace	39	273	0.2	370	0.09	0.39	0.2	2
	Yoghurt:																	
71	Made from partially skimmed milk	1 cup	245	89	125	8	4	2	1	Trace	13	294	0.1	170	0.10	0.44	0.2	2
72	Made from whole milk	1 cup	245	88	150	7	8	5	3	Trace	12	272	0.1	340	0.07	0.39	0.2	2
	Eggs																	
	Eggs, large, 24 ounces per dozen: Raw or cooked in shell or with nothing added:																	
73	Whole, without shell	1 egg	50	74	80	6	6	2	3	Trace	Trace	27	1.1	590	0.05	0.15	Trace	0
74	White of egg	1 white	33	88	15	4	Trace	—	—	—	Trace	3	Trace	0	Trace	0.09	Trace	0
75	Yolk of egg	1 yolk	17	51	60	3	5	2	2	Trace	Trace	24	0.9	580	0.04	0.07	Trace	0
76	Scrambled with milk and fat	1 egg	64	72	110	7	8	3	3	Trace	1	51	1.1	690	0.05	0.18	Trace	0
	Meat, Poultry, Fish, Shellfish; Related Products																	
77	Bacon (20 slices per lb raw), broiled or fried crisp	2 slices	15	8	90	5	8	3	4	1	1	2	0.5	0	0.08	0.05	0.8	—
	Beef, cooked: Cuts braised, simmered, or pot-roasted:																	
78	Lean and fat	3 ounces	85	53	245	23	16	8	7	Trace	0	10	2.9	30	0.04	0.18	3.5	—

No.	Item																
79	Lean only — 2.5 ounces	72	62	140	22	5	2	2	Trace	0	10	2.7	10	0.04	0.16	3.3	—
	Hamburger (ground beef), broiled:																
80	Lean — 3 ounces	85	60	185	23	10	5	4	Trace	0	10	3.0	20	0.08	0.20	5.1	—
81	Regular — 3 ounces	85	54	245	21	17	8	8	Trace	0	9	2.7	30	0.07	0.18	4.6	—
	Roast, oven-cooked, no liquid added:																
	Relatively fat, such as rib:																
82	Lean and fat — 3 ounces	85	40	375	17	34	16	15	1	0	8	2.2	70	0.05	0.13	3.1	—
83	Lean only — 1.8 ounces	51	57	125	14	7	3	3	Trace	0	6	1.8	10	0.04	0.11	2.6	—
	Relatively lean, such as heel of round:																
84	Lean and fat — 3 ounces	85	62	165	25	7	3	3	Trace	0	11	3.2	10	0.06	0.19	4.5	—
85	Lean only — 2.7 ounces	78	65	125	24	3	1	1	Trace	0	10	3.0	Trace	0.06	0.18	4.3	—
	Steak, broiled:																
	Relatively fat, such as sirloin:																
86	Lean and fat — 3 ounces	85	44	330	20	27	13	12	1	0	9	2.5	50	0.05	0.16	4.0	—
87	Lean only — 2.0 ounces	56	59	115	18	4	2	2	Trace	0	7	2.2	10	0.05	0.14	3.6	—
	Relatively lean, such as round:																
88	Lean and fat — 3 ounces	85	55	220	24	13	6	6	Trace	0	10	3.0	20	0.07	0.19	4.8	—
89	Lean only — 2.4 ounces	68	61	130	21	4	2	2	Trace	0	9	2.5	10	0.06	0.16	4.1	—
	Beef, canned:																
90	Corned beef — 3 ounces	85	59	185	22	10	5	4	Trace	0	17	3.7	20	0.01	0.20	2.9	—
91	Corned beef hash — 3 ounces	85	67	155	7	10	5	4	Trace	9	11	1.7	—	0.01	0.08	1.8	—
92	Beef, dried or chipped — 2 ounces	57	48	115	19	4	2	2	Trace	0	11	2.9	—	0.04	0.18	2.2	—
93	Beef and vegetable stew — 1 cup	235	82	210	15	10	5	4	Trace	15	28	2.8	2,310	0.13	0.17	4.4	15
94	Beef potpie, baked, 4 1/4-inch diam., weight before baking about 8 ounces — 1 pie	227	55	560	23	33	9	20	2	43	32	4.1	1,860	0.25	0.27	4.5	7
	Chicken, cooked:																
95	Flesh only, broiled — 3 ounces	85	71	115	20	3	1	1	1	0	8	1.4	80	0.05	0.16	7.4	—
	Breast, fried, 1/2 breast:																
96	With bone — 3.3 ounces	94	58	155	25	5	1	1	1	1	9	1.3	70	0.04	0.17	11.2	—
97	Flesh and skin only — 2.7 ounces	76	58	155	25	5	1	1	1	1	9	1.3	70	0.04	0.17	11.2	—
	Drumstick, fried:																
98	With bone — 2.1 ounces	59	55	90	12	4	1	1	1	Trace	6	0.9	50	0.03	0.15	2.7	—
99	Flesh and skin only — 1.3 ounces	38	55	90	12	4	1	1	1	Trace	6	0.9	50	0.03	0.15	2.7	—
100	Chicken, canned, boneless — 3 ounces	85	65	170	18	10	3	4	2	0	18	1.3	200	0.03	0.11	3.7	3
101	Chicken potpie, baked 4 1/4-inch diam., weight before baking about 8 ounces — 1 pie	227	57	535	23	31	10	15	3	42	68	3.0	3,020	0.25	0.26	4.1	5
	Chili con carne, canned:																
102	With beans — 1 cup	250	72	335	19	15	7	7	Trace	30	80	4.2	150	0.08	0.18	3.2	—
103	Without beans — 1 cup	255	67	510	26	38	18	17	1	15	97	3.6	380	0.05	0.31	5.6	—
104	Heart, beef, lean, braised — 3 ounces	85	61	160	27	5	—	—	—	1	5	5.0	20	0.21	1.04	6.5	1
	Lamb,[3] cooked:																
105	Chop, thick, with bone, broiled — 4.8 ounces	137	47	400	25	33	18	12	1	0	10	1.5	—	0.14	0.25	5.6	—
106	Lean and fat — 4.0 ounces	112	47	400	25	33	18	12	1	0	10	1.5	—	0.14	0.25	5.6	—
107	Lean only — 2.6 ounces	74	62	140	21	6	3	2	Trace	0	9	1.5	—	0.11	0.20	4.5	—
	Leg, roasted:																
108	Lean and fat — 3 ounces	85	54	235	22	16	9	6	Trace	0	9	1.4	—	0.13	0.23	4.7	—
109	Lean only — 2.5 ounces	71	62	130	20	5	3	2	Trace	0	9	1.4	—	0.12	0.21	4.4	—
	Shoulder, roasted:																
110	Lean and fat — 3 ounces	85	50	285	18	23	13	8	1	0	9	1.0	—	0.11	0.20	4.0	—
111	Lean only — 2.3 ounces	64	61	130	17	6	3	2	Trace	0	8	1.0	—	0.10	0.18	3.7	—
112	Liver, beef, fried — 2 ounces	57	57	130	15	6	2	1	Trace	3	6	5.0	30,280	0.15	2.37	9.4	15

[2]Contributed largely from beta-carotene used for coloring.
[3]Outer layer of fat on the cut was removed to within approximately 1/2-inch of the lean. Deposits of fat within the cut were not removed.

	Food, Approximate Measure, and Weight (in grams)		gm	Water per cent	Food Energy calories	Protein gm	Fat gm	Fatty Acids Saturated (total) gm	Unsaturated Oleic gm	Unsaturated Linoleic gm	Carbohydrate gm	Calcium mg	Iron mg	Vitamin A Value I.U.	Thiamine mg	Riboflavin mg	Niacin mg	Ascorbic Acid mg
	Pork, cured, cooked:																	
113	Ham, light cure, lean and fat, roasted	3 ounces	85	54	245	18	19	7	8	2	0	8	2.2	0	0.40	0.16	3.1	—
	Luncheon meat:																	
114	Boiled ham, sliced	2 ounces	57	59	135	11	10	4	4	1	0	6	1.6	0	0.25	0.09	1.5	—
115	Canned, spiced or unspiced	2 ounces	57	55	165	8	14	5	6	1	1	5	1.2	0	0.18	0.12	1.6	—
	Pork, fresh, cooked:																	
116	Chop, thick, with bone	1 chop, 3.5 ounces	98	42	260	16	21	8	9	2	0	8	2.2	0	0.63	0.18	3.8	—
117	Lean and fat	2.3 ounces	66	42	260	16	21	8	9	2	0	8	2.2	0	0.63	0.18	3.8	—
118	Lean only	1.7 ounces	48	53	130	15	7	2	3	1	0	7	1.9	0	0.54	0.16	3.3	—
	Roast, oven-cooked, no liquid added:																	
119	Lean and fat	3 ounces	85	46	310	21	24	9	10	2	0	9	2.7	0	0.78	0.22	4.7	—
120	Lean only	2.4 ounces	68	55	175	20	10	3	4	1	0	9	2.6	0	0.73	0.21	4.4	—
	Cuts, simmered:																	
121	Lean and fat	3 ounces	85	46	320	20	26	9	11	2	0	8	2.5	0	0.46	0.21	4.1	—
122	Lean only	2.2 ounces	63	60	135	18	6	2	3	1	0	8	2.3	0	0.42	0.19	3.7	—
	Sausage:																	
123	Bologna, slice, 3-in diam. by 1/8 inch	2 slices	26	56	80	3	7	—	—	—	Trace	2	0.5	—	0.04	0.06	0.7	—
124	Braunschweiger, slice 2-in diam. by 1/4 inch	2 slices	20	53	65	3	5	—	—	—	Trace	2	1.2	1,310	0.03	0.29	1.6	—
125	Deviled ham, canned	1 tbsp	13	51	45	2	4	2	2	Trace	0	1	0.3	—	0.02	0.01	0.2	—
126	Frankfurter, heated (8 per lb purchased pkg)	1 frank	56	57	170	7	15	—	—	—	1	3	0.8	—	0.08	0.11	1.4	—
127	Pork links, cooked (16 links per lb raw)	2 links	26	35	125	5	11	4	5	1	Trace	2	0.6	0	0.21	0.09	1.0	—
128	Salami, dry type	1 oz	28	30	130	7	11	—	—	—	Trace	4	1.0	—	0.10	0.07	1.5	—
129	Salami, cooked	1 oz	28	51	90	5	7	—	—	—	Trace	3	0.7	—	0.07	0.07	1.2	—
130	Vienna, canned (7 sausages per 5-oz can)	1 sausage	16	63	40	2	3	—	—	—	Trace	1	0.3	—	0.01	0.02	0.4	—
	Veal, medium fat, cooked, bone removed:																	
131	Cutlet	3 oz	85	60	185	23	9	5	4	Trace	—	9	2.7	—	0.06	0.21	4.6	—
132	Roast	3 oz	85	55	230	23	14	7	6	Trace	0	10	2.9	—	0.11	0.26	6.6	—
	Fish and shellfish:																	
133	Bluefish, baked with table fat	3 oz	85	68	135	22	4	—	—	—	0	25	0.6	40	0.09	0.08	1.6	—
	Clams:																	
134	Raw, meat only	3 oz	85	82	65	11	1	—	—	—	2	59	5.2	90	0.08	0.15	1.1	8
135	Canned, solids and liquid	3 oz	85	86	45	7	1	—	—	—	2	47	3.5	—	0.01	0.09	0.9	—
136	Crabmeat, canned	3 oz	85	77	85	15	2	—	—	—	1	38	0.7	—	0.07	0.07	1.6	—
137	Fish sticks, breaded, cooked, frozen; stick 3 3/4 by 1 by 1/2 inch	10 sticks or 8 oz pkg.	227	66	400	38	20	5	4	10	15	25	0.9	—	0.09	0.16	3.6	—
138	Haddock, breaded, fried	3 oz	85	66	140	17	5	1	3	Trace	5	34	1.0	—	0.03	0.06	2.7	2
139	Ocean perch, breaded, fried	3 oz	85	59	195	16	11	—	—	—	6	28	1.1	—	0.08	0.09	1.5	—
140	Oysters, raw, meat only (13–19 med. selects)	1 cup	240	85	160	20	4	—	—	—	8	226	13.2	740	0.33	0.43	6.0	—

516

Item No.	Food, approximate measure, and weight	Grams	Water (%)	Food energy (cal)	Protein (g)	Fat (g)	Saturated (total) (g)	Oleic (g)	Linoleic (g)	Carbohydrate (g)	Calcium (mg)	Iron (mg)	Vitamin A (I.U.)	Thiamin (mg)	Riboflavin (mg)	Niacin (mg)	Ascorbic acid (mg)
141	Salmon, pink, canned — 3 oz	85	71	120	17	5	1	1	Trace	0	167[4]	0.7	60	0.03	0.16	6.8	—
142	Sardines, Atlantic, canned in oil, drained solids — 3 oz	85	62	175	20	9	—	—	—	0	372	2.5	190	0.02	0.17	4.6	—
143	Shad, baked with table fat and bacon — 3 oz	85	64	170	20	10	—	—	—	0	20	0.5	20	0.11	0.22	7.3	—
144	Shrimp, canned, meat — 3 oz	85	70	100	21	1	—	—	—	1	98	2.6	50	0.01	0.03	1.5	—
145	Swordfish, broiled with butter or margarine — 3 oz	85	65	150	24	5	—	—	—	0	23	1.1	1,750	0.03	0.04	9.3	—
146	Tuna, canned in oil, drained solids — 3 oz	85	61	170	24	7	2	1	1	0	7	1.6	70	0.04	0.10	10.1	—
	Mature Dry Beans and Peas, Nuts, Peanuts; Related Products																
147	Almonds, shelled, whole kernels — 1 cup	142	5	850	26	77	6	52	15	28	332	6.7	0	0.34	1.31	5.0	Trace
	Beans, dry: Common varieties as Great Northern, navy and others: Cooked, drained:																
148	Great Northern — 1 cup	180	69	210	14	1	—	—	—	38	90	4.9	0	0.25	0.13	1.3	0
149	Navy (pea) — 1 cup	190	69	225	15	1	—	—	—	40	95	5.1	0	0.27	0.13	1.3	0
	Canned, solids and liquid: White with—																
150	Frankfurters (sliced) — 1 cup	255	71	365	19	18	—	—	—	32	94	4.8	330	0.18	0.15	3.3	Trace
151	Pork and tomato sauce — 1 cup	255	71	310	16	7	3	3	1	49	138	4.6	330	0.20	0.08	1.5	5
152	Pork and sweet sauce — 1 cup	255	66	385	16	12	4	5	1	54	161	5.9	—	0.15	0.10	1.3	—
153	Red kidney — 1 cup	255	76	230	15	1	—	—	—	42	74	4.6	10	0.13	0.10	1.5	—
154	Lima, cooked, drained — 1 cup	190	64	260	16	1	—	—	—	49	55	5.9	—	0.25	0.11	1.3	—
155	Cashew nuts, roasted — 1 cup	140	5	785	24	64	11	45	4	41	53	5.3	140	0.60	0.35	2.5	—
	Coconut, fresh, meat only:																
156	Pieces, approx. 2 by 2 by 1/2 inch — 1 piece	45	51	155	2	16	14	1	Trace	4	6	0.8	0	0.02	0.01	0.2	1
157	Shredded or grated, firmly packed — 1 cup	130	51	450	5	46	39	3	Trace	12	17	2.2	0	0.07	0.03	0.7	4
158	Cowpeas or blackeye peas, dry, cooked — 1 cup	248	80	190	13	1	—	—	—	34	42	3.2	20	0.41	0.11	1.1	Trace
159	Peanuts, roasted, salted, halves — 1 cup	144	2	840	37	72	16	31	21	27	107	3.0	—	0.46	0.19	24.7	0
160	Peanut butter — 1 tbsp	16	2	95	4	8	2	4	2	3	9	0.3	—	0.02	0.02	2.4	0
161	Peas, split, dry, cooked — 1 cup	250	70	290	20	1	—	—	—	52	28	4.2	100	0.37	0.22	2.2	—
162	Pecans, halves — 1 cup	108	3	740	10	77	5	48	15	16	79	2.6	140	0.93	0.14	1.0	2
163	Walnuts, black or native, chopped — 1 cup	126	3	790	26	75	4	26	36	19	Trace	7.6	380	0.28	0.14	0.9	—
	Vegetables and Vegetable Products																
	Asparagus, green: Cooked, drained:																
164	Spears, 1/2-in. diam. at base — 4 spears	60	94	10	1	Trace	—	—	—	2	13	0.4	540	0.10	0.11	0.8	16
165	Pieces, 1 1/2 to 2-in. lengths — 1 cup	145	94	30	3	Trace	—	—	—	5	30	0.9	1,310	0.23	0.26	2.0	38
166	Canned, solids and liquid — 1 cup	244	94	45	5	1	—	—	—	7	44	4.1	1,240	0.15	0.22	2.0	37

³Outer layer of fat on the cut was removed to within approximately 1/2-inch of the lean. Deposits of fat within the cut were not removed.

⁴If bones are discarded, value will be greatly reduced.

	Food, Approximate Measure, and Weight (in grams)		gm	Water per cent	Food Energy calories	Pro-tein gm	Fat gm	Fatty Acids			Carbo-hy-drate gm	Cal-cium mg	Iron mg	Vita-min A Value I.U.	Thia-mine mg	Ribo-flavin mg	Niacin mg	Ascor-bic Acid mg
								Satu-rated (total) gm	Unsaturated Oleic gm	Lin-oleic gm								
	Beans:																	
167	Lima, immature seeds, cooked, drained	1 cup	170	71	190	13	1	—	—	—	34	80	4.3	480	0.31	0.17	2.2	29
	Snap:																	
	Green:																	
168	Cooked, drained	1 cup	125	92	30	2	Trace	—	—	—	7	63	0.8	680	0.09	0.11	0.6	15
169	Canned, solids and liquid	1 cup	239	94	45	2	Trace	—	—	—	10	81	2.9	690	0.07	0.10	0.7	10
	Yellow or wax:																	
170	Cooked, drained	1 cup	125	93	30	2	Trace	—	—	—	6	63	0.8	290	0.09	0.11	0.6	16
171	Canned, solids and liquid	1 cup	239	94	45	2	1	—	—	—	10	81	2.9	140	0.07	0.10	0.7	12
172	Sprouted mung beans, cooked, drained	1 cup	125	91	35	4	Trace	—	—	—	7	21	1.1	30	0.11	0.13	0.9	8
	Beets:																	
	Cooked, drained, peeled:																	
173	Whole beets, 2-in. diam.	2 beets	100	91	30	1	Trace	—	—	—	7	14	0.5	20	0.03	0.04	0.3	6
174	Diced or sliced	1 cup	170	91	55	2	Trace	—	—	—	12	24	0.9	30	0.05	0.07	0.5	10
175	Canned, solids and liquid	1 cup	246	90	85	2	Trace	—	—	—	19	34	1.5	20	0.02	0.05	0.2	7
176	Beet greens, leaves and stems, cooked, drained	1 cup	145	94	25	3	Trace	—	—	—	5	144	2.8	7,400	0.10	0.22	0.4	22
	Blackeye peas. See Cowpeas																	
	Broccoli, cooked, drained:																	
177	Whole stalks, medium size	1 stalk	180	91	45	6	1	—	—	—	8	158	1.4	4,500	0.16	0.36	1.4	162
178	Stalks cut into 1/2-in pieces	1 cup	155	91	40	5	1	—	—	—	7	136	1.2	3,880	0.14	0.31	1.2	140
179	Chopped, yield from 10-oz frozen pkg	1 3/8 cups	250	92	65	7	1	—	—	—	12	135	1.8	6,500	0.15	0.30	1.3	143
180	Brussels sprouts, 7–8 sprouts (1 1/4 to 1 1/2 in diam.) per cup, cooked	1 cup	155	88	55	7	1	—	—	—	10	50	1.7	810	0.12	0.22	1.2	135
	Cabbage:																	
	Common varieties:																	
	Raw:																	
181	Coarsely shredded or sliced	1 cup	70	92	15	1	Trace	—	—	—	4	34	0.3	90	0.04	0.04	0.2	33
182	Finely shredded or chopped	1 cup	90	92	20	1	Trace	—	—	—	5	44	0.4	120	0.05	0.05	0.3	42
183	Cooked	1 cup	145	94	30	2	Trace	—	—	—	6	64	0.4	190	0.06	0.06	0.4	48
184	Red, raw, coarsely shredded	1 cup	70	90	20	1	Trace	—	—	—	5	29	0.6	30	0.06	0.04	0.3	43
185	Savoy, raw, coarsely shredded	1 cup	70	92	15	2	Trace	—	—	—	3	47	0.6	140	0.04	0.06	0.2	39
186	Cabbage, celery or Chinese raw, cut in 1-in pieces	1 cup	75	95	10	1	Trace	—	—	—	2	32	0.5	110	0.04	0.03	0.5	19
187	Cabbage, spoon (or pakchoy), cooked	1 cup	170	95	25	2	Trace	—	—	—	4	252	1.0	5,270	0.07	0.14	1.2	26
	Carrots:																	
	Raw:																	
188	Whole, 5 1/2 by 1 inch, (25 thin strips)	1 carrot	50	88	20	1	Trace	—	—	—	5	18	0.4	5,500	0.03	0.03	0.3	4

No.	Food	Measure	Weight (g)	Water (%)	Food energy	Protein	Fat				Carbohydrate	Calcium	Iron	Vit. A				Ascorbic acid
189	Grated	1 cup	110	88	45	1	Trace	—	—	—	11	41	0.8	12,100	0.06	0.06	0.7	9
190	Cooked, diced	1 cup	145	91	45	1	Trace	—	—	—	10	48	0.9	15,220	0.08	0.07	0.7	9
191	Canned, strained or chopped (baby food)	1 ounce	28	92	10	Trace	Trace	—	—	—	2	7	0.1	3,690	0.01	0.01	0.1	1
192	Cauliflower, cooked, flowerbuds	1 cup	120	93	25	3	Trace	—	—	—	5	25	0.8	70	0.11	0.10	0.7	66
	Celery, raw:																	
193	Stalk, large outer, 8 by about 1 1/2 inches, at root end	1 stalk	40	94	5	Trace	Trace	—	—	—	2	16	0.1	100	0.01	0.01	0.1	4
194	Pieces, diced	1 cup	100	94	15	1	Trace	—	—	—	4	39	0.3	240	0.03	0.03	0.3	9
195	Collards, cooked	1 cup	190	91	55	5	1	—	—	—	9	289	1.1	10,260	0.27	0.37	2.4	87
	Corn sweet:																	
196	Cooked, ear 5 by 1 3/4 inches[5]	1 ear	140	74	70	3	1	—	—	—	16	2	0.5	[6]310	0.09	0.08	1.0	7
197	Canned, solids and liquid	1 cup	256	81	170	5	2	—	—	—	40	10	1.0	[6]690	0.07	0.12	2.3	13
198	Cowpeas, cooked immature seeds	1 cup	160	72	175	13	1	—	—	—	29	38	3.4	560	0.49	0.18	2.3	28
	Cucumbers, 10-ounce; 7 1/2 by about 2 inches:																	
199	Raw, pared	1 cucumber	207	96	30	1	Trace	—	—	—	7	35	0.6	Trace	0.07	0.09	0.4	23
200	Raw, pared, center slice 1/8-inch thick	6 slices	50	96	5	Trace	Trace	—	—	—	2	8	0.2	Trace	0.02	0.02	0.1	6
201	Dandelion greens, cooked	1 cup	180	90	60	4	1	—	—	—	12	252	3.2	21,060	0.24	0.29	—	32
202	Endive, curly (including escarole)	2 ounces	57	93	10	1	Trace	—	—	—	2	46	1.0	1,870	0.04	0.08	0.3	6
203	Kale, leaves including stems, cooked	1 cup	110	91	30	4	1	—	—	—	4	147	1.3	8,140	—	—	—	68
	Lettuce, raw:																	
204	Butterhead, as Boston types; head, 4-inch diameter	1 head	220	95	30	3	Trace	—	—	—	6	77	4.4	2,130	0.14	0.13	0.6	18
205	Crisphead, as Iceberg; head, 4 3/4 inch diameter	1 head	454	96	60	4	Trace	—	—	—	13	91	2.3	1,500	0.29	0.27	1.3	29
206	Looseleaf, or bunching varieties, leaves	2 large	50	94	10	1	Trace	—	—	—	2	34	0.7	950	0.03	0.04	0.2	9
207	Mushrooms, canned, solids and liquid	1 cup	244	93	40	5	Trace	—	—	—	6	15	1.2	Trace	0.04	0.60	4.8	4
208	Mustard greens, cooked	1 cup	140	93	35	3	1	—	—	—	6	193	2.5	8,120	0.11	0.19	0.9	68
209	Okra, cooked, pod 3 by 5/8 inch	8 pods	85	91	25	2	Trace	—	—	—	5	78	0.4	420	0.11	0.15	0.8	17
	Onions: Mature:																	
210	Raw, onion 2 1/2-inch diameter	1 onion	110	89	40	2	Trace	—	—	—	10	30	0.6	40	0.04	0.04	0.2	11
211	Cooked	1 cup	210	92	60	3	Trace	—	—	—	14	50	0.8	80	0.06	0.06	0.4	14
212	Young green, small, without tops	6 onions	50	88	20	1	Trace	—	—	—	5	20	0.3	Trace	0.02	0.02	0.2	12
213	Parsley, raw, chopped	1 tablespoon	4	85	Trace	Trace	Trace	—	—	—	Trace	8	0.2	340	Trace	0.01	Trace	7
214	Parsnips, cooked	1 cup	155	82	100	2	1	—	—	—	23	70	0.9	50	0.11	0.12	0.2	16
	Peas, green:																	
215	Cooked	1 cup	160	82	115	9	1	—	—	—	19	37	2.9	860	0.44	0.17	3.7	33
216	Canned, solids and liquid	1 cup	249	83	165	9	1	—	—	—	31	50	4.2	1,120	0.23	0.13	2.2	22
217	Canned, strained (baby food)	1 ounce	28	86	15	1	Trace	—	—	—	3	3	0.4	140	0.02	0.02	0.4	3

[5]Measure and weight apply to entire vegetable or fruit including parts not usually eaten.
[6]Based on yellow varieties; white varieties contain only a trace of cryptoxanthin and carotenes, the pigments in corn that have biologic activity.

No.	Food, Approximate Measure, and Weight (in grams)		Weight gm	Water per cent	Food Energy calories	Protein gm	Fat gm	Fatty Acids Saturated (total) gm	Unsaturated Oleic gm	Unsaturated Linoleic gm	Carbohydrate gm	Calcium mg	Iron mg	Vitamin A Value I.U.	Thiamine mg	Riboflavin mg	Niacin mg	Ascorbic Acid mg
218	Peppers, hot, red, without seeds, dried (ground chili powder, added seasonings)	1 tablespoon	15	8	50	2	2	—	—	—	8	40	2.3	9,750	0.03	0.17	1.3	2
	Peppers, sweet:																	
	Raw, about 5 per pound:																	
219	Green pod without stem and seeds	1 pod	74	93	15	1	Trace	—	—	—	4	7	0.5	310	0.06	0.06	0.4	94
220	Cooked, boiled, drained	1 pod	73	95	15	1	Trace	—	—	—	3	7	0.4	310	0.05	0.05	0.4	70
	Potatoes, medium (about 3 per pound raw):																	
221	Baked, peeled after baking	1 potato	99	75	90	3	Trace	—	—	—	21	9	0.7	Trace	0.10	0.04	1.7	20
	Boiled:																	
222	Peeled after boiling	1 potato	136	80	105	3	Trace	—	—	—	23	10	0.8	Trace	0.13	0.05	2.0	22
223	Peeled before boiling	1 potato	122	83	80	2	Trace	—	—	—	18	7	0.6	Trace	0.11	0.04	1.4	20
	French-fried, piece 2 by 1/2 by 1/2 inch:																	
224	Cooked in deep fat	10 pieces	57	45	155	2	7	2	2	4	20	9	0.7	Trace	0.07	0.04	1.8	12
225	Frozen, heated	10 pieces	57	53	125	2	5	1	1	2	19	5	1.0	Trace	0.08	0.01	1.5	12
	Mashed:																	
226	Milk added	1 cup	195	83	125	4	1	—	—	—	25	47	0.8	50	0.16	0.10	2.0	19
227	Milk and butter added	1 cup	195	80	185	4	8	4	3	Trace	24	47	0.8	330	0.16	0.10	1.9	18
228	Potato chips, medium, 2-inch diameter	10 chips	20	2	115	1	8	2	2	4	10	8	0.4	Trace	0.04	0.01	1.0	3
229	Pumpkin, canned	1 cup	228	90	75	2	1	—	—	—	18	57	0.9	14,590	0.07	0.12	1.3	12
230	Radishes, raw, small, without tops	4 radishes	40	94	5	Trace	Trace	—	—	—	1	12	0.4	Trace	0.01	0.01	0.1	10
231	Sauerkraut, canned, solids and liquid	1 cup	235	93	45	2	Trace	—	—	—	9	85	1.2	120	0.07	0.09	0.4	33
	Spinach:																	
232	Cooked	1 cup	180	92	40	5	1	—	—	—	6	167	4.0	14,580	0.13	0.25	1.0	50
233	Canned, drained solids	1 cup	180	91	45	5	1	—	—	—	6	212	4.7	14,400	0.03	0.21	0.6	24
	Squash:																	
	Cooked:																	
234	Summer, diced	1 cup	210	96	30	2	Trace	—	—	—	7	52	0.8	820	0.10	0.16	1.6	21
235	Winter, baked, mashed	1 cup	205	81	130	4	1	—	—	—	32	57	1.6	8,610	0.10	0.27	1.4	27
	Sweetpotatoes: Cooked, medium, 5 by 2 inches, weight raw about 6 ounces:																	
236	Baked, peeled after baking	1 sweetpotato	110	64	155	2	1	—	—	—	36	44	1.0	8,910	0.10	0.07	0.7	24
237	Boiled, peeled after boiling	1 sweetpotato	147	71	170	2	1	—	—	—	39	47	1.0	11,610	0.13	0.09	0.9	25
238	Candied, 3 1/2 by 2 1/4 inches	1 sweetpotato	175	60	295	2	6	2	3	1	60	65	1.6	11,030	0.10	0.08	0.8	17
239	Canned, vacuum or solid pack	1 cup	218	72	235	4	Trace	—	—	—	54	54	1.7	17,000	0.10	0.10	1.4	30
	Tomatoes:																	
240	Raw, approx. 3-in diam. 2 1/8 in high; wt. 7 oz	1 tomato	200	94	40	2	Trace	—	—	—	9	24	0.9	1,640	0.11	0.07	1.3	742
241	Canned, solids and liquid	1 cup	241	94	50	2	1	—	—	—	10	14	1.2	2,170	0.12	0.07	1.7	41

Fruits and Fruit Products

No.	Food, approximate measure, and weight	Measure	Grams	Water (%)	Food energy (Cal.)	Protein (g)	Fat (g)	Saturated (g)	Oleic (g)	Linoleic (g)	Carbohydrate (g)	Calcium (mg)	Iron (mg)	Vitamin A (I.U.)	Thiamine (mg)	Riboflavin (mg)	Niacin (mg)	Ascorbic acid (mg)
242	Tomato catsup: Cup	1 cup	273	69	290	6	1	—	—	—	69	60	2.2	3,820	0.25	0.19	4.4	41
243	Tablespoon	1 tbsp.	15	69	15	Trace	Trace	—	—	—	4	3	0.1	210	0.01	0.01	0.2	2
244	Tomato juice, canned: Cup	1 cup	243	94	45	2	Trace	—	—	—	10	17	2.2	1,940	0.12	0.07	1.9	39
245	Glass (6 fl oz)	1 glass	182	94	35	2	Trace	—	—	—	8	13	1.6	1,460	0.09	0.05	1.5	29
246	Turnips, cooked, diced	1 cup	155	94	35	1	Trace	—	—	—	8	54	0.6	Trace	0.06	0.08	0.5	34
247	Turnip greens, cooked	1 cup	145	94	30	3	Trace	—	—	—	5	252	1.5	8,270	0.15	0.33	0.7	68
248	Apples, raw (about 3 per lb)[5]	1 apple	150	85	70	Trace	Trace	—	—	—	18	8	0.4	50	0.04	0.02	0.1	3
249	Apple juice, bottled or canned	1 cup	248	88	120	Trace	Trace	—	—	—	30	15	1.5	—	0.02	0.05	0.2	2
250	Applesauce, canned: Sweetened	1 cup	255	76	230	1	Trace	—	—	—	61	10	1.3	100	0.05	0.03	0.1	3
251	Unsweetened or artificially sweetened	1 cup	244	88	100	1	Trace	—	—	—	26	10	1.2	100	0.05	0.02	0.1	2
252	Apricots: Raw (about 12 per lb)[5]	3 apricots	114	85	55	1	Trace	—	—	—	14	18	0.5	2,890	0.03	0.04	0.7	11
253	Canned in heavy syrup	1 cup	259	77	220	2	Trace	—	—	—	57	28	0.8	4,510	0.05	0.06	0.9	10
254	Dried, uncooked (40 halves per cup)	1 cup	150	25	390	8	1	—	—	—	100	100	8.2	16,350	0.02	0.23	4.9	19
255	Cooked, unsweetened, fruit and liquid	1 cup	285	76	240	5	1	—	—	—	62	63	5.1	8,550	0.01	0.13	2.8	8
256	Apricot nectar, canned	1 cup	251	85	140	1	Trace	—	—	—	37	23	0.5	2,380	0.03	0.03	0.5	8[8]
257	Avocados, whole fruit, raw:[5] California (mid- and late-winter; diam. 3 1/8 in)	1 avocado	284	74	370	5	37	7	17	5	13	22	1.3	630	0.24	0.43	3.5	30
258	Florida (late summer, fall; diam. 3 5/8 in)	1 avocado	454	78	390	4	33	7	15	4	27	30	1.8	880	0.33	0.61	4.9	43
259	Bananas, raw, medium size[5]	1 banana	175	76	100	1	Trace	—	—	—	26	10	0.8	230	0.06	0.07	0.8	12
260	Banana flakes	1 cup	100	3	340	4	1	—	—	—	89	32	2.8	760	0.18	0.24	2.8	7
261	Blackberries, raw	1 cup	144	84	85	2	1	—	—	—	19	46	1.3	290	0.05	0.06	0.5	30
262	Blueberries, raw	1 cup	140	83	85	1	1	—	—	—	21	21	1.4	140	0.04	0.08	0.6	20
263	Cantaloups, raw; medium; 5-inch diameter about 1 2/3 pounds[5]	1/2 melon	385	91	60	1	Trace	—	—	—	14	27	0.8	9,240[9]	0.08	0.06	1.2	63
264	Cherries, canned, red, sour, pitted, water pack	1 cup	244	88	105	2	Trace	—	—	—	26	37	0.7	1,660	0.07	0.05	0.5	12
265	Cranberry juice cocktail, canned	1 cup	250	83	165	Trace	Trace	—	—	—	42	13	0.8	Trace	0.03	0.03	0.1	40[10]
266	Cranberry sauce, sweetened, canned, strained	1 cup	277	62	405	Trace	1	—	—	—	104	17	0.6	60	0.03	0.03	0.1	6
267	Dates, pitted, cut	1 cup	178	22	490	4	1	—	—	—	130	105	5.3	90	0.16	0.17	3.9	0
268	Figs, dried, large, 2 by 1 in	1 fig	21	23	60	1	Trace	—	—	—	15	26	0.6	20	0.02	0.02	0.1	0
269	Fruit cocktail, canned, in heavy syrup	1 cup	256	80	195	1	Trace	—	—	—	50	23	1.0	360	0.05	0.03	1.3	5
270	Grapefruit: Raw, medium, 3 3/4-in diam.[5] White	1/2 grapefruit	241	89	45	1	Trace	—	—	—	12	19	0.5	10	0.05	0.02	0.2	44
271	Pink or red	1/2 grapefruit	241	89	50	1	Trace	—	—	—	13	20	0.5	540	0.05	0.02	0.2	44
272	Canned, syrup pack	1 cup	254	81	180	2	Trace	—	—	—	45	33	0.8	30	0.08	0.05	0.5	76

[5] Measure and weight apply to entire vegetable or fruit including parts not usually eaten.

[7] Year-round average. Samples marketed from November through May, average 20 milligrams per 200-gram tomato; from June through October, around 52 milligrams.

[8] This is the amount from the fruit. Additional ascorbic acid may be added by the manufacturer. Refer to the label for this information.

[9] Value for varieties with orange-colored flesh; value for varieties with green flesh would be about 540 I.U.

[10] Value listed is based on products with label stating 30 mg per 6-fl-oz serving.

	Food, Approximate Measure, and Weight (in grams)		gm	Water per cent	Food Energy calories	Protein gm	Fat gm	Fatty Acids			Carbohydrate gm	Calcium mg	Iron mg	Vitamin A Value I.U.	Thiamine mg	Riboflavin mg	Niacin mg	Ascorbic Acid mg
								Saturated (total) gm	Unsaturated Oleic gm	Linoleic gm								
	Grapefruit juice:																	
273	Fresh	1 cup	246	90	95	1	Trace	—	—	—	23	22	0.5	(11)	0.09	0.04	0.4	92
	Canned, white:																	
274	Unsweetened	1 cup	247	89	100	1	Trace	—	—	—	24	20	1.0	20	0.07	0.04	0.4	84
275	Sweetened	1 cup	250	86	130	1	Trace	—	—	—	32	20	1.0	20	0.07	0.04	0.4	78
	Frozen, concentrate, unsweetened:																	
276	Undiluted, can, 6 fluid ounces	1 can	207	62	300	4	1	—	—	—	72	70	0.8	60	0.29	0.12	1.4	286
277	Diluted with 3 parts water, by volume	1 cup	247	89	100	1	Trace	—	—	—	24	25	0.2	20	0.10	0.04	0.5	96
278	Dehydrated crystals	4 oz	113	1	410	6	1	—	—	—	102	100	1.2	80	0.40	0.20	2.0	396
279	Prepared with water (1 pound yields about 1 gallon)	1 cup	247	90	100	1	Trace	—	—	—	24	22	0.2	20	0.10	0.05	0.5	91
	Grapes, raw:[5]																	
280	American type (slip skin)	1 cup	153	82	65	1	1	—	—	—	15	15	0.4	100	0.05	0.03	0.2	3
281	European type (adherent skin)	1 cup	160	81	95	1	Trace	—	—	—	25	17	0.6	140	0.07	0.04	0.4	6
	Grapejuice:																	
282	Canned or bottled	1 cup	253	83	165	1	Trace	—	—	—	42	28	0.8	—	0.10	0.05	0.5	Trace
	Frozen concentrate, sweetened:																	
283	Undiluted, can, 6 fluid ounces	1 can	216	53	395	1	Trace	—	—	—	100	22	0.9	40	0.13	0.22	1.5	(12)
284	Diluted with 3 parts water, by volume	1 cup	250	86	135	1	Trace	—	—	—	33	8	0.3	10	0.05	0.08	0.5	(12)
285	Grapejuice drink, canned	1 cup	250	86	135	Trace	Trace	—	—	—	35	8	0.3	—	0.03	0.03	0.3	(12)
286	Lemons, raw, 2 1/8-in diam., size 165.[5] Used for juice	1 lemon	110	90	20	1	Trace	—	—	—	6	19	0.4	10	0.03	0.01	0.1	39
287	Lemon juice, raw	1 cup	244	91	60	1	Trace	—	—	—	20	17	0.5	50	0.07	0.02	0.2	112
	Lemonade concentrate:																	
288	Frozen, 6 fl oz per can	1 can	219	48	430	Trace	Trace	—	—	—	112	9	0.4	40	0.04	0.07	0.7	66
289	Diluted with 4 1/3 parts water, by volume	1 cup	248	88	110	Trace	Trace	—	—	—	28	2	Trace	Trace	Trace	0.02	0.2	17
	Lime juice:																	
290	Fresh	1 cup	246	90	65	1	Trace	—	—	—	22	22	0.5	20	0.05	0.02	0.2	79
291	Canned, unsweetened	1 cup	246	90	65	1	Trace	—	—	—	22	22	0.5	20	0.05	0.02	0.2	52
	Limeade concentrate, frozen:																	
292	Undiluted, can, 6 fluid ounces	1 can	218	50	410	Trace	Trace	—	—	—	108	11	0.2	Trace	0.02	0.02	0.2	26
293	Diluted with 4 1/3 parts water, by volume	1 cup	247	90	100	Trace	Trace	—	—	—	27	2	Trace	Trace	Trace	Trace	Trace	5
294	Oranges, raw, 2 5/8-in diam., all commercial varieties[5]	1 orange	180	86	65	1	Trace	—	—	—	16	54	0.5	260	0.13	0.05	0.5	66
295	Orange juice, fresh, all varieties	1 cup	248	88	110	2	Trace	—	—	—	26	27	0.5	500	0.22	0.07	1.0	124
296	Canned, unsweetened	1 cup	249	87	120	2	Trace	—	—	—	28	25	1.0	500	0.17	0.05	0.7	100
	Frozen concentrate:																	
297	Undiluted, can, 6 fluid ounces	1 can	213	55	360	5	Trace	—	—	—	87	75	0.9	1,620	0.68	0.11	2.8	360

Item	Food, approximate measure	Measure	Grams	Water (%)	Food energy (cal)	Protein (g)	Fat (g)	Saturated fatty acids (g)	Oleic (g)	Linoleic (g)	Carbohydrate (g)	Calcium (mg)	Iron (mg)	Vitamin A (I.U.)	Thiamine (mg)	Riboflavin (mg)	Niacin (mg)	Ascorbic acid (mg)
298	Diluted with 3 parts water, by volume	1 cup	249	87	120	2	Trace	—	—	—	29	25	0.2	550	0.22	0.02	1.0	120
299	Dehydrated crystals	4 oz	113	1	430	6	2	—	—	—	100	95	1.9	1,900	0.76	0.24	3.3	408
300	Prepared with water (1 pound yields about 1 gallon)	1 cup	248	88	115	2	1	—	—	—	27	25	0.5	500	0.20	0.07	1.0	109
301	Orange-apricot juice drink	1 cup	249	87	125	1	Trace	—	—	—	32	12	0.2	1,440	0.05	0.02	0.5	[10]40
	Orange and grapefruit juice: Frozen concentrate:																	
302	Undiluted, can, 6 fluid ounces	1 can	210	59	330	4	1	—	—	—	78	61	0.8	800	0.48	0.06	2.3	302
303	Diluted with 3 parts water, by volume	1 cup	248	88	110	1	Trace	—	—	—	26	20	0.2	270	0.16	0.02	0.8	102
304	Papayas, raw, 1/2-inch cubes	1 cup	182	89	70	1	Trace	—	—	—	18	36	0.5	3,190	0.07	0.08	0.5	102
	Peaches: Raw:																	
305	Whole, medium, 2-inch diameter, about 4 per pound[5]	1 peach	114	89	35	1	Trace	—	—	—	10	9	0.5	[13]1,320	0.02	0.05	1.0	7
306	Sliced	1 cup	168	89	65	1	Trace	—	—	—	16	15	0.8	[13]2,230	0.03	0.08	1.6	12
	Canned, yellow-fleshed, solids and liquid: Syrup pack, heavy:																	
307	Halves or slices	1 cup	257	79	200	1	Trace	—	—	—	52	10	0.8	1,100	0.02	0.06	1.4	7
308	Water pack	1 cup	245	91	75	1	Trace	—	—	—	20	10	0.7	1,100	0.02	0.06	1.4	7
309	Dried, uncooked	1 cup	160	25	420	5	1	—	—	—	109	77	9.6	6,240	0.02	0.31	8.5	28
310	Cooked, unsweetened, 10–12 halves and juice	1 cup	270	77	220	3	1	—	—	—	58	41	5.1	3,290	0.01	0.15	4.2	6
	Frozen:																	
311	Carton, 12 ounces, not thawed	1 carton	340	76	300	1	Trace	—	—	—	77	14	1.7	2,210	0.03	0.14	2.4	[14]135
	Pears:																	
312	Raw, 3 by 2 1/2-inch diameter[5]	1 pear	182	83	100	1	1	—	—	—	25	13	0.5	30	0.04	0.07	0.2	7
	Canned, solids, and liquid: Syrup pack, heavy:																	
313	Halves or slices	1 cup	255	80	195	1	1	—	—	—	50	13	0.5	Trace	0.03	0.05	0.3	4
	Pineapple:																	
314	Raw, diced	1 cup	140	85	75	1	Trace	—	—	—	19	24	0.7	100	0.12	0.04	0.3	24
	Canned, heavy syrup pack, solids and liquids:																	
315	Crushed	1 cup	260	80	195	1	Trace	—	—	—	50	29	0.8	120	0.20	0.06	0.5	17
316	Sliced, slices and juice	2 small or 1 large	122	80	90	Trace	Trace	—	—	—	24	13	0.4	50	0.09	0.03	0.2	8
317	Pineapple juice, canned	1 cup	249	86	135	1	Trace	—	—	—	34	37	0.7	120	0.12	0.04	0.5	[8]22
	Plums, all except prunes:																	
318	Raw, 2-inch diameter, about 2 ounces[5]	1 plum	60	87	25	Trace	Trace	—	—	—	7	7	0.3	140	0.02	0.02	0.3	3
	Canned, syrup pack (Italian prunes):																	
319	Plums (with pits) and juice[5]	1 cup	256	77	205	1	Trace	—	—	—	53	22	2.2	2,970	0.05	0.05	0.9	4

[5] Measure and weight apply to entire vegetable or fruit including parts not usually eaten.

[8] This is the amount from the fruit. Additional ascorbic acid may be added by the manufacturer. Refer to the label for this information.

[10] Value listed is based on product with label stating 30 milligrams per 6-fl-oz serving.

[11] For white-fleshed varieties value is about 20 I.U. per cup; for red-fleshed varieties, 1,080 I.U. per cup.

[12] Present only if added by the manufacturer. Refer to the label for this information.

[13] Based on yellow-fleshed varieties; for white-fleshed varieties value is about 50 I.U. per 114-gm peach and 80 I.U. per cup of sliced peaches.

[14] This value includes ascorbic acid added by manufacturer.

| | | | | | | Fatty Acids | | | | | | | | | | |
| | | | | | | | Unsaturated | | | | | | | | | |
Food, Approximate Measure, and Weight (in grams)	gm	Water per cent	Food Energy calories	Pro-tein gm	Fat gm	Satu-rated (total) gm	Oleic gm	Lin-oleic gm	Carbo-hy-drate gm	Cal-cium mg	Iron mg	Vita-min A Value I.U.	Thia-mine mg	Ribo-flavin mg	Niacin mg	Ascor-bic Acid mg
Prunes, dried, "softenized," medium:																
320 Uncooked[5]	4 prunes	32	28	70	1	Trace	—	—	18	14	1.1	440	0.02	0.04	0.4	1
321 Cooked, unsweetened, 17–18 prunes and 1/3 cup liquid[5]	1 cup	270	66	295	2	1	—	—	78	60	4.5	1,860	0.08	0.18	1.7	2
322 Prune juice, canned or bottled	1 cup	256	80	200	1	Trace	—	—	49	36	10.5	—	0.03	0.03	1.0	85
Raisins, seedless:																
323 Packaged, 1/2 oz or 1 1/2 tbsp per pkg.	1 pkg	14	18	40	Trace	Trace	—	—	11	9	0.5	Trace	0.02	0.01	0.1	Trace
324 Cup, pressed down	1 cup	165	18	480	4	Trace	—	—	128	102	5.8	30	0.18	0.13	0.8	2
Raspberries, red:																
325 Raw	1 cup	123	84	70	1	1	—	—	17	27	1.1	160	0.04	0.11	1.1	31
326 Frozen, 10-ounce carton, not thawed	1 carton	284	74	275	2	1	—	—	70	37	1.7	200	0.06	0.17	1.7	59
327 Rhubarb, cooked, sugar added	1 cup	272	63	385	1	Trace	—	—	98	212	1.6	220	0.06	0.15	0.7	17
Strawberries:																
328 Raw, capped	1 cup	149	90	55	1	1	—	—	13	31	1.5	90	0.04	0.10	1.0	88
329 Frozen, 10-ounce carton, not thawed	1 carton	284	71	310	1	1	—	—	79	40	2.0	90	0.06	0.17	1.5	150
330 Tangerines, raw, medium, 2 3/8-in diam., size 176[5]	1 tangerine	116	87	40	1	Trace	—	—	10	34	0.3	360	0.05	0.02	0.1	27
331 Tangerine juice, canned, sweetened	1 cup	249	87	125	1	1	—	—	30	45	0.5	1,050	0.15	0.05	0.2	55
332 Watermelon, raw, wedge, 4 by 8 inches (1/16 of 10 by 16-inch melon, about 2 pounds with rind)[5]	1 wedge	925	93	115	2	1	—	—	27	30	2.1	2,510	0.13	0.13	0.7	30
Grain Products																
Bagel, 3-in diam.:																
333 Egg	1 bagel	55	32	165	6	2	—	—	28	9	1.2	30	0.14	0.10	1.2	0
334 Water	1 bagel	55	29	165	6	2	—	—	30	8	1.2	0	0.15	0.11	1.4	0
335 Barley, pearled, light, uncooked	1 cup	200	11	700	16	2	Trace	1	1	158	32	4.0	0	0.24	0.10	6.2	0
336 Biscuits, baking powder from home recipe with enriched flour, 2-in diam.	1 biscuit	28	27	105	2	5	1	2	1	13	34	0.4	Trace	0.06	0.06	0.1	Trace
337 Biscuits, baking powder from mix, 2-in diam.	1 biscuit	28	28	90	2	3	1	1	1	15	19	0.6	Trace	0.08	0.07	0.6	Trace
338 Bran flakes (40% bran), added thiamine and iron	1 cup	35	3	105	4	1	—	—	28	25	12.3	0	0.14	0.06	2.2	0
339 Bran flakes with raisins, added thiamine and iron	1 cup	50	7	145	4	1	—	—	40	28	13.5	Trace	0.16	0.07	2.7	0
Breads:																
340 Boston brown bread, slice 3 by 3/4 in	1 slice	48	45	100	3	1	—	—	22	43	0.9	0	0.05	0.03	0.6	0
Cracked-wheat bread:																
341 Loaf, 1 lb	1 loaf	454	35	1,190	40	10	2	5	2	236	399	5.0	Trace	0.53	0.41	5.9	Trace
342 Slice, 18 slices per loaf	1 slice	25	35	65	2	1	—	—	13	22	0.3	Trace	0.03	0.02	0.3	Trace

No.	Food, approximate measure	Measure	Weight (g)	Water (%)	Food energy (cal)	Protein (g)	Fat (g)	Saturated (total) (g)	Unsaturated Oleic (g)	Unsaturated Linoleic (g)	Carbo-hydrate (g)	Calcium (mg)	Iron (mg)	Vitamin A (IU)	Thiamine (mg)	Riboflavin (mg)	Niacin (mg)	Ascorbic acid (mg)
	French or Vienna bread:																	
343	Enriched, 1-lb loaf	1 loaf	454	31	1,315	41	14	3	8	2	251	195	10.0	Trace	1.27	1.00	11.3	Trace
344	Unenriched, 1-lb loaf	1 loaf	454	31	1,315	41	14	3	8	2	251	195	3.2	Trace	0.36	0.36	3.6	Trace
	Italian bread:																	
345	Enriched, 1-lb loaf	1 loaf	454	32	1,250	41	4	Trace	1	2	256	77	10.0	0	1.32	0.91	11.8	0
346	Unenriched, 1-lb loaf	1 loaf	454	32	1,250	41	4	Trace	1	2	256	77	3.2	0	0.41	0.27	3.6	0
	Raisin bread:																	
347	Loaf, 1 lb	1 loaf	454	35	1,190	30	13	3	8	2	243	322	5.9	Trace	0.23	0.41	3.2	Trace
348	Slice, 18 slices per loaf	1 slice	25	35	65	2	1	—	—	—	13	18	0.3	Trace	0.01	0.02	0.2	Trace
	Rye bread:																	
	American, light (1/3 rye, 2/3 wheat):																	
349	Loaf, 1 lb	1 loaf	454	36	1,100	41	5	—	—	—	236	340	7.3	0	0.82	0.32	6.4	0
350	Slice, 18 slices per loaf	1 slice	25	36	60	2	Trace	—	—	—	13	19	0.4	0	0.05	0.02	0.4	0
351	Pumpernickel, loaf, 1 lb	1 loaf	454	34	1,115	41	5	—	—	—	241	381	10.9	0	1.04	0.64	5.4	0
	White bread, enriched:[15]																	
	Soft-crumb type																	
352	Loaf, 1 lb	1 loaf	454	36	1,225	39	15	3	8	2	229	381	11.3	Trace	1.13	0.95	10.9	Trace
353	Slice, 18 slices per loaf	1 slice	25	36	70	2	1	—	—	—	13	21	0.6	Trace	0.06	0.05	0.6	Trace
354	Slice, toasted	1 slice	22	25	70	2	1	—	—	—	13	21	0.6	Trace	0.05	0.05	0.6	Trace
355	Slice, 22 slices per loaf	1 slice	20	36	55	2	1	—	—	—	10	17	0.5	Trace	0.05	0.04	0.5	Trace
356	Slice, toasted	1 slice	17	25	55	2	1	—	—	—	10	17	0.5	Trace	0.04	0.04	0.5	Trace
357	Loaf, 1 1/2 lb	1 loaf	680	36	1,835	59	22	5	12	3	343	571	17.0	Trace	1.70	1.43	16.3	Trace
358	Slice, 24 slices per loaf	1 slice	28	36	75	2	1	—	—	—	14	24	0.7	Trace	0.07	0.06	0.7	Trace
359	Slice, toasted	1 slice	24	25	75	2	1	—	—	—	14	24	0.7	Trace	0.07	0.06	0.7	Trace
360	Slice, 28 slices per loaf	1 slice	24	36	65	2	1	—	—	—	12	20	0.6	Trace	0.06	0.05	0.6	Trace
361	Slice, toasted	1 slice	21	25	65	2	1	—	—	—	12	20	0.6	Trace	0.06	0.05	0.6	Trace
	Firm-crumb type:																	
362	Loaf, 1 lb	1 loaf	454	35	1,245	41	17	4	10	2	228	435	11.3	Trace	1.22	0.91	10.9	Trace
363	Slice, 20 slices per loaf	1 slice	23	35	65	2	1	—	—	—	12	22	0.6	Trace	0.06	0.05	0.6	Trace
364	Slice, toasted	1 slice	20	24	65	2	1	—	—	—	12	22	0.6	Trace	0.06	0.05	0.6	Trace
365	Loaf, 2 lb	1 loaf	907	35	2,495	82	34	8	20	4	455	871	22.7	Trace	2.45	1.81	21.8	Trace
366	Slice, 34 slices per loaf	1 slice	27	35	75	2	1	—	—	—	14	26	0.7	Trace	0.07	0.05	0.6	Trace
367	Slice, toasted	1 slice	23	35	75	2	1	—	—	—	14	26	0.7	Trace	0.07	0.05	0.6	Trace
	Whole-wheat bread, soft-crumb type:																	
368	Loaf, 1 lb	1 loaf	454	36	1,095	41	12	2	6	2	224	381	13.6	Trace	1.36	0.45	12.7	Trace
369	Slice, 16 slices per loaf	1 slice	28	36	65	3	1	—	—	—	14	24	0.8	Trace	0.09	0.03	0.8	Trace
370	Slice, toasted	1 slice	24	24	65	3	1	—	—	—	14	24	0.8	Trace	0.09	0.03	0.8	Trace
	Whole-wheat bread, firm-crumb type:																	
371	Loaf, 1 lb	1 loaf	454	36	1,100	48	14	3	6	3	216	449	13.6	Trace	1.18	0.54	12.7	Trace
372	Slice, 18 slices per loaf	1 slice	25	36	60	3	1	—	—	—	12	25	0.8	Trace	0.06	0.03	0.7	Trace
373	Slice, toasted	1 slice	21	24	60	3	1	—	—	—	12	25	0.8	Trace	0.06	0.03	0.7	Trace
374	Breadcrumbs, dry, grated	1 cup	100	6	390	13	5	1	2	1	73	122	3.6	Trace	0.22	0.30	3.5	Trace
375	Buckwheat flour, light, sifted	1 cup	98	12	340	6	1	—	—	—	78	11	1.0	0	0.08	0.04	0.4	0
376	Bulgur, canned, seasoned	1 cup	135	56	245	8	4	—	—	—	44	27	1.9	0	0.08	0.05	4.1	0
	Cakes made from cake mixes:																	
	Angel food:																	
377	Whole cake	1 cake	635	34	1,645	36	1	—	—	—	377	603	1.9	0	0.03	0.70	0.6	0
378	Piece, 1/12 of 10-in diam. cake	1 piece	53	34	135	3	Trace	—	—	—	32	50	0.2	0	Trace	0.06	0.1	0

[5]Measure and weight apply to entire vegetable or fruit including parts not usually eaten.

[8]This is the amount from the fruit. Additional ascorbic acid may be added by the manufacturer. Refer to the label for this information.

[15]Values for iron, thiamine, riboflavin, and niacin per pound of unenriched white bread would be as follows:

	Iron mg	Thiamine mg	Riboflavin mg	Niacin mg
Soft crumb	3.2	.31	.39	5.0
Firm crumb	3.2	.32	.59	4.1

Food, Approximate Measure, and Weight (in grams)		gm	Water per cent	Food Energy calories	Protein gm	Fat gm	Fatty Acids			Carbohydrate gm	Calcium mg	Iron mg	Vitamin A Value I.U.	Thiamine mg	Riboflavin mg	Niacin mg	Ascorbic Acid mg
							Saturated (total) gm	Unsaturated									
								Oleic gm	Linoleic gm								
Cakes made from cake mixes (cont.)																	
Cupcakes, small, 2 1/2 in diam.:																	
379	Without icing 1 cupcake	25	26	90	1	3	1	1	1	14	40	0.1	40	0.01	0.03	0.1	Trace
380	With chocolate icing 1 cupcake	36	22	130	2	5	2	2	1	21	47	0.3	60	0.01	0.04	0.1	Trace
Devil's food, 2-layer, with chocolate icing:																	
381	Whole cake 1 cake	1,107	24	3,755	49	136	54	58	16	645	653	8.9	1,660	0.33	0.89	3.3	1
382	Piece, 1/16 of 9-in diam. cake 1 piece	69	24	235	3	9	3	4	1	40	41	0.6	100	0.02	0.06	0.2	Trace
383	Cupcake, small, 2 1/2-in diam 1 cupcake	35	24	120	2	4	1	2	Trace	20	21	0.3	50	0.01	0.03	0.1	Trace
Gingerbread:																	
384	Whole cake 1 cake	570	37	1,575	18	39	10	19	9	291	513	9.1	Trace	0.17	0.51	4.6	2
385	Piece, 1/9 of 8-in square cake 1 piece	63	37	175	2	4	1	2	1	32	57	1.0	Trace	0.02	0.06	0.5	Trace
White, 2-layer, with chocolate icing:																	
386	Whole cake 1 cake	1,140	21	4,000	45	122	45	54	17	716	1,129	5.7	680	0.23	0.91	2.3	2
387	Piece, 1/16 of 9-in diam. cake 1 piece	71	21	250	3	8	3	3	1	45	70	0.4	40	0.01	0.06	0.1	Trace
Cakes made from home recipes:[16]																	
388	Boston cream pie; piece 1/12 of 8-in diam. 1 piece	69	35	210	4	6	2	3	1	34	46	0.3	140	0.02	0.08	0.1	Trace
Fruitcake, dark, made with enriched flour:																	
389	Loaf, 1 lb 1 loaf	454	18	1,720	22	69	15	37	13	271	327	11.8	540	0.59	0.64	3.6	2
390	Slice, 1/30 of 8-in loaf 1 slice	15	18	55	1	2	Trace	1	Trace	9	11	0.4	20	0.02	0.02	0.1	Trace
Plain sheet cake:																	
Without icing:																	
391	Whole cake 1 cake	777	25	2,830	35	108	30	52	21	434	497	3.1	1,320	0.16	0.70	1.6	2
392	Piece, 1/9 of 9-in square cake 1 piece	86	25	315	4	12	3	6	2	48	55	0.3	150	0.02	0.08	0.2	Trace
393	With boiled white icing, piece, 1/9 of 9-in square cake 1 piece	114	23	400	4	12	3	6	2	71	56	0.3	150	0.02	0.08	0.2	Trace
Pound:																	
394	Loaf, 8 1/2 by 3 1/2 by 3 in 1 loaf	514	17	2,430	29	152	34	68	17	242	108	4.1	1,440	0.15	0.46	1.0	0
395	Slice, 1/2-in thick 1 slice	30	17	140	2	9	2	4	1	14	6	0.2	80	0.01	0.03	0.1	0
Sponge:																	
396	Whole cake 1 cake	790	32	2,345	60	45	14	20	4	427	237	9.5	3,560	0.40	1.11	1.6	Trace
397	Piece, 1/12 of 10-in diam. cake 1 piece	66	32	195	5	4	1	2	Trace	36	20	0.8	300	0.03	0.09	0.1	Trace
Yellow, 2-layer, without icing:																	
398	Whole cake 1 cake	870	24	3,160	39	111	31	53	22	506	618	3.5	1,310	0.17	0.70	1.7	2
399	Piece, 1/16 of 9-in diam. cake 1 piece	54	24	200	2	7	2	3	1	32	39	0.2	80	0.01	0.04	0.1	Trace
Yellow, 2-layer, with chocolate icing:																	
400	Whole cake 1 cake	1,203	21	4,390	51	156	55	69	23	727	818	7.2	1,920	0.24	0.96	2.4	Trace
401	Piece, 1/16 of 9-in diam. cake 1 piece	75	21	275	3	10	3	4	1	45	51	0.5	120	0.02	0.06	0.2	Trace
Cake icings. See Sugars, Sweets																	

No.	Food	Measure																
	Cookies:																	
	Brownies with nuts:																	
402	Made from home recipe with enriched flour	1 brownie	20	10	95	1	6	1	3	1	10	8	0.4	40	0.04	0.02	0.1	Trace
403	Made from mix	1 brownie	20	11	85	1	4	1	2	1	13	9	0.4	20	0.03	0.02	0.1	Trace
	Chocolate chip:																	
404	Made from home recipe with enriched flour	1 cookie	10	3	50	1	3	1	1	1	6	4	0.2	10	0.01	0.01	0.1	Trace
405	Commercial	1 cookie	10	3	50	1	2	1	1	Trace	7	4	0.2	10	Trace	Trace	Trace	Trace
406	Fig bars, commercial	1 cookie	14	14	50	1	1	Trace	1	—	11	11	0.2	20	Trace	0.01	0.1	Trace
407	Sandwich, chocolate or vanilla, commercial	1 cookie	10	2	50	1	2	1	1	Trace	7	2	0.1	0	Trace	Trace	0.1	0
	Corn flakes, added nutrients:																	
408	Plain	1 cup	25	4	100	2	Trace	—	—	—	21	4	0.4	0	0.11	0.02	0.5	0
409	Sugar-covered	1 cup	40	2	155	2	Trace	—	—	—	36	5	0.4	0	0.16	0.02	0.8	0
	Corn (hominy) grits, degermed, cooked:																	
410	Enriched	1 cup	245	87	125	3	Trace	—	—	—	27	2	0.7	[17]150	0.10	0.07	1.0	0
411	Unenriched	1 cup	245	87	125	3	Trace	—	—	—	27	2	0.2	[17]150	0.05	0.02	0.5	0
	Cornmeal:																	
412	Whole-ground, unbolted, dry	1 cup	122	12	435	11	5	1	2	2	90	24	2.9	[17]620	0.46	0.13	2.4	0
413	Bolted (nearly whole-grain) dry	1 cup	122	12	440	11	4	Trace	1	2	91	21	2.2	[17]590	0.37	0.10	2.3	0
	Degermed, enriched:																	
414	Dry form	1 cup	138	12	500	11	2	—	—	—	108	8	4.0	[17]610	0.61	0.36	4.8	0
415	Cooked	1 cup	240	88	120	3	1	—	—	—	26	2	1.0	[17]140	0.14	0.10	1.2	0
	Degermed, unenriched:																	
416	Dry form	1 cup	138	12	500	11	2	—	—	—	108	8	1.5	[17]610	0.19	0.07	1.4	0
417	Cooked	1 cup	240	88	120	3	1	—	—	—	26	2	0.5	[17]140	0.05	0.02	0.5	0
418	Corn muffins, made with enriched degermed cornmeal and enriched flour; muffin 2 3/8-in diam.	1 muffin	40	33	125	3	4	2	2	Trace	19	42	0.7	[17]120	0.08	0.09	0.6	Trace
419	Corn muffins, made with mix, egg, and milk; muffin 2 3/8-in diam.	1 muffin	40	30	130	3	4	1	2	1	20	96	0.6	100	0.07	0.08	0.6	Trace
420	Corn, puffed, presweetened, added nutrients	1 cup	30	2	115	1	Trace	—	—	—	27	3	0.5	0	0.13	0.05	0.6	0
421	Corn, shredded, added nutrients	1 cup	25	3	100	2	Trace	—	—	—	22	1	0.6	0	0.11	0.05	0.5	0
	Crackers:																	
422	Graham, 2 1/2-in square	4 crackers	28	6	110	2	3	—	—	—	21	11	0.4	0	0.01	0.06	0.4	0
423	Saltines	4 crackers	11	4	50	1	1	—	—	—	8	2	0.1	0	Trace	Trace	0.1	0
	Danish pastry, plain (without fruit or nuts):																	
424	Packaged ring, 12 ounces	1 ring	340	22	1,435	25	80	24	37	15	155	170	3.1	1,050	0.24	0.51	2.7	Trace
425	Round piece, approx. 4 1/4-in diam. by 1 in	1 pastry	65	22	275	5	15	5	7	3	30	33	0.6	200	0.05	0.10	0.5	Trace
	Doughnuts, cake type:																	
426	Ounce	1 oz	28	22	120	2	7	2	3	1	13	14	0.3	90	0.02	0.04	0.2	Trace
427	Doughnuts, cake type	1 doughnut	32	24	125	1	6	1	4	1	16	13	[18]0.4	30	[18]0.05	[18]0.05	[18]0.4	Trace
428	Farina, quick-cooking, enriched, cooked	1 cup	245	89	105	3	Trace	—	—	—	22	147	[19]0.7	0	[19]0.12	[19]0.07	[19]1.0	0

[16]Unenriched cake flour used unless otherwise specified.

[17]This value is based on product made from yellow varieties of corn; white varieties contain only a trace.

[18]Based on product made with enriched flour. With unenriched flour, approximate values per doughnut are:iron, 0.2 mg; thiamine, 0.01 mg; riboflavin, 0.03 mg; niacin, 0.2 mg.

[19]Iron, thiamine, riboflavin, and niacin are based on the minimum levels of enrichment specified in standards of identity promulgated under the Federal Food, Drug, and Cosmetic Act.

527

#	Food, Approximate Measure, and Weight (in grams)	gm	Water per cent	Food Energy calories	Protein gm	Fat gm	Fatty Acids Saturated (total) gm	Fatty Acids Unsaturated Oleic gm	Fatty Acids Unsaturated Linoleic gm	Carbo-hydrate gm	Calcium mg	Iron mg	Vitamin A Value I.U.	Thiamine mg	Riboflavin mg	Niacin mg	Ascorbic Acid mg
	Macaroni, cooked:																
	Enriched:																
429	Cooked, firm stage (undergoes additional cooking in a food mixture) 1 cup	130	64	190	6	1	—	—	—	39	14	[19]1.4	0	[19]0.23	[19]0.14	[19]1.8	0
430	Cooked until tender 1 cup	140	72	155	5	1	—	—	—	32	8	[19]1.3	0	[19]0.20	[19]0.11	[19]1.5	0
	Unenriched:																
431	Cooked, firm stage (undergoes additional cooking in a food mixture) 1 cup	130	64	190	6	1	—	—	—	39	14	0.7	0	0.03	0.03	0.5	0
432	Cooked until tender 1 cup	140	72	155	5	1	—	—	—	32	11	0.6	0	0.01	0.01	0.4	0
433	Macaroni (enriched) and cheese, baked 1 cup	200	58	430	17	22	10	9	2	40	362	1.8	860	0.20	0.40	1.8	Trace
434	Canned 1 cup	240	80	230	9	10	4	3	1	26	199	1.0	260	0.12	0.24	1.0	Trace
435	Muffins, with enriched white flour; muffin, 3-inch diam. 1 muffin	40	38	120	3	4	1	2	1	17	42	0.6	40	0.07	0.09	0.6	Trace
	Noodles (egg noodles), cooked:																
436	Enriched 1 cup	160	70	200	7	2	1	1	Trace	37	16	[19]1.4	110	[19]0.22	[19]0.13	[19]1.9	0
437	Unenriched 1 cup	160	70	200	7	2	1	1	Trace	37	16	1.0	110	0.05	0.03	0.6	0
438	Oats (with or without corn) puffed, added nutrients 1 cup	25	3	100	3	1	—	—	—	19	44	1.2	0	0.24	0.04	0.5	0
439	Oatmeal or rolled oats, cooked 1 cup	240	87	130	5	2	—	—	1	23	22	1.4	0	0.19	0.05	0.2	0
	Pancakes, 4-inch diam.:																
440	Wheat, enriched flour (home recipe) 1 cake	27	50	60	2	2	Trace	1	Trace	9	27	0.4	30	0.05	0.06	0.4	Trace
441	Buckwheat (made from mix with egg and milk) 1 cake	27	58	55	2	2	1	1	Trace	6	59	0.4	60	0.03	0.04	0.2	Trace
442	Plain or buttermilk (made from mix with egg and milk) 1 cake	27	51	60	2	2	1	1	Trace	9	58	0.3	70	0.04	0.06	0.2	Trace
	Pie (piecrust made with unenriched flour): Sector, 4-in, 1/7 of 9-in-diam. pie:																
443	Apple (2-crust) 1 sector	135	48	350	3	15	4	7	3	51	11	0.4	40	0.03	0.03	0.5	1
444	Butterscotch (1-crust) 1 sector	130	45	350	6	14	5	6	3	50	98	1.2	340	0.04	0.13	0.3	Trace
445	Cherry (2-crust) 1 sector	135	47	350	4	15	4	7	3	52	19	0.4	590	0.03	0.03	0.7	Trace
446	Custard (1-crust) 1 sector	130	58	285	8	14	5	6	2	30	125	0.8	300	0.07	0.21	0.4	0
447	Lemon meringue (1-crust) 1 sector	120	47	305	4	12	4	6	2	45	17	0.6	200	0.04	0.10	0.2	1
448	Mince (2-crust) 1 sector	135	43	365	3	16	4	8	3	56	38	1.4	Trace	0.09	0.05	0.5	4
449	Pecan (1-crust) 1 sector	118	20	490	6	27	16	8	5	60	55	3.3	190	0.19	0.08	0.4	1
450	Pineapple chiffon (1-crust) 1 sector	93	41	265	6	11	3	5	2	36	22	0.8	320	0.04	0.08	0.4	1
451	Pumpkin (1-crust) 1 sector	130	59	275	5	15	5	6	2	32	66	0.7	3,210	0.04	0.13	0.7	Trace
	Piecrust, baked shell for pie made with:																
452	Enriched flour 1 shell	180	15	900	11	60	16	28	12	79	25	3.1	0	0.36	0.25	3.2	0
453	Unenriched flour 1 shell	180	15	900	11	60	16	28	12	79	25	0.9	0	0.05	0.05	0.9	0

No.	Food, approximate measure	Grams	Water (%)	Food energy (cal.)	Protein (g)	Fat (g)	Saturated (g)	Oleic (g)	Linoleic (g)	Carbohydrate (g)	Calcium (mg)	Iron (mg)	Vitamin A (I.U.)	Thiamin (mg)	Riboflavin (mg)	Niacin (mg)	Ascorbic acid (mg)
454	Piecrust mix including stick form: Package, 10 oz, for double crust — 1 pkg.	284	9	1,480	20	93	23	46	21	141	131	1.4	0	0.11	0.11	2.0	0
455	Pizza (cheese) 5 1/2-in sector; 1/8 of 14-in diam. pie — 1 sector	75	45	185	7	6	2	3	Trace	27	107	0.7	290	0.04	0.12	0.7	4
	Popcorn, popped:																
456	Plain, large kernel — 1 cup	6	4	25	1	Trace	—	Trace	Trace	5	1	0.2	—	—	0.01	0.1	0
457	With oil and salt — 1 cup	9	3	40	1	2	1	—	1	5	1	0.2	—	—	0.01	0.2	0
458	Sugar coated — 1 cup	35	4	135	2	1	—	—	—	30	2	0.5	—	—	0.02	0.4	0
	Pretzels:																
459	Dutch, twisted — 1 pretzel	16	5	60	2	1	—	—	—	12	4	0.2	0	Trace	Trace	0.1	0
460	Thin, twisted — 1 pretzel	6	5	25	1	Trace	—	—	—	5	1	0.1	0	Trace	Trace	Trace	0
461	Sticks, small 2 1/4 inches — 10 sticks	3	5	10	Trace	Trace	—	—	—	2	1	Trace	0	Trace	Trace	Trace	0
462	Stick, regular, 3 1/8 inches — 5 sticks	3	5	10	Trace	Trace	—	—	—	2	1	Trace	0	Trace	Trace	Trace	0
	Rice, white: Enriched:																
463	Raw — 1 cup	185	12	670	12	1	—	—	—	149	44	[20]5.4	0	[20]0.81	[20]0.06	[20]6.5	0
464	Cooked — 1 cup	205	73	225	4	Trace	—	—	—	50	21	[20]1.8	0	[20]0.23	[20]0.02	[20]2.1	0
465	Instant, ready to serve — 1 cup	165	73	180	4	Trace	—	—	—	40	5	[20]1.3	0	[20]0.21	[20]—	[20]1.7	0
466	Unenriched, cooked — 1 cup	205	73	225	4	Trace	—	—	—	50	21	0.4	0	0.04	[20]—	0.8	0
467	Parboiled, cooked — 1 cup	175	73	185	4	Trace	—	—	—	41	33	[20]1.4	0	[20]0.19	0.02	[20]2.1	0
468	Rice, puffed, added nutrients — 1 cup	15	4	60	1	Trace	—	—	—	13	3	0.3	0	0.07	0.01	0.7	0
	Rolls, enriched: Cloverleaf or pan:																
469	Home recipe — 1 roll	35	26	120	3	3	1	1	Trace	20	16	0.7	30	0.09	0.09	0.8	Trace
470	Commercial — 1 roll	28	31	85	2	2	Trace	1	Trace	15	21	0.5	Trace	0.08	0.05	0.6	Trace
471	Frankfurter or hamburger — 1 roll	40	31	120	3	2	1	1	Trace	21	30	0.8	Trace	0.11	0.07	0.9	Trace
472	Hard, round or rectangular — 1 roll	50	25	155	5	2	Trace	1	Trace	30	24	1.2	Trace	0.13	0.12	1.4	Trace
473	Rye wafers, whole-grain, 1 7/8 by 3 1/2 inches — 2 wafers	13	6	45	2	Trace	—	—	—	10	7	0.5	0	0.04	0.03	0.2	0
474	Spaghetti, cooked, tender stage, enriched — 1 cup	140	72	155	5	1	—	—	—	32	11	[19]1.3	0	[19]0.20	[19]0.11	[19]1.5	0
	Spaghetti with meat balls, and tomato sauce:																
475	Home recipe — 1 cup	248	70	330	19	12	4	6	4	39	124	3.7	1,590	0.25	0.30	4.0	22
476	Canned — 1 cup	250	78	260	12	10	2	3	2	28	53	3.3	1,000	0.15	0.18	2.3	5
	Spaghetti in tomato sauce with cheese:																
477	Home recipe — 1 cup	250	77	260	9	9	2	5	2	37	80	2.3	1,080	0.25	0.18	2.3	13
478	Canned — 1 cup	250	80	190	6	2	1	1	1	38	40	2.8	930	0.35	0.28	4.5	10
479	Waffles, with enriched flour, 7-in diam. — 1 waffle	75	41	210	7	7	2	4	1	28	85	1.3	250	0.13	0.19	1.0	Trace
480	Waffles, made from mix, enriched, egg and milk added, 7-in diam. — 1 waffle	75	42	205	7	8	3	3	1	27	179	1.0	170	0.11	0.17	0.7	Trace
481	Wheat, puffed, added nutrients — 1 cup	15	3	55	2	Trace	—	—	—	12	4	0.6	0	0.08	0.03	1.2	0
482	Wheat, shredded, plain — 1 biscuit	25	7	90	2	1	—	—	—	20	11	0.9	0	0.06	0.03	1.1	0
483	Wheat flakes, added nutrients — 1 cup	30	4	105	3	Trace	—	—	—	24	12	1.3	0	0.19	0.04	1.5	0
	Wheat flours:																
484	Whole wheat, from hard wheats, stirred — 1 cup	120	12	400	16	2	Trace	1	1	85	49	4.0	0	0.66	0.14	5.2	0

[19] Iron, thiamine, riboflavin, and niacin are based on the minimum levels of enrichment specified in standards of identity promulgated under the Federal Food, Drug, and Cosmetic Act.

[20] Iron, thiamine, and niacin are based on the minimum levels of enrichment specified in standards of identity promulgated under the Federal Food, Drug, and Cosmetic Act. Riboflavin is based on unenriched rice. When the minimum level of enrichment specified in the standards of identity becomes effective the value will be 0.12 mg per cup of parboiled rice and of white rice.

	Food, Approximate Measure, and Weight (in grams)		Weight gm	Water per cent	Food Energy calories	Protein gm	Fat gm	Saturated (total) gm	Unsaturated Oleic gm	Linoleic gm	Carbohydrate gm	Calcium mg	Iron mg	Vitamin A Value I.U.	Thiamine mg	Riboflavin mg	Niacin mg	Ascorbic Acid mg
	Wheat flours (cont.)																	
	All-purpose or family flour, enriched:																	
485	Sifted	1 cup	115	12	420	12	1	—	—	—	88	18	193.3	0	190.51	190.30	194.0	0
486	Unsifted	1 cup	125	12	455	13	1	—	—	—	95	20	193.6	0	190.55	190.33	194.4	0
487	Self-rising, enriched	1 cup	125	12	440	12	1	—	—	—	93	331	193.6	0	190.55	190.33	194.4	0
488	Cake or pastry flour, sifted	1 cup	96	12	350	7	1	—	—	—	76	16	0.5	0	0.03	0.03	0.7	0
	Fats, Oils																	
	Butter:																	
	Regular, 4 sticks per pound:																	
489	Stick	1/2 cup	113	16	810	1	92	51	30	3	1	23	0	213,750	—	—	—	0
490	Tablespoon (approx. 1/8 stick)	1 tbsp.	14	16	100	Trace	12	6	4	Trace	Trace	3	0	21470	—	—	—	0
491	Pat (1-in sq. 1/3-in high; 90 per lb)	1 pat	5	16	35	Trace	4	2	1	Trace	Trace	1	0	21170	—	—	—	0
	Whipped, 6 sticks or 2, 8-oz containers per pound:																	
492	Stick	1/2 cup	76	16	540	1	61	34	20	2	Trace	15	0	212,500	—	—	—	0
493	Tablespoon (approx. 1/8 stick)	1 tbsp.	9	16	65	Trace	8	4	3	Trace	Trace	2	0	21310	—	—	—	0
494	Pat (1 1/4-in sq 1/3-in high; 120 per lb)	1 pat	4	16	25	Trace	3	2	1	Trace	Trace	1	0	21130	—	—	—	0
	Fats, cooking:																	
495	Lard	1 cup	205	0	1,850	0	205	78	94	20	0	0	0	0	0	0	0	0
496		1 tbsp.	13	0	115	0	13	5	6	1	0	0	0	0	0	0	0	0
497	Vegetable fats	1 cup	200	0	1,770	0	200	50	100	44	0	0	0	—	0	0	0	0
498		1 tbsp	13	0	110	0	13	3	6	3	0	0	0	—	0	0	0	0
	Margarine:																	
	Regular, 4 sticks per pound:																	
499	Stick	1/2 cup	113	16	815	1	92	17	46	25	1	23	0	223,750	—	—	—	0
500	Tablespoon (approx. 1/8 stick)	1 tbsp	14	16	100	Trace	12	2	6	3	Trace	3	0	22470	—	—	—	0
501	Pat (1-in sq 1/3-in high; 90 per lb)	1 pat	5	16	35	Trace	4	1	2	1	Trace	1	0	22170	—	—	—	0
	Whipped, 6 sticks per pound:																	
502	Stick	1/2 cup	76	16	545	1	61	11	31	17	Trace	15	0	222,500	—	—	—	0
	Soft, 2 8-oz tubs per pound:																	
503	Tub	1 tub	227	16	1,635	1	184	34	68	68	1	45	0	227,500	—	—	—	0
504	Tablespoon	1 tbsp	14	16	100	Trace	11	2	4	4	Trace	3	0	22470	—	—	—	0
	Oils, salad or cooking:																	
505	Corn	1 cup	220	0	1,945	0	220	22	62	117	0	0	0	—	0	0	0	0
506		1 tbsp	14	0	125	0	14	1	4	7	0	0	0	—	0	0	0	0
507	Cottonseed	1 cup	220	0	1,945	0	220	55	46	110	0	0	0	—	0	0	0	0
508		1 tbsp	14	0	125	0	14	4	3	7	0	0	0	—	0	0	0	0
509	Olive	1 cup	220	0	1,945	0	220	24	167	15	0	0	0	—	0	0	0	0
510		1 tbsp	14	0	125	0	14	2	11	1	0	0	0	—	0	0	0	0
511	Peanut	1 cup	220	0	1,945	0	220	40	103	64	0	0	0	—	0	0	0	0
512		1 tbsp	14	0	125	0	14	3	7	4	0	0	0	—	0	0	0	0

Sugars, Sweets

No.	Food	Measure	Grams	Water (%)	Food energy (cal)	Protein (g)	Fat (g)	Saturated (g)	Oleic (g)	Linoleic (g)	Carbohydrate (g)	Calcium (mg)	Iron (mg)	Vitamin A (I.U.)	Thiamine (mg)	Riboflavin (mg)	Niacin (mg)	Ascorbic acid (mg)
513	Safflower	1 cup	220	0	1,945	0	220	18	37	165	0	0	0	—	0	0	0	0
514		1 tbsp	14	0	125	0	14	1	2	10	0	0	0	—	0	0	0	0
515	Soybean	1 cup	220	0	1,945	0	220	33	44	114	0	0	0	—	0	0	0	0
516		1 tbsp	14	0	125	0	14	2	3	7	0	0	0	—	0	0	0	0
	Salad dressing:																	
517	Blue cheese	1 tbsp	15	32	75	1	8	2	2	4	1	12	Trace	30	Trace	0.02	Trace	Trace
	Commercial, mayonnaise type:																	
518	Regular	1 tbsp	15	41	65	Trace	6	1	1	3	3	2	Trace	30	Trace	Trace	Trace	—
519	Special dietary, low calorie	1 tbsp	16	81	20	Trace	2	Trace	Trace	1	2	3	Trace	40	Trace	Trace	Trace	—
	French:																	
520	Regular	1 tbsp	16	39	65	Trace	6	1	1	3	Trace	2	0.1	—	—	—	—	—
521	Special dietary, low fat with artificial sweeteners	1 tbsp	15	95	Trace	Trace	Trace	—	—	—	2	2	0.1	—	—	—	—	—
522	Home cooked, boiled	1 tbsp	16	68	25	1	2	—	1	Trace	2	14	0.1	80	0.01	0.03	Trace	Trace
523	Mayonnaise	1 tbsp	14	15	100	Trace	11	2	2	6	Trace	3	0.1	40	Trace	0.01	Trace	—
524	Thousand island	1 tbsp	16	32	80	Trace	8	1	2	4	2	2	0.1	50	Trace	Trace	Trace	Trace
	Cake icings:																	
525	Chocolate made with milk and table fat	1 cup	275	14	1,035	9	38	21	14	1	185	165	3.3	580	0.06	0.28	0.6	1
526	Coconut (with boiled icing)	1 cup	166	15	605	3	13	11	1	Trace	124	10	0.8	0	0.02	0.07	0.3	0
527	Creamy fudge from mix with water only	1 cup	245	15	830	7	16	5	8	3	183	96	2.7	Trace	0.05	0.20	0.7	Trace
528	White, boiled	1 cup	94	18	300	1	0	—	—	—	76	2	Trace	0	Trace	0.03	Trace	0
	Candy:																	
529	Caramels, plain or chocolate	1 oz	28	8	115	1	3	2	1	Trace	22	42	0.4	Trace	0.01	0.05	0.1	Trace
530	Chocolate, milk, plain	1 oz	28	1	145	2	9	5	3	Trace	16	65	0.3	80	0.02	0.10	0.1	Trace
531	Chocolate-coated peanuts	1 oz	28	1	160	5	12	3	6	2	11	33	0.4	0	0.10	0.05	2.1	Trace
532	Fondant; mints, uncoated; candy corn	1 oz	28	8	105	Trace	1	—	—	—	25	4	0.3	Trace	Trace	Trace	Trace	0
533	Fudge, plain	1 oz	28	8	115	1	4	2	1	Trace	21	22	0.3	Trace	0.01	0.03	0.1	Trace
534	Gum drops	1 oz	28	12	100	Trace	Trace	—	—	—	25	2	0.1	0	0	Trace	0	0
535	Hard	1 oz	28	1	110	0	Trace	—	—	—	28	6	0.5	0	0	0	Trace	0
536	Marshmallows	1 oz	28	17	90	1	Trace	—	—	—	23	5	0.5	0	0	Trace	Trace	0
	Chocolate-flavored syrup or topping:																	
537	Thin type	1 fl oz	38	32	90	1	1	Trace	Trace	Trace	24	6	0.6	Trace	0.01	0.03	0.2	0
538	Fudge type	1 fl oz	38	25	125	2	5	3	2	Trace	20	48	0.5	60	0.02	0.08	0.2	Trace
	Chocolate-flavored beverage powder (approx. 4 heaping teaspoons per oz):																	
539	With nonfat dry milk	1 oz	28	2	100	5	1	Trace	Trace	Trace	20	167	0.5	10	0.04	0.21	0.2	1
540	Without nonfat dry milk	1 oz	28	1	100	1	1	Trace	Trace	Trace	25	9	0.6	0	0.01	0.03	0.1	0
541	Honey, strained or extracted	1 tbsp	21	17	65	Trace	0	—	—	—	17	1	0.1	0	Trace	0.01	0.1	Trace
542	Jams and preserves	1 tbsp	20	29	55	Trace	Trace	—	—	—	14	4	0.2	Trace	Trace	0.01	Trace	Trace
543	Jellies	1 tbsp	18	29	50	Trace	Trace	—	—	—	13	4	0.3	Trace	Trace	0.01	Trace	1
	Molasses, cane:																	
544	Light (first extraction)	1 tbsp	20	24	50	—	—	—	—	—	13	33	0.9	—	0.01	0.01	Trace	—
545	Blackstrap (third extraction)	1 tbsp	20	24	45	—	—	—	—	—	11	137	3.2	—	0.02	0.04	0.4	—
	Syrups:																	
546	Sorghum	1 tbsp	21	23	55	—	—	—	—	—	14	35	2.6	—	—	0.02	Trace	—

[19]Iron, thiamine, riboflavin, and niacin are based on the minimum levels of enrichment specified in standards of identity promulgated under the Federal Food, Drug, and Cosmetic Act.

[21]Year-round average.

[22]Based on the average vitamin A content of fortified margarine. Federal specifications for fortified margarine require a minimum of 15,000 I.U. of vitamin A per pound.

Syrups (cont.)

Food, Approximate Measure, and Weight (in grams)		Water per cent	Food Energy calories	Protein gm	Fat gm	Saturated (total) gm	Oleic gm	Linoleic gm	Carbohydrate gm	Calcium mg	Iron mg	Vitamin A Value I.U.	Thiamine mg	Riboflavin mg	Niacin mg	Ascorbic Acid mg
547	Table blends, chiefly corn, light and dark 1 tbsp 21	24	60	0	0	—	—	—	15	9	0.8	0	0	0	0	0
	Sugars:															
548	Brown, firm packed 1 cup 220	2	820	0	0	—	—	—	212	187	7.5	0	0.02	0.07	0.4	0
	White:															
549	Granulated 1 cup 200	Trace	770	0	0	—	—	—	199	0	0.2	0	0	0	0	0
550	1 tbsp 11	Trace	40	0	0	—	—	—	11	0	Trace	0	0	0	0	0
551	Powdered, stirred before measuring 1 cup 120	Trace	460	0	0	—	—	—	119	0	0.1	0	0	0	0	0

Miscellaneous Items

Food, Approximate Measure, and Weight (in grams)		Water per cent	Food Energy calories	Protein gm	Fat gm	Saturated (total) gm	Oleic gm	Linoleic gm	Carbohydrate gm	Calcium mg	Iron mg	Vitamin A Value I.U.	Thiamine mg	Riboflavin mg	Niacin mg	Ascorbic Acid mg
552	Barbecue sauce 1 cup 250	81	230	4	17	2	5	9	20	53	2.0	900	0.03	0.03	0.8	13
	Beverages, alcoholic:															
553	Beer 12 fl oz 360	92	150	1	0	—	—	—	14	18	Trace	—	0.01	0.11	2.2	—
	Gin, rum, vodka, whiskey:															
554	80 proof 1 1/2 fl oz jigger 42	67	100	—	—	—	—	—	Trace	—	—	—	—	—	—	—
555	86 proof 1 1/2 fl oz jigger 42	64	105	—	—	—	—	—	Trace	—	—	—	—	—	—	—
556	90 proof 1 1/2 fl oz jigger 42	62	110	—	—	—	—	—	Trace	—	—	—	—	—	—	—
557	94 proof 1 1/2 fl oz jigger 42	60	115	—	—	—	—	—	Trace	—	—	—	—	—	—	—
558	100 proof 1 1/2 fl oz jigger 42	58	125	—	—	—	—	—	Trace	—	—	—	—	—	—	—
	Wines:															
559	Dessert 3 1/2 fl oz glass 103	77	140	Trace	0	—	—	—	8	8	—	—	0.01	0.02	0.2	—
560	Table 3 1/2 fl oz glass 102	86	85	Trace	0	—	—	—	4	9	0.4	—	Trace	0.01	0.1	—
	Beverages, carbonated, sweetened, nonalcoholic:															
561	Carbonated water 12 fl oz 366	92	115	0	0	—	—	—	29	—	—	0	0	0	0	0
562	Cola type 12 fl oz 369	90	145	0	0	—	—	—	37	—	—	0	0	0	0	0
563	Fruit-flavored sodas and Tom Collins mixes 12 fl oz 372	88	170	0	0	—	—	—	45	—	—	0	0	0	0	0
564	Ginger ale 12 fl oz 366	92	115	0	0	—	—	—	29	—	—	0	0	0	0	0
565	Root beer 12 fl oz 370	90	150	0	0	—	—	—	39	—	—	0	0	0	0	0
566	Bouillon cubes, approx.1/2 in 1 cube 4	4	5	1	Trace	—	—	—	Trace	—	—	—	—	—	—	—
	Chocolate:															
567	Bitter or baking 1 oz 28	2	145	3	15	8	6	Trace	8	22	1.9	20	0.01	0.07	0.4	0
568	Semisweet, small pieces 1 cup 170	1	860	7	61	34	22	1	97	51	4.4	30	0.02	0.14	0.9	0
	Gelatin:															
569	Plain, dry powder in envelope 1 envelope 7	13	25	6	Trace	—	—	—	0	—	—	—	—	—	—	—
570	Dessert powder, 3-oz package 1 pkg 85	2	315	8	0	—	—	—	75	—	—	—	—	—	—	—
571	Gelatin dessert, prepared with water 1 cup 240	84	140	4	0	—	—	—	34	—	—	—	—	—	—	—

No.	Food	Measure	Grams	Water (%)	Food energy (cal)	Protein (g)	Fat (g)	Saturated (g)	Oleic (g)	Linoleic (g)	Carbohydrate (g)	Calcium (mg)	Iron (mg)	Vitamin A (IU)	Thiamin (mg)	Riboflavin (mg)	Niacin (mg)	Ascorbic acid (mg)
	Olives, pickled:																	
572	Green	4 medium or 3 extra large or 2 giant	16	78	15	Trace	2	Trace	2	Trace	Trace	8	0.2	40	—	—	—	—
573	Ripe: Mission	3 small or 2 large	10	73	15	Trace	2	Trace	2	Trace	Trace	9	0.1	10	Trace	Trace	Trace	—
	Pickles, cucumber:																	
574	Dill, medium, whole, 3 3/4 in long, 1 1/4 in. diam.	1 pickle	65	93	10	1	Trace	—	—	—	1	17	0.7	70	Trace	0.01	Trace	4
575	Fresh, sliced, 1 1/2 in diam., 1/4 in thick	2 slices	15	79	10	Trace	Trace	—	—	—	3	5	0.3	20	Trace	Trace	Trace	1
576	Sweet, gherkin, small, whole, approx. 2 1/2 in long, 3/4 in diam.	1 pickle	15	61	20	Trace	Trace	—	—	—	6	2	0.2	10	Trace	Trace	Trace	1
577	Relish, finely chopped, sweet	1 tbsp	15	63	20	Trace	Trace	—	—	—	5	3	0.1	—	Trace	—	—	—
	Popcorn. See Grain Products																	
578	Popsicle, 3-fl oz size	1 popsicle	95	80	70	Trace	0	0	0	0	18	0	Trace	0	0	0	0	0
	Pudding, home recipe with starch base:																	
579	Chocolate	1 cup	260	66	385	8	12	7	4	Trace	67	250	1.3	390	0.05	0.36	0.3	1
580	Vanilla (blanc mange)	1 cup	255	76	285	9	10	5	3	Trace	41	298	Trace	410	0.08	0.41	0.3	2
581	Pudding mix, dry form, 4-oz package	1 pkg	113	2	410	3	2	1	1	Trace	103	23	1.8	Trace	0.02	0.08	0.5	0
582	Sherbet	1 cup	193	67	260	2	2	—	—	—	59	31	Trace	120	0.02	0.06	Trace	4
	Soups:																	
	Canned, condensed, ready-to-serve:																	
	Prepared with an equal volume of milk:																	
583	Cream of chicken	1 cup	245	85	180	7	10	3	3	3	15	172	0.5	610	0.05	0.27	0.7	2
584	Cream of mushroom	1 cup	245	83	215	7	14	4	4	5	16	191	0.5	250	0.05	0.34	0.7	1
585	Tomato	1 cup	250	84	175	7	7	3	2	1	23	168	0.8	1,200	0.10	0.25	1.3	15
	Prepared with an equal volume of water:																	
586	Bean with pork	1 cup	250	84	170	8	6	1	2	2	22	63	2.3	650	0.13	0.08	1.0	3
587	Beef broth, bouillon consommé	1 cup	240	96	30	5	0	—	—	—	3	Trace	0.5	Trace	Trace	0.02	1.2	—
588	Beef noodle	1 cup	240	93	70	4	3	1	1	1	7	7	1.0	50	0.05	0.07	1.0	Trace
589	Clam chowder, Manhattan type (with tomatoes, without milk)	1 cup	245	92	80	2	3	—	—	—	12	34	1.0	880	0.02	0.02	1.0	—
590	Cream of chicken	1 cup	240	92	95	3	6	1	2	3	8	24	0.5	410	0.02	0.05	0.5	Trace
591	Cream of mushroom	1 cup	240	90	135	2	10	1	3	5	10	41	0.5	70	0.02	0.12	0.7	Trace
592	Minestrone	1 cup	245	90	105	5	3	—	—	—	14	37	1.0	2,350	0.07	0.05	1.0	—
593	Split pea	1 cup	245	85	145	9	3	1	2	Trace	21	29	1.5	440	0.25	0.15	1.5	1
594	Tomato	1 cup	245	90	90	2	3	Trace	1	1	16	15	0.7	1,000	0.05	0.05	1.2	12
595	Vegetable beef	1 cup	245	92	80	5	2	—	—	—	10	12	0.7	2,700	0.05	0.05	1.0	—
596	Vegetarian	1 cup	245	92	80	2	2	—	—	—	13	20	1.0	2,940	0.05	0.05	1.0	—
	Dehydrated, dry form:																	
597	Chicken noodle (2-oz package)	1 pkg	57	6	220	8	6	2	3	1	33	34	1.4	190	0.30	0.15	2.4	3
598	Onion mix (1 1/2-oz package)	1 pkg	43	3	150	6	5	1	2	1	23	42	0.6	30	0.05	0.03	0.3	6
599	Tomato vegetable with noodles (2 1/2-oz pkg)	1 pkg	71	4	245	6	6	2	3	1	45	33	1.4	1,700	0.21	0.13	1.8	18
	Frozen, condensed:																	
	Clam chowder, New England type (with milk, without tomatoes):																	
600	Prepared with equal volume of milk	1 cup	245	83	210	9	12	—	—	—	16	240	1.0	250	0.07	0.29	0.5	Trace

	Food, Approximate Measure, and Weight (in grams)		gm	Water per cent	Food Energy calories	Protein gm	Fat gm	Fatty Acids			Carbohydrate gm	Calcium mg	Iron mg	Vitamin A Value I.U.	Thiamine mg	Riboflavin mg	Niacin mg	Ascorbic Acid mg
								Saturated (total) gm	Unsaturated Oleic gm	Linoleic gm								
	Soups, frozen (cont.)																	
	Clam chowder, New England type																	
601	Prepared with equal volume of water	1 cup	240	89	130	4	8	—	—	—	11	91	1.0	50	0.05	0.10	0.5	—
	Cream of potato:																	
602	Prepared with equal volume of milk	1 cup	245	83	185	8	10	5	3	Trace	18	208	1.0	590	0.10	0.27	0.5	Trace
603	Prepared with equal volume of water	1 cup	240	90	105	3	5	3	2	Trace	12	58	1.0	410	0.05	0.05	0.5	—
	Cream of shrimp:																	
604	Prepared with equal volume of milk	1 cup	245	82	245	9	16	—	—	—	15	189	0.5	290	0.07	0.27	0.5	Trace
605	Prepared with equal volume of water	1 cup	240	88	160	5	12	—	—	—	8	38	0.5	120	0.05	0.05	0.5	—
	Oyster stew:																	
606	Prepared with equal volume of milk	1 cup	240	83	200	10	12	—	—	—	14	305	1.4	410	0.12	0.41	0.5	Trace
607	Prepared with equal volume of water	1 cup	240	90	120	6	8	—	—	—	8	158	1.4	240	0.07	0.19	0.5	—
608	Tapioca, dry, quick cooking	1 cup	152	13	535	1	Trace	—	—	—	131	15	0.6	0	0	0	0	0
	Tapioca desserts:																	
609	Apple	1 cup	250	70	295	1	Trace	—	—	—	74	8	0.5	30	Trace	Trace	Trace	Trace
610	Cream pudding	1 cup	165	72	220	8	8	4	3	Trace	28	173	0.7	480	0.07	0.30	0.2	2
611	Tartar sauce	1 tbsp	14	34	75	Trace	8	1	1	Trace	1	3	0.1	30	Trace	Trace	Trace	Trace
612	Vinegar	1 tbsp	15	94	Trace	Trace	0	—	—	—	1	1	0.1	—	—	—	—	—
613	White sauce, medium	1 cup	250	73	405	10	31	10	10	1	22	288	0.5	1,150	0.10	0.43	0.5	2
	Yeast:																	
614	Bakers', dry, active	1 pkg	7	5	20	3	Trace	—	—	—	3	3	1.1	Trace	0.16	0.38	2.6	Trace
615	Brewers', dry	1 tbsp	8	5	25	3	Trace	—	—	—	3	17	1.4	Trace	1.25	0.34	3.0	Trace
	Yogurt. See Milk, Cheese, Cream, Imitation Cream																	

Sources for Nutrition Information and Education Materials

Professional Organizations

These organizations provide the following services: publish pamphlets and other types of educational materials, professional journals, and may be contacted concerning the authenticity of nutrition information.

The American Dietetic Association
430 North Michigan Avenue
Chicago, Illinois 60611

The American Home Economics Association
2010 Massachusetts Avenue, N.W.
Washington, D.C. 20036

The American Public Health Association
1015 Eighteenth Street N.W.
Washington, D.C. 20036

Society for Nutrition Education
2140 Shattuck Avenue, Suite 1110
Berkeley, California 94704

Nutrition Today Society
P.O. Box 2375
Baltimore, Maryland 21203

Governmental Agencies

These agencies offer technical reports, research findings, pamphlets for the public, films, filmstrips, posters, charts, and other educational materials. They may be consulted according to their function about the accuracy of nutrition information.

United States Department of Agriculture, which includes

Economic Research Service
Agricultural Research Service
Office of Experiment Stations
Cooperative Extension Service
Consumer and Food Economics Research Division
Food and Nutrition Service

United States Department of Health, Education and Welfare, which includes

Children's Bureau
Office of Education
Public Health Service
Food and Drug Administration

Other governmental agencies that have a special concern with protecting the public against misleading and false information are

Federal Communications Commission
Federal Trade Commission
United States Post Office

All these governmental agencies are located in Washington, D.C. Publications of these agencies may be purchased from the Superintendent of Documents, U.S. Government Printing Office, Washington, D.C. 20402

Individuals may be placed on the mailing list to receive a biweekly notice of all government publications.

Nongovernmental Agencies

American Red Cross
17th and D Streets N.W.
Washington, D.C. 20006

Chapters are found in many local communities which are concerned with present-day problems, such as disaster relief and civilian defense feeding. Educational materials are available such as pamphlets, posters, films, and filmstrips.

Food and Nutrition Board
National Academy of Sciences—National
 Research Council
2101 Constitution Avenue S.W.
Washington, D.C. 20025

This agency is a privately financed unit whose objective is a concern with the protection of human health. Publications are largely for professional personnel, such as reviews and symposiums. Establish the Recommended Daily Dietary Allowances periodically.

Consumers Union of U.S., Inc.
256 Washington Street
Mount Vernon, New York 10550

Nonprofit organization that is the publisher of *Consumer Reports* which provides consumers with information on consumer goods and services and also publishes reprints of books that are nutrition-oriented.

Foundations

These organizations were established by industry, public-spirited citizens, or other groups to carry on research and to prepare educational materials. In some instances, nutrition programs have been developed.

The Nutrition Foundation, Inc.
99 Park Avenue
New York, New York 10016

The Rockefeller Foundation
111 West 50th Street
New York, New York 10019

Industry-Sponsored Organizations

Some industries and life insurance companies support organizations that offer a number of services, such as sponsoring nutrition leaders, preparing many types of publications, and distributing educational materials.

Cereal Institute, Inc.
135 South LaSalle Street
Chicago, Illinois 60603

Metropolitan Life Insurance Company
1 Madison Avenue
New York, New York 10010

National Dairy Council
111 North Canal Street
Chicago, Illinois 60601

National Livestock and Meat Board
407 South Dearborn Street
Chicago, Illinois 60605

Recommended Daily Nutrient Intakes (Canada)

Recommended Daily Nutrient Intakes (Canada)

Age (years)	Sex	Weight (k j)	Height (cm)	Energy (Cal)	Protein (g)	Vit. A₁ (µg RE)	Vit. D (µg)	Vit. E (mg)	Thiamin (mg)	Niacin (mg)
0–6 mos.	Both	6	–	kg × 117	kg × 2.2(2.0)	400	10	3	0.3	5
7–11 mos.	Both	9	–	kg × 108	k × 1.4	400	10	3	0.5	6
1–3	Both	13	90	1400	22	400	10	4	0.7	9
4–6	Both	19	110	1800	27	500	5	5	0.9	12
7–9	M	27	129	2200	33	700	2.5	6	1.1	14
	F	27	128	2000	33	700	2.5	6	1.0	13
10–12	M	36	144	2500	41	800	2.5	7	1.2	17
	F	38	145	2300	40	800	2.5	7	1.1	15
13–15	M	51	162	2800	52	1000	2.5	9	1.4	19
	F	49	159	2200	43	800	2.5	7	1.1	15
16–18	M	64	172	3200	54	1000	2.5	10	1.6	21
	F	54	161	2100	43	800	2.5	6	1.1	14
19–35	M	70	176	3000	56	1000	2.5	9	1.5	20
	F	56	161	2100	41	800	2.5	6	1.1	14
36–50	M	70	176	2700	56	1000	2.5	8	1.4	18
	F	56	161	1900	41	800	2.5	6	1.0	13
51 +	M	70	176	2300	56	1000	2.5	8	1.4	18
	F	56	161	1800	41	800	2.5	6	1.0	13
Pregnant				+300	+20	+100	+2.5	+1	+0.2	+2
Lactating				+500	+24	+400	+2.5	+2	+0.4	+7

DEFINITIONS:
Cal—calorie
cm —centimetre, 1 centimetre = .39 inches
g —gram
kg —kilogram, 1 kilogram = 2.2 pounds
mg —milligram
µg —microgram

SOURCE: Health and Welfare Canada. Committee for Revision of the Canadian Dietary Standard, Bureau of Nutritional Sciences, Ottawa (Revised 1974)

Ribo-flavin (mg)	Vit. B_6 (mg)	Folate (μg)	Vit. B_{12} (μg)	As-corbic Acid (mg)	Cal-cium (mg)	Phos-phorus (mg)	Mag-nesium (mg)	Iodine (μg)	Iron (mg)	Zinc (mg)
0.4	0.3	40	0.3	20	500	250	50	35	7	4
0.6	0.4	60	0.3	20	500	400	50	50	7	5
0.8	0.8	100	0.4	20	500	500	75	70	8	5
1.1	1.3	100	1.5	20	500	500	100	90	9	6
1.3	1.6	100	1.5	30	700	700	150	110	10	7
1.2	1.4	100	1.5	30	700	700	150	100	10	7
1.5	1.8	100	3.0	30	900	900	175	130	11	8
1.4	1.5	100	3.0	30	1000	1000	200	120	11	9
1.7	2.0	200	3.0	30	1200	1200	250	140	13	10
1.4	1.5	200	3.0	30	800	800	250	110	14	10
2.0	2.0	200	3.0	30	1000	1000	300	160	14	12
1.3	1.5	200	3.0	30	700	700	250	110	14	11
1.8	2.0	200	3.0	30	800	800	300	150	10	10
1.3	1.5	200	3.0	30	700	700	250	110	14	9
1.7	2.0	200	3.0	30	800	800	300	140	10	10
1.2	1.5	200	3.0	30	700	700	250	100	14	9
1.7	2.0	200	3.0	30	800	800	300	140	10	10
1.2	1.5	200	3.0	30	700	700	250	100	9	9
+0.3	+0.5	+50	+1.0	+20	+500	+500	+25	+15	+1	+3
+0.6	+0.6	+50	+0.5	+30	+500	+500	+75	+25	+1	+7

Index

Thiamin, 49, 95, 127, 138, 142, 163
  absorption, 165
  for adolescents, 336
  for adults, 346
  carbohydrates and, 164
  in cereals, 403
  chemistry, 164
  as coenzyme, 164
  consumption, 168
  content of selected foods, 167t
  deficiency, 165
  discovery, 163
  food preparation and, 167
  functions, 163
  metabolism and storage, 165
  in milk, 388, 389t
  nervous system and, 165
  nutritional status, 166
  nutritive needs, 165
  for pregnancy, 377
  recommended dietary allowances, 166t
  sources, 166, 167t
  in vegetables, 396
Thyroid hormone, 72, 178
Thyroxine, 75, 203, 229–30
Tocopherols, 157, 158, 159
  see also Vitamin E
Toddler
  avoiding food problems, 299–300
  feeding habits, 298–99
  foods included in the daily diet, 297t
  nutritive needs, 294–97, 297t
  snacks, 299
  suggested menu, 298
Trace elements, 202, 220–37
Transketolase, 164
Triglycerides, 63, 68, 351, 388
Trypsin, 92
Tryptophan, 71, 74, 79, 172–74, 175, 178, 352, 388
  see also Niacin
Tuberculosis, 173
Tyrosine, 73, 230

Undernourishment, 11
Undernutrition, 113, 205
  in children, 310–11
  in infants, 285
Underweight, 131–32
UNICEF program, 11, 287
United States Department of Agriculture, 11, 14, 48, 59, 138, 316, 320, 321–22, 323–25, 337, 364, 365, 387, 426, 431
  Child Nutrition Programs, 315–16
  Commodity Distribution Program, 325–26
  Consumer and Marketing Service, 438
  Food Stamps, 325

Household Food Consumption Survey, 48, 79, 337
  Nutrient Data Bank, 386–87
Unsaturated fatty acids, 8, 63

Vegetables, 19, 47, 59, 127, 188, 279, 318, 365, 393, 418
  buying, 449
  calcium in, 211
  folacin in, 185
  iron in, 226, 394
  magnesium in, 216
  nutrients in, 398t
  processing and preservation, 397
  protein in, 79
  storage, 397
  thiamin in, 166
  vitamin A in, 152, 395–96
  vitamin C in, 197, 394–95, 395t
  vitamin E in, 159
  vitamin K in, 160
Vegetarianism, 257, 304, 340, 421–23
  additional nutrients and kcalories, 423
  anemia and, 425
  evaluation of menus, 423
  malnutrition, 425
  nutritional evaluation, 424
  nutritional status, 424
  suggested menus, 423
Vitamin A, 21, 47, 49, 135, 138, 139, 141, 142, 145–53, 209
  absorption, transport, and storage, 148–49
  for adolescents, 336
  for adults, 348
  chemical and physical properties, 145
  deficiency, 147
  dental health and, 252
  discovery and early investigation, 145
  fat soluble, 145
  functions, 146
  in milk, 388, 389t
  nutritional status, 151–52
  nutritive needs, 149–51
  for pregnancy, 377
  sources, 152
  in vegetables, 394t
Vitamin B, 140, 398
Vitamin B$_2$, 168
Vitamin B$_6$, 64, 138, 177–80
  in cereals, 403
  chemical and physical properties, 177
  consumption, 180
  deficiencies, 178
  discovery, 177
  endocrine activities and, 177
  functions, 177